# In-Vitro Fertilization

**Fourth Edition**

# In-Vitro Fertilization

**Fourth Edition**

**Kay Elder**
Bourn Hall Clinic, Cambridge

**Brian Dale**
Centre for Assisted Reproduction, Naples

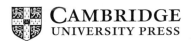

# CAMBRIDGE
## UNIVERSITY PRESS

University Printing House, Cambridge CB2 8BS, United Kingdom

One Liberty Plaza, 20th Floor, New York, NY 10006, USA

477 Williamstown Road, Port Melbourne, VIC 3207, Australia

314–321, 3rd Floor, Plot 3, Splendor Forum, Jasola District Centre, New Delhi – 110025, India

79 Anson Road, #06–04/06, Singapore 079906

Cambridge University Press is part of the University of Cambridge.

It furthers the University's mission by disseminating knowledge in the pursuit of education, learning, and research at the highest international levels of excellence.

www.cambridge.org
Information on this title: www.cambridge.org/9781108441810
DOI: 10.1017/9781108611633

© Kay Elder and Brian Dale 2020

This edition published by Cambridge University Press 2020
Third edition published by Cambridge University Press 2011
Second edition published by Cambridge University Press 2000
First edition published by Cambridge University Press 1997

Printed in Singapore by Markono Print Media Pte Ltd

*A catalogue record for this publication is available from the British Library.*

*Library of Congress Cataloging-in-Publication Data*
Names: Elder, Kay, 1946–
Title: In-vitro fertilization / Kay Elder, Bourn Hall Clinic,
   Cambridge, Brian Dale, Centre for Assisted Reproduction, Naples.
Description: Cambridge, United Kingdom ; New York, NY :
   Cambridge University  Press, 2020. | Includes bibliographical
   references and index.
Identifiers: LCCN 2019009973 | ISBN 9781108441810
   (paperback : alk. paper)
Subjects: LCSH: Fertilization in vitro, Human. | Fertilization (Biology)
Classification: LCC RG135 .I5555 2019 | DDC 618.1/780599–dc23
LC record available at https://lccn.loc.gov/2019009973

ISBN 978-1-108-44181-0 Paperback

# Contents

v

# Preface

The union of male and female gametes during the process of fertilization marks the creation of a completely new individual, a unique event that ensures genetic immortality by transferring information from one generation to the next. It also creates variation, which introduces the effects of evolutionary forces. During the first half of the nineteenth century, fertilization and the creation of early embryos were studied in a variety of marine, amphibian and mammalian species, and by the early 1960s had been successfully achieved in rabbits (Chang, 1959), the golden hamster (Yanagimachi and Chang, 1964) and mice (Whittingham, 1968). Following a decade of extensive research in mouse, rat and rabbit reproductive biology and genetics, Robert Edwards began to study in-vitro maturation of human oocytes in the early 1960s (Edwards, 1965). On February 15, 1969, the journal *Nature* published a paper authored by R.G. Edwards, B.D. Bavister and P.C. Steptoe: "Early stages of fertilization in vitro of human oocytes matured in vitro" (Edwards *et al.*, 1969). The paper scandalized the international community; reporters and camera crews from all around the world fought to gain entry to the Physiological Laboratory in Cambridge, where Edwards and his team were based. It drew fierce criticism from Nobel Laureates and much of the scientific, medical and religious establishment in the United Kingdom and elsewhere, being regarded as tampering with the beginning of a human life: religious, ethical and moral implications were numerous. In-vitro fertilization (IVF) is now accepted completely as a clinical procedure; in the quest for improvements via new technology we should not be disheartened or surprised by irrational criticism, but draw courage from the pioneering work of Bob Edwards and his colleagues, whose brave perseverance opened up an entirely new field of interdisciplinary study that embraces science, medicine, ethics, the law and social anthropology.

Half a century later, the creation of new life via human IVF continues to attract debate and discussion, prompting many governments to define "the beginning of a human life" in formulating legislation surrounding assisted reproductive technologies (ART). Not surprisingly, these definitions vary from country to country and often reflect the theological beliefs of the nations involved. Scientifically, a number of basic facts regarding fertilization and embryo development must be considered in defining the "beginning of life." Both in vivo and in vitro, gametes and preimplantation embryos are produced in great excess, with only a tiny proportion surviving to implant and produce offspring; human gametes are certainly error-prone, and the majority are never destined to begin a new life. Some female gametes may undergo fertilization, but subsequently fail to support further development due to deficiencies in the process of oogenesis. Once gametes are selected, their successful interaction is probably one of the most difficult steps on the way to the formation of a new life. At this stage the two genomes have not yet mixed, and numerous developmental errors can still occur, with failures in oocyte activation, sperm decondensation or in the patterns of signals that are necessary for the transition to early stages of embryo development. A fertilized ovum is a totipotent cell that initially divides into a few cells that are equally totipotent, but for a brief period of time these cells can give rise to one (a normal pregnancy), none (a blighted ovum or anembryonic vesicular mole) or even several (monozygotic twinning) individuals. Although fertilization is necessary for the life of a being, it is not the only critical event, as preimplantation embryo development can be interrupted at any stage by lethal processes or simple mistakes in the developmental program. A series of elegantly programmed events begins at gametogenesis and continues through to parturition, involving a myriad of synchronized interdependent mechanisms, choreographed such that each must function at the right time during embryogenesis. Combinations of both physiological and chromosomal factors result in a continuous reduction, or "selection" of conception products throughout the stages that lead to the potential implantation of an embryo in the uterus. Preimplantation embryogenesis might be described as a type of Darwinian filter where only the fittest embryos survive, and the survival of these is initially determined during gametogenesis.

It may be argued that the task of elaborating and defining the concept of a "new individual" belongs to philosophers and moralists. For some, the beginning of human life coincides with the formation of a diploid body in which the male and female chromosomes are brought together. For others, true human life only occurs after implantation of the embryo in the uterine mucosa. Many believe that a new individual is formed only after differentiation of the neural tube, whilst others believe that life begins when a fetus can live outside the uterus. In its most extreme form, some philosophers consider the acquisition of self- awareness of the newborn to define a new life. Most scientists would probably agree that life is a continuous cyclical process, with the gametes merely bridging the gap between adult stages. Science, one of the bases of human intellect and curiosity, is generally impartial and often embraces international and religious boundaries; ethicists, philosophers and theologians cannot proceed without taking into account the new information and realities that are continuously generated in the fields of biology and embryology. Advances in the expanding range and sensitivity of molecular biology techniques, in particular genomics, epigenomics and proteomics, continue to further our understanding of reproductive biology, at the same time adding further levels of complexity to this remarkable process of creating a new life.

The first edition of this book was written two decades ago; the field of human IVF has undergone significant transformation in many different ways, with accelerated expansion since publication of the third edition in 2010. IVF is now practiced in most countries of the world, and the number of babies born is estimated as approaching 8–10 million.

Further scientific knowledge gained from the use of sophisticated technology has expanded our understanding of clinical and laboratory variables that can influence human preimplantation development; management of patients and treatment cycles has also been influenced by commercial pressures as well as legislative issues. The rapid expansion in both numbers of cycles and range of treatments offered has introduced a need for more rigorous control and discipline in the IVF laboratory routine, and it is especially important that IVF laboratory personnel have a good basic understanding of the science that underpins our attempts to create the potential beginning of a new life.

A vast and comprehensive collection of published literature covers clinical and scientific procedures and protocols, as well as information gained from modern molecular biology techniques. Many books are now available that cover single chapters (and in some cases individual paragraphs) of this edition. The range and variety of media, equipment and supplies available specifically for use in human IVF continues to expand, and the commercial companies involved have evolved and merged to provide an ever-increasing range of products. For this reason, we have tried to avoid mention of specific equipment and supplies. IVF is successfully carried out with numerous adaptations in individual labs, and specific detailed protocols are no longer appropriate; protocols and procedures supplied by individual companies should be carefully studied and followed, in the perspective of the relevant basic scientific principles provided in this book. As with previous editions, our aim in preparing this fourth edition was to try to distill large bodies of information relevant to human IVF into a comprehensive background of physiological, biochemical and physical principles that provide the scientific foundation for well-established protocols in current use, together with an extensively updated list of references.

This book is dedicated to Bob Edwards, who embraced and inspired all who were blessed with the experience of knowing him ... we salute and honor his infinite vision and endless optimism:

> There wasn't any limit, no boundary at all to the future . . . and it would be so that a man wouldn't have room to store such happiness. . .
> (James Dickey, American poet and novelist, 1923–1997)

# Further Reading

Braude P, Bolton V, Moore S (1988) Human gene expression first occurs between the four- and eight-cell stages of preimplantation development. *Nature* 333: 459–461.

Carp H, Toder V, Aviram A, Daniely M, Mashiach S, Barkai G (2001) Karyotype of the abortus in recurrent miscarriages. *Fertility and Sterility* 75: 678–682.

Chang MC (1959) Fertilization of rabbit ova in vitro. *Nature* 184: 406.

Edwards RG (1965) Maturation in vitro of human ovarian oocytes. *Lancet* ii: 926–929.

Edwards RG (1965) Meiosis in ovarian oocytes of adult mammals. *Nature* 196: 446–450.

Edwards RG (1965) Maturation in vitro of mouse, sheep, cow, pig, rhesus monkey and human ovarian oocytes. *Nature* 208: 349–351.

Edwards RG (1972) Control of human development. In: Austin CR, Short RV (eds.) *Artificial Control of Reproduction, Reproduction in Mammals*, Book 5, Cambridge University Press. Cambridge, pp. 87–113.

Edwards RG (1989) *Life Before Birth: Reflections on the Embryo Debate.* Hutchinson, London.

Edwards RG, Hansis C (2005) Initial differentiation of blastomeres in 4-cell human embryos and its significance for early embryogenesis and implantation. *Reproductive Biomedicine Online* 2: 206–218.

Edwards RG, Bavister BD, Steptoe PC (1969) Early stages of fertilization in vitro of human oocytes matured in vitro. *Nature* 221: 632–635.

Hassold T, Chiu D (1985) Maternal age-specific rates of numerical chromosome abnormalities with special reference to trisomy. *Human Genetics* 70: 11–17.

Hassold T, Chen N, Funkhouser J, *et al.* (1980) A cytogenetic study of 1000 spontaneous abortuses. *Annals of Human Genetics* 44: 151–178.

Jacobs PA, Hassold TJ (1987) Chromosome abnormalities: origin and etiology in abortions and live births. In: Vogal F, Sperling K (eds.) *Human Genetics.* Springer-Verlag, Berlin, pp. 233–244.

Márquez C, Sandalinas M, Bahçe M, Alikani M, Munné S (2000) Chromosome abnormalities in 1255 cleavage-stage human embryos. *Reproductive Biomedicine Online* 1: 17–27.

Munné S, Cohen J (1998) Chromosome abnormalities in human embryos. *Human Reproduction Update* 4: 842–855.

Nothias JY, Majumder S, Kaneko KJ, *et al.* (1995) Regulation of gene expression at the beginning of mammalian development. *Journal of Biological Chemistry* 270: 22077–22080.

Steptoe PC, Edwards RG (1978) Birth after the re-implantation of a human embryo. [Letter] *Lancet* 2: 366.

Warner C (2007) Immunological aspects of embryo development. In: Elder K, Cohen J (eds.) *Human Preimplantation Embryo Evaluation and Selection.* Informa Healthcare, London, pp. 155–168.

Whittingham DG (1968) Fertilization of mouse eggs in vitro. *Nature* 200: 281–282.

Yanagimachi R, Chang MC (1964) IVF of golden hamster ova. *Journal of Experimental Zoology* 156: 361–376.

# Acknowledgments

We are deeply indebted to the colleagues who patiently advised, reviewed and revised new material for this fourth edition of the book. Rusty Poole gave us a starting point by offering invaluable suggestions for updates required for every chapter, and we are immensely grateful for the expert advice, review and revision on specific topics offered by:

Yves Ménézo (overall basic biochemistry, metabolism, metabolic pathways, oxidative stress and DNA methylation)

Melina Schuh and Bianka Seres (meiosis in human oocytes, including figures; new oocyte images supplied by Julia Uraji)

Kathy Niakan and Helen O'Neill (genome editing)

Elisabetta Tosti and Alessandra Gallo (sperm–oocyte interaction, including new figure)

Marc van den Bergh (the IVF laboratory and quality management)

Charles Cornwell (micromanipulation)

Tereza Cindrova-Davies (implantation and early placental development)

Special and very sincere thanks to Zuzana Holubcova for help in obtaining images for the cover, to Alejandra Elder Ontiveros for her help in creating new illustrations, and to Mike Macnamee and all of the friends and colleagues at Bourn Hall Clinic who continue to offer endless encouragement and support.

# Chapter 1

# Review of Cell and Molecular Biology

Gametogenesis, embryo development, implantation and in-vitro culture involve numerous complex pathways and interactions at the cellular and molecular level; a true understanding of their significance requires fundamental knowledge of the underlying principles. This chapter therefore provides a condensed overview and review of basic terminology and definitions, with particular emphasis on aspects relevant to reproductive biology and in-vitro fertilization.

## Mammalian Cell Biology

In 1839, two German scientists, Matthias Jakob Schleiden and Theodor Schwann, introduced the 'cell theory,' the proposal that all higher organisms are made up of a single fundamental unit as a building block. In 1855, Rudolf Virchow extended this cell theory with a suggestion that was highly controversial at the time: '*Omnis cellulae e celula*' (all living cells arise from pre-existing cells). This statement has become known as the 'biogenic law.' The cell theory is now accepted to include a number of principles:

1. All known living things are made up of cells.
2. The cell is the structural and functional unit of all living things.
3. All cells come from pre-existing cells by division (spontaneous generation does not occur).
4. Cells contain hereditary information that is transmitted from cell to cell during cell division.
5. The chemical composition of all cells is basically the same.
6. The energy flow (metabolism and biochemistry) of life occurs within cells.

Although these features are common to all cells, the expression and repression of genes dictate individual variation, resulting in a large number of different types of variegated but highly organized cells, with convoluted intracellular structures and interconnected elements. The average size of a somatic cell is around 20 μm; the oocyte is the largest cell in the body, with a diameter of approximately 120 μm in its final stages of growth (Figure 1.1). The basic elements and organelles in an individual cell vary in distribution and number according to the cell type. Bacterial cells differ from mammalian cells in that they have no distinct nucleus, mitochondria or endoplasmic reticulum. Their cell membrane has numerous attachments, and their ribosomes are scattered throughout the cytoplasm.

Cell **membranes** are made up of a bimolecular layer of polar lipids, coated on both sides with protein films. Some proteins are buried in the matrix, others float independently of each other in or on the membrane surface, forming a fluid mosaic of different functional units that are highly selective and specialized in different cells. Cells contain many different

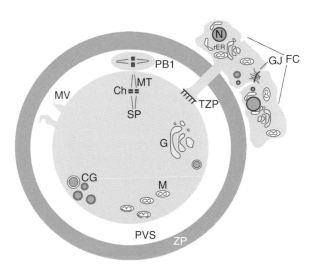

**Figure 1.1** Schematic diagram of oocyte ultrastructure showing the zona pellucida (ZP) and the perivitelline space (PVS), first polar body (PB1), microvilli (MV), rough endoplasmic reticulum (rER), chromosomes (Ch) on the spindle (SP), Golgi complex (G), cortical granules (CG), two follicle cells (FC) attached to the oocyte and to each other via gap junctions (GJ). TZP = transzonal process, MT = microtubules, M = mitochondria, N = nucleus.

types of membrane, and each one encloses a space that defines an organelle, or a part of an organelle. The function of each organelle is determined largely by the types of protein in the membranes and the contents of the enclosed space. Membranes are important in the control of selective permeability, active and passive transport of ions and nutrients, contractile properties of the cell, and recognition of/ association with other cells.

Cellular membranes always arise from pre-existing membranes, and the process of assembling new membranes is carried out by the endoplasmic reticulum (ER, see below). The synthesis and metabolism of fatty acids and cholesterol is important in membrane composition, and fatty acid oxidation (e.g., by the action of reactive oxygen species, ROS) can cause the membranes to lose their fluidity, as well as have an effect on transport mechanisms.

**Microvilli** are extensions of the plasma membrane that increase the cell surface area; they are abundant in cells with a highly absorptive capacity, such as the brush border of the intestinal lumen. Microvilli are present on the surface of oocytes, zygotes and early cleavage stage embryos in many species, and in some species (but not humans) their distribution is thought to be important in determining the site of sperm entry.

Cell **cytoplasm** is a fluid space, containing water, ions, enzymes, nutrients and macromolecules; the cytoplasm is permeated by the cell's architectural support, the cytoskeleton.

**Microtubules** are hollow polymer tubes made up of alpha–beta dimers of the protein tubulin. They are part of the cytoskeletal structure and are involved in intracellular transport, for example, the movement of mitochondria. Specialized structures such as centrioles, basal bodies, cilia and flagella are made up of microtubules. During prophase of mitosis or meiosis, microtubules form the spindle for chromosome attachment and movement.

**Microfilaments** are threads of actin protein, usually found in bundles just beneath the cell surface; they play a role in cell motility, ionic regulation and in endo- and exocytosis.

Centrioles are a pair of hollow tubes at right angles to each other, just outside the nucleus. These structures organize the nuclear spindle in preparation for the separation of chromatids during nuclear division. When the cell is about to divide by mitosis, one of the centrioles migrates to the antipode of the nucleus so that one lies at each end. The microtubule

fibers in the spindle are contractile, and they pull the chromosomes apart during cell division.

The **nucleus** of each cell is surrounded by a layered membrane, with a thickness of 7.5 nm. The outer layer of this membrane is connected to the ER, and the outer and inner layers are connected by 'press studs,' creating pores in the nuclear membrane that allow the passage of ions, RNA and other macromolecules between the nucleus and the cell cytoplasm. These pores have an active role in the regulation of DNA synthesis, since they control the passage of DNA precursors and thus allow only a single duplication of the pre-existing DNA during each cell cycle. The inner surface of the membrane has nuclear lamina, a regular network of three proteins that separate the membrane from peripheral chromatin. DNA is distributed throughout the nucleoplasm wound around spherical clusters of histones to form nucleosomes, which are strung along the DNA like beads. These are then further aggregated into the chromatin fibers of approximately 30 nm diameter. The nucleosomes are supercoiled within the fibers in a cylindrical or solenoidal structure to form chromatin, and the nuclear lamina provide anchoring points for chromosomes during interphase (Figure 1.2):

- Active chromatin = euchromatin – less condensed
- Inactive (turned off ) = heterochromatin – more condensed
- Before and during cell division, chromatin becomes organized into chromosomes.

Three types of cell lose their nuclei as part of normal differentiation, and their nuclear contents are broken down and recycled:

- Red blood cells (RBCs)
- Squamous epithelial cells
- Platelets.

Other cells may be multinuclear: syncytia in muscle and giant cells (macrophages), syncytiotrophoblast.

Nuclear RNA is concentrated in nucleoli, which form dense, spherical particles within the nucleoplasm (Figure 1.3); these are the sites where ribosome subunits, ribosomal RNA and transfer RNA are manufactured. RNA polymerase I rapidly transcribes the genes for ribosomal RNA from large loops of DNA, and the product is packed in situ with ribosomal proteins to generate new ribosomes (RNP: ribonucleoprotein particles).

**Mitochondria** are the site of aerobic respiration. Each cell contains 40–1000 mitochondria, and they

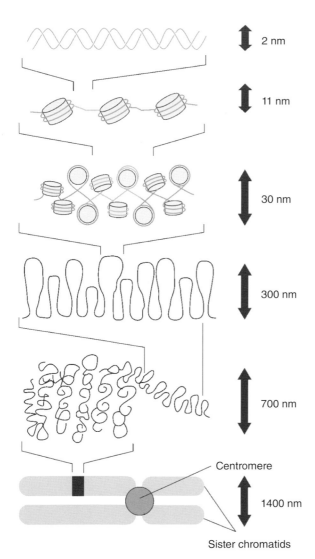

2 nm

11 nm

30 nm

300 nm

700 nm

Centromere

1400 nm

Sister chromatids

**Figure 1.2** Levels of chromatin packaging. From the top: DNA double helix, nucleosome 'beads on a string,' chromatin fiber of packed nucleosomes, section of extended chromosome, condensed chromosome and finally the entire chromosome.

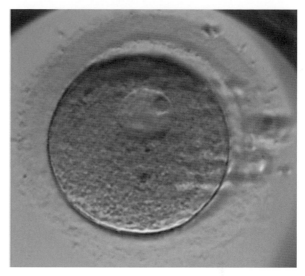

**Figure 1.3** Human oocyte at germinal vesicle stage, showing prominent nucleolus.

are most abundant in cells that are physically and metabolically active. They are elliptical, 0.5–1 μm in size, with a smooth outer membrane, an intermembranous space, and a highly organized inner membrane that forms cristae (crests) with elementary particles attached to them, 'F1-F0 lollipops,' which act as molecular dynamos. The cristae are packed with proteins, some in large complexes: the more active the tissue, the more cristae in the mitochondria. Cristae are the site of intracellular energy production and transduction, via the Krebs (TCA) cycle, as well as processes of oxidation, dehydrogenation, fatty acid oxidation, peroxidation, electron transport chains and oxidative phosphorylation.

They also act as a $Ca^{2+}$ store and are important in calcium regulation. Mitochondria contain their own double-stranded DNA that can replicate independently of the cell, but the information for their assembly is coded for by nuclear genes that direct the synthesis of mitochondrial constituents in the cytoplasm. These are transported into the mitochondria for integration into its structures.

A number of rare diseases are caused by mutations in mitochondrial DNA, and the tissues primarily affected are those that most rely on respiration, i.e., the brain and nervous system, muscles, kidneys and the liver. All the mitochondria in the developing human embryo come from the oocyte, and therefore all mitochondrial diseases are maternally inherited, transmitted exclusively from mother to child. In the sperm, mitochondria are located in the midpiece, providing the metabolic energy required for motility; there are no mitochondria in the sperm head.

- Oocytes contain 100 000–1 000 000 mitochondria.
- Sperm contain 70–100 mitochondria, in the midpiece of each sperm. These are incorporated into the oocyte cytoplasm, but do not contribute to the zygote mitochondrial population – they are eliminated at the four- to eight-cell stage.
- All of the mitochondria of an individual are descendants of the mitochondria of the zygote,

3

which contains mainly oocyte mitochondria, i.e. mitochondria are maternal in origin.

. Paternal mtDNA has been identified in a few exceptional cases, transmitted with an unusual autosomal dominant-like inheritance (Luo *et al.*, 2018).

### The Human Mitochondrial Genome

The sequence of human mitochondrial DNA was published by Fred Sanger in 1981, who shared the 1980 Nobel Prize in Chemistry with Paul Berg and Walter Gilbert, 'for their contributions concerning the determination of base sequences in nucleic acids.' The mitochondrial genome has:

- Small double-stranded circular DNA molecule (mtDNA) 16 568 bp in length.
- 37 genes that code for:

    2 ribosomal RNAs

    22–23 tRNAs

    10–13 proteins associated with the inner mitochondrial membrane, involved in energy production.

Other mitochondrial proteins are encoded by nuclear DNA and specifically transported to the mitochondria.

Mitochondrial DNA is much less tightly packed and protected than nuclear DNA and is therefore more susceptible to ROS damage that can cause mutations.

As it is inherited only through the maternal line, mutations can be clearly followed through generations and are used as 'markers' in forensic science and archaeology, as well as in tracking different human populations and ethnic groups.

Mitochondria can be seen in different distributions during early development (Figure 1.4); they do not begin to replicate until the blastocyst stage, and therefore an adequate store of active mitochondria in the mature oocyte is a prerequisite for early development.

- Germinal vesicle oocyte: homogeneous clusters associated with ER
- Metaphase I oocyte: polarized toward the spindle
- Metaphase II oocyte: perinuclear ring and polar body
- Embryos at 1c, 2c, 4c stages: perinuclear ring
- Cytoplasmic fragments in cleavage stage embryos contain large amounts of active mitochondria

The **endoplasmic reticulum** (ER) is an interconnected lipoprotein membrane network of tubules, vesicles and flattened sacs that extends from the nuclear membrane outwards to the plasma membrane, held together by the cytoskeleton. The ER itself is a membrane-enclosed organelle that carries out complex biosynthetic processes, producing proteins, lipids and polysaccharides. As new lipids and proteins are made, they are inserted into the existing ER membrane and the space enclosed by it. **Smooth ER** (**sER**) is involved in metabolic processes, including synthesis and metabolism of lipids, steroids and carbohydrates, as well as regulation of calcium levels. The surface of **rough ER** (**rER**) is studded with ribosomes, the units of protein synthesis machinery. Membrane-bound vesicles shuttle proteins between the rER and the **Golgi apparatus**, another part of the membrane system. The Golgi apparatus is important in modifying, sorting and packaging macromolecules for secretion from the cell; it is also involved in transporting lipids around the cell, and in making lysosomes.

## Rough Endoplasmic Reticulum (rER)

- Has attached 80S ribonucleoprotein particles, the ribosomes (bacterial ribosomes are 70S), which are made in the nucleus and then travel out to the cytoplasm through nuclear pores.
- Ribosomes are composed of two subunits: 40 s and 60 s (bacteria: 30S and 50S); the association between the subunits is controlled by $Mg^{2+}$ concentration.
- Polysomes are several ribosomes which move along a single strand of mRNA creating several copies of the same protein.

## Smooth Endoplasmic Reticulum (sER)

- A series of flattened sacs and sheets, site of lipid and steroid synthesis.
- Cells that make large amounts of steroids have extensive sER.

The **Golgi apparatus** was first observed by Camillo Golgi in 1898, using a novel silver staining technique to observe cellular structures under the light microscope; he was awarded the 1906 Nobel Prize in Physiology or Medicine for his studies on the structure of the nervous system. The Golgi apparatus consists of a fine, compact network of tubules near the cell nucleus, a collection of closely associated compartments with

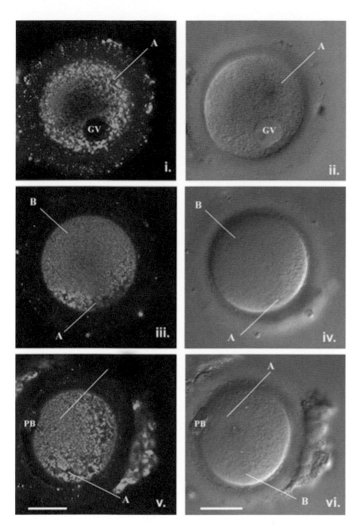

**Figure 1.4** Mitochondrial aggregation patterns in a germinal vesicle (GV) oocyte (top), an MI oocyte (center) and an MII oocyte (bottom). Frames to the left are in fluorescence using the potential sensitive dye JC-1 to show the mitochondria; frames on the right are transmitted light images. The two mitochondrial patterns, A (granular-clumped) and B (smooth), are shown. From Wilding *et al.*, 2001. See color plate section.

stacked arrays of smooth sacs and variable numbers of cisternae, vesicles or vacuoles. It is connected to rER, linked to vacuoles that can develop into secretory granules, which contain and store the proteins produced by the rER. All of the proteins exported from the ER are funneled through the Golgi apparatus, and every protein passes in a strict sequence through each of the compartments (cis, medial, trans). This process consists of three stages:

1. 'Misdirected mail' – sends back misdirected proteins (cis).
2. 'Addressing' – (medial) stacks of cisternae that modify lipid and sugar moieties, giving them 'tags' for subsequent sorting.
3. 'Sorting and delivering' (trans): proteins and lipids are identified, sorted and sent to their proper destination.

Transport occurs via vesicles, which bud from one compartment and fuse with the next. The Golgi apparatus will move to different parts of the cell according to the ongoing metabolic processes at the time; it is very well developed in secretory cells (e.g., in the pancreas).

The Golgi apparatus also makes lysosomes, which contain hydrolytic enzymes that digest worn-out organelles and foreign particles, acting as 'rubbish bins' and providing a recycling apparatus for intracellular digestion; they contain at least 50 different enzymes, and 'leaky' lysosomes can damage and kill cells. Macromolecules inside the cell are transported to lysosomes, those from outside the cell reach them by pinocytosis or phagocytosis; phagocytosis only occurs in specialized cells (e.g., white blood cells).

**Peroxisomes** are microbody vesicles that contain oxidative enzymes such as catalase; they dispose of toxic hydrogen peroxide and are important in cell aging.

# Fundamental Principles of Molecular Biology

## Nucleic Acids

The nucleic acids, DNA (deoxyribose nucleic acid; Figure 1.5) and RNA (ribose nucleic acid), are made up of:

1. Nucleotides: organic compounds containing a nitrogenous base
2. Sugar: deoxyribose in DNA, ribose in RNA
3. Phosphate group.

Nucleotides are purines and pyrimidines, determined by the structure of the nitrogenous base.

|  | DNA | RNA |
|---|---|---|
| Purines (double ring) | Adenine (A) | Adenine (A) |
|  | Guanine (G) | Guanine (G) |
| Pyrimidines (single ring) | Cytosine (C) | Cytosine (C) |
|  | Thymine (T = methylated U) | Uracil (U) |

Methylation of cytosine is important in gene silencing and imprinting processes.

Nucleotides also function as important cofactors in cell signaling and metabolism: coenzyme A (CoA), flavin adenine dinucleotide (FAD), flavin mononucleotide, adenosine triphosphate (ATP), nicotinamide adenine dinucleotide phosphate (NADP).

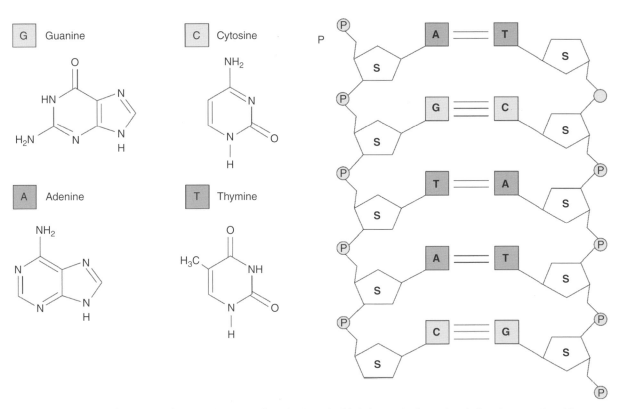

**Figure 1.5** Structure of DNA. Complementary base pairs form the DNA double helix; two hydrogen bonds form between A and T, three hydrogen bonds form between G and C. The two polynucleotide chains must be antiparallel to each other to allow pairing. S= sugar, P= phosphate group.

## DNA

- Double-stranded helix with paired bases to form complementary strands.
- G=C or A=T.
- Pentose deoxyribose – phosphate backbone.
- Stabilized by H bonds between purines and pyrimidines, on the inside of the helix.
- Each pitch of the double helix has 10 base pairs.

## DNA Replication

DNA copies itself by semi-conservative replication: each strand acts as a template for synthesis of a complementary strand.

1. Free nucleotides are made in the cytoplasm and are present in the nucleoplasm before replication begins.
2. The double helix unwinds and hydrogen bonds, holding the two DNA strands together, break. This leaves unpaired bases exposed on each strand.
3. The sequence of unpaired bases serves as a template on which to arrange the free nucleotides from the nucleoplasm.
4. DNA polymerase moves along the unwound parts of the DNA, pairing complementary nucleotides from the nucleoplasm with each exposed base.
5. The same enzyme connects the nucleotides together to form a new strand of DNA, hydrogen bonded to the old strand:
   - DNA polymerase forms new hydrogen bonds on the $5'3'$ strand.
   - DNA ligase acts on the $3'5'$ strand.
   - Several replication points appear along the strand, which eventually join.
6. DNA is then mounted on 'scaffolding proteins,' histones – and this is then wrapped around non-histones to form chromatin. Histones are basic proteins that bind to nuclear DNA and package it into nucleosomes; the regulation of gene expression involves histone acetylation and deacctylation. There are two ATP-dependent remodeling complexes and acetyltransferases that preferentially bind activated states and fix chromatin configurations:
   - Histone acetyltransferase coactivator complex
   - Histone deacetylase corepressor complex.

Methylation of protamines and histones is a crucial component of imprinting processes: an association has been found between Beckwith–Wiedemann syndrome and epigenetic alterations of LitI and H19 during in-vitro fertilization (DeBaum et al., 2003).

Each mammalian cell contains around 1.8 m of DNA, of which only 10% is converted into specific proteins; the noncoding part of the DNA still carries genetic information and probably functions in regulatory control mechanisms.

### The Genetic Code: The Biochemical Basis of Heredity

In 1968, the Nobel Prize in Physiology or Medicine was awarded to Robert Holland, Ghobind Khorana and Marshall Nirenberg 'for their interpretation of the genetic code and its function in protein synthesis':

- DNA transfers information to mRNA in the form of a code defined by a sequence of nucleotide bases.
- The code is triplet, unpunctuated and nonoverlapping.
- Three bases are required to specify each amino acid, there are no gaps between codons and codons do not overlap.
- Since RNA is made up of four types of nucleotides (A, C, G, U), the number of triplet sequences (codons) that are possible is $4 \times 4 \times 4 = 64$; three of these are 'stop codons' that signal the termination of a polypeptide chain.
- The remaining 61 codons can specify 20 different amino acids, and more than one codon can specify the same amino acid. (Only methionine [Met] and tryptophan [Trp] are specified by a single codon).
- Since the genetic code thus has more information than it needs, it is said to be 'degenerate.'
- A mutation in a single base can alter the coding for an amino acid, resulting in an error in protein synthesis: translated RNA will incorporate a different amino acid into the protein, which may then be defective in function. (Sickle cell anemia and phenylketonuria are examples of single-gene defects.)

## Regulation of Transcription

- A **homeobox** is a DNA sequence that codes for a 60-amino-acid protein domain known as the **homeodomain**.
- A **homeodomain** acts as a switch that controls gene transcription.
- **Homeobox genes**, first discovered in 1983, are a highly conserved family of transcription factors that switch on cascades of other genes:

  - Are involved in the regulation of embryonic development of virtually all multicellular animals, playing a crucial role from the earliest steps in embryogenesis to the latest stages of differentiation
  - Are arranged in clusters in the genome.

- **POU factors** are a class of transcriptional regulators, required for high-affinity DNA binding, that are important in tissue-specific gene regulation; they are named after three proteins in the group: **P** it-l (also known as GHF-1), **O** ct-l and **U** nc-86.

- Genes = chief functional unit of DNA
- Exons = regions that contain information for the amino acid sequence of a protein (coding sequence)
- Introns = noncoding regions in between exons
- Codon = a group of three nucleotide bases which code for one amino acid

## RNA

- Paired bases are G–C and A–U.
- Pentose sugar = ribose.
- Basic structure in mammalian cells is single-stranded, but most biologically active forms contain self-complementary sequences that allow parts of the RNA to fold and pair with itself to form double helices, creating a specific tertiary structure.
- RNA molecules have a negative charge, and metal ions such as $Mg^{2+}$ and $Zn^{2+}$ are needed to stabilize many secondary and tertiary structures.
- Hydroxyl groups on the deoxyribose ring make RNA less stable than DNA because it is more prone to hydrolysis.

There are many different types of RNA, each with a different function:

- Transcription, translation/protein synthesis: mRNA, rRNA, tRNA
- Post-transcriptional modification or DNA replication: small nuclear RNA (snRNA), small nucleolar RNA (snoRNA), guide RNA (gRNA), ribonuclease P, ribonuclease MRP, etc.
- Gene regulation: microRNA (miRNA), small interfering RNA (siRNA), etc.
- microRNAs are increasingly recognized as 'master regulators' of gene expression, regulating large networks of genes by chopping up or inhibiting the expression of protein-coding transcripts.

### Ribosomal RNA

Makes up 80% of total RNA.

- Made in the nucleolus, then moved out into the nucleoplasm and then to the cytoplasm to be incorporated into ribosomes.

### Transfer RNA (4S RNA)

Makes up 10–15% of total RNA.

- Single strand, 75–90 nucleotides wound into a clover leaf shape; each tRNA molecule transfers an amino acid to a growing polypeptide chain during translation.

A three-base anticodon sequence on the 'tail' is complementary to a codon on mRNA; an amino acid is attached at the $3'$ terminal site of the molecule, via a covalent link that is catalyzed by an aminoacyl tRNA synthetase. Each type of tRNA molecule can be attached to only one type of amino acid; however, multiple codons in DNA can specify the same amino acid, and therefore the same amino acid can be carried by tRNA molecules that have different three-base anticodons.

- Methionyl tRNA has a critical function, required for the initiation of protein synthesis.

### Messenger RNA

This makes up 3–5% of total cellular RNA (exception: sperm cells contain approximately 40% mRNA and very little rRNA)

The mRNA molecules are single-stranded, complementary to one strand of DNA (coding strand) and identical to the other. DNA is transcribed into mRNA molecules, which carry coding information to the ribosomes for translation into proteins.

### Transcription

- DNA information is transcribed to mRNA in the nucleus, starting from a promoter sequence on the DNA at the $5'$ end, and finishing at the $3'$ end.

- All of the exons and introns in the DNA are transcribed; stop and start sequences are encoded in the gene.
- The product, nuclear mRNA precursor (HnRNA, heterogeneous nuclear RNA) is processed into mature cytoplasmic mRNA by splicing at defined base pairs to remove the introns and join the exons together.
- A cap of 7-methylG is added at the 5′ end.
- A string of polyA is added at 3′ end = polyA tail, 50–300 residues.
- The polyA tail adds stability to mRNA molecules, making them less susceptible to degradation, and also has a role in transporting mRNA from the nucleus to the cytoplasm.

A **promoter** is a specific DNA sequence that signals the site for RNA polymerase to initiate transcription; this process needs an orchestrated interaction between proteins binding to specific DNA sequences, as well as protein–protein interactions. DNA methylation is involved in the regulation of transcription. Gene sequences that lie 5′ to the promoter sequence bind specific proteins that influence the rate of transcription from a promoter:

- A TATA box aligns RNA polymerase II with DNA by interacting with transcription initiation factors (TFs).
- Proteins that bind to a CAAT box determine the rate at which transcription is initiated, bringing RNA polymerase II into the area of the start site in order to assemble the transcriptional machinery. The tertiary structure of the DNA (bends and folds) is important in making sure that all components are correctly aligned.
- Enhancers, silencers and hormone response elements (steroid receptors) are important in determining the tissue-specific expression or physiological regulation of a gene; these factors respond to signals such as cAMP levels.

### Transcription in Oocytes

- Transcription takes place during oocyte growth and stops before ovulation.
- The mRNA turnover begins before ovulation: mRNA molecules must be protected from premature translation.
- Oocytes contain mechanisms that remove histone H1 from condensed chromatin.

- Differential acetylation profiles of core histone H4 and H3 for parental genomes during the first G1 phase may be important in establishing early zygotic 'memory.'
- The timing of transcriptional events during the first zygotic cell cycle will have an effect on further developmental potential.

### Translation (Protein Synthesis)

During protein synthesis, ribosomes move along the mRNA molecule and 'read' its sequence three nucleotides at a time, from the 5′ end to the 3′ end. Each amino acid is specified by the mRNA's codon, and then pairs with a sequence of three complementary nucleotides carried by a particular tRNA (anticodon). The translation of mRNA into polypeptide chains involves three phases: initiation, elongation and termination. Messenger RNA binds to the small (40 s) subunit of the ribosome on rER in the cytoplasm, and six bases at a time are exposed to the large (60 s) subunit. The endpoint is specified by a 'stop' codon: UAA, UAG or UGA.

1. *Initiation:* The first three bases (codon) are always AUG, and the initiation complex locates this codon at the 5′ end of the mRNA molecule. A methionyl-tRNA molecule with UAC on its coding site forms hydrogen bonds with AUG, and the complex associates with the small ribosome subunit (methionine is often removed after translation, so that not every protein has methionine as its first amino acid). Some mRNAs contain a supernumerary AUG and associated short coding region upstream and independent of the main AUG coding region; these upstream open reading frames (uORFs) can regulate the translation of the downstream gene.

The large ribosome subunit has a P site which binds to the growing peptide chain, and an A site which binds to the incoming aa-tRNA.

2. *Elongation:* the unbound tRNA may now leave the P site, and the ribosome moves along the mRNA by one codon.

   - A peptide bond is formed, and the aa-tRNA bond is hydrolyzed to release the free tRNA.
   - A second tRNA molecule, bringing another amino acid, bonds with the next three exposed bases. The two amino acids are held closely

together, and peptidyl transferase in the small ribosomal subunit forms a peptide bond between them.

- The ribosome moves along the mRNA, exposing the next three bases on the ribosome, and a third tRNA molecule brings a third amino acid, which joins to the second one.

3. *Termination:* The polypeptide chain continues to grow until a stop codon (UAA, UAC or UGA) is exposed on the ribosome. The stop codon codes for a releasing factor instead of another aa-tRNA; the completed peptide is released, and components of the translation complex are disassembled.

## DNA Methylation

DNA methylation plays an important role in regulating gene expression, generally preventing ('silencing') gene expression. The addition and removal of methyl groups on DNA and histone proteins controls three-dimensional chromatin structure to allow or prevent binding of transcriptional promoters; interaction between DNA methylation and other proteins that modify nucleosomes results in a mechanism that regulates gene expression so that the correct genes are expressed at the appropriate time.

DNA is methylated by adding a methyl group ($-CH_3$) covalently to the base cytosine (C), usually within the dinucleotide 5′-CpG-3′; methylated cytosine residues are sometimes referred to as the 'fifth nucleotide.' The CpG sequence in DNA represents a cytosine base (C) linked to a guanine base (G) by a phosphate bond. The majority (70–80%) of CpG dinucleotides in the human genome are methylated. Those that are unmethylated are usually clustered together in 'CpG islands,' sequences of at least 200 base pairs that contain a higher number of CpG sites than expected. They are usually found upstream of many mammalian genes, in regions that facilitate transcription, the 'promoter' sites. More than 98% of DNA methylation in somatic cells is found within CpG islands, usually concentrated within central cores of nucleosomes rather than internucleosomal regions. However, in embryonic stem (ES) cells around 25% of methylation appears in non-CpG regions. The promoter regions of important genes that are expressed in most cells ('housekeeping genes') are mainly protected from methylation, allowing continued transcription of genes that maintain basic cellular homeostasis. Methylation of CpG islands blocks transcription, silencing expression of the related gene(s) (Figure 1.6).

The addition of methyl groups is controlled at several different levels by a family of DNA methyltransferase enzymes (DNMTs); DNMT1, DNMT3a

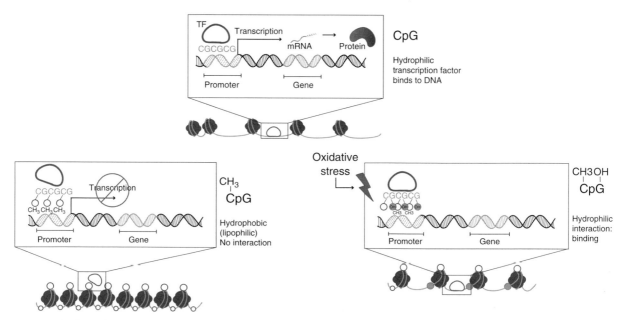

**Figure 1.6** Effect of oxidation on epigenetic regulation of gene expression. Simplified scheme outlining the effect of DNA methylation on transcription. The transcription factor (TF) binds to CpG promoter islands via a hydrophilic interaction, allowing downstream gene expression. The addition of a methyl group to CpG converts the molecule to one that is hydrophobic, silencing gene expression by preventing TF binding. Oxidation of guanine (G) at methylated CpG sites modifies the interaction to one that is again hydrophilic, restoring affinity between TF and DNA to allow gene expression. Modified with permission from Ménézo *et al.* 2016, with thanks to Alejandra Ontiveros.

and DNMT3b establish and maintain DNA methylation patterns. Variants in genes encoding DNMTs have been identified as risk factors for disease (Tollefsbol, 2017).

- DNMT1 appears to maintain established patterns.
- DNMT3a and DNMT3b mediate new or *de novo* patterns.
- DNMT2 and DNMT3L may also have more specialized roles.

*Demethylation*, i.e., removal of methyl groups, is essential for epigenetic reprogramming of genes and is also directly involved in disease mechanisms that cause cell transformation to malignant states. The process can be passive, active or a combination of both.

- Passive: usually takes place via DNMT1 during rounds of replication, on newly synthesized DNA strands, with a downstream 'dilution' effect during subsequent replication rounds.

- Active: can be carried out by two different mechanisms:
  1. Cytosine deaminases convert 5mC to thymine, followed by T–G mismatch repair that specifically replaces thymine with cytosine.
  2. A family of ten-eleven translocation (TET) hydroxylases bind to CpG-rich regions to prevent DNMT activity, and convert 5mC to oxidized bases: 5-hmC, 5hmC to 5-formylcytosine (5fc), and 5-fc to 5-carboxylcytosine (5-caC) through hydroxylase activity. These oxidized 5mC bases can be actively removed by base excision repair (BER) to regenerate cytosine (Figure 1.7).

The TET proteins have been shown to participate in activating and repressing transcription (TET1), tumor suppression (TET2), and DNA methylation reprogramming (TET3). Oxidation by TET appears to be

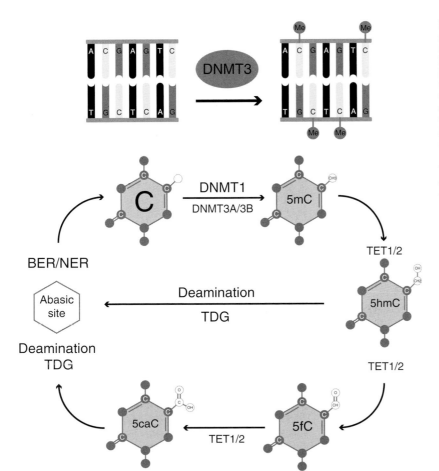

**Figure 1.7** DNA methylation in mammalian cells. The nucleotide cytosine (C) is methylated at the 5th carbon either by de novo DNA methyltransferases DNMT3A or DNMT3B, or by the DNA maintenance methyltransferase 1 (DNMT1) during DNA replication; active demethylation of 5-methylcytosine (5mC) takes place through repeated oxidation by ten-eleven translocation proteins (TET1/2), producing 5-hydroxymethylcytosine (5hmC). This is further oxidized to 5-formylcytosine (5fC) and lastly 5-carboxylcytosine (5caC). By an alternative route, not only 5caC, but also 5hmC, are deaminated to thymine and excised by thymine DNA glycosylase (TDG). The mismatched bases are then repaired by the base excision and/or nucleotide excision repair machinery (BER/NER). Adapted by Alejandra Ontiveros from fig 1 in Hoffmann A, Sportelli V, Ziller M, Spengler D (2017) Epigenomics of major depressive disorders and schizophrenia: early life decides. *International Journal of Molecular Sciences* 18: 1711, licensed under CC BY 4.0.

important in preventing the accumulation of 5mC at CpG islands and other promoter sites. TET deficiency affects methylation, with downregulation of the related genes.

Demethylation is a crucial process during development, and dysregulation of methylation processes contributes to numerous disease states, including cancer; it also occurs due to adverse environmental influences and as a function of aging. Methylation capacity/activity usually decreases with age (Richardson, 2003).

The distribution of DNA methylation marks on the genome encodes important biological information that is crucial for early development. DNA analysis technology has progressed significantly during the last decade, and this has revealed that the dynamics of DNA methylation/demethylation during early preimplantation development are highly complex and intricate with respect to removal and re-establishment of imprinting marks (Okamoto *et al.*, 2015). The establishment of methylation patterns in the zygote is a highly dynamic process, involving both active and passive demethylation, in tandem with *de novo* and maintenance methylation: methylation and demethylation processes are counterbalanced. By the time of implantation, imprinting marks from the parent gametes have been removed, and the entire genome undergoes methylation at specific sites, while CpG islands are protected. This results in global repression, but with continued expression of cellular housekeeping genes, which have a unique CpG island promoter structure that remains unmethylated in every cell. Further stage- and tissue-specific changes in methylation then mold epigenetic patterns for each individual cell type during postimplantation development, and these are maintained through cell division. Many factors regulate and contribute to determining the precise methylation/demethylation patterns, and perturbation of one process is likely to affect other processes in the chain, with downstream effects on cell fate conversion. Figure 1.6 describes the effects of oxidative stress on gene expression (Ménézo *et al.*, 2016).

## Metabolism in the Mammalian Cell

Four basic factors influence the metabolic activity of a cell:

1. Spatial: compartmentation, permeability, transport, interactions.
2. Temporal: products become substrates, positive and negative feedback.

3. Intensity/concentrations: precise amounts of reactants/substrates/products.
4. Determinants that specify the structure of enzymes and direct their formation/activation.

Molecules that are important in the biology/metabolism of the cell include carbohydrates, fats, lipids and proteins.

### Carbohydrates

Carbohydrates are made up of carbon (C), hydrogen (H) and oxygen (O), with the molecular ratio $C_x(H_2O)_y$.

- Monosaccharides: pentose – 5 C's (ribose, deoxyribose); hexose – 6 C's (glucose, fructose).
- Disaccharides: two monosaccharides (sucrose, maltose, lactose).
- Oligosaccharides: combine with proteins and lipids to form glycoproteins and glycolipids, important in cell–cell recognition and the immune response.
- Polysaccharides: polymers, insoluble, normally contain 12 to 10 000 monosaccharides (starch, cellulose, glycogen)
  - Also form complexes with lipids and phosphate.

### Fats and Lipids

Fatty acids (FAs) have a long hydrocarbon chain ending in a carboxyl group:

- Saturated FAs have single bonds between carbon atoms.
- Unsaturated FAs have some double bonds between carbon atoms.

Lipids are made up of FAs plus water:

- Phospholipids are important in membranes.
- Glycolipids are important in receptors.

### Proteins

The primary structure of a protein is a sequence of amino acids with peptide bonds:

–CONH–

Amino acids have at least one amino and one carboxyl group; they are amphoteric and form dipolar zwitterions in solution. Proteins have secondary structures; they can be folded into a helix or form beta sheets that are held together by hydrogen bonds:

- Alpha helix – tends to be soluble (most enzymes).
- Beta sheets – insoluble – fibrous tissue.

Proteins also have a three-dimensional *tertiary structure*, which is formed by folding of the secondary structure, held in place by different types of bond to form a more rigid structure: disulfide bonds, ionic bonds, intermolecular bonds (van der Waals – non-polar side chains attracted to each other).

High temperatures and extremes of pH denature proteins, destroying their tertiary structure and their functional activity.

Some proteins have a *quaternary structure*, with several tertiary structures fitted together; e.g., collagen consists of a triple-stranded helix.

**Enzymes** are proteins that catalyze a large number of biologically important actions, including anabolic and catabolic processes, and transfer of groups (e.g., methylase, kinase, hydroxylase, dehydrogenase). Some enzymes are isolated in organelles, others are free in the cytoplasm; there are more than 5000 enzymes in a typical mammalian cell.

- Kinases: add a phosphate group, key enzymes in many activation pathways.
- Methylases: add a methyl group. DNA methylation is important in modifications that are involved in imprinting, lipid methylation is important for membrane stability, and proteins are also stabilized by methylation.

Most enzymes are conjugated proteins, with an active site that has a definite shape; a substrate fits into the active site or may induce a change of shape so that it can fit.

- The rate of an enzymatic reaction is affected by temperature, pH, substrate concentration, enzyme concentration.
- Enzymes can be activated by removal of a blocking peptide, maintaining the S–H groups, or by the presence of a cofactor.
- The active site of an enzyme is often linked to the presence of an amino acid OH– group (serine, threonine). Mutations at this level render the enzymes inactive.

Enzyme inhibitors can be:

- Competitive – structurally similar
- Noncompetitive – no similarity, form an enzyme/inhibitor complex that changes the shape of the protein so that the active site is distorted
- Irreversible: heavy metal ions combine with –SH causing the protein to precipitate. Lead ($Pb^{2+}$) and cadmium ($Cd^{2+}$) are the most hazardous; these

cations can also replace zinc ($Zn^{2+}$), which is usually a stabilizer of tertiary structures.

Allosteric enzymes are regulated by compounds that are not their substrate, but which bind to the enzyme away from the active site in order to modify activity. The compounds can be activators or inhibitors, increasing or decreasing the affinity of the enzyme for the substrate. These interactions help to regulate metabolism by end-product inhibition/feedback mechanisms.

For example, low levels of ATP activate the enzyme phosphofructokinase (PFK), and high levels of ATP then inhibit the reaction

**Km** is the substrate concentration that sustains half the maximum rate of reaction. Two or more enzymes may catalyze the same substrate, but in different reactions; if the reserves of substrate are low, then the enzyme with the lowest Km will claim more of the substrate.

### Cytokines

- Cytokines are proteins, peptides or peptidoglycan molecules that are involved in signaling pathways. They represent a large and diverse family of regulatory molecules that are produced by many different types of cell, and are used extensively in cellular communication:
  - Colony stimulating factors
  - Growth and differentiation factors
  - Immunoregulatory and proinflammatory cytokines function in the immune system (interferon, interleukins, tumor necrosis factors).

- Each cytokine has a unique cell surface receptor that conducts a cascade of intracellular signaling that may include upregulation and/or downregulation of genes and their transcription factors.
- They can amplify or inhibit their own expression via feedback mechanisms:
  - Type 1 cytokines enhance cellular immune responses:
    - Interleukin-2 (IL-2), gamma interferon (IFN-γ), TGF-β, TNF-β, etc.
  - Type 2 favor antibody responses:
    - IL-4, IL-5, IL-6, IL-10, IL-13, etc.
  - Type 1 and type 2 cytokines can regulate each other.

## HeLa Cells

The majority of our knowledge about fundamental principles of cell and molecular biology has been gained from model systems, particularly in yeast and bacteria, as well as human cell lines maintained in tissue culture. The first human cell line to be propagated and grown continuously in culture as a permanent cell line is the HeLa cell, an immortal epithelial line: knowledge of almost every process that takes place in human cells has been obtained through the use of HeLa cells, and the many other cell lines that have since been isolated.

The cells were cultured from biopsy of a cervical cancer taken from Henrietta Lacks, a 31-year-old African American woman from Baltimore, in 1951. George Gey, the head of the cell culture laboratory at Johns Hopkins Hospital, cultivated and propagated the cells; Henrietta died from her cancer 8 months later. Gey and his wife Margaret continued to propagate the cells, and sent them to colleagues in other laboratories. In 1954, Jonas Salk used HeLa cells to develop the first vaccine for polio, and they have been used continually since then for research into cancer, AIDS, gene mapping, toxicity testing and numerous other research areas; they even went up in the first space missions to see what would happen to cells in zero gravity.

HeLa cells attained 'immortality' because they have an active version of the enzyme telomerase, which prevents telomere shortening that is associated with aging and eventual cell death. They adapt readily to different growth conditions in culture, and can be difficult to control: their growth is so aggressive that slight contamination by these cells can take over and overwhelm other cell cultures. Many other in-vitro cell lines used in research (estimates range from 1 to 10% of established cell lines) have been shown to have HeLa cell contamination. Twenty-five years after Henrietta's death, many cell cultures thought to be from other tissue types, including breast and prostate cells, were discovered to be in fact HeLa cells, a finding that unleashed a huge controversy and led to questions about published research findings. Further investigation revealed that HeLa cells could float on dust particles in the air and travel on unwashed hands to contaminate other cultures.

The cells were established in culture without the knowledge of her family, who discovered their 'fame' accidentally 24 years after her death; they were contacted for DNA samples that could be used to map Henrietta's genes in order to resolve the contamination problem (Skoot, 2010).

# Ion Regulation in Cells

All cells maintain a different cytoplasmic ionic constitution with respect to their environment, regulated by the hydrophobic lipid membrane bilayer and by ion channels and transporters associated with the membrane. A major proportion of cellular energy is dedicated to ionic homeostasis, and loss of membrane-controlled ionic imbalance is one of the first manifestations of cell death. Although the cell cytoplasm is electrically neutral, i.e., it contains equal quantities of positive and negative charges, the differential distribution of ions across the cell membrane forms an electrochemical gradient that creates potential energy. Approximately 15–30% of all membrane proteins are involved in ion transport, via two mechanisms:

1. Ion channels form a narrow hydrophilic pore that allows passive movement of small inorganic ions.
2. Transporters actively transport specific molecules across membranes; these may be coupled to an energy source.

## Ion Transport

### Ion Channels

Ions can be transferred thousands of times faster through an ion channel than via transporters: $10^8$ ions can pass through an open channel in one second. This 'passive' transport through channels is not directly linked to energy sources and is often specific for a particular type of ion. Ion channels are not continuously open; they are opened or 'gated,' in response to a change in voltage, mechanical stress or the binding of a ligand. The activity of many ion channels is also regulated by protein phosphorylation and dephosphorylation.

The resting potential of a cell membrane can be calculated from the ratio of internal to external ion concentrations, using the Nernst equation:

$$V_{Eq} = RT/zF \ln \{[X]_{out}/[X]_{in}\}$$

$R$ = universal gas constant, 8.314 J K$^{-1}$ mol$^{-1}$ (joules per kelvin per mole).

$T$ = temperature in kelvin (K =°C + 273.15).

$z$ = valence of the ion, e.g., $z$ = +1 for Na$^+$ and K$^+$, +2 for Ca$^{2+}$, −1 for Cl$^-$, etc.

$F$ = Faraday's constant, 96485 C mol$^{-1}$ (coulombs per mole).

$[X]_{out}$ = extracellular ion (X) concentration in mM.

$[X]_{in}$ = intracellular ion (X) concentration in mM.

The resting potential depends mainly on the $K^+$ gradient across the membrane, as well as the characteristics of its $K^+$ ion channels. The plasma membrane of many cells also contains voltage-gated cation channels, which are responsible for depolarizing the plasma membrane, creating a less negative value inside the cell. Voltage-gated $Na^+$ channels allow a small amount of $Na^+$ to enter the cell down its electrochemical gradient; this then depolarizes the membrane further, opening more $Na^+$ channels that may continue to open by auto-amplification. Voltage-gated sodium channels are primarily responsible for propagating action potential in neurons. Ion channels are specific for particular ions:

1. The sodium channel family consists of nine members, each with two subunits ($\alpha$ and $\beta$) as well as several membrane-spanning regions.
2. Potassium channels have a tetrameric structure consisting of four subunits.
3. Voltage-gated calcium channels are complex, with $\alpha_1$, $\alpha_2\delta$, $\beta_{1-4}$ and $\gamma$ subunits, and these form four common types: L-type, N-type, P/Q type, R-type and T-type.
4. Voltage-gated chloride channels also exist, and these play a role in resetting the action potential caused by the opening of other voltage-gated channels.

Another gene family embraces $Cl^-$ channels and a class of ligand-gated channels activated by ATP. Ligand-gated ion channels are relatively insensitive to the membrane potential and therefore cannot by themselves produce a self-amplifying depolarization. The acetylcholine receptor is the best example of a ligand-gated ion channel; this was the first channel to be sequenced. The acetylcholine receptor of skeletal muscle is composed of five transmembrane polypeptides encoded by four separate genes, and is non-specific for ion selectivity. $Na^+$, $K^+$ and $Ca^{2+}$ may pass through the acetylcholine-gated channel.

### Transporters or Pumps

Transporters are long polypeptide chains that cross the lipid bilayer several times and transfer bound solutes across the membrane either passively or actively. Transporters are often called pumps since they are able to 'pump' certain solutes across the membrane against their electrochemical gradients. This active transport is tightly coupled to a source of metabolic energy such as an ion gradient or ATP hydrolysis. The solute binding sites are exposed alternately on one side of the membrane and then on the other. There are three categories of transporters:

1. Uniporters move a solute from one side of the membrane to the other.
2. Symporters simultaneously transport two solutes in the same direction.
3. Antiporters transfer two solutes, in opposite directions.

### Antiporters, pH and $Ca^{2+}$ Regulation

Enzymes in mammalian and marine cells require a pH of around 7.2 in order to function correctly, and the correct cellular pH is maintained via one or more $Na^+$-driven antiporters in the plasma membrane; these use energy stored in the $Na^+$ gradient to pump excess H across the membrane:

1. The $Na^+/H^+$ exchanger couples an influx of $Na^+$ to an efflux of $H^+$.
2. The $Na^+$-driven $Cl^-/HCO_3^-$ exchanger couples an influx of $Na^+$ and $HCO_3^-$ to an efflux of $Cl^-$ and $H^+$.

Free cytosolic calcium must be maintained at very low levels in all cells, and $Ca^{2+}$ is actively pumped out of the cell by $Ca^{2+}$ ATPase and a $Na^+/Ca^{2+}$ exchanger.

### The $Na^+/K^+$ Pump

The concentration of $K^+$ is typically 20 times higher inside cells than outside, whereas the reverse is true for $Na^+$. The $Na^+/K^+$ pump maintains these concentration differences by actively pumping $Na^+$ out of the cell against its steep electrochemical gradient and pumping $K^+$ inside. This pump is vital for survival: it has been estimated that 30% of cellular energy is devoted to maintaining its activity. The pump is an enzyme, and it can work in reverse to produce ATP. Electrochemical gradients for $Na^+$ and $K^+$ together with relative concentrations of ATP, ADP and phosphate in the cell determine whether ATP is synthesized or $Na^+$ is pumped out of the cell. This pump is also involved in regulating osmolarity.

### Calcium Regulation

Extracellular fluids contain millimolar quantities of calcium, whereas the cytoplasm contains nanomolar levels; therefore, calcium ions tend to enter cells by diffusion. Several pumps operate to maintain low cytoplasmic $Ca^{2+}$ levels:

1. A 110-kDa $Ca^{2+}$-transport ATPase on the endoplasmic reticulum (ER) membrane lowers cytoplasmic calcium.
2. A $Na^+/Ca^{2+}$ exchanger on the cell plasma membrane pumps calcium ions out of the cell.
3. Calcium is also sequestered into the mitochondrial matrix.

Calcium is stored on the ER bound to several proteins, including calsequestrins and calreticulin. In order to use intracellular calcium gradients as messengers for signaling, cells must employ two further mechanisms:

1. A mechanism that enables a short burst of calcium to be released into the cytoplasm in response to other signals.
2. A mechanism that can 'read' these signals and translate them into cellular signals: receptor-operated calcium channels on the calcium stores and proteins that respond to calcium signals cause a cascade of phosphorylation/dephosphorylation reactions that translate into specific activities.

Four groups of calcium channels have been recognized thus far:

1. Voltage-gated calcium channels were discovered in cardiac and neuronal cells; major groups in this category are L- and T-type voltage-dependent calcium channels. Voltage-dependent calcium channels are found in the oocyte plasma membrane.
2. Receptor-operated calcium channels include the N-methyl-D-aspartate (NMDA) receptor found in neuronal tissue and the ATP receptor found in smooth muscle.
3. Second messenger-operated calcium channels include the inositol trisphosphate ($IP_3$) and calcium-induced calcium release (CICR)-activated group of channels.
4. Calcium channels have been found that are sensitive to physical forces and stretching; these may regulate cell size and response to injury.

The $IP_3$ and CICR receptors are of major interest in fertilization and early development.

A receptor-operated calcium channel known as the ryanodine-sensitive calcium release channel (due to its sensitivity to the plant alkaloid ryanodine) was discovered in skeletal muscle. This receptor consists of a tetrameric unit with 450-kDa protein monomers and a ryanodine-binding site, a $Ca^{2+}$-release channel and a membrane-spanning domain. The activity of the channel is enhanced by caffeine, adenine nucleotides and calcium itself; ruthenium red and procaine act as inhibitors. The ryanodine-sensitive calcium channel is thought to be responsible for $IP_3$-insensitive calcium-induced calcium release in many systems, suggesting a further sensitivity to calcium itself.

The inositol trisphosphate ($IP_3$)-sensitive calcium release channel is found in nonmuscle cells, discovered initially as a channel gated by hormone–ligand interactions on the cell surface. The $IP_3$ receptor is a tetramer of 260-kDa subunits, and $IP_3$ receptors are found in the oocytes of many species, as well as in neurons. The $IP_3$ receptor releases calcium in response to $IP_3$ and related molecules. Heparin is a known inhibitor of $IP_3$-induced calcium release. Interestingly, both the $IP_3$ receptor and the ryanodine channel show a bell-type sensitivity to calcium: the channel is first sensitized, and then desensitized in the presence of increasing amounts of $Ca^{2+}$. These data suggest that a small amount of calcium release has a positive feedback effect on further calcium release, which eventually stops through both emptying of stores and channel desensitization. This property of calcium channels helps to explain the 'calcium spike' phenomenon observed in many cell types.

Oocytes, in common with other cells, have three fundamental calcium release mechanisms:

1. Calcium influx from the external milieu can be regulated through voltage-dependent calcium channels in the plasma membrane.
2. Inositol trisphosphate produced within the cell binds to a receptor-operated calcium channel on the ER, causing calcium to be released from internal stores.
3. The CICR mechanism in which calcium itself causes a further release of calcium, either by sensitizing the $IP_3$ receptor to IICR or through the action of a third channel, the ryanodine receptor.

The potent calcium-releasing activity of cyclic ADP-ribose (cADPr) was initially discovered in sea urchin oocytes, and in 1989 cADPr was found to be the natural ligand for the ryanodine receptor in nonmuscle cells. cADPr is a metabolite of $NAD^+$ and has now been shown to be an active calcium-releasing metabolite in many species. However, other calcium-releasing metabolites such as $NAADP^+$, derived from

$NADP^+$, have also been shown to possess calcium-releasing properties, suggesting that metabolites of nicotinamide form a family of calcium-releasing second messengers. cADPr is produced through the activity of adenosine diphosphate-ribosyl cyclases, which are in turn regulated by levels of cyclic guanosine monophosphate (cGMP), and may be produced in response to hormonal stimulation in some cell types such as pancreatic β-cells.

Calcium transients or 'spikes' in the cell cytoplasm were first measured in the 1970s using calcium-sensitive aquaporin proteins that released light in the presence of calcium together with calcium-sensitive fluorescence dyes such as Fura-2 and Fluo 3. These proteins clearly demonstrated transient increases in intracellular calcium but gave little information on the properties of these spikes. The introduction of two-dimensional cell imaging such as photo-imaging detectors and confocal microscopy allowed the properties of calcium peaks to be observed in many cell types. Calcium spikes are now known to either remain localized to distinct regions of the cell cytoplasm or cross the cytoplasm in the form of a wave. Waves of calcium release are common to many cell types and are especially common in oocytes of many species during fertilization. Interestingly, calcium increases simultaneously throughout the whole cytoplasm in some cells, and different species have distinct mechanisms for the formation of calcium waves or the simultaneous increase in calcium. However, one common feature underlies the calcium transients: they are produced either by $IP_3$-induced mechanisms, CICR-induced mechanisms – or both.

Calcium spikes regulate cell activities through the action of two major proteins: calmodulin and calcium/calmodulin-dependent protein kinase II (CaMKII). Calmodulin is a 16-kDa ubiquitous calcium-binding protein that mediates a host of cell processes in many cell types in response to a calcium signal. Most cellular proteins are unable to bind to calcium itself, and therefore calmodulin acts as the primary messenger of calcium signals. Calmodulin has four sites for calcium binding and undergoes a conformational change when calcium is bound. Its function does not depend on all four sites being occupied, suggesting that different levels of cytoplasmic calcium can activate diverse processes. The relevance of calmodulin during the cell cycle is inferred from its spatial localization: during interphase it is localized throughout the cytoplasm but migrates to the mitotic apparatus during M-phase.

The calcium/calmodulin-dependent protein kinases (CaM kinases) are a series of serine/threonine protein kinases activated by calmodulin. These kinases are oligomeric proteins with diverse subunits of approximately 50–60 kDa that form a complex of between 300 and 600 kDa, depending on cell type. The CaM kinase is characterized by a 'memory' effect, i.e., the activation of the kinase supersedes the presence of $Ca^{2+}$/calmodulin. Two types of CaM kinase exist:

1. Specialized CaM kinases, e.g., myosin light chain kinase (MLCK), involved in muscle contraction.
2. Multifunctional CaM kinases, e.g., CaM kinase II, involved in a variety of cellular processes; it is relatively nonspecific for substrates, leading to the question of how it can manage to organize specific cell processes.

A calcium spike can trigger specific activities in a cell. The calcium spike at fertilization is probably designed to be a large, nonspecific signal that causes several major effects including degrading cell cycle blocks, release of cortical granules, upregulation of metabolism, decondensation of the sperm head and activating a developmental program. However, calcium spikes can also trigger specific mechanisms, often achieved through spatial localization of calcium signals, e.g., in sea urchin oocytes after activation. Localized calcium spikes appear in many classes of cells such as neurons, pancreatic cells and embryos.

## Metabolic Pathways

Each metabolic pathway is a series of reactions, organized such that the products of one reaction become substrates for the next (Figure 1.8). The reactants in a pathway may be modified in a series of small steps, so that energy is released in controlled amounts, or minor adjustments can be made to the structure of molecules.

**Anabolic** pathways require energy to synthesize complex molecules from smaller units.

**Catabolic** pathways break molecules up into smaller units which can then be used to generate energy.

Each step in a pathway is catalyzed by a specific enzyme, and each enzyme represents a point for control of the overall pathway. The steps of the pathway may be spatially arranged, so that the product of one reaction is in the right place to become the substrate of the next enzyme. This allows high local concentrations of

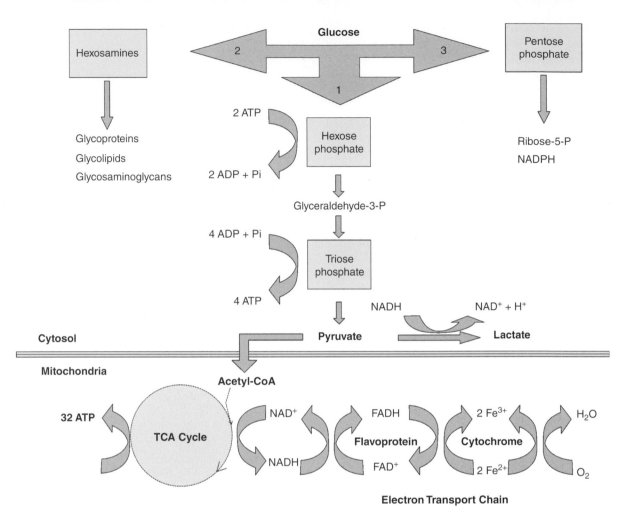

**Figure 1.8** Pathways that metabolize glucose in a mammalian cell. Pi = inorganic phosphate.

substrate molecules to build up and biochemical reactions to proceed rapidly. A pathway arranged in this manner may be catalyzed by a multienzyme complex.

- **Glycolysis,** which breaks glucose down into pyruvate, takes place in the cell cytoplasm; pyruvate enters mitochondria to be further metabolized.
- **Fatty acid oxidation** and the **Krebs cycle** (TCA or citric acid cycle) take place in the mitochondrial matrix.

The Krebs cycle is part of a metabolic pathway that converts carbohydrates, fats and proteins into $CO_2$ and ATP, which is generated by a process of oxidative phosphorylation. ATP is exported from the mitochondria for use in protein synthesis, DNA replication, etc.: all energy-requiring processes of life are coupled to the cleavage of ATP:

$$ATP \longleftrightarrow ADP + Phosphate + Energy$$

ATP is exported from the mitochondria in exchange for ADP arising from the ATP that has been broken down to drive cellular metabolism.

**Redox reactions:** oxidation and reduction are electron-transfer processes, involving NAD–NADH.

- NADP(H) is generally used for anabolic reactions.
- NAD(H) is used for catabolic reactions.

These reactions need ubiquinone and cytochrome C, cytochrome oxidase (inhibited by cyanide).

- Oxidation: loss of electrons; reduction: gain of electrons.
- An oxidizing agent removes electrons and is itself reduced.
- A reducing agent gains electrons and is itself oxidized.

# Reactive Oxygen Species (ROS, Oxygen Radicals)

ROS are molecules that contain the oxygen ion or peroxide; the presence of unpaired valence electrons makes them highly reactive. They are formed as a by-product of oxygen metabolism, and have an important role in cell signaling mechanisms. However, high levels of ROS (i.e., oxidative stress) can cause oxidative damage to nucleic acids, proteins and lipids, as well as inactivate enzymes by oxidation of cofactors.

ROS also play fundamental roles in physiology; they are involved in signal transduction pathways, and more than 10 redox-sensitive transcription factors have thus far been identified. Through effects on kinase enzymes, they can influence cell growth, differentiation, migration, mitosis and other cellular processes. Cellular homeostasis maintains ROS concentrations at optimal, physiologically low levels, regulated by the overall antioxidant status. An imbalance that leads to an excess creates high-grade oxidative stress, with effects on DNA, proteins and lipids. A stressful imbalance can be caused by malfunction of endogenous pro- and antioxidants, as well as by various exogenous factors: smoking, inappropriate nutrition and other environmental and lifestyle-related factors. Antioxidants such as ascorbic acid (vitamin C), tocopherol (vitamin E), glutathione, hypotaurine, pyruvic acid, uric acid and albumin are important in cellular defense mechanisms against ROS damage (Figure 1.9).

ROS can cause damage to DNA in oocytes, sperm and embryos, with important consequences for fertilization and embryo development (Guerin *et al.*, 2001; Ménézo *et al.*, 2017). Oocytes are

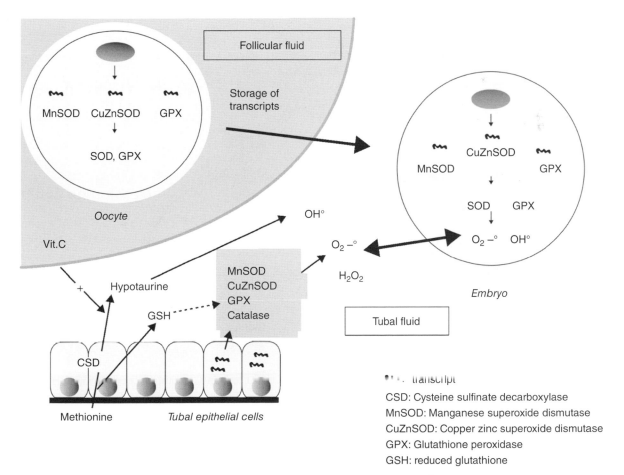

**Figure 1.9** Mechanisms in oocytes and embryos that protect against ROS damage. Courtesy of Y. Ménézo.

particularly susceptible during the final stages of follicular growth, and ROS damage to sperm DNA has been strongly linked to male infertility (Evenson, 2016). Most significantly, there is a strong correlation between oxidative stress and DNA methylation, via an influence on the one-carbon cycle; oxidative stress can induce inappropriate gene expression.

### Superoxide Dismutase (SOD)

SOD enzymes catalyze the dismutation of superoxide into oxygen and hydrogen peroxide, an important defense against potential ROS damage. Three SOD enzymes are present in mammalian cells:

- SOD1: dimer, present in the cytoplasm, contains $Cu^{2+}$ and $Zn^{2+}$
- SOD2: tetramer, mitochondrial enzyme, contains $Mn^{2+}$
- SOD3: tetramer, extracellular, contains $Cu^{2+}$ and $Zn^{2+}$.

## The One-Carbon Cycle

The one-carbon cycle (1-CC), also known as the methionine or methylation cycle, is a network of metabolic pathways that transfer stable one-carbon groups in a series of inter-related biochemical reactions surrounding folate, methionine and choline (Figure 1.10). Carbon units from amino acids (serine, glycine) are cycled to a variety of outputs, including generation of active methyl groups, synthesis of purines and thymidine and maintenance of redox potential via generation of NADPH (anabolic pathways), NADH (catabolic pathways) and antioxidant molecules. Generation of S-adenosylmethionine (SAM), the universal methyl donor required for methylation of DNA and histones, is one of the most important functions of the 1-CC. Vitamins B3, B6, B9, B12 and zinc are mandatory cofactors in maintaining the integrity of the 1-CC, and any deficiency in their supply, transport and metabolism will lead to problems associated with methylation.

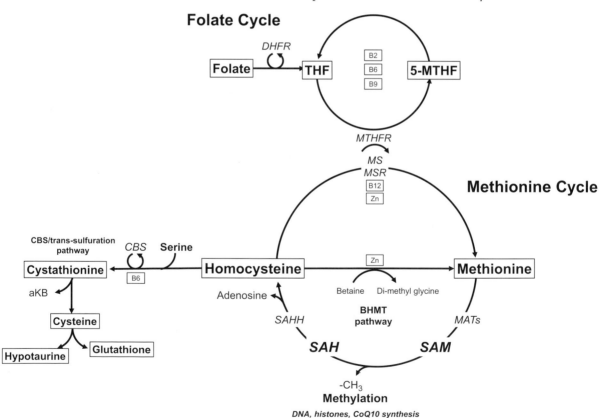

**Figure 1.10** The one-carbon cycle Two separate pathways that revolve around methionine and folate interact to produce outputs that are important in the metabolism of nucleotides, proteins, lipids and substrates for methylation reactions and in generating reducing power to maintain appropriate redox potential. Homocysteine recycling is an important feature of these pathways. Courtesy of A. Ontiveros.

## The One-Carbon Cycle

The 1-CC can be outlined in two separate but interacting pathways that revolve around methionine and folate, respectively. The outputs from these two cycles are important in the metabolism of nucleotides, proteins, lipids and substrates for methylation reactions and in generating reducing power to maintain appropriate redox potential. Homocysteine recycling is an important feature of these pathways.

### The Methionine Cycle

- Methionine is activated by conversion to S-adenosylmethionine (SAM) through the action of methionine adenosyltransferases.
- SAM is an active methyl (–CH$_3$) donor, necessary for methylation of DNA/histones, RNA, hormones, neurotransmitters, membrane lipids, proteins, etc. It is required for chromatin-mediated regulation of gene expression, and for the synthesis of spermine and spermidine, which are essential for sperm DNA stability; it is also required for synthesis of the ubiquitous coenzyme Q10, an important component of the mitochondrial electron transport chain in generating cellular energy in the form of ATP.
- After releasing its methyl group, SAM forms S-adenosylhomocysteine (SAH); deadenylation by S-adenosylhomocysteine hydrolase (SAHH) releases homocysteine (Hcy) and adenosine, completing a full turn of the methionine cycle.
- Activity of the methionine cycle is dependent upon the folate cycle.

### The Folate Cycle

- Dietary folate is converted to active tetrahydrofolate (THF) by the enzyme dihydrofolate reductase (DHFR).
- Methylene tetrahydrofolate reductase (MTHFR) converts THF to 5-methyl-tetrahydrofolate (5-MTHF).
- Demethylation of MTHFR donates the carbon into the methionine cycle through methylation of Hcy via methionine synthase (MS, also known as MTR) and methionine synthase reductase (MSR, also known as MTRR) and its cofactor, vitamin B12.
- Tetrahydrofolate (THF) is released and will be recycled to 5-MTHF by DHFR.

## The One-Carbon Cycle (continued)

### Homocysteine recycling

Homocysteine must be recycled to methionine by the addition of a methyl group, and this can be accomplished via different pathways:

1. Methylation via methionine synthase (MS/MTR): Hcy accepts the carbon from the folate pool through 5-MTHF to generate methionine (Met).
2. Betaine homocysteine methyl transferase (BHMT) pathway (less active).
3. Cystathionine beta synthase (CBS)/ transsulfuration pathway:

   - Hcy can condense with serine to generate cystathione, via CBS
   - Cystathione is cleaved to generate alpha-ketobutyrate (aKB) and cysteine
   - Cysteine sulfonate decarboxylase can shunt cysteine into glutathione production and hypotaurine synthesis (Guerin et al., 2001). Both glutathione and hypotaurine are major antioxidants and potent neutralizers of ROS; they are found in high concentrations in the environment of the preimplantation embryo.

Successful reproduction and embryonic/fetal development are crucially dependent upon maintaining the correct function of the 1-CC: deficiencies or defects in this cycle during development can affect the integrity of the epigenome, with both prenatal and postnatal consequences. An adequate supply of folic acid for the folate pathway is of paramount importance. The human oocyte has very high levels of folate receptor (300× background) and folate transporter 1 (660× background) expression, indicating a high level of trafficking of this molecule (Benkhalifa et al., 2010). Zinc, folic acid (vitamin B9), and vitamins B12 (cobalamin), B6 and B2 act as coenzymes in the 1-CC; deficiencies of these nutrients can disrupt molecular rearrangement reactions in pathways involved in methylation, with an impact on the establishment of epigenetic/imprinting marks in gametes and early embryos.

This is of particular concern in assisted reproduction: ovarian stimulation increases the homocysteine concentration in follicular fluid, which passes into the oocyte. Hcy is a neurotoxic compound; it competes with methionine for the same amino acid transporter, restricting methionine entry into any cell. Reduced intracellular methionine creates an imbalance in the methionine cycle that will inhibit methylation reactions (Ménézo *et al.*, 1989; Ebisch *et al.*, 2006, 2007; Berker *et al.*, 2009). Methionyl transfer RNA (Met tRNA) is also important as the initiator molecule for protein synthesis. Human oocytes cannot recycle homocysteine via the transsulfuration pathway, due to the fact that cystathione synthase (CBS) is not expressed and cystathionase (CT) is very weakly expressed, both in the oocyte and in the preimplantation embryo. Homocysteine is therefore both a cause and a consequence of oxidative stress, acting as a link between oxidative stress and imprinting problems (Ménézo *et al.*, 2011, 2014, 2016).

Placental development is highly susceptible to changes in epigenetic status (Tunster *et al.*, 2013); methylation is also important for trophoblast formation and differentiation, under paternal control. Defects in the 1-CC affect the availability of methyl groups for epigenetic regulation of genes that affect placental formation and function; this can lead to altered programming in the fetus with the potential of increasing risk for metabolic disease in later life (Padmanabhan & Watson, 2013). Abnormal folate metabolism has been shown to cause transgenerational effects, probably through epigenetic inheritance, suggesting that effects of disrupted 1-CC metabolism might have effects on the health of future progeny (Padmanabhan *et al.*, 2013).

Environmental endocrine-disrupting chemicals (EDCs), including bisphenol A (BPA), induce DNA methylation errors and oxidative stress, with an impact on fertility. Animal studies have demonstrated that supporting the 1-CC with appropriate dietary supplements can reduce the effects of EDCs on critical metabolic pathways: couples who are attending for infertility treatment can benefit from nutritional support that is capable of activating and sustaining the 1-CC (Cornet *et al.*, 2015).

Although it is now clear that methyl donor deficiency or abnormal folate metabolism can disrupt epigenetic profiles, the majority of ART media currently available for embryo culture does not contain methyl donors, including folate, methionine and *S*-adenosylmethionine (SAM).

## Genetic Variation in Components of the 1-CC

Genetic polymorphism in genes encoding the enzymes involved in the 1-CC can have important functional consequences, with links now established to fertility, pregnancy outcomes, Down's syndrome, neural tube defects, cancers, cardiovascular disease and neuropsychiatric syndromes (see Tollefsbol, 2017 for review). The downstream consequences of disruption in the 1-CC are complex and include changes to genomic DNA methylation and imbalance in Hcy levels. Numerous genetic variants have been identified, of which a few are listed below:

1. Mutations in the gene encoding methylenetetrahydrofolate reductase (MTHFR) are common, reaching a prevalence of 50% in some populations. At least 30 different mutations have been identified (Rozen, 2004); two of the most common variants, C677T and A1298C, have been widely studied and are known to result in decreased enzyme activity that limits the supply of 5-MTHF into the 1-CC, with downstream effects on methionine synthase (MTR) in particular. Individuals who are homozygous for these mutations (especially C677T) often show increased levels of serum Hcy, and an association between the C677T isoform and the risk of autism spectrum disorders has been observed (Sener *et al.*, 2014).

   Recent evidence suggests that defective methylation linked to MTHFR may contribute to male infertility, via increased sperm fragmentation (SDI). Patients with high levels of fragmentation measured by a sperm DNA integrity (SDI) assay should be tested for MTHFR isoforms, and accordingly recommended treatment with its downstream metabolite, 5-MTHF, when appropriate (Ménézo *et al.*, 2017).

2. Serinehydroxymethyltransferase (SHMT), which allows the synthesis of methyleneTHF, has a C1420T variant that leads to hyperhomocysteinemia (Wernimont *et al.*, 2011).

3. Variant P1173L of the MTR gene that encodes methionine synthase causes megaloblastic anemia and developmental delay; the A2756G variant generates hyperhomocysteinemia, especially in homozygotes (Watkins *et al.*, 2002).

4. The defective variant A66G of methionine synthase reductase (MTRR) is almost as prevalent as MTHFR variants, is clinically linked to hyperhomocysteinemia and may be associated with male infertility (Xu *et al.*, 2017).

Mutations in the BHMT pathway induce neural tube defects and/or hyperhomocysteinemia (Cao *et al.*, 2018).

# Cellular Replication

## The Cell Cycle

Replication of individual cells is the fundamental basis of growth and reproduction for all living organisms: each cell grows and then divides to produce daughter cells. Cells can divide by using one of two different mechanisms – mitosis or meiosis. During mitosis, the cellular DNA that represents the cell's entire diploid genome is replicated into two copies, and the two cells produced after division each contain this same diploid genome. Meiosis, or 'reduction division,' splits the DNA in the diploid genome in half, so that the daughter cells are haploid, with a single copy of each gene. This is the process that leads to the generation of the germ cells, sperm and oocyte.

However, true haploidy is only reached after two meiotic divisions: the two sister chromatids of the remaining chromosomes are not identical before the second meiotic division, so that some genes are still present as two different variants. The female pronucleus in the zygote is truly haploid only for a short time period, between anaphase II and the point at which zygotic DNA replication is initiated (zygote gene activation).

The sequence of growth, replication and division that produces a new cell is known as the cell cycle; in human cells, the **mitotic** cell cycle takes from 8 to 24 hours to complete. The mitotic cell cycle is divided into phases, G1, S, G2 (**interphase**) and M (Figure 1.11):

- **G1**: cell growth, a period of high metabolic activity when new proteins are synthesized; rRNA, mRNA, tRNA are produced in the nucleolus, and new organelles are formed.

- **S**: synthesis of DNA and duplication of the centrosome. Each new DNA double helix is surrounded by histones to form chromatids, which are held together at the centromere.

- **G2**: centrioles replicate, and the cell prepares for mitosis.

- **M**: mitosis has four phases, during which the replicated DNA is distributed to the two new daughter cells:

  - prophase, metaphase, anaphase, telophase.

(i) *Early prophase*: the two replicated chromosomes condense, the nuclear membrane dissociates, centrioles divide and migrate to different poles, microtubules form an aster shape around the centrioles, and form the spindle. Spindle fibers attach to the centromeres at the kinetochore.

(ii) *Metaphase*: chromosomes are lined up on the equatorial spindle plate.

(iii) *Anaphase*: chromatids separate and are pulled by the spindle fibers to opposite poles.

(iv) *Telophase*: chromatids have reached opposite poles, and a nuclear membrane forms around them. The chromosomes uncoil to become indistinct, spindle fibers disintegrate and the nucleolus reforms.

During **cytokinesis**, the cytoplasm divides to form two daughter cells. A ring of microfilaments develops around the cell, usually near the equator. These microfilaments are attached to the cell membrane and contract when division takes place to pull the cell in (like a drawstring), creating a division furrow.

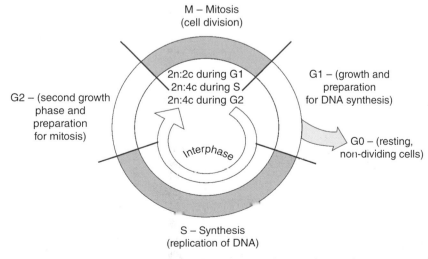

**Figure 1.11** Phases of the cell cycle. n = chromosome number; c = chromatid (DNA copy) number.

**G0:** a cell can leave the cell cycle, temporarily or permanently during G1, and enter a 'resting' phase known as G0, where its designated function will continue (e.g., secretion, immune functions). Some G0 cells may be terminally differentiated and will never re-enter the cell cycle to continue dividing. Others can be stimulated to re-enter at G1 and proceed to new rounds of cell division (e.g., lymphocytes encountering a new antigen). A G0 phase requires active repression of the genes required for mitosis – cancer cells cannot enter G0, and they continue to divide indefinitely.

The duration of the cell cycle varies considerably, ranging from a few hours in early embryonic development to an average of 2 to 5 days for epithelial cells. Specialized cells such as cortical neurons or cardiac muscle cells that are terminally differentiated may remain in G0 indefinitely. The time that each cell spends in each phase of the cell cycle also varies. Human cells that are dividing in culture with a 24-hour cell cycle spend approximately 9 hours in G1, 10 hours in S and 4.5 hours in G2, and the M-phase lasts approximately 30 minutes. During human preimplantation development, the cycle in which the zygote genome is activated is the longest. The timing of events in the cell cycle can be initiated by external events, such as a hormonal trigger, cell density or other extracellular signals; a highly sophisticated and carefully orchestrated series of internal control mechanisms regulates each phase/stage of the cycle via fluctuating levels of a number of proteins and cofactors within the cell.

## Cell Cycle Checkpoints

When a cell receives a signal to divide, a cascade of internal events takes place to regulate its progress into interphase. The daughter cells produced must be exact duplicates, containing the same cellular DNA of its diploid genome – mistakes in the duplication or distribution of the chromosomes lead to mutations that will be subsequently carried to new cells. Every parameter required during each phase of the cycle must be correctly met before the cell can continue, and precisely timed internal checkpoint mechanisms act to prevent compromised cells from continuing to divide:

**G1 checkpoint:** checks the integrity of DNA, and determines whether cell size and protein reserves are sufficient for the cell to irreversibly commit to mitosis.

**G2 checkpoint:** ensures that all of the chromosomes have been replicated; if DNA damage is detected, the cycle is halted and the cell attempts to repair the damaged DNA or complete DNA replication. This checkpoint can block entry into mitosis if conditions are not met.

**M checkpoint**, also known as the **spindle checkpoint**: ensures correct attachment of all the sister chromatids to the spindle microtubules. The cycle will only proceed if the kinetochores of each pair of sister chromatids are attached to at least two spindle fibers arising from opposite poles of the cell. This checkpoint inhibits the anaphase-promoting complex (APC) until the chromosomes are correctly attached to spindle fibers.

Cell cycle checkpoints consist of positive and negative regulator molecules that interact: in order for the cell to move past each checkpoint, all positive regulators must be 'turned on,' and negative regulators 'turned off.'

Positive regulators are driven by *cyclin-dependent kinases* (CDKs), serine/threonine protein kinases that phosphorylate key substrates to promote the DNA synthesis that will lead to mitosis. Cyclin proteins bind to CDKs and induce conformational changes that promote kinase activity, and this initiates a positive feedback loop that increases CDK activity. The cyclin/CDK complex induces transcriptional changes that allow synthesis of proteins to regulate downstream cell cycle events that will commit the cell to division. Levels of CDK proteins are relatively stable throughout the cell cycle, but the levels of cyclin proteins fluctuate; this determines when the cyclin/CDK complexes form, which acts to regulate different checkpoints. The cyclins that were active in the previous cell cycle stage are degraded in the next stage. The cell cycle can progress through the checkpoints only in the presence of a specific concentration of fully activated cyclin/CDK.

Molecules that are known to have a negative (inhibitory) function include retinoblastoma protein (Rb), p53 and p21; these proteins have a primary role at the G1 checkpoint. *Rb* functions in monitoring cell size, through binding to transcription factors (most commonly E2F). When active (dephosphorylated) Rb binds to E2F, transcription is blocked. As cell size increases, Rb is slowly phosphorylated until it becomes inactivated, releasing E2F which can now turn on the genes required for G1/S transition.

*p53* has a role in detecting damaged DNA. If DNA damage is detected duing G1, p53 halts the cell cycle and recruits enzymes to repair the DNA. If the DNA cannot be repaired, p53 can trigger apoptosis, preventing the duplication of damaged chromosomes.

Production of *p21* is triggered by rising levels of p53, and this molecule binds to and inhibits the activity of the CDK/cyclin complexes, enforcing a block initiated by p53 to prevent G1/S transition. Cells that are exposed to stress accumulate higher levels of p53 and p21, repressing the transition into S-phase.

The *anaphase-promoting complex/cyclosome* (APC/C) is a large multi-subunit E3 ubiquitin ligase that is important in controlling entry into S-phase; it also has a role in regulating meiosis. APC/C becomes activated at the onset of mitosis, interacting with cyclin proteins to control cyclin/CDK activity. CDK activity inhibits separase, a protease that functions in allowing sister chromatid segregation; APC/C sustains low levels of mitotic CDK activity during G1, allowing the cell to disassemble the mitotic spindle as a prelude to a new round of DNA replication in S-phase.

## Definitions

**Chromosomes**: The repository of genetic information, molecules of DNA complexed with specific proteins.

**Chromatin**: The protein/DNA complex that makes up the chromosome.

**Chromatids**: Pairs of identical DNA molecules formed after DNA replication, joined at the centromere.

**Centromere**: Constricted region in a chromosome which divides it into two 'arms.' It serves as an attachment site for sister chromatids and spindle fibers, allowing chromosomes to be pulled to different poles. Normally located centrally, but in some species found near the end (pericentric), at the end (telocentric) or spread all over the chromosomes (holocentric).

**Diploid**: Two pairs of each chromosome in a cell.

**Haploid**: One of each pair of chromosomes in a cell.

**Aneuploid**: Incorrect number of chromosomes; e.g., trisomy (three copies), monosomy (one copy).

**Univalent**: abnormal chromosome that contains a pair of nonidentical sister chromatids, formed when a bivalent splits before anaphase I into a pair of chromosomes. A correct metaphase II chromosome can also be referred to as 'univalent.'

## Cytoplasmic Organelles Involved in Mitosis and Meiosis

**Spindle apparatus**: barrel-shaped structure responsible for separating sister chromatids during cell division; contains condensed chromosomes, microtubules and associated proteins including the 'molecular motors' kinesis and dynein.

**Centriole**: nine triplets of microtubules arranged in a pinwheel shape to form a cylinder; contains centrin, connexin and tektin.

**Centrosome**: two centrioles positioned at right angles to each other, surrounded by dense pericentriolar material; acts as the microtubule-organizing center (MTOC) of the cell, regulating progression of the cell cycle. It is usually associated with the nuclear membrane during prophase, when centrosomes migrate to opposite poles of the cell. The spindle apparatus forms between the two centrosomes; each daughter cell receives one centrosome after cell division, and this is duplicated during S-phase of the next cell cycle.

- The meiotic spindle in human oocytes lacks centrosomes.

**Pericentriolar material** (PCN): amorphous mass of >100 proteins that nucleate and anchor the microtubules; include γ-tubulin, pericentrin and ninein.

**Spindle fibers**: clusters of microtubules that grow out from each centrosome toward the metaphase plate, guiding chromosomes so that sister chromatids are at opposite poles.

**Kinetochore**: a protein complex that assembles on centromeres, acting as a molecular bridge between the chromosomes and microtubule filaments. Kinetochores assemble, disassemble and reassemble during different stages of meiosis. Microtubule clusters (spindle fibers, 'K fibers') attach to kinetochores during cell division to pull sister chromatids apart. Kinetochore–microtubule attachments can be:

*Amphitelic*: sister kinetochores of each chromosome are attached to a single pole of the spindle, so that chromosomes can be correctly separated during anaphase.

*Monotelic*: one kinetochore is unattached.

*Syntelic*: both sister kinetochores are attached to K-fibers from the same pole.

*Merotelic*: a sister kinetochore is attached to both spindle poles instead of being attached to a single spindle pole only; the chromatid will be pulled from both sides during anaphase leading to lagging chromosomes.

(See Figure 1.12)

25

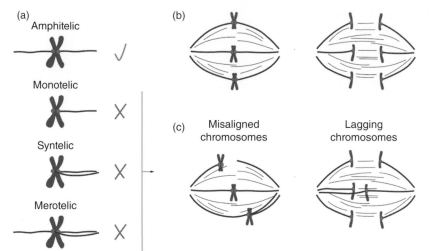

**Figure 1.12** Kinetochore–microtubule attachments. (a) Correct attachment (tick, amphitelic). Incorrect attachments (**X**): monotelic, one kinetochore is unattached; syntelic, both sister kinetochores attached to K-fibers from the same pole; merotelic, one of the kinetochores attached to K-fibers from opposite poles. (b) Balanced, amphitelic attachment: chromosomes are aligned, and sister chromatid separation is synchronized. (c) Incorrect attachments can lead to unbalanced tension and chromosome alignment defects (misaligned chromosomes) or lagging chromosomes during anaphase. Reproduced with kind permission of Bianka Seres, from 'Characterisation of a novel spindle domain in mammalian meiosis,' PhD thesis, University of Cambridge. See color plate section.

Reproduction is based upon transmission of half of each parent's chromosomes to the next generation. This is carried out by setting aside a special population of germ cells that are destined to form the gametes, i.e., spermatozoa and oocytes. Successful completion of meiosis, a specialized form of cell division, is a fundamental part of gametogenesis, and a detailed understanding of this process is a crucial background.

## Mitosis and Meiosis

Meiosis differs from mitosis in a number of ways, as summarized below (see also Figure 1.13).

### Mitosis

- Occurs in all tissues.
- Involves one round of DNA replication for each cell division.
- Produces genetically identical diploid somatic (body) cells.
- Is a rapid process.
- The daughter cells are genetically identical to the parent cell and have the same number of chromosomes.
- This type of cell division takes place during growth of an organism (e.g., embryonic growth), healing and the development of new cells, and is also important for maintaining populations of cells, replacing those that die.

### Meiosis

- Occurs only in the ovary (oocytes) and the testis (spermatozoa).

- Involves one round of DNA replication and two cell divisions, thus generating haploid products.
- Involves pairing of specific chromosome homologues that then exchange pieces of DNA (genetic recombination), which results in daughter cells that are genetically different from the original germ cells.
- Completion of this cell division may take years.

## Principles of Meiosis

In humans, meiosis is initiated during the first trimester of gestation in females, and following puberty in males. Meiosis allows the exchange of DNA between overlapping sister chromatids, with subsequent recombination into two 'new' chromatids – new, but related, gene combinations can be created, facilitating genetic diversity. This occurs during the 'crossing over' stage of prophase I after homologous chromosomes have been paired, as illustrated in Figure 1.14. In the middle diagram, the sister chromatids crossover at a single cross-over point. In the diagram on the bottom, this leads to an equal and reciprocal exchange of chromatin. The cross-over point occurs between two DNA duplexes that contain four DNA strands (see Figure 1.14). The strands in fact switch their pairing at the joining point to form a crossed-strand junction, a mechanism that was first proposed by Robin Holliday in 1964 and is known as a Holliday structure/junction. Heteroduplexes are regions on recombinant DNA molecules where the two strands are not exactly complementary, and Holliday carried out experiments that detected heteroduplex regions in

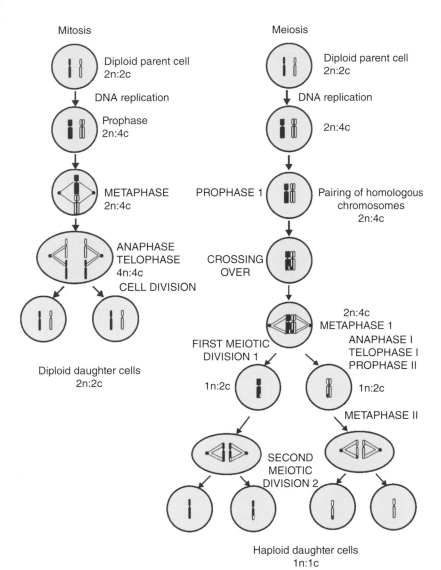

**Figure 1.13** Comparison of mitosis and meiosis; mitosis generates two identical diploid daughter cells, and meiosis generates four chromosomally unique haploid cells from each diploid cell.

both strands of recombining DNA. In Figure 1.14, the junction is magnified to reveal its structure.

Meiosis differs from mitosis in terms of:

1. Checkpoint controls
2. DNA replication
3. Dependence on external stimuli
4. Regulation of cell cycle control proteins.

As described above, cell cycle checkpoints control the order and timing of cell cycle transition, ensuring that critical events such as DNA replication and chromosome separation are completed correctly; one process must be completed before another starts. During meiotic division, recombination must be completed before the beginning of cell division so that a correct segregation of homologous chromosomes is obtained. Several genes have been identified in yeast that are responsible for blocking meiosis when double-strand DNA breaks are not repaired. A spindle assembly checkpoint (SAC) ensures that anaphase I does not begin until paired chromosomes are correctly attached to the spindle. However, the SAC cannot detect some incorrect attachments during meiosis, such as merotelic attachments. Fulka *et al.* (1998) carried out a series of experiments to test DNA-responsive cell cycle checkpoints in bovine and mouse oocytes, using ultraviolet (UV) irradiation to induce DNA damage or chemical treatment to prevent chromosome

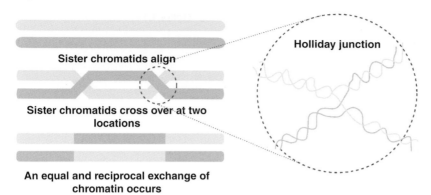

**Figure 1.14** Exchange of genetic material during chromosomal crossing-over; a cross-over point is magnified to illustrate the Holliday junction.

condensation. Their results suggest that replication-dependent checkpoints may be either inactive or highly attenuated in fully grown mammalian oocytes; this should be borne in mind when considering the effects of endocrine or in-vitro manipulations carried out during assisted reproduction cycles, or the in-vitro maturation of oocytes. Although resumption of meiosis apparently has no cell cycle checkpoint, the first cell cycle does, as does each embryonic cell cycle. Micromanipulation experiments in spermatocytes show that tension on the spindle generated by attached homologues acts as a checkpoint. If this tension is eliminated by experimental manipulation, anaphase is prevented. A major difference between the mitotic and meiotic cell cycles lies in the fact that during meiosis the oocyte can be blocked at precise phases of the cell cycle, until a specific stimulus (e.g., hormone or sperm) removes the block.

On completion of MI, oocytes prevent parthenogenetic activation via the activity of cytostatic factor (CSF), which arrests their cell cycle at metaphase of MII (MetII). CSF blocks metaphase II exit until sperm break the arrest, via a cytoplasmic $Ca^{2+-}$ signal that induces MII completion. An egg-specific protein Emi2 (or Early mitotic inhibitor 1-related protein 1; Erp1) has been identified, which inhibits the APC/C. Emi2 degradation is $Ca^{2+}$–dependent and probably functions to establish and then maintain low CSF activity by inhibiting APC/C.

Meiotic blocks differ from the G0 phase in somatic cells in terms of cell cycle regulation and the activity of the key kinases that maintain the arrest. In oocytes, progression from the first to the second meiotic arrest is usually referred to as **oocyte maturation**, and the oocyte is now ready to be ovulated,

i.e., expelled from the ovary. Shortly after ovulation, fertilization occurs; removal of the second meiotic block at fertilization is called **oocyte activation**.

- In the female, only one functional cell is produced from the two meiotic divisions. The three remaining smaller cells are called polar bodies.
- In the male, four functional spermatozoa are produced from each primary cell (Figure 1.15).

## Meiosis in Human Oocytes

Human oocytes begin their process of development in the fetal ovary (see Chapter 3); primary oocytes undergo DNA synthesis, and around the twelfth week of gestation homologous paternal and maternal chromosomes are paired and linked by meiotic recombination as they enter into meiosis I. The sister kinetochores of each chromosome are fused, so that they act as a single kinetochore in what is now called a bivalent chromosome (2n:4c, Figure 1.14). Unlike mitosis, during meiosis the oocyte segregates entire chromosomes instead of sister chromatids. Chromosome alignment and orientation is facilitated by kinetochores fusing into a single unit, with a cohesion complex acting as a 'glue' between chromosomes. At around 16 weeks of gestation, primordial follicles form and primary oocytes arrest at the dictyate stage of prophase 1; homologous bivalent chromosomes are still paired together in a nucleus called the germinal vesicle (GV). This stage persists until just before ovulation, when oocyte growth and maturation resume under the hormonal control of the menstrual cycle. Thus, primary oocytes remain arrested in meiosis I for up to 50 years. During this period, the

GV may undergo degenerative changes that prevent the chromosomes from separating correctly: incorrect chromosome segregation during first or second meiotic divisions results in aneuploidy. With autosomes this is usually lethal; sex chromosome aneuploidy can lead to anomalies of sexual development. Sometimes pairs of chromosomes fail to rejoin after crossing-over at diplotene and are lost from the gamete – they may become attached to another chromosome to produce a partial trisomy, or a balanced translocation.

Meiosis in human oocytes is highly prone to errors in chromosome segregation, resulting in aneuploid oocytes that can lead to either pregnancy loss or genetic disorders (Hassold & Hunt, 2001; Table 1.1).

Human oocytes, like most animal oocytes, lack centrosomes; in the mouse, the function of the centrosome is carried out by MTOCs (Schuh & Ellenberg, 2007); however, meiotic spindles in human oocytes do not have detectable MTOCs, and the spindle is assembled very slowly over a period of several hours (Figure 1.16).

**Table 1.1** Frequency of segregation errors in different types of cells

| Cell type | Frequency of segregation errors |
|---|---|
| Normal mitotic cells | <1% (Knouse *et al.*, 2014) |
| Human spermatocytes | 1–2% (Templado *et al.*, 2011) |
| Oocytes from young women | Approx. 10–25% (Kuliev *et al.*, 2011) |
| Oocytes from women >38 yrs | 50% or higher (Kuliev *et al.*, 2011) |

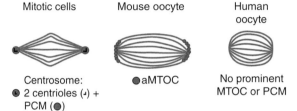

**Figure 1.16** Examples of different types of spindle morphology and location of spindle poles. Bipolar mitotic cell spindles are organized by centrosomes (two centrioles in orthogonal arrangement surrounded by the pericentriolar material [PCM]) with sharp, pointed spindle poles. The barrel-shaped meiotic spindle in mouse oocytes is organized by the coalescence of multiple acentrosomal microtubule-organizing centers made up of PCM components (aMTOCs). The small, barrel-shaped spindle in human oocytes does not contain prominent MTOCs or foci of PCM. Modified from Bennabi *et al.*, 2016 [CC license BY-NC-SA 3.0], with thanks to Bianka Seres. See color plate section.

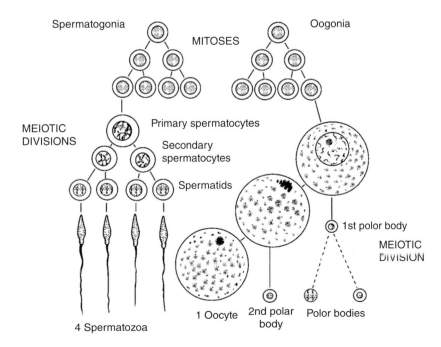

**Figure 1.15** Gametogenesis. Gametogenesis in the male gives rise to four functional spermatozoa; in the female only one of the four daughter cells becomes a functional oocyte. Modified from Dale [1983].

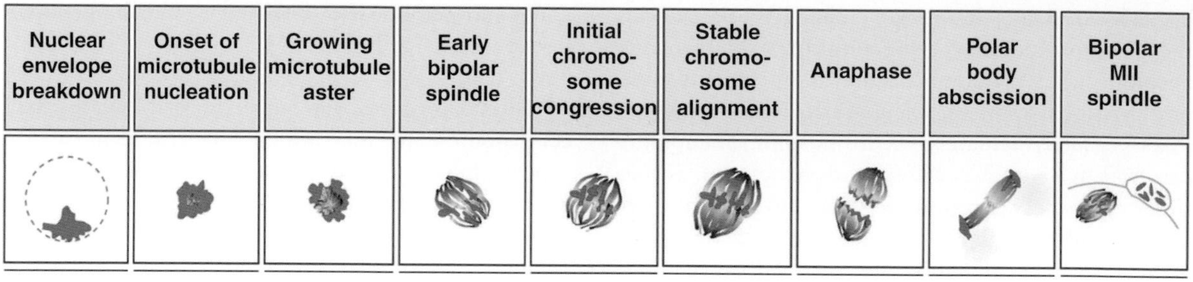

| Nuclear envelope breakdown | Onset of microtubule nucleation | Growing microtubule aster | Early bipolar spindle | Initial chromo-some congression | Stable chromo-some alignment | Anaphase | Polar body abscission | Bipolar MII spindle |
|---|---|---|---|---|---|---|---|---|
| | | | | | | | | |

**Figure 1.17** Schematic representation of the stages of meiosis in human oocytes. Adapted from Holubcova *et al.*, 2015, with permission. See color plate section.

Holubcova *et al.* (2015) observed that microtubules are nucleated on chromosomes during spindle assembly, with spindle fibers extending from kinetochores. This process is driven by a small GTPase enzyme, Ran, which releases spindle assembly factors with the help of a chromatin-bound GTP exchange factor RCC1. The spindle gradually increases in volume over approximately 16 hours to form a structure of loosely clustered bundles of microtubules. The oocytes then progress into anaphase to eliminate half of the chromosomes into the first polar body (Figure 1.17).

Mitotic and meiotic spindles in other species such as mouse usually form a stable bipolar spindle before cell division; homologous chromosomes are simultaneously separated during anaphase so that they are evenly distributed to form euploid cells after cytokinesis. However, the spindle in human oocytes sometimes rounds up to become apolar, or shows several poles (multipolar), suggesting that the structure may be unstable during the period between microtubule nucleation (5 hours) and chromosome alignment on a bipolar spindle (Holubcova *et al.*, 2015; see Figure 1.16). The period of instability lasts for an average of $7.5 \pm 3.1$ hours, but eventually most of the oocytes progress into anaphase with bipolar spindles to extrude the first polar body. However, oocytes with unstable spindles tend to have chromosomes that segregate more slowly, lagging behind the others during anaphase so that they are likely to be 'left behind,' thus increasing the chance of aneuploidy after cell division. These oocytes are also more likely to have defects in chromosome alignment. Oocytes with a stable spindle do not show persistent lagging chromosomes. Further analysis to investigate kinetochore–microtubule attachment revealed that around 80% of kinetochores were correctly attached to microtubules, linked to a single spindle pole

(amphitelic attachment); 20% remained attached to both spindle poles (meritelic attachment), increasing the chance of incorrect chromosomal segregation (Figure 1.13).

The authors of this study suggest that the mechanism of spindle assembly in human oocytes, involving Ran-GTP and chromosomes, is less efficient than the mechanisms used in other species that involve MTOCs. As a result, the meiotic spindle is intrinsically unstable: accurate kinetochore–microtubule attachment is more difficult, and abnormalities in this attachment lead to a greater chance of errors during chromosome segregation. This may provide at least one explanation for the high frequency of aneuploidy found in human oocytes compared with other species.

Kinetochore fusion is important in keeping paired homologous chromosomes together as bivalents. A subsequent study by the same group (Zielinska *et al.*, 2015) revealed that many (60%) sister kinetochores in human oocytes could be seen as three or four discrete spots, separated by significant gaps: 90% of these were attached to separate fibers, so that sister kinetochores were positioned at different locations on the spindle poles. The spindle then recognized the split kinetochores as independent units (meritelic attachment). This separation allows bivalents to rotate on the spindle, with each of their sister kinetochores facing opposite spindle poles: a chromosome will be pulled from two sides during anaphase, leading it to lag behind and result in aneuploidy when the chromosomes are partitioned during cell division. Furthermore, the number and degree of separation between sister kinetochores increased with advanced maternal age, and the incidence of meritelic kinetochore-microtubule attachments was greater in oocytes from older women: 7% in women <30, around 21% in women>35. Univalent chromosomes were observed in more than 40% of oocytes from women >35 years;

it is possible that bivalents may disintegrate precociously into univalents with advancing maternal age. In addition, repeated rounds of microtubule attachment and detachment during spindle reorganization may increase the likelihood that sister kinetochores will split, causing strain on cohesion between the chromosome arms and allowing bivalents to twist or prematurely dissociate into univalents, promoting defects in chromosome segregation

### Meiosis in Human Oocytes

- Human oocytes have no centrosomes or detectable MTOCs.
- Microtubules nucleate on chromosomes with spindle fibers extending from kinetochores.
- Spindle assembly takes place over approximately 16 hrs: apolar and multipolar spindles can appear during assembly, suggesting that the process is unstable.
- Oocytes with unstable/transient multipolar spindles are more likely to have chromosomes that 'lag behind' or are misaligned, leading to aneuploidy.
- Many sister kinetochores in human oocytes are separated and do not behave as a single functional unit during the first meiotic division.
- More than 20% of kinetochores are wrongly attached to both spindle poles close to anaphase, and abnormal kinetochore–microtubule attachments lead to lagging chromosomes.
- Sister kinetochore separation increases with age during both meiosis I and meiosis II.
- Onset and progression into anaphase are not affected by the presence of lagging chromosomes or defects in chromosome alignment.

## Genome Editing: CRISPR Sequences

Molecular biology tools and technologies are now available that can add, remove or alter genetic material at specific locations in the genome: this is known as 'genome (or gene) editing.' Making changes in a specific sequence of DNA creates mutations that can change the effect of a gene, and this allows the function of particular genes to be studied. Several methods for manipulating/editing gene function have been tried thus far, including homologous recombination and RNA interference (RNAi). Zinc finger nucleases (ZFNs) and transcription-activator-like effector nucleases (TALENs) can introduce site-specific

double-stranded breaks in DNA, that in turn activate repair pathways. However, these approaches are time-consuming and have been limited by the need for specialist knowledge to use them effectively, as well as difficulties in their assembly.

### Definitions

**CRISPR**: Clustered Regularly Interspaced Short Palindromic Repeats. Sections of DNA containing short repeats of base sequences followed by spacer DNA segments.

**Palindromic repeat**: a sequence of nucleotides that is the same in both directions (e.g., TCCACCT).

**Cas9**: CRISPR-associated protein 9, an enzyme that acts as 'molecular scissors' to cut a piece of double-stranded DNA at a specific location in the genome, allowing new DNA to be inserted.

**crRNA**: CRISPR RNA, made up of a spacer RNA (approximately 20 bp) that is complementary to a DNA sequence; it targets the Cas9 nuclease specifically and makes the tracrRNA sequence complementary to the DNA sequence.

**tracrRNA**: Transactivating crRNA, provides the stem loop structure that is bound by the Cas9 nuclease.

**gRNA**: Guide RNA, made up of the crRNA, tracrRNA and a linker region. Altogether the gRNA informs Cas9 which DNA site should be cut.

**sgRNA**: Single-guide RNA.

**DSB**: Double-strand DNA break.

**NHEJ**: Non-homology end-joining.

**INDELS**: Small insertions or deletions.

**RuvC**: Domain on Cas9 endonuclease that cleaves the non-complementary strand (named for an *Escherichia coli* enzyme involved in DNA repair).

**HNH**: Endonuclease domain containing histidine and arginine residues that cleaves the complementary DNA strand.

**PAM**: Protospacer-associated motif; short conserved sequence (NGG, where N = any nucleotide) at the 3′ end of crRNA, required so that Cas9 can recognize the DNA sequence.

**Targeting efficiency**: The percentage of desired mutation achieved.

**Off-target mutations**: Mutations that may appear in sites other than the target, usually in sites that differ from the target by only a few nucleotides.

The research potential of genome editing has been revolutionized by a gene editing tool known as CRISPR-Cas9; this mechanism has been refined to provide an efficient, effective and reliable system that can change a single nucleotide within a DNA sequence. The method is accurate, as well as simpler, faster, cheaper and more versatile than previous techniques.

CRISPR DNA sequences were first identified in *E. coli* during the 1980s. Their function was later recognized to be a type of prokaryotic immune system, a defense mechanism that allows certain bacteria to acquire selective immunity/resistance to invading plasmids/viruses (Barrangou *et al.*, 2007). The invading foreign DNA is cut into small fragments, and these are incorporated into a CRISPR array of around 20-bp repeats on the bacterial genome. If the virus attacks again, these arrays are transcribed and processed into small RNAs (crRNA). These molecules then guide nuclease (Cas9) enzymes to DNA sequences on the invading genome that are complementary, where they cleave double-stranded foreign DNA sequences and disable the virus attack.

At least three different CRISPR systems have been identified, one of which (type II) functions via a single Cas9 protein (Figure 1.18). In type II CRISPR systems, a primary crRNA transcript forms a duplex with 'transactivating' trRNA, and this guides Cas9 to its target. The target site must have a specific but common short sequence (3-bp nucleotides) at its $3'$ end, known as a protospacer-associated motif (PAM). Cas9 cuts the DNA at precise positions 3 nucleotides upstream of the PAM and will ignore even fully complementary DNA sequences in the absence of a PAM (Sternberg *et al.*, 2014). Cas9 has two nuclease domains: RuvC at the N-terminus and HNH in the mid-region. The HNH domain cuts the complementary strand, and RuvC cuts the non-complementary strand (Jinek *et al.*, 2012).

This type II system has been engineered so that a single-guide RNA (sgRNA) and Cas9 form a ribonucleoprotein (RNP) complex that can be targeted to any desired DNA sequence. In order to use this complex as a gene editing research tool, it has been adapted and refined by combining crRNA + trRNA into a small piece of synthetic RNA with a short, engineered 'guide' sequence (sgRNA). The sgRNA is designed to be complementary to a specific DNA sequence, and it guides Cas9 to cut the two DNA strands at the target site, creating a DSB. The cell recognizes that DNA has been damaged and activates its own DNA repair machinery. Cellular nonhomologous end-joining (NHEJ) pathways repair the DSB, inserting and/or deleting nucleic acid bases that modify the targeted site (INDELS). The DSB can also be repaired by the homology-directed repair (HDR) pathway if a donor template homologous to the targeted DNA is added. Errors can occur during the repair, leading to small mutations that inactivate ('knockout') or modify the gene: for example, a mutation in the coding region can prevent the product of the gene from being made. However, a mutation in the coding region does not necessarily abolish gene function, and the guides must first be screened to see how effective they are in inducing a mutation. For example, targeting the first exon of a gene may result in a cryptic splicing, generating a functional transcript; however, if the DSB repair results in a 3-bp deletion or insertion, the gene will still be 'in frame': unless the amino acids affected are critical for protein function, the end product may still be functional. Such mutations are often the desired outcome of the experiment, as they facilitate further study of gene function.

Harnessing the true capacity of these innate systems requires a deep understanding of the CRISPR toolbox. Major research goals have focused on re-engineering Cas-9 nucleases in attempts to (a) reduce the size of Cas9 nucleases, (b) increase their fidelity and (c) expand the targeting scope of Cas9 variants. Reducing size has been of limited success, but several groups have successfully altered the PAM requirements and the targeting specificity of Cas9 in gene editing protocols:

1. **Wild-type (WT) Cas9** cleaves double-stranded DNA at specific sites, and this activates DSB repair machinery. This may generate an INDEL mutation, of variable size; the outcome is difficult to predict without testing each guide RNA. Large deletions or rearrangements (inversions or translocations) can be made by using a pair of gRNA-directed Cas9 nucleases.

2. **Cas9D10A** is a mutant form of Cas9, which has only nickase activity and cleaves a single DNA strand. NHEJ is not activated, and reduced INDEL mutations are produced when the break is repaired via the high-fidelity HDR pathway in the presence of a homologous DNA template. Paired Cas9 complexes can be designed to generate adjacent DNA nicks, which increases target specificity and precision.

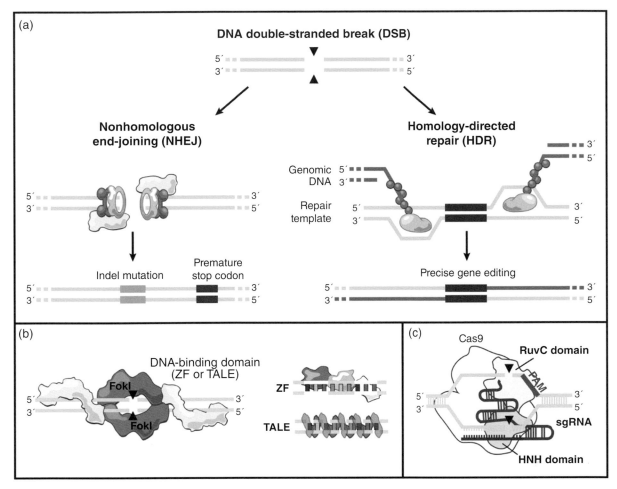

**Figure 1.18** CRISPR. (a) DNA double-strand breaks (DSBs) are repaired by nonhomologous end-joining (NHEJ) or homology-directed repair (HDR). In the error-prone NHEJ pathway, Ku heterodimers bind to DSB ends and serve as a molecular scaffold for associated repair proteins. Indels are introduced when the complementary strands undergo end resection and misaligned repair due to microhomology, eventually leading to frameshift mutations and gene knockout. Alternatively, Rad51 proteins may bind DSB ends during the initial phase of HDR, recruiting accessory factors that direct genomic recombination with homology arms on an exogenous repair template. Bypassing the matching sister chromatid facilitates the introduction of precise gene modifications. (b) Zinc finger (ZF) proteins and transcription-activator-like effectors (TALEs) are naturally occurring DNA-binding domains that can be modularly assembled to target specific sequences. ZF and TALE domains each recognize 3 bp and 1 bp of DNA, respectively. Such DNA-binding proteins can be fused to the FokI endonuclease to generate programmable site-specific nucleases. (c) The Cas9 nuclease from the microbial CRISPR adaptive immune system is localized to specific DNA sequences via the guide sequence on its guide RNA (dark gray), directly base-pairing with the DNA target. Binding of a protospacer-adjacent motif (PAM, light gray) downstream of the target locus helps to direct Cas9-mediated DSBs. Reproduced with permission from Hsu *et al.*, 2014, fig 1.

3. **Nuclease-deficient Cas9 (dCas9):** the Cas9 nuclease catalytic site has been mutated so that it cannot generate DSBs, while still allowing DNA binding. dCas9 can be used to target proteins that activate gene expression, and thus the system can be adapted to turn genes on or off (Perez-Pinera *et al.*, 2013; Mali *et al.*, 2013; Cheng *et al.*, 2013). dCas9 can be used to block other proteins (e.g., RNA polymerase) and prevent transcription: the gene is switched off, without changing the DNA sequence. A similar strategy has been used to add acetyl groups to histones in order to manipulate epigenetic marks and study downstream gene expression (Hilton *et al.*, 2015). dCas9 can also be used to visualize DNA sequences by fusing the enzyme to a fluorescent protein (Chen *et al.*, 2013).

4. **Base editors:** a partially catalytic mutation in Cas9 allows it to break single strands of DNA, and this promotes a mismatch repair pathway. Adding

a uracil glycosylase inhibitor blocks the uracil DNA glycosylase-mediated base excision repair pathway, and cytosine is converted to uridine. This is ultimately resolved via cytosine to thymine (or guanine to adenine) base pair substitution (Komor *et al.*, 2016).

Other CRISPR systems are currently being explored in order to identify effector proteins similar to Cas9 that may have preferential sizes, PAM requirements and substrate affinities. The use and effectiveness of naturally occurring Cas9 variants is limited by their size: SpCas9 protein has 1,366 amino acids, and such large proteins are difficult to package for delivery into different cell types via Lenti- or adeno-associated viruses (AAV). This challenge has led to the use of smaller Cas9 variants such as:

- Cas9 from *Neisseria meningitides* (NmCas9)
- From *Staphylococcus aureus* (SaCas9)
- From *Campylobacter jejuni* (CjCas9)

(Hou *et al.*, 2013; Ran *et al.*, 2015; Friedland *et al.*, 2015; Kim *et al.*, 2017).

More than 10 different Cas proteins have thus far been identified and re-purposed for genome editing. Cas9 isolated from *Staphylococcus pyogenes* is the most commonly used cutting tool at present, but advantages have been demonstrated by using proteins with a single effector nuclease, e.g.:

- Cpf1 or Cas12a (CRISPR from *Prevotella* and *Francisella*1): whereas Cas9 produces blunt ends when cutting and requires two short RNAs, Cpf1 cuts DNA 3′ downstream of the PAM sequence in a staggered mechanism that generates a 5′ overhang (Zetsche *et al.*, 2015; Yamano *et al.*, 2016; Fonfara *et al.*, 2016). Importantly, this variant of the CRISPR system has been demonstrated to bind to single-stranded DNA without any sequence specificity, once the enzyme becomes activated (Chen *et al.*, 2018). This has allowed unique new diagnostic methods to be developed.
- C2c1, C2c2 and C2c3 effector nucleases and AsCpf1 (CRISPR from *Acidaminococcus* spp.) (Shmakov *et al.*, 2015; Abudayyeh *et al.*, 2016; Liu *et al.*, 2017).

### Efficiency and Off-Target Mutation

Nuclease cutting can sometimes 'miss' targeted sites, and DNA repair may be inaccurate, with an impact on the efficiency and precision of the system. If there is a sequence similar to the target DNA sequence somewhere else in the genome, the sgRNA might be guided to this locus as well as, or instead of, the target. Cas9 can then cut at the wrong site ('off target'), introducing a mutation in a separate location. This can potentially have an effect on transcription of other genes in the genome. The sgRNA 'seed sequence,' which is 12 bp upstream of the PAM site, is critical; if there is a sequence similar to this sequence in another region of the genome, there is a chance of off-target editing, and this sgRNA should not be selected. A nucleotide difference within the seed sequence lowers the probability of off-target mutations, especially if the differences are located in the 3–4 bp upstream of the PAM (Hu *et al.*, 2018).

A number of methods exist to check the efficiency of a cut (Sentmanat *et al.*, 2018); however, off-target mutations can be very difficult to detect, and can only be completely ruled out by sequencing the whole genome. The chance of creating off-target effects can be decreased by using bioinformatics resources to identify repetitive sequences and avoid their selection as a target (Moreno-Mateos *et al.*, 2015). Methods such as CIRCLE-seq, Digenome-seq and others can also be used to experimentally predict putative off-target sites or to screen for off-target editing in primary cells (Kim *et al.*, 2015; Tsai *et al.*, 2017).

## Germline Editing

Gene editing that will create permanent changes in the DNA of gametes and embryos which will be inherited through subsequent generations is referred to as 'germline editing.' Theoretically, this approach might be used to prevent devastating inherited monogenic disease by altering defective genes in the patients' gametes or embryos, which would subsequently be used for assisted reproduction. Alternatively, IVF embryos identified by preimplantation genetic diagnosis (PGD) as carrying a disease might be repaired before embryo transfer.

However, these approaches are fraught with a range of practical and technical difficulties, as well as concerns regarding safety/off-target effects. The results of this kind of manipulation could not be analyzed for long periods of time, possibly generations. In addition, it is now clear that gene expression is influenced through epigenetic changes, many of which are associated with environmental factors through mechanisms that are still unclear. Altering gene expression via germline modification is only one small component of a very complex picture and could have dangerous consequences. Much more basic research is needed to understand the consequences of genome editing in human embryos, off-target mutations that may be inadvertently induced, changes at the on-target site that are not precise and the repair mechanisms that may or may not operate at this unique stage of human development. Applying this kind of gene editing technology is currently illegal in many countries; it raises a number of ethical questions and challenges that have been discussed and summarized in several publications as well as international consensus documents (Lander, 2015; Friedmann *et al.*, 2015; Ishii, 2017). The Hinxton Group, an international consensus on stem cells, ethics and law, concluded in 2015 that germline editing for potential clinical application is currently premature and unacceptable (www .hinxtongroup.org/Hinxton2015_Statement.pdf).

In 2017, the National Academies of Sciences and National Academy of Medicine published a detailed report covering the science, ethics and governance of human genome editing (National Academies of Sciences, Engineering and Medicine, 2017). The Nuffield Council for Bioethics spent two years gathering evidence from scientists, patients, lawyers, bioethicists and the public, producing an extensive report in July 2018: 'Genome editing and human reproduction: social and ethical issues.' Amongst their conclusions was the statement 'The use of heritable genome editing interventions would only be ethically acceptable if carried out in accordance with principles of social justice and solidarity.' Attempts at germline editing are therefore premature and irresponsible, without a great deal more substantial basic research into a variety of cell types and organisms as well as in human embryos. A case reported in China during December 2018 was widely condemned, provoking an immense international outcry (see Cyranoski & Ledford, 2018); the scientist's research activities were immediately suspended by the Chinese authorities.

## Summary

Genome editing technology has emerged as a tremendously valuable basic research tool toward understanding the function of specific genes, elucidating fundamental processes in developmental biology, and in discovering the differences and similarities between human and nonhuman biology. Models of human disease can potentially be generated, in order to characterize molecular and biochemical bases for pathogenesis. Further nonclinical research is needed in order to understand and improve the efficiency and precision of the technique, to generate preliminary data for developing potential applications, and to discover whether safe application in human reproductive technologies is likely to be plausible. However, the fundamental research required is limited by the practical and ethical difficulties involved in obtaining human gametes and embryos for basic research.

---

**Theoretical Applications for Gene Editing Technology**

1. Model disease mutations – knockin/knockout animal models for detailed study of a disease.
2. Modify gene expression in cell lines: activation/repression to identify function and effects.
3. Study gene function via gene labeling for cell lineage tracking.
4. Create transgenic organisms.
5. Target gene mutation: In-vivo repair of somatic cell gene mutations associated with specific diseases, e.g.:

   - Inactivate mutant allele in retinal cell gene to treat progressive blindness caused by dominant form of retinitis pigmentosa.
   - Edit blood stem cells to treat sickle cell anemia, hemophilia, hemoglobinopathies.

     – practical application of this kind of strategy is limited by technical problems associated with incomplete or inaccurate editing, off-target mutations, epigenetic changes, etc.

---

## Further Reading

### Books and Reviews

Barnum KJ, O'Connell MJ (2014). Cell cycle regulation by checkpoints. *Methods in Molecular Biology* 1170: 29–40.

Barrangou R, Fremaux C, Deveau H, *et al.* (2007) CRISPR provides acquired resistance against viruses in prokaryotes. *Science* 315(5819). 1709–1712.

Berg JM, Tymoczko JL, Stryer L (eds.) (2002) *Biochemistry*, 5th edn. W H Freeman & Co., New York.

Biointeractive. CRISPR-Cas9 Mechanisms and Applications. www.hhmi.org/bioizteractive/crispr-cas-9-mechanism-applications

Dale B (1983) *Fertilization in Animals* (Studies in Biology). Hodder, London.

Dale B (2018) *Fertilization: The Beginning of Life.* Cambridge University Press, Cambridge.

Hamilton G (2015) The mitochondria mystery. *Nature* 525: 444–446.

Hassold T, Hunt P (2001) To err (meiotically) is human: the genesis of human aneuploidy. *Nature Reviews Genetics* 2: 280–291.

Hassold T, Hall H, Hunt P (2007) The origin of human aneuploidy: where we have been, where we are going. *Human Molecular Genetics* 16(R2): R203–R208.

Hoffman A, Sportelli V, Ziller M, Spengler D (2017) Epigenomics of major depressive illness and schizophrenia: early life decides (Review). *International Journal of Molecular Science* 18(8): 1711.

Hsu PD, Lander ES, Zhang F (2014) Development and applications of CRISPR-Cas9 for genome engineering. *Cell* 157(6): 1262–1278.

Johnson MH (2017) *Essential Reproduction*, 7th edn. Blackwell Publishing, Oxford.

Lodish H, Berk A, Zipursky SL, Matsudaira P, Baltimore D, Darnell J (eds.) (2000) *Molecular Cell Biology*, 4th edn. W H Freeman & Co., New York.

Ménézo Y (2017) *Oxidative Stress and Women's Health.* Editions Eska, Paris, France.

Ménézo Y, Dale B, Cohen M (2010) DNA damage and repair in human oocytes and embryos: a review. *Zygote* 18: 357–365.

Nagaoka SI, Hassold TJ, Hunt PA (2012) Human aneuploidy: mechanisms and new insights into an age-old problem. *Nature Reviews Genetics* 13(7): 493–504.

National Academies of Sciences, Engineering and Medicine (2017) *Human Genome Editing: Science, Ethics and Governance.* The National Academies Press, Washington DC.

Nuffield Council on Bioethics (2018) *Genome Editing and Human Reproduction: Social and Ethical Issues.* Nuffield Council on Bioethics, London.

Richardson B (2003) Impact of aging on DNA methylation. *Ageing Research Reviews* 2(3): 245–261.

Rozen R (2004) Folate and genetics. *Journal of Food Science and Technology* 69(1): SNQ65–SNQ67.

Skoot R (2010) *The Immortal Life of Henrietta Lacks.* Crown Publishing Group, New York.

Tollefsbol T (ed.) (2017) *Handbook of Epigenetics: The New Molecular and Medical Genetics.* 2nd edn. Academic Press, USA.

Van Blerkom J (2004) Mitochondria in human oogenesis and preimplantation embryogenesis: engines of metabolism, ionic regulation and developmental competence. *Reproduction* 128: 269–280.

Webster A & Schuh M (2017) Mechanisms of aneuploidy in human eggs (Review). *Trends in Cell Biology* 27(1): 55–68.

## Research Publications

Abudayyeh OO, Gootenberg JS, Konermann S, *et al* (2016) C2c2 is a single-component programmable RNA-guided RNA-targeting CRISPR effector. *Science* 353: aaf5573.

Akera T, Lampson MA (2016) Chromosome segregation: freewheeling sisters cause problems. *eLife* e13788. DOI: 10.7554/eLife.13788.

Amar E, Cornet D, Cohen M, Menezo Y (2015) Treatment for high levels of sperm DNA fragmentation and nuclear decondensation: sequential treatment with a potent antioxidant followed by stimulation of the one-carbon cycle vs. one-carbon cycle back-up alone. *Austin Journal of Reproductive Medicine and Infertility* 2(1): 1006.

Barrangou R, Horvath P (2017) A decade of discovery: CRISPR functions and applications. *Nature Microbiology* 2: 17092. DOI: 10.1038/nmicrobiol.2017.92.

Barrit J, Kokot T, Cohen J, *et al.* (2002) Quantification of human ooplasmic mitochondria. *Reproductive BioMedicine Online* 4: 243–237.

Benkhalifa M, Montjean D, Cohen-Bacrie P, Menezo Y (2010) Imprinting: RNA expression for homocysteine recycling in the human oocyte. *Fertility and Sterility* 93: 1585-1590.

Bennabi I, Terret M-E, Verlhac M-H (2016) Meiotic spindle assembly and chromosome segregation in oocytes. *Journal of Cell Biology* 215(5): 611–619.

Berker B, Kaya C, Aytac R, *et al.* (2009) Homocysteine concentrations in follicular fluid are associated with poor oocyte and embryo qualities in polycystic ovary syndrome patients undergoing assisted reproduction. *Human Reproduction* 24: 2293–2302.

Cao L, Wang Y, Zhang R, *et al.* (2018). Association of neural tube defects with gene polymorphisms in one-carbon metabolic pathway. *Child's Nervous System* 34(2): 277–284.

Cappell SD, Chung M, Jaimovich A, Spencer SL, Meyer T (2016) Irreversible APC (Cdh1) inactivation underlies the point of no return for cell-cycle entry. *Cell* 166: 167–180.

Chen B, Gilbert LA, Cimini BA, *et al.* (2013) Dynamic imaging of genomic loci in living human cells by an optimized CRISPR/Cas system. *Cell* 155(7): 1479–1491.

Cheng AW, Wang H, Yang H, *et al.* (2013) Multiplexed activation of endogenous genes by CRISPR-on, an RNA-guided transcriptional activator system. *Cell Research* 23: 1163–1171.

Chen JS, Ma E, Harrington LB, *et al.* (2018) CRISPR-Cas12a target binding unleashes indiscriminate single-stranded DNase activity. *Science* 360(6387): 436–439.

Cornet D, Amar E, Cohen M, Menezo Y (2015) Clinical evidence for the importance of 1-Carbon support in subfertile couples. *Austin Journal of Reproductive Medicine and Infertility* 2(2): 1011.

Cummins JM (2002) The role of maternal mitochondria during oogenesis, fertilization and embryogenesis. *Reproductive BioMedicine Online* 4: 176–182.

Cyranoski D, Ledford H (2018) Genome-edited baby provokes international outcry. *Nature* 563 (7733): 607–608.

DeBaum M, Niemitz E, Feinberg A (2003) Association of in vitro fertilization with Beckwith-Wiedemann syndrome and epigenetic alterations of LitI and H19. *American Journal of Human Genetics* 72: 156–160.

Ebisch IM, Peters WH, Thomas CM, *et al.* (2006) Homocysteine, glutathione and related thiols affect fertility parameters in the (sub) fertile couple. *Human Reproduction* 21: 1725–1733.

Ebisch IM, Thomas CM, Peters WH (2007) The importance of folate, zinc and anti-oxidants in the pathogenesis and prevention of subfertility. *Human Reproduction Update* 13: 163–174.

Evenson DP (2016) The sperm chromatin structure assay (SCSA) and other sperm DNA fragmentation tests for evaluation of sperm nuclear DNA integrity as related to fertility. *Animal Reproduction Science* 169: 56-75.

Evenson DP, Darzynkiewicz Z, Melamed MR (1980) Relation of mammalian sperm chromatin heterogeneity to fertility. *Science* 210: 1131–1133.

Fonfara I, Richter H, Bratovic M, Le Rhun A, Charpentier E (2016) The CRISPR-associated DNA-cleaving enzyme Cpf1 also processes precursor CRISPR RNA. *Nature* 532: 517–521.

Friedland AE, Baral B, Singhai P, *et al.* (2015) Characterization of Staphylococcus aureus Cas9: a smaller Cas9 for all-in-one adeno-associated virus delivery and paired nickase applications. *Genome Biology* 16: 257.

Friedmann T, Jonlin EC, King NMP, *et al.* (2015) ASGCT and JSGT Joint Position Statement on Human Genomic Editing. *Molecular Therapy* 23(8): 1282.

Fulka J Jr., First N, Moor RM (1998) Nuclear and cytoplasmic determinants involved in the regulation of mammalian oocyte maturation. *Molecular Human Reproduction* 4(1): 41–49.

Guerin P, El Mouatassim S, Ménézo Y (2001) Oxidative stress and protection against reactive oxygen species in the pre-implantation embryo and its surroundings. *Human Reproduction Update* 7: 175–189.

Hays FA, Watson J, Shing Ho (2003) Caution! DNA crossing: crystal structures of Holliday junctions. *Journal of Biological Chemistry* 278(50): 49663–49666.

Hernando-Herrasez I, Garcia-Perez R, Sharp AJ, Marques-Bonet T (2015) DNA methylation: insights into human evolution. *PLoS Genetics* 11(12): 31005661.

Hilton IB, D'Ippolito AM, Vockley CM, *et al.* (2015) Epigenome editing by a CRISPR-Cas9-based acetyltransferase activates genes from promoters and enhancers. *Nature Biotechnology* 33(5): 510–517.

Holubcova Z, Blayney M, Elder K, Schuh M (2015) Error-prone chromosome-mediated spindle assembly favors chromosome segregation defects in human oocytes. *Science* 348: 1143–1147.

Hou Z, Zhang Y, Propson NE, *et al.* (2013) Efficient genome engineering in human pluripotent stem cells using Cas9 from Neisseria meningitidis. *Proceedings of the National Academy of Sciences USA* 110: 15644–15649.

Hu JH, Miller SM, Geurts MH, Tang W, *et al.* (2018) EvolvedCas9 variants with broad PAM compatibility and high DNA specificity. *Nature* 556(7699): 57–63.

Huarte J, Stutz A, O'Connell ML, *et al.* (1992) Transient translational silencing by reversible mRNA deadenylation. *Cell* 69: 1021–1030.

Ishii, T (2017) Reproductive medicine involving genome editing: clinical uncertainties and embryological needs. *Reproductive BioMedicine Online* 34: 27–31.

Jinek M, Chylinski K, Fonfara I, *et al.* (2012) A programmable dual RNA-guided DNA endonuclease in adaptive bacterial immunity. *Science* 337(6096): 816–821.

Kim D, Bae S, Park J, *et al.* (2015) Digenome-seq: genome-wide profiling of CRISPR-Cas9 off-target effects in human cells. *Nature Methods* 12: 237–243.

Kim E, Koo T, Park SW, *et al.* (2017) In vivo genome editing with a small Cas9 orthologue derived from Campylobacter jejuni. *Nature Communications* 8: 14500.

Knouse KA, Wu J, Whittaker CA, Amon A (2014) Single cell sequencing reveals low levels of aneuploidy across mammalian tissues. *Proceedings of the National Academy of Sciences USA* 111: 13409–13414.

Komor AC, Kim YB, Packer MS, Zuris JA, Liu DR (2016) Programmable editing of a target base in genomic DNA without double-stranded DNA cleavage. *Nature* 533(7603): 420–424.

Kuliev A, Zlatopolsky Z, Kirillova I, Spivakova J, Cieslak Janzen J (2011) Meiosis errors in over 20,000 oocytes studied in the practice of preimplantation aneuploidy testing. *Reproductive BioMedicine Online* 22: 2–8.

Lander ES (2015) Brave new genome. *New England Journal of Medicine* 373: 5–8.

Liu L, Chen P, Wang M, *et al.* (2017) C2c1–sgRNA complex structure reveals RNA-guided DNA cleavage mechanism. *Molecular Cell* 65: 310–322.

Luo C, Valencia CA, Zhang J, *et al.* (2018) Biparental inheritance of mitochondrial DNA in humans. Proceedings of the National Academy of Sciences USA 115(51): 13039–13044.

Mali P, Aach J, Guell M, *et al.* (2013) RNA-guided human genome engineering via Cas9. *Science* 339(6121): 823–826.

Marucci GH, Zampieri BL, Biselli JM, *et al.* (2012) Polymorphism C1420T of serine hydroxymethyltransferase gene on maternal risk for Down syndrome. *Molecular Biology Reports* 39(3): 2561–2566.

Ménézo Y, Khatchadourian C, Gharib A, *et al.* (1989) Regulation of S-adenosyl methionine synthesis in the mouse embryo. *Life Sciences* 44: 1601–1609.

Ménézo YJR, Russo G, Tosti E, *et al.* (2007) Expression profile of genes coding for DNA repair in human oocytes using pangenomic microarrays, with a special focus on ROS linked decays. *Journal of Assisted Reproduction and Genetics* 24: 513–520.

Ménézo Y, Mares P, Cohen M, *et al.* (2011) Autism, imprinting and epigenetic disorders: a metabolic syndrome linked to anomalies in homocysteine recycling starting in early life? *Journal of Assisted Reproduction and Genetics* 28: 1143–1145.

Ménézo Y, Entezami F, Lichtblau I, *et al.* (2014) Oxidative stress and fertility: incorrect assumptions and ineffective solutions? *Zygote* 22: 80–90.

Ménézo Y, Silvestris E, Dale B, Elder K (2016) Oxidative stress and alterations in DNA methylation: two sides of the same coin in reproduction. *Reproductive BioMedicine Online* 33(6): 668–683.

Ménézo Y, Cornet D, Cohen M, *et al.* (2017) Association between the MTHFR-C677T isoform and structure of sperm DNA. *Journal of Assisted Reproduction and Genetics* 34(10): 1283–1288.

Moreno-Mateos MA, Vejnar CE, Beauddoin JD, *et al.* (2015) CRISPRscan: designing highly efficient sgRNAs for CRISPR-Cas9 targeting in vivo. *Nature Methods* 12(10): 982–988.

Okamoto Y, Yoshidda N, Suzuki T, *et al.* (2015) DNA methylation dynamics in mouse preimplantation embryos revealed by mass spectrometry. *Scientific Reports* 6: 19134. DOI: 10.1038/srep19134.

Padmanabhan N, Watson ED (2013) Lessons from the one-carbon metabolism: passing it along to the next generation. *Reproductive BioMedicine Online* 27: 637–643.

Padmanabhan N, Jia D, Geary-Joo C, *et al.* (2013) Mutation in folate metabolism causes epigenetic instability and transgenerational effects on development. *Cell* 155(1): 81–93.

Perez-Pinera P, Kocak DD, Vockley CM, *et al.* (2013) RNA-guided gene activation by CRISPR-Cas9-based transcription factors. *Nature Methods* 10(10): 973–976.

Ran FA, Cong L, Yan WX, *et al.* (2015) In vivo genome editing using Staphylococcus aureus Cas9. *Nature* 520: 186–191.

Sakakibara Y, Hashimoto S, Nakaoka Y, Kouznetsova A, Höög C, Kitajima TS (2015) Bivalent separation into univalents precedes age-related meiosis I errors in oocytes. *Nature Communications* 6: 7550.

Sakkas D, Urner F, Bizzaro D, *et al.* (1998) Sperm nuclear DNA damage and altered chromatin structure: effect on fertilization and embryo development. *Human Reproduction* 13(Suppl 4): 11–19.

Schuh M, Ellenberg J (2007) Self-organization of MTOCs replaces centrosome function during acentrosomal spindle assembly in live mouse oocytes. *Cell* 130: 484–498.

Sener EF, Oztop DB, Ozkui Y (2014) MTHFR gene C677T polymorphism in autism spectrum disorders. *Genetics Research International* Art ID: 698574.

Sentmanat MF, Peters ST, Florian CP, Connelly JP, Pruett-Miller SM (2018) A survey of validation strategies for CRISPR-Cas9 editing. *Scientific Reports* 8: Art No. 888.

Shmakov S, Abudayyeh OO, Makarova KS, *et al.* (2015) Discovery and functional characterization of diverse class 2 CRISPR-Cas systems. *Molecular Cell* 60: 385–397.

Sternberg SH, Redding S, Jinek M, *et al.* (2014) DNA interrogation by the CRISPR RNA-guided endonuclease Cas9. *Nature* 506(7490): 62–67.

Sutovsky P, Navara CS, Schatten G (1996) Fate of the sperm mitochondria, and the incorporation, conversion, and disassembly of the sperm tail structures during bovine fertilization. *Biology of Reproduction* 55: 1195–1205.

Templado C, Vidal F, Estop A (2011) Aneuploidy in human spermatozoa. *Cytogenetic and Genome Research* 133: 91–99.

Tsai SQ, Nguyen NT, Malagon-Lopez J, Topkar VV, Aryee MJ, Joung LK (2017) CIRCLE-seq: a highly sensitive *in vitro* screen for genome-wide CRISPR–Cas9 nuclease off-targets. *Nature Methods* 14: 607–614.

Tunster SJ, Jensen AB, John RM (2013) Imprinted genes in mouse placental development and the regulation of fetal energy stores. *Reproduction* 145(5): R117–R137.

Vassena R, Heindrycks R, Peco R, *et al.* (2016) Genome engineering through CRISPR/Cas9 technology in the human germline and pluripotent stem cells. *Human Reproduction Update* 22(4): 411–419.

Verlhac MH, Terret ME (2016) Oocyte maturation and development. *F1000Research* 5 (F1000 Faculty Rev): 309. DOI: 10.12688/f1000research.7892.1.

Ward WS (1993) Deoxyribonucleic acid loop domain tertiary structure in mammalian spermatozoa. *Biology of Reproduction* 48(6): 1193–1201.

Watkins D, Ru M, Hwang H-Y, *et al.* (2002) Hyperhomocysteinemia due to methionine synthase deficiency, cbIG: structure of the MTR gene, genotype diversity, and recognition of a common mutation, P1173L. *American Journal of Human Genetics* 71(1): 143–153.

Wernimont SM, Raiszadeh F, Stover PJ, *et al.* (2011) Polymorphisms in serine hydroxymethyltransferase 1 and methylenetetrahydrofolate reductase interact to increase cardiovascular disease risk in humans. *Journal of Nutrition* 141(2): 255–260.

Wilding M, Dale B, Marino M, *et al.* (2001) Mitochondrial aggregation patterns and activity in human oocytes and preimplantation embryos. *Human Reproduction* 16(5): 909–917.

Xu W, Zhang L, Wu X, Jin F (2017) Association between methionine synthase reductase A66G polymorphism and male infertility: a meta-analysis. *Critical Reviews Eukaryotic Gene Expression* 27(1): 37–46.

Yamano T, Nishimasu H, Zetsche B, *et al.* (2016) Crystal structure of Cpf1 in complex with guide RNA and target DNA. *Cell* 165: 949–962.

Zemach A, McDaniel IE, Silva P, Zilberman D (2010) Genome-wide evolutionary analysis of eukaryotic DNA methylation. *Science* 328(5980): 916–919.

Zetsche B, Gootenberg JS, Abudayyeh OO, *et al.* (2015) Cpf1 is a single RNA-guided endonuclease of a class 2 CRISPR-Cas system. *Cell* 163: 759–771.

Zielinska AP, Holubcova Z, Blayney M, Elder K, Schuh M (2015) Sister kinetochore splitting and precocious disintegration of bivalents could explain the maternal age effect. *eLife* 4: e11389.

# Endocrine Control of Reproduction
## Controlled Ovarian Hyperstimulation for ART

## Introduction

Synchrony is essential for gametogenesis and correct embryo development, and a basic knowledge of reproductive endocrinology is fundamental to understanding synchrony in reproductive physiology. Although sexual arousal, erection and ejaculation in the male are obviously under cerebral control, it is less obvious that the ovarian and testicular cycles are also coordinated by the brain. For many years after the discovery of the gonadotropic hormones follicle-stimulating hormone (FSH) and luteinizing hormone (LH), the anterior pituitary gland was considered to be an autonomous organ, until animal experiments in which lesions were induced in the hypothalamus clearly demonstrated that reproductive processes were mediated by the nervous system. The hypothalamus is a small inconspicuous part of the brain lying between the midbrain and the forebrain; unlike any other region of the brain, it not only receives sensory inputs from almost every other part of the central nervous system (CNS), but also sends nervous impulses to several endocrine glands and to pathways governing the activity of skeletal muscle, the heart and smooth muscle (Figure 2.1). Via a sophisticated network of neural signals and hormone release, the hypothalamus controls sexual cycles, growth, pregnancy, lactation and a wide range of other basic and emotional reactions. Each hypothalamic function is associated with one or more small areas that consist of aggregations of neurons called hypothalamic nuclei. In the context of reproduction, several groups of hypothalamic nuclei are connected to the underlying pituitary gland by neural and vascular connections.

### Functions of the Hypothalamus in Reproduction

The hypothalamus links the nervous system to the pituitary gland by receiving signals from:

- The central nervous system (CNS)
- Neurons from other parts of the brain, including the amygdala (involved in emotional response), the visual cortex and the olfactory cortex
- Endocrine factors from the testis, ovary and other endocrine glands.

It then releases factors into the hypothalamic–hypophyseal portal veins that stimulate or inhibit synthesis and release of hormones by the pituitary, including (but not only):

- Gonadotropin-releasing hormone (GnRH): releases FSH and LH
- Thyroid-releasing hormone (TRH): releases thyroid-stimulating hormone (TSH)
- Corticotropin-releasing hormone/corticotropin-releasing factor (CRH/CRF): releases adrenocorticotropic hormone (ACTH)
- Growth hormone-releasing hormone (GHRH): releases growth hormone (GH).

Gonadotropin-releasing hormone (GnRH) is secreted by groups of hypothalamic nuclei and transported to the anterior pituitary through the portal vessels. GnRH, a decapeptide with the structure (Pyr)-Glu-His-Trp-Ser-Tyr-Gly-Leu-Arg-Pro-Gly-NH2, is the most important mediator of reproduction by the CNS. Any abnormality in its synthesis, storage, release or action will cause partial or complete failure of gonadal function. GnRH is secreted in pulses and binds to specific receptors on the plasma membrane of the gonadotroph cells in the pituitary, triggering the inositol triphosphate second messenger system within these cells. This signal induces the movement of secretory granules toward the plasma membrane and eventually stimulates the pulsatile secretion of LH and FSH. Alterations in the output of LH and FSH may be achieved by changing the amplitude or frequency of GnRH, or by modulating the response of the gonadotroph cells.

The anterior pituitary secretes LH, FSH and TSH, which are heterodimeric glycoprotein molecules that

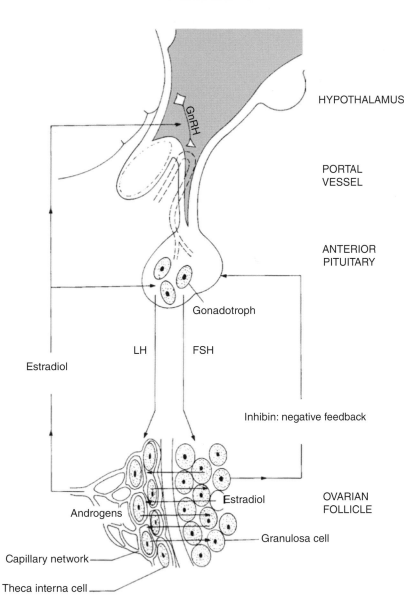

**Figure 2.1** Hypothalamic–pituitary–gonadal (HPG) axis. Schematic summary of the endocrine control of reproduction in mammals. Adapted with permission from Johnson (2018).

HYPOTHALAMUS

GnRH

PORTAL VESSEL

ANTERIOR PITUITARY

Gonadotroph

LH        FSH

Estradiol

Inhibin: negative feedback

Estradiol

Androgens

OVARIAN FOLLICLE

Granulosa cell

Capillary network

Theca interna cell

share a common alpha-subunit (also shared by human chorionic gonadotropin [hCG]) and differ by their unique beta-subunit. Only the heterodimers have biological activity. The specific functions of FSH have been studied with targeted deletions in 'knockout' mice: FSH-deficient male mice have a decrease in testicular size and epididymal sperm count, but remain fertile. In contrast, homozygous females with the mutation are infertile: their ovaries show normal primordial and primary follicles, with no abnormalities in oocytes, granulosa or theca cells, but the follicles fail to develop beyond the preantral stage. The ovaries also lack corpora lutea, and serum progesterone levels were decreased by 50% compared with normal mice. These studies indicate that, in mice, whereas spermatogenesis can continue in the absence of FSH, follicle maturation beyond the preantral stage is FSH-dependent.

At the onset of puberty, increased activity of the GnRH pulse generator induces maturation of the pituitary–gonadal axis. A progressive increase in the release of gonadotropins from the pituitary stimulates a subsequent rise in gonadal steroid hormones. In males, FSH released in response to the GnRH pulses acts on Sertoli–Leydig cells to initiate spermatogenesis, and LH acts on the Leydig cells to stimulate testosterone production. In females, FSH initiates follicular maturation and estrogen production, and LH stimulates theca cell steroidogenesis and triggers ovulation.

# Male Reproductive Endocrinology

The neuroendocrine mechanisms that regulate testicular function are fundamentally similar to those that regulate ovarian activity. The male hypothalamo–pituitary unit is responsible for the secretion of gonadotropins that regulate the endocrine and spermatogenic activities of the testis, and this gonadotropin secretion is subject to feedback regulation. A major difference between male and female reproductive endocrinology is the fact that gamete and steroid hormone production in the male is a continuous process after puberty, and not cyclical as in the female. This is reflected in the absence of a cyclical positive feedback control of gonadotropin release by testicular hormones. The hypothalamus integrates all of these signals and relays a response via the release of the peptide hormone GnRH. The hormone is released in pulses, with peaks every 90–120 minutes, and travels to the anterior pituitary gland, where it stimulates the synthesis and episodic release of gonadotropic hormones to regulate sperm production in the testes. Interestingly and paradoxically, after the pituitary is initially stimulated to produce these gonadotropins, exposure to constant GnRH (or a GnRH agonist) occupies the receptors so that the signaling pathway is disrupted, and gonadotropin release is inhibited.

The process of spermatogenesis is a 'two-cell' process, dependent on cross-talk between the Leydig (equivalent to ovarian theca) and Sertoli (equivalent to granulosa) cells via their respective gonadotropin receptors, LH and FSH. Sertoli cells respond to pituitary FSH and secrete androgen-binding proteins (ABPs). Pituitary LH stimulates the interstitial cells of Leydig to produce testosterone, which combines with ABP in the seminiferous tubules, and testosterone controls LH secretion by negative feedback to the hypothalamus, maintaining the high intratesticular testosterone that is appropriate for normal spermatogenesis. Sertoli cells also produce inhibin, which exerts a negative feedback effect on pituitary FSH secretion. It probably also has a minor controlling influence on the secretion of LH.

Although the role of inhibin is less clear in the male than in the female, inhibin-like molecules have also been found in testicular extracts, which presumably also regulate FSH secretion. In humans, failure of spermatogenesis is correlated with elevated serum FSH levels, perhaps through reduced inhibin secretion by the testis. In the testis, LH acts on Leydig cells, and FSH on Sertoli cells; males are very sensitive to changes in activity of LH and are relatively resistant to changes in FSH activity.

---

**Gonadotropins in the Male**

1. Follicle-stimulating hormone (FSH): acts on the germinal epithelium to initiate spermatogenesis; receptors are found on Sertoli cells.

   - Sertoli cells secrete inhibin, which regulates FSH secretion.

2. Luteinizing hormone (LH): stimulates the Leydig (interstitial) cells to produce testosterone.

---

Gonadotropic stimulation of the testes regulates the release of hormones (androgens) that are required for the development of puberty, and then to initiate and maintain male reproductive function and spermatogenesis. Testosterone is the major secretory product of the testes, responsible for male sexual characteristics such as facial hair growth, distribution of body fat/muscle and other 'masculine' features. Testosterone is metabolized in peripheral tissue to the potent androgen dihydrotestosterone, or to the potent estrogen estradiol. These androgens and estrogens act independently to modulate LH secretion. In the testis, the androgen receptor is found on Sertoli cells, Leydig and peritubular myoid cells. Ablating the androgen receptor inhibits spermatogenesis.

Feedback mechanisms are an important part of the reproductive axis; testosterone inhibits LH secretion, while inhibin (secreted by Sertoli cells in the testes) regulates FSH secretion. If negative feedback is reduced, the pituitary responds by increasing its FSH secretion, similar to the situation in women reaching the menopause. Serum FSH levels in the male therefore act as an indicator of testicular germinal epithelial function – i.e., they are broadly correlated with spermatogenesis. Testosterone levels indicate Leydig cell function, and reflect the presence of 'masculine' characteristics:

- Low levels in boys and castrates ($<4$ nm/L).
- Varies throughout the day in adult males – highest in the morning.
- Levels decrease in older men.

Serum LH level is difficult to assess, because it is released in pulses. Prolactin also interacts with LH and FSH in a complex manner, via inhibition of GnRH release from the hypothalamus. In males with hyperprolactinemia, inhibition of GnRH decreases LH secretion and testosterone production; elevated prolactin levels may also have a direct effect on the CNS.

---

**Male Sexual Maturity and Reproductive Function Depends upon Appropriate Secretion of Hormones**

- Gonadotropin-releasing hormone (GnRH)
- Luteinizing hormone (LH)
- Follicle-stimulating hormone (FSH)
- Testosterone (T)
- Inhibin

---

**Serum Endocrinology in the Male**

An endocrine profile should be performed in men with oligospermia, or if there are signs or symptoms to suggest androgen deficiency or endocrine disease.

1. Testosterone: normal range is 10–35 nmol/L, but serum levels undergo diurnal variation, with highest levels in the morning. Therefore, the time of the test is important, and borderline levels should be compared with other measurements taken on different days.
2. FSH and LH: normal serum levels of both are <10 IU/L (but normal ranges for specific laboratories should be noted).

    - Azoospermia with normal T, FSH and LH indicates mechanical obstruction to the passage of sperm.
    - Elevated FSH indicates germinal cell insufficiency.
    - Elevated FSH and LH, low T indicates primary testicular failure.
    - Low FSH, LH and T indicates hypothalamic or pituitary insufficiency.

# Female Reproductive Endocrinology

In females, gonadotropin output is regulated by the ovary.

1. Low circulating levels of estradiol exert a negative feedback control on LH and FSH secretion, and high maintained levels of estradiol exert a positive feedback effect.
2. High plasma levels of progesterone enhance the negative feedback effects of estradiol and keep FSH and LH secretion down to a low level.

3. The secretion of FSH, but not LH, is also regulated by nonsteroidal high-molecular-weight (around 30 000 kDa) proteins called inhibins found in follicular fluid: inhibins are found at high levels in late follicular phase plasma of fertile women, and although they have been used as a relative marker of ovarian reserve, the direct correlation is not clear.

In an ovulatory cycle, FSH stimulates the growth of follicles and increases the rate of granulosa cell production, and stimulates the aromatization of androgenic precursors and the appearance of receptors for LH/hCG on granulosa cells. Estrogens enhance the action of LH on the follicle, and also exert a negative feedback effect on the hypothalamus and pituitary to inhibit further release of gonadotropins. The levels of estrogen produced by the granulosa cells increase throughout the follicular phase until a threshold is reached where a separate positive feedback mechanism elicits the LH surge and overrides the negative feedback on gonadotropin secretion; this is the trigger for ovulation.

Inhibin is also secreted by the ovary and reduces pituitary FSH secretion.

LH stimulates theca cells to secrete androgens, which are converted to estrogens by the granulosa cells, and also influences granulosa cell differentiation, i.e., limits their replication and causes luteinization. LH stimulates the formation of progesterone directly from cholesterol in both granulosa and theca cells, and after ovulation the follicle changes rapidly from estrogen to progesterone dominance within a short period of time. Two common genetic variants in the LH beta-chain have been described that affect the molecule's biological properties (Lamminen and Huhtaniemi, 2001), with potential effects on ovarian steroidogenesis as well as response to hormonal stimulation.

## FSH Receptors

FSH acts by binding to a specific receptor in the granulosa cell plasma membrane (FSHR), and normal function of FSHR is crucial for female fertility: FSHR knockout mice are infertile. Binding leads to the elevation of intracellular cAMP through a G-protein-coupled signal transduction mechanism that activates adenylate cyclase (Simoni et al., 2000).

## FSHR Polymorphism

The FSHR gene has been localized to chromosome 2p21 and spans 54 kbp. Although naturally occurring mutations in this gene are rare, at least three common single-nucleotide polymorphisms (SNPs) have been found in the receptor: one in its promoter, and two on exon 10. FSH receptor mRNA also undergoes extensive alternative splicing, potentially giving rise to a number of different isoforms. The FSHR genotype is important in determining the action of FSH, and SNPs, either single or in various combinations, can modify endocrine feedback systems and the effects of other hormones. Thus, polymorphism in the FSHR gene results in a variable response to FSH among individuals, ranging from normal function to infertility, and these variations can affect how the ovary responds to FSH stimulation (Perez-Mayorga et al., 2000): follicles cannot grow and mature when FSH action is disrupted. Reduced expression of FSHR on granulosa cells is associated with poor ovarian response (Cai et al., 2007), and women with an FSHR polymorphism may require larger doses of FSH during controlled ovarian stimulation (COS) to achieve an adequate response during ART.

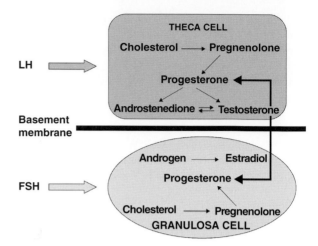

**Figure 2.2** Two-cell two-gonadotropin hypothesis.

## Anti-Müllerian Hormone (AMH)

AMH is a glycoprotein composed of two identical monomers linked by disulfide bridges, and the hormone circulates as a dimer. It is a member of the transforming growth factor-beta (TGF-beta) superfamily of molecules involved in tissue growth and differentiation. AMH was first identified as a key factor in male sex differentiation, and owes its name to the role it plays in this process (see Chapter 3). At 7–8 weeks' gestation, Sertoli cells in the fetal testis secrete AMH, which induces regression of the Müllerian ducts. In the early female fetus, the absence of AMH allows these ducts to develop into uterus, fallopian tubes and the upper part of the vagina.

In women, AMH is produced by granulosa cells from growing preantral and antral follicles. It is secreted into the blood and therefore can be measured in serum. Levels are almost undetectable in female babies, and they then gradually increase during the first 2 to 4 years of life, after which they remain stable until onset of puberty. Serum AMH declines gradually through reproductive life as the follicular reserve is depleted, and it is undetectable after menopause. Serum AMH levels reflect the follicular ovarian pool: a reduction in the number of small growing follicles is followed by a reduction in circulating AMH, and this strong correlation may be used to predict the onset of menopause. If the ovaries are surgically removed, AMH is undetectable within 3–5 days, indicating that it is produced only by cells in the ovary (La Marca et al., 2005). This also makes it a useful biomarker

---

### Two-Cell Two-Gonadotropin Theory

The 'two-cell two-gonadotropin' theory suggests that both FSH and LH are required for estrogen biosynthesis, and this requires the cooperation of both theca and granulosa cells, with coordinated expression of a cytochrome P450 enzyme triad: cholesterol side-chain cleavage cytochrome P450, 17-alpha hydroxylase cytochrome P450 and aromatase cytochrome P450.

1. The surface of theca interna cells expresses LH receptors, and LH binding to these receptors initiates a G-protein-cell signaling pathway that leads to production of cAMP. cAMP in turn stimulates the synthesis of androgens from acetate and cholesterol precursors.
2. Androstenedione is released from the thecal cell and enters the mural granulosa cells, where P450 aromatase converts it to estradiol (E2), which is released into the follicular fluid and the bloodstream. This reaction is enhanced by FSH.

The secreted estradiol is required for follicle maturation and subsequent follicle survival, and these follicles are referred to as 'gonadotropin-dependent,' since they require both LH and FSH in order to carry out their steroid biosynthesis (Figure 2.2).

in post-ovariectomy follow-up of ovarian cancer patients: granulosa cell tumors have a high incidence of recurrence, and AMH monitoring allows their early detection.

Experiments in the rat show that AMH alters the expression of several hundred genes regulating cellular pathways that inhibit the development of primordial follicles; early stages of follicular development are inhibited via a transmembrane serine/threonine kinase type II receptor signaling pathway (Nilsson et al., 2007).

During the menstrual cycle, the granulosa cells of the growing antral follicles secrete AMH under the influence of pituitary FSH. When a follicle reaches the size and stage of differentiation that determines its dominance prior to ovulation, AMH is no longer expressed (Weenen et al., 2004). In the human, this occurs in antral follicles of 4–6 mm; growing follicles are more sensitive to FSH in the absence of AMH, and the transition from primordial into growing follicles is enhanced in its absence (Durlinger et al., 2001; Visser & Themmen, 2005). It is not expressed in atretic follicles or in theca cells. Polymorphisms in the AMH gene or in its receptor seem to be related to follicular fluid and follicular phase serum estradiol levels, suggesting that it may also have a role in FSH-induced steroidogenesis in the ovary (Kevenaar et al., 2007).

Several studies have investigated variation in serum AMH levels throughout the menstrual cycle. For clinical purposes, the variation between and within cycles appears to be sufficiently low so that basal measurements can be carried out at any time in the cycle (La Marca et al, 2006, 2010). Serum levels are not affected by pregnancy, GnRH agonist administration or short-term oral contraceptive treatment. During COS with gonadotropins, AMH levels in follicular fluid have been found to be threefold higher in small than in large follicles (Fanchin et al., 2005), confirming that AMH production by granulosa cells declines during final follicular maturation, as follicles grow to a stage where AMH is no longer expressed (La Marca et al., 2004).

## AMH as a Biomarker of Ovarian Function

The correlation between circulating AMH levels and the number of early antral follicles has led to its measurement as a biomarker of ovarian function in assessing functional ovarian reserve. Very low or undetectable serum levels are found in women with early ovarian aging and premature ovarian failure, and AMH is now used routinely as a basal measurement prior to COS for assisted reproduction. Studies indicate that serum AMH is more useful in predicting ovarian response than the age of the patient or serum Day 3 FSH, estradiol and inhibin B. One of its advantages over the other hormonal markers is that it can be measured at any time of the cycle, since levels seem to have very low inter- and intracycle variation. Levels decrease during FSH stimulation, and therefore assessment must be carried out before starting FSH treatment. Ovarian reserve as measured by AMH level does not appear to be related to the probability of achieving a pregnancy (Steiner et al., 2017).

## Polycystic Ovary Syndrome and Ovarian Hyperstimulation Syndrome

Women with polycystic ovary syndrome (PCOS) characteristically have increased development of antral follicles. Histologically, the number of primordial follicles in PCO ovaries is normal compared to that in non-PCO ovaries, but the number of developing follicles is at least doubled (Webber et al., 2003). Circulating AMH levels in women with PCOS are significantly higher than in healthy controls, and this can be used as a diagnostic marker for PCO. Levels are even higher in women with insulin-resistant PCOS and may correlate with the severity of the syndrome. Significantly elevated basal AMH levels are associated with a risk of hyper-response to gonadotropins and ovarian hyperstimulation syndrome (OHSS): treatment can be individualized in order to avoid OHSS by modifying FSH dosage during ART (Pigny et al., 2006). Women with high AMH levels should be informed of their risk of developing OHSS.

## Poor Responders

AMH assessment is less reliable for the prediction of a poor response to stimulation, due to the incidence of false positive and false negative results at lower serum levels. Different laboratories have different cut-off points, and therefore predictive performance for 'poor response,' depending on the proportion of older patients in their population as well as the definition of poor response, varies widely in different settings.

Many patients described as 'poor responders' on the basis of AMH levels go on to achieve pregnancy and live birth; it seems that young poor responders have a different prognosis compared with those in the older age group. AMH measurements should be used with very low cut-off values in order to minimize the incidence of false positive tests, and low AMH values should not be used to exclude couples from IVF without consideration of other markers of ovarian reserve, such as age, basal FSH and estradiol. Nutritional supplements that support the one-carbon cycle (1-CC) can have a positive effect on ovarian reserve, with an increase in circulating AMH levels (Silvestris *et al.*, 2017). Similar observations have been made in a mouse model (Ben-Meir *et al.*, 2015).

### Obesity

Obese women have similar antral follicle counts to those of women of the same age with normal weight, but their serum AMH levels are lower. This suggests that there may be physiological factors in obese women that have an effect on circulating AMH (Su *et al.*, 2008). Smoking, alcohol use and race or ethnicity have also been found to have an effect on circulating AMH (La Marca *et al.*, 2010).

## AMH as Predictor of Treatment Outcome

Although many studies have shown a positive correlation between basal serum AMH and the number of oocytes retrieved (La Marca *et al.*, 2010), a correlation with fertilization rate, embryo morphology and chance of successful pregnancy has not been clearly defined. It appears that follicular fluid AMH levels may have some predictive value (Wunder *et al.*, 2008), but circulating peripheral levels have not been found to be useful in this respect.

In conclusion, serum AMH levels are relatively stable and consistent, and this measurement has become an important and relevant tool in patient assessment prior to ART. High levels allow patients to be counseled about their risk of OHSS, and permit stimulation regimes to be individualized in order to minimize this risk. Similarly, women with low AMH levels may be given the option of using an antagonist protocol, with a higher starting dose of FSH.

**Table 2.1** Serum AMH levels

| Age range | Median (ng/mL) (95% reference interval) | Median (pmol/L) (95% reference interval) |
|---|---|---|
| 18–25 | 3.71 (0.96–13.34) | 26.49 (6.82–95.22) |
| 26–30 | 2.27 (0.17–7.37) | 16.21 (1.22–52.66) |
| 31–35 | 1.88 (0.07–7.35) | 13.43 (0.53–52.48) |
| 36–40 | 1.62 (0.03–7.15) | 11.60 (0.20–51.03) |
| 41–45 | 0.29 (0.00–3.27) | 2.05 (0.00–23.35) |
| ≥46 | 0.01 (0.00–1.15) | 0.06 (0.00–8.19) |
| **Males >18 yrs** | 4.87 (0.73–16.05) | 34.77 (5.20–114.60) |

Adapted with permission from Beckman Coulter Access AMH Immunoassay system.

## AMH Assay

Serum AMH can be quantitatively determined using immunoassay systems, and a number of different kits are available. Results are reported as either ng/mL, or pmol/L (conversion factor = 7.1), and may vary according to the assay kit used, as well as with the demographics of patient populations (Table 2.1). Current automatic assays appear to have improved sensitivity and reproducibility compared with the older manual ELISA kits. However, every IVF unit should establish its own reference ranges and cut-off points, without relying on data from published work. Individual erroneous results can occur in patients who have received immunotherapy, as they may have antibodies that interfere with the immunoassay. Rheumatoid factor, fibrin, endogenous alkaline phosphatase and proteins that can bind to alkaline phosphatase can also interfere with the assay leading to anomalous results. In addition, polymorphisms that can affect ovarian response have been identified in all of the peptide hormones and receptors of the hypothalamo–pituitary–gonadal axis (Cargill *et al.*, 1999), and the predictive value of AMH may be limited in individuals with genetic polymorphisms.

## Serum Endocrinology in the Female

A baseline endocrine profile should be performed during the first 3 days of the menstrual cycle; if the patient has amenorrhea or oligomenorrhea, a random blood sample must be used for the profile.

| Hormone | Normal range |
| --- | --- |
| Follicle-stimulating hormone (FSH) | <8 IU/L |
| Luteinizing hormone (LH) | <10 IU/L |
| Estradiol: Early follicular | 50–200 pmol/L |
| Mid-cycle | 50–1000 pmol/L |
| Luteal | 250–1000 pmol/L |
| Progesterone mid-luteal | >30 nmol/L |
| Testosterone (T) | 0.5–3.0 nmol/L |
| Sex hormone-binding globulin (SHBG) | 16–119 nmol/L |
| Free androgen index (FAI) (T × 100)/SHBG | <5 |
| TSH | 0.5–5.5 mU/L |
| Total thyroxine | 60–160 nmol/L |
| Prolactin | <600 mIU/L |

- Serum FSH levels >15 IU/L indicate poor ovarian activity, and levels >25 IU/L suggest menopause or premature ovarian failure.
- Elevated serum LH suggests the presence of polycystic ovarian disease.
- Serum level of progesterone >30 nmol/L is indicative of ovulation.
- Amenorrhea with very low levels of FSH and LH (<2 IU/L) suggests pituitary failure or hypogonadotropic hypogonadism.
- The most usual cause of elevated serum testosterone is polycystic ovary syndrome (PCOS), but levels >5 nmol/L should be investigated to exclude other causes (congenital adrenal hyperplasia, Cushing's syndrome, androgen-secreting tumors).
- Mild elevations in serum prolactin are associated with stress and can occur simply as a result of having blood taken.

# Controlled Ovarian Hyperstimulation (COH) for ART

Ovarian stimulation with gonadotropins, 'superovulation,' in order to increase the number of oocytes available for IVF is now an established routine. The concept was first extensively studied in mice by Fowler and Edwards (1957), who showed a dose–response relationship between the amount of FSH administered and the number of small antral follicles developing. FSH suppresses apoptosis in the granulosa cells, preventing their atresia.

During COH for assisted reproduction, GnRH agonists are used to suppress pituitary release of both LH and FSH. Follicle growth and development can be achieved by the administration of pure FSH alone, in the absence of exogenous LH. However, in women with hypogonadotropic hypogonadism, who lack both LH and FSH, administration of FSH alone promotes follicular growth, but the oocytes apparently lack developmental competence. The difference between these two patient populations has been attributed to the fact that downregulation with a GnRH agonist leaves sufficient residual LH secretion to support FSH-induced follicular development. The response to FSH in downregulated ART patients is independent of serum LH levels at the time of starting FSH administration. Granulosa cells synthesize estradiol in response to FSH and LH, and estradiol levels per retrieved oocyte appear to be correlated to developmental competence of the oocytes. Women who are at risk of hyper-response to FSH and subsequent OHSS should be given lower doses of FSH; this does not affect their chance of a live birth (Oudshoom et al., 2017).

Follicular fluid contains high levels of steroids and enzymes, and aspiration of follicles during ART procedures removes this milieu from its natural environment after follicle rupture in vivo; in addition, follicle flushing removes the cells which would have been incorporated into the new corpus luteum. It is possible that this artifactual procedure leads to luteal insufficiency or other subtle consequences on ovarian physiology that are not presently obvious. Progesterone is usually administered to support the luteal phase in downregulated ART cycles.

GnRH analogs have been used in COH protocols since the mid-1980s, when high tonic levels of LH during the follicular phase were found to be detrimental to oocyte competence, decreasing fertilization and pregnancy rates (Howles et al., 1986). GnRH agonists were used to suppress and control the LH surge, thus regulating the timing of ovulation. Their use then led to the development of programmed COH protocols, which provide a convenient and effective means of scheduling and organizing a clinical IVF program: oocyte retrievals can be scheduled for specific days of the week, or in 'batches.' GnRH analogs have substitutions in their peptide sequence that increase their bioavailability over that of native GnRH, and they bind to receptors on the anterior pituitary so that the receptors are fully occupied, blocking release of FSH and LH. Two types of analogs are currently used in ART protocols:

1. GnRH agonists: Continuous administration initially causes LH and FSH hypersecretion (flare-up), and after a period of about 10 days, the pituitary store of gonadotropins is depleted. The pituitary is desensitized so that secretion of LH and FSH is suppressed, preventing ovarian steroidogenesis and follicular growth, creating an artificial but reversible menopausal state. Different GnRH agonist preparations can be administered by depot injection (Decapeptyl, Zoladex), daily subcutaneous injection (buserelin) or daily intranasal sniff (nafarelin, Synarel).

2. GnRH antagonists bind to and immediately block receptors on the pituitary; there is no initial hypersecretion of gonadotropins, but their release is instead immediately and rapidly suppressed. A third generation of these compounds (cetrorelix, ganirelix) is now used to suppress LH secretion after follicular growth has been first stimulated by gonadotropin administration on Day 1 or 2 of a menstrual cycle (or withdrawal bleed after oral contraceptive pill administration). The antagonist is administered by daily subcutaneous injection from approximately Day 6 of stimulation, or when the largest follicle size reaches 14 mm, and continued until the day of hCG administration. Due to the fact that LH suppression is more complete than with agonist administration, some protocols advocate compensating by simultaneously 'adding back' recombinant LH (Luveris) during the period of antagonist treatment.

Several protocols using GnRH analogs have been devised, and individual ART programs apply the same strategy with a variety of different drugs and schedules. Downregulation with a GnRH agonist may begin either in the luteal or the follicular phase ('long protocol') of the previous menstrual cycle and can be administered with any preparation of choice. It may also be administered from Day 1 of the treatment cycle and continued until ovulation induction with hCG ('short protocol,' sometimes also known as 'flare-up protocol'). The 'ultrashort protocol' uses only three doses

of the agonist, on Days 2, 3 and 4 of the treatment cycle. Treatment cycles can also be scheduled by programming menstruation using an oral contraceptive preparation, such as norethisterone 5 mg three times a day, and inducing a withdrawal bleed. The 'standard' protocols are not always suitable for every patient, and every treatment regimen should be tailored according to the patient's medical history and response to any previous ovarian stimulation. Patients with suspected PCO and those with limited ovarian reserve ('poor responders') require careful management and individualized treatment regimens.

The use of GnRH antagonists is thought to be more physiological ('natural'), since there is no initial suppression of pituitary FSH; however, antagonist cycles require more meticulous monitoring of the cycle in order to prevent a premature LH surge.

Original protocols for ovarian stimulation involved oral administration of clomifene citrate (Clomid), which acts as both an agonist and an antagonist by competitively binding to receptors on the hypothalamus and pituitary. It displaces endogenous estrogen and eliminates feedback inhibition, which stimulates FSH release from the pituitary. Clomid is administered at a dose of 50–100 mg twice daily for 5 days from Days 2 to 6 of the menstrual cycle, and FSH injections are commenced on Day 3. This protocol has the disadvantage that it does not block the LH surge, and therefore the cycle must be carefully monitored in order to detect and intercede before an LH surge induces ovulation. However, it may sometimes be useful for patients who have failed to respond to agonist or antagonist protocols.

With any of the COH protocols, a baseline assessment may be is normally conducted prior to starting gonadotropin stimulation, in order to ensure that the ovaries are quiescent and the endometrial lining has been shed, as well as to exclude any pathologies that might jeopardize the treatment cycle.

Oocyte retrieval (OCR) procedures are performed by vacuum aspirating follicles under vaginal ultrasound guidance using disposable OCR needles, and collecting aspirates into heated 15-mL Falcon tubes. Oocyte retrieval can be safely carried out as an outpatient procedure, using paracervical block for local anesthesia, intravenous sedation or light general anesthesia. An experienced operator can collect an average number of oocytes (i.e., 8–12) in a 5- to 10-minute time period, and the patient can usually be discharged within 2–3 hours of a routine oocyte collection.

## Stimulation Protocols for IVF

1. **Clomifene citrate (CC)/gonadotropins:**

   - CC 100 mg from Day 2, for 5 days.

   - Gonadotropin stimulation from Day 3 or 4 until day of hCG.

2. **Long GnRH agonist protocols:**

   a. *Luteal phase start (7 days after presumed ovulation, approx. Day 21):*

      - GnRH agonist from Day 21 until menses.
      - Start gonadotropins after baseline assessment, continue to day of hCG.
      - Reduce GnRH agonist dose after start of stimulation, continue until day of hCG.

   b. *Follicular phase start:*

      - Start GnRH agonist Day 2 after menses.
      - Continue until downregulation, usually at least 14 days.
      - Start gonadotropin stimulation.
      - Reduce GnRH dose after start of stimulation, continue to day of hCG.

3. **Short GnRH agonist protocol:**

   - Start GnRH agonist on Day 2 after menses, continue until day of hCG.
   - Gonadotropin stimulation from Day 3 until day of hCG.

4. **Ultrashort GnRH agonist protocol:**

   - Start GnRH agonist on Day 2 after menses, continue for 3 days.
   - Gonadotropin stimulation from Day 3 until day of hCG.

5. **GnRH antagonist protocol:**

   - Gonadotropin stimulation from Day 2 until day of hCG.
   - Start antagonist after 6 days of stimulation, or when largest follicle size = 14 mm.
   - Continue antagonist until day of hCG.

## Baseline Assessment: Ultrasound

- Ovaries: size, position
- Shape, texture
- Cysts
- Evidence of PCO
- Uterus: endometrial size, shape, texture and thickness

- Fibroids
- Congenital or other anomalies/abnormalities
- Hydrosalpinges, loculated fluid

## Baseline Assessment: Endocrinology

- Estradiol: $<50$ pg/mL
- LH: $<5$ IU/L
- Progesterone: $<2$ ng/mL

If any values are elevated:

- continue GnRH agonist treatment
- withhold stimulation
- reassess 3–7 days later.

If LH remains elevated:

- withhold stimulation
- increase dose of GnRH agonist.

(FSH: $<10$ IU/L without downregulation.)

## Ovarian Stimulation

Pure FSH (Gonal F, Puregon, Menopur) by subcutaneous self-injection. Starting dose according to age and/or history:

- age 35 or younger: 150 IU/day
- age over 35: 225 IU/day
- depending on previous response, up to 300–450 IU daily.

A long-acting chimeric preparation of human recombinant FSH, corifollitropin alpha, has a half-life of 4 days and has been shown to initiate and sustain multifollicular growth for 7 days: a single injection can replace seven daily injections of conventional FSH.

Begin monitoring after 7 days of stimulation (*adjusted according to history and baseline assessment*).

## Cycle Monitoring

Assess follicular growth after 6–8 days of gonadotropin stimulation.

- Ultrasound assessment:

  . Follicle size 14 mm or less: review in 2 or 3 days
  . Follicle size 16 mm or greater: review daily

- Plasma estradiol
- Plasma LH

  . Review as necessary

49

**Induction of Ovulation**

hCG (Profasi) 10 000 IU or r-hCG (Ovitrelle/Ovidrel 6500 IU) by subcutaneous injection when:

- Leading follicle is at least 17–18 mm in diameter
- Two or more follicles >14 mm in diameter
- Endometrium: at least 8 mm in thickness with trilaminar 'halo' appearance
- Estradiol levels approx. 100–150 pg/mL per large follicle
- Oocyte retrieval scheduled for 34–36 hours post hCG.

## Luteal Phase Support

Hormonal support of the luteal phase is felt to be necessary following pituitary downregulation with GnRH agonist treatment and is usually also used in antagonist cycles. Progesterone supplementation may be introduced on the evening following oocyte retrieval:

- Cyclogest pessaries per vaginam, 200–400 mg twice a day
- Utrogestan capsules per vaginam, 100–200 mg three times a day
- Crinone gel per vaginam, once daily application
- Gestone 50–100 mg daily by intramuscular injection
- Oral dydrogesterone 10 mg three times a day.

## In-Vitro Maturation Protocols

'In-Vitro Maturation' techniques are now successfully used as an alternative to COH in selected patient groups, particularly in those with PCOS who have large numbers of small antral follicles. Immature (GV) oocytes are recovered from antral follicles and cultured in vitro until they resume meiosis and reach metaphase II.

Protocols include initial priming of the ovaries with low doses of rFSH (100–150 IU) for 3–6 days with or without administration of hCG or a GnRH agonist. FSH priming generates GV stage oocytes that can undergo meiosis in vitro; in endocrinologically normal patients, small to mid-size antral follicles do not respond to the LH surge, and these will not respond to hCG in the same manner as larger pre-ovulatory follicles. Therefore, protocols that include hCG administration can produce some oocytes that may have been matured 'in vivo,' as well as those that will mature in vitro. However, follicles from polycystic ovaries prematurely express functionally active LH

receptors, and protocols that include hCG triggering are in widespread use, especially for PCOS patients (Chang *et al.*, 2014; Chian and Cao, 2014).

## Further Reading

### Books

Allahbadia GN, Morimoto Y (2016) *Ovarian Stimulation Protocols*. Springer, India.

Austin CT, Short RV (1972) *Reproduction in Mammals*. Cambridge University Press, Cambridge, UK.

Balen A (2014) *Infertility in Practice*. Informa Healthcare, London.

Carr BR, Blackwell RE, Azziz R (2005) *Essential Reproductive Medicine*. McGraw Hill, New York.

Johnson MH (2018) *Essential Reproduction*, 8th edn. Wiley-Blackwell, Oxford.

### Publications

Ben-Meir A, Burstein E, Borrego-Alvarez A, *et al.* (2015) Coenzyme Q10 restores oocyte mitochondrial function and fertility during reproductive aging. *Aging Cell* 14: 887–895.

Bourgain C, Devroey P (2003) The endometrium in stimulated cycles for IVF. *Human Reproduction Update* 9(6): 515–522.

Brinsden P (2005) Superovulation strategies in assisted conception. In: Brinsden P (ed.) *A Textbook of In Vitro Fertilization and Assisted Reproduction*, 3rd edn. Taylor-Francis, London, pp. 177–188.

Broer SL, Dólleman M, Opmeer BC, *et al.* (2011) AMH and AFC as predictors of excessive response in controlled ovarian hyperstimulation: a meta-analysis. *Human Reproduction Update* 17(1): 46–54.

Cai J, Lou H-Y, Dong M-Y, *et al.* (2007) Poor ovarian response to gonadotropin stimulation is associated with low expression of follicle-stimulating hormone receptor in granulosa cells. *Fertility and Sterility* 87(6): 1350–1356.

Cargill M, Altshuler D, Ireland J, *et al.* (1999) Characterization of single-nucleotide polymorphisms in coding regions of human genes. *Nature Genetics* 22: 231–238.

Chang EM, Song HS, Lee DR, *et al.* (2014) *In vitro maturation of human oocytes: its role in infertility treatment and new possibilities. Clinical Experiments in Reproductive Medicine* 41(2): 41–46.

Chian RC, Cao YX (2014) In vitro maturation of immature human oocytes for clinical application. *Methods in Molecular Biology* 1154: 271–288.

Conway GS (1996) Clinical manifestations of genetic defects affecting gonadotrophins and their receptors. *Clinical Endocrinology* 45: 657–663.

Cortvrindt R, Smitz J, Van Steirteghem AC (1997) Assessment of the need for follicle stimulating hormone in early preantral mouse follicle culture in vitro. *Human Reproduction* 12: 759–768.

Desai AS, Achrekar AK, Paranjape SR, *et al.* (2013) Association of allelic combinations of FSHR gene polymorphisms with ovarian response. *Reproductive BioMedicine Online* 27: 400–406.

Devroey P, Boostanfar R, Koper NP, Mannaerts BM, Ijzerman-Boon PC, Fauser BC (2009) A double-blind, non-inferiority RCT comparing corifollitropin alfa and recombinant FSH during the first seven days of ovarian stimulation using a GnRH antagonist protocol. *Human Reproduction* 24: 3063–3072.

Durlinger AL, Gruijters MJ, Kramer P, *et al.* (2001) Anti-Müllerian hormone attenuates the effects of FSH on follicle development in the mouse ovary. *Endocrinology* 142: 4891–4899.

Fanchin R, Louafi N, Mendez Lozano DH, Frydman N, Frydman R, Taieb J (2005) Per-follicle measurements indicate that anti-mullerian hormone secretion is modulated by the extent of follicular development and luteinization and may reflect qualitatively the ovarian follicular status. *Fertility and Sterility* 84: 167–173.

Fowler RE, Edwards RG (1957) Induction of superovulation and pregnancy in mature mice by gonadotrophins. *Journal of Endocrinology* 15: 374–384.

Hillier SG (1991) Regulatory functions for inhibin and activin in human ovaries. *Journal of Endocrinology* 131: 171–175.

Hillier SG (2009) The science of ovarian ageing: How might knowledge be translated into practice? In: Bewley S, Ledger W, Nikolaou D (eds.) *Reproductive Ageing.* RCOG Press, London, pp. 75–87.

Howles CM, Macnamee MC, Edwards RG (1987) Follicular development and early luteal function of conception and non-conceptual cycles after human in vitro fertilization. *Human Reproduction* 2: 17–21.

Howles CM, Macnamee MC, Edwards RG, Goswamy R, Steptoe PC (1986) Effect of high tonic levels of luteinizing hormone on outcome of in vitro fertilization. *Lancet* 2: 521–522.

Kevenaar ME, Themmen AP, Laven JS, *et al.* (2007) Anti-Müllerian hormone and anti-Müllerian hormone type II receptor polymorphisms are associated with follicular phase estradiol levels in normo-ovulatory women. *Human Reproduction* 22: 1547–1554.

Kumar TR, Wang Y, Lu N, Matzuk MM (1997) Follicle stimulating hormone is required for ovarian follicle maturation but not male fertility. *Nature Genetics* 15: 201–203.

La Marca A, De Leo V, Giulini S, *et al.* (2005) Anti-Mullerian hormone in premenopausal women and after spontaneous or surgically induced menopause. *Journal of the Society for Gynecological Investigation* 12(7): 545–548.

La Marca A, Malmusi S, Giulini S, *et al.* (2004) Anti-Mullerian hormone plasma levels in spontaneous menstrual cycle and during treatment with FSH to induce ovulation. *Human Reproduction* 19(12): 2738–2741.

La Marca A, Sighinolfi G, Radi D, *et al.* (2010) Anti-Müllerian hormone (AMH) as a predictive marker in assisted reproductive technology. *Human Reproduction Update* 16(2): 113–130.

La Marca A, Stabile G, Artensio AC, Volpe A (2006) Serum anti-Müllerian hormone throughout the human menstrual cycle. *Human Reproduction* 21: 3103–3107.

Lamminen T, Huhtaniemi I (2001) A common genetic variant of luteinizing hormone: relation to normal and aberrant pituitary-gonadal function. *European Journal of Pharmacology* 414: 1–7.

Loumaye E, Engrand P, Howles CM, O'Dea L (1997) Assessment of the role of serum luteinizing hormone and estradiol response to follicle-stimulating hormone on in vitro fertilization outcome. *Fertility and Sterility* 67: 889–899.

Macnamee MC, Howles CM, Edwards RG, *et al.* (1989) Short term luteinising hormone agonist treatment: prospective trial of a novel ovarian stimulation regimen for in vitro fertilisation. *Fertility and Sterility* 52: 264–269.

Nilsson E, Rogers N, Skinner MK (2007) Actions of anti-Mullerian hormone on the ovarian transcriptome to inhibit primordial to primary follicle transition. *Reproduction* 134(2): 209–221.

Oudshoom SC, van Tilborg TC, Eijkemans MJC, *et al.* (2017) Individualized versus standard FSH dosing in women starting IVF/ICSI: an RCT. Part 2: The predicted hyper responder. *Human Reproduction* 32(12): 2506–2514.

Perez-Mayorga M, Gromoll J, Behre HM, *et al.* (2000). Ovarian response to follicle-stimulating hormone (FSH) stimulation depends on the FSH receptor genotype. *Journal of Clinical Endocrinology and Metabolism* 85(9): 3365–3369.

Pigny P, Jonard S, Robert Y, Dewailly D (2006) Serum Anti-Müllerian Hormone as a surrogate for antral follicle count for definition of the Polycystic Ovary Syndrome. *Journal of Clinical Endocrinology and Metabolism* 91: 941–945.

Regan L, Owen EJ, Jacobs HS (1990) Hypersecretion of luteinising hormone, infertility, and miscarriage. *Lancet* 336: 1141–1144.

Shenfield F (1996) FSH: what is its role in infertility treatments, and particularly in IVF? *Medical Dialogue* 471: 1–4.

Silvestris E, Cohen M, Cornet D, *et al.* (2017) Supporting the One-Carbon Cycle restores ovarian reserve in subfertile women: absence of correlation with urinary Bisphenol A concentration. *BioResearch Open Access* 6(1). DOI: 10.1089/biores.2017.0016.

Simoni M, Nieschlag E, Gromoll J (2002) Isoforms and single nucleotide polymorphisms of the FSH receptor gene: implications for human reproduction. *Human Reproduction Update* 8(5): 413–421.

Steiner AZ, Pritchard D, Stanczyk FZ, *et al.* (2017) Association between biomarkers of ovarian reserve and infertility among older women of reproductive age. *Journal of the American Medical Association* 318(14): 1367–1376.

Su HI, Sammel MD, Freeman EW, *et al.* (2008) Body size affects measures of ovarian reserve in late reproductive age women. *Menopause* 15: 857–861.

Tavaniotou A, Smitz J, Bourgain C, Devroey P (2001) Ovulation induction disrupts luteal phase function. *Annals of the New York Academy of Sciences* 943: 55–63.

Telfer EE (1996) The development of methods for isolation and culture of preantral follicles from bovine and porcine ovaries. *Theriogenology* 45: 101–110.

Tohlob D, Hshem EA, Gharreb N, *et al.* (2016) Association of a promoter polymorphism in FSHR with ovarian reserve and response to ovarian stimulation in women undergoing assisted reproductive treatment. *Reproductive BioMedicine Online* 33: 391–397.

Tournaye H, Sukhikh GT, Kahler E, Griesinger G (2017) A Phase III randomized controlled trial comparing the efficacy, safety and tolerability of oral dydrogesterone versus micronized vaginal progesterone for luteal support in in vitro fertilization. *Human Reproduction* 32(5): 1019–1027.

Ulug U, Ben-Shlomo I, Turan E, Erden HF, Akman MA, Bahceci M (2003) Conception rates following assisted reproduction in poor responder patients: a retrospective study in 300 consecutive cycles. *Reproductive BioMedicine Online* 6: 439–443.

Visser JA, Themmen AP (2005) Anti-Müllerian hormone and folliculogenesis. *Molecular and Cellular Endocrinology* 234: 81–86.

Webber LJ, Stubbs S, Stark J, *et al.* (2003) Formation and early development of follicles in the polycystic ovary. *Lancet* 362: 1017–1021.

Weenen C, Laven JS, Von Bergh AR, *et al.* (2004) Anti-Mullerian hormone expression pattern in the human ovary: potential implications for initial and cyclic follicle recruitment. *Molecular Human Reproduction* 10: 77–83.

Wunder DM, Bersinger NA, Yared M, Kretschmer R, Birkhauser MH (2008). Statistically significant changes of anti-mullerian hormone and inhibin levels during the physiologic menstrual cycle in reproductive age women. *Fertility and Sterility* 89: 927–933.

# Gametes and Gametogenesis

**Chapter 3**

## Gamete Precursor Cells: Primordial Germ Cells

After a blastocyst has implanted in the uterus and begins to differentiate into the three primary germ layers, a special population of cells develops as primordial germ cells (PGCs). These are destined to become the gametes of the new individual: future reproduction of the organism is absolutely dependent upon the correct development of these unique populations of cells. They originate immediately behind the primitive streak in the extraembryonic mesoderm of the yolk sac; toward the end of gastrulation they move into the embryo via the allantois, and temporarily settle in the mesoderm and endoderm of the primitive streak. In humans, PGCs can be identified at about 3 weeks of gestation, close to the yolk sac

endoderm at the root of the allantois. These cells have many special properties in terms of morphology, behavior and gene expression, and undergo a number of unique biological processes:

- Lengthy migration through the developing embryo to the gonadal ridge
- Erasure of epigenetic information from the previous generation
- Reactivation of the X chromosome that has been silenced (Barr body) in XX cells.

## Migration of Primordial Germ Cells

PGCs proliferate by mitosis, and begin to migrate through the embryonic tissue, completing approximately six mitotic divisions by the time they colonize the future gonad (Figure 3.1).

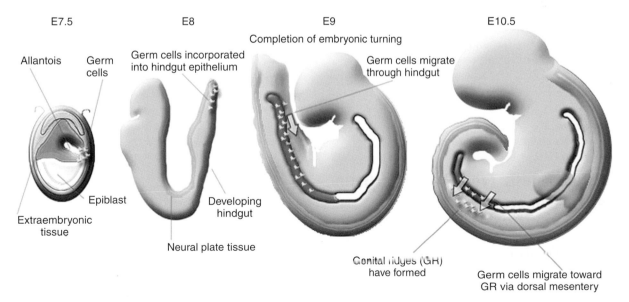

E7.5     E8     E9     E10.5

Completion of embryonic turning

Allantois — Germ cells

Germ cells incorporated into hindgut epithelium

Germ cells migrate through hindgut

Epiblast

Extraembryonic tissue

Developing hindgut

Neural plate tissue

Gonital ridges (GR) have formed

Germ cells migrate toward GR via dorsal mesentery

**Figure 3.1** Migration of primordial germ cells in the mouse. PGCs arise at the start of gastrulation, around embryonic Days 7–7.25 (E7–7.5) at the border of the extraembryonic tissue and the epiblast, at the root of the allantois. The PGCs can be identified and distinguished from the surrounding somatic cells by their positive staining for alkaline phosphatase. Expression of the OCT4 transcription factor becomes restricted to PGCs around day E8 and is used as a PGC marker. See color plate section. Adapted diagram courtesy of J. Huntriss, University of Leeds. Modified from Starz-Gaiano & Lehmann, 2001, with permission from Elsevier Ltd.

Proliferation and migration continue for 3–4 weeks in humans, and during their migration the germ cells and the somatic cells interact together via a number of different types of signals. The PGCs move to the inside of the embryo along with the gut to embed in the connective tissue of the hindgut, migrate through the dorsal mesentery along the hindgut a few days later, and then finally populate the gonadal ridge to form the embryonic gonad. The tissue of the gonadal ridge makes up the somatic (nongamete) part of the gonads. In humans, PGCs can be seen in the region of the developing kidneys (the mesonephros) approximately 4 weeks after fertilization (gestational age 5–6 weeks), and their migration is completed by 6 weeks of gestation. Primordial gonads can be identified on either side of the central dorsal aorta between 37 and 42 days after fertilization (gestational age 8–9 weeks) as a medial thickening of the mesodermal epithelium that lines the coelom (body cavity).

### PGCs in the Mouse

- During their migration in the mouse, the population of PGCs increases from around 100 cells to 25 000 cells by stage 13.5 of embryonic development (E13.5).
- The genital ridges may secrete a chemotactic substance (probably SDF-1, stromal cell derived factor 1 and its receptor CXCR4) that attracts the PGCs: primordial gonadal tissue grafted into abnormal sites within a mouse embryo attracts germ cells to colonize it.
- Experiments using gene knockout animal models have identified a number of genes involved in regulating the establishment and migration of PGCs, the signals involved in their movement and their renewal properties (see MacLaren, 2003).

# Gonadogenesis: From Primordial Germ Cells to Gametes

The primordial gonadal ridges develop on the posterior wall of the lower thoracic and upper lumbar regions, and in both sexes this undifferentiated mesenchymal tissue forms the basic matrices of the testes and ovaries. At approximately 6 weeks of gestation the developing gonad appears identical in male and female embryos, and remains sexually undifferentiated for a period of 7–10 days. During this period, groups of cells derived from the columnar coelomic (germinal) epithelium surrounding the genital ridge migrate into the undifferentiated tissue as columns to colonize the gonad; these are known as the primitive sex cords. Key morphological changes then start to take place in the gonads, which depend upon whether or not the Sex-determining Region Y (SRY) gene on a Y chromosome is expressed in the cells of the sex cords. These morphological changes result in the formation of:

1. Genital ducts
   - Wolffian duct = male, precursor of the vas deferens and epididymis
   - Müllerian duct = female, precursor of the uterus, the upper parts of the vagina and the oviducts.
2. Urogenital sinus.

Knockout mouse technology has identified a number of genes involved in these early stages of gonadogenesis, some of which are outlined in Figure 3.2, and summarized here:

1. SRY expression is upregulated by only one isoform of Wilms' tumor gene product WT1 (–KTS).
2. The WT1(–KTS) isoform also upregulates DAX1 expression (which antagonizes development of Sertoli cells). The WT1(–KTS) isoform is therefore considered essential for development of both the male and the female gonad.
3. The WT1(+KTS) isoform increases the number of SRY transcripts and is required for formation of the male gonad.
4. WNT4 acts to repress migration of mesonephric endothelial and steroidogenic cells in the XX gonad, preventing the formation of a male-specific coelomic blood vessel and the production of steroids. WNT4 expression is downregulated after sex determination in the XY gonad.
5. DAX1 may inhibit SRY indirectly by inhibiting expression of male-specific genes that are activated by SF1.
6. SRY upregulates expression of a related transcription factor, SOX9. SOX9 is required for activation of anti-Müllerian hormone (AMH)/Müllerian inhibitory substance (MIS), which causes regression of the female Müllerian duct.
7. Dmrt1 is thought to interfere with the action of SOX9. Dmrt1 is a candidate sex-determining gene in birds, carried on their Z chromosome.

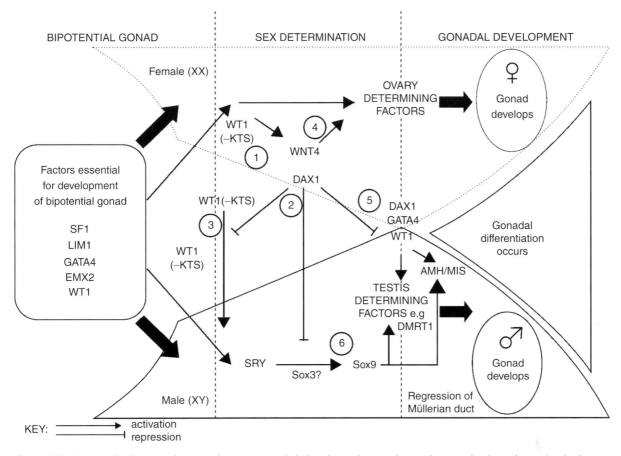

**Figure 3.2** Genes involved in gonadogenesis; key points are circled, outlining the complex regulatory molecular pathways involved. Adapted with permission from Clarkson & Harley, 2002.

## Sex Determination

A classic experiment by Alfred Jost in the 1940s demonstrated that mammalian embryos castrated prior to differentiation of the testis appear to develop phenotypically as females. This established that the female route of sexual development is the default differentiation pathway, and led the authors to propose the existence of a testis-determining factor (TDF). This has now been established by experiments on early embryos, and by molecular experiments. Genetic studies also suggest that ovarian differentiation and development may be regulated by certain 'anti-testis' factors:

- In XY humans who carry a duplication of part of the small arm of the X chromosome (Xp21) (and in XY mice of certain genetic backgrounds), overexpression of the DAX1 gene causes sex reversal; i.e., these human or mouse individuals develop as females. Therefore, DAX1 can apparently antagonize SRY in a dosage-sensitive manner to cause sex reversal.
- Wnt4 is also required for female development. Genetic studies in the mouse show that:

  . Wnt4 is initially required for the formation of the Müllerian duct in both sexes.
  . In the developing ovary, Wnt4 suppresses the development of Leydig cells.
  . In Wnt4 mutants, the Müllerian duct is absent, and the Wolffian duct develops further.

Wnt4-mutant females activate testosterone biosynthesis and become masculinized.

Knock-outs of SF1, Lim-9 and Wnt1 genes develop as phenotypic females, in support of Jost's proposal.

55

# Development of the Testis

After the mesonephros has been populated with primordial germ cells to form the genital ridge, the coelomic epithelium proliferates at a faster rate in male than in female gonads, and the cells penetrate deep into the medullary mesenchyme to form the testis cords. Two different testicular compartments are formed: the testicular cords and the interstitial region. Expression of the SRY gene initiates differentiation of Sertoli cells, and the developing Sertoli cells produce a growth factor, fibroblast growth factor 9 (FGF-9), that is necessary for formation of the testicular cords. At 7–8 weeks of gestation, the testicular cords (precursor of the seminiferous tubules) can be seen in histological sections as protrusions of the cortical epithelium into the medulla; animal experiments indicate that germ cells are not involved in this process.

- Sertoli cells cluster around the germ cells; peritubular myoid cells surround the clusters and deposit the basal lamina.
- Sertoli cells secrete AMH/MIS, which suppresses the default pathway that would develop Müllerian ducts as precursors of female sexual anatomy. The Sertoli cells continue to secrete AMH throughout fetal and postnatal life until the time of puberty, when the levels drop sharply.
- Leydig cells remain in the interstitial region, close to blood and lymphatic systems, and they actively secrete androgens from at least 8–10 weeks of gestation. This capacity to secrete testosterone is essential for continued testicular development and, ultimately, for the establishment of the male phenotype.
- Testosterone causes growth and differentiation of the Wolffian duct structures (precursor of the male sexual anatomy).
- Dihydrotestosterone (a metabolite of testosterone) induces virilization of the urogenital sinus and the external genitalia.

The Müllerian duct then regresses, and the Wolffian duct develops further.

By 16–20 weeks of fetal life, Sertoli cells and relatively quiescent prospermatogonial cells lie on a basement membrane within seminiferous cords; these are within a vascularized stroma that also contains condensed Leydig cells, and the entire structure is enclosed within a fibrous capsule, the tunica albuginea.

The testes gradually increase in size until the time of puberty, and with the onset of puberty they begin to rapidly enlarge:

- The solid cords canalize to give rise to tubules, which eventually connect to the rete testis, the vasa efferentia and then the epididymis.
- Leydig cells significantly increase their endocrine secretion, and intratubular Sertoli cells also increase in size and activity.
- Prospermatogonial PGCs (gonocytes) in the cords now line the seminiferous tubules as spermatogenic epithelium and begin to divide by mitosis.

After the population has been expanded, the prospermatogonia enter a quiescent non-proliferative phase; they are initially located toward the center of the seminiferous cords, but then migrate to a niche in the periphery where they can begin to function as spermatogenic stem cells (SSC), known as as type A spermatogonia. This SSC population must both self-renew to maintain its numbers and generate progenitor cells that then enter spermatogenesis to produce mature sperm.

## Genetic Control

- SRY, SOX9, WT1, XH2, SF1 and DAX1 are known to be involved in the control of testis determination. Many of these genes have been identified through analysis of cases of sex reversal.
- The SRY gene is a key switch in male sexual differentiation; it acts only briefly in male embryos to initiate differentiation of the Sertoli cells in the somatic cells of the genital ridge.
- SRY may function either:

  - As a transcriptional repressor to repress activation of the genes that cause differentiation of the ovary.
  - As a repressor of the factors that repress testis development.
  - Synergistically with SF1 to activate SOX9.

## Testicular Descent

The testes develop initially in the upper lumbar region of the embryo and gradually migrate during fetal life through the abdominal cavity and over the pelvic brim. This descent is influenced by hormones secreted by the Leydig cells and involves two ligamentous structures: the suspensory ligament at the superior pole and the gubernaculum at the inferior pole of the testis. As the fetal body grows in size, the suspensory ligament elongates and the gubernaculum does not, so that the position of the testis becomes localized to the pelvis. Between weeks 25 and 28 of pregnancy, the testes migrate over the pubic bone, and reach the scrotum via the inguinal canal by weeks 35–40. As a result of their external position outside the body cavity, the temperature of the testes is approximately 2°C below body temperature, which is optimal for spermatogenesis.

The adult testes contain approximately 200 m of seminiferous tubules, forming the bulk of the volume of the testis. These tubules are the site of spermatogenesis. The round tubules are separated from each other by a small amount of connective tissue that contains, in addition to blood vessels, a few lymphocytes, plasma cells and clumps of interstitial Leydig cells. The tubules are lined by spermatogenic epithelium, which is made up of spermatogonia at different stages of maturation; a cross-section of any normal seminiferous tubule reveals four or five distinct generations of germ cells. The younger generation cells are on the basement membrane, and the more differentiated cells approach the lumen of the tubule. This growth pattern has a wavelike cycle with intermingling of different stages that lie close to each other; any single cross-section of the tubule does not always reveal all generations of spermatogenesis. The tubules rest on a delicate anuclear basement membrane that in turn lies on a connective tissue layer, the tunica propria. The supporting Sertoli cells, which are believed to nourish the germ cells, form a continuous layer connected by tight junctions. These large polymorphous cells have large, pale nuclei and abundant cytoplasm that extends from the periphery of the tubule to the lumen, stretching through the layers of developing germ cells. Mature spermatozoa can be seen attached to and surrounding the Sertoli cells prior to their release (Figure 3.3). A wave of spermatogenesis passes along the tubule, and the process of development from spermatogonium to spermatozoon takes approximately 65 days. A transverse cross-section through the human testis shows tubules containing cells at many different stages in spermatogenesis (in contrast to the rat testis, where every tubule has cells at the same stage). In humans, many seminiferous tubules can be seen that are apparently without spermatocytes and spermatids, a phenomenon that may contribute to the relatively poor efficiency of spermatogenesis.

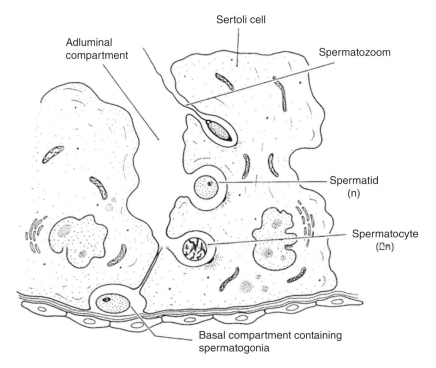

**Figure 3.3** Spermatogenesis in the mammal. Maturation and modeling of the male gamete is regulated by the Sertoli cell. Modified with permission from Johnson [2018].

Sertoli cell

Adluminal compartment

Spermatozoom

Spermatid (n)

Spermatocyte ($2n$)

Basal compartment containing spermatogonia

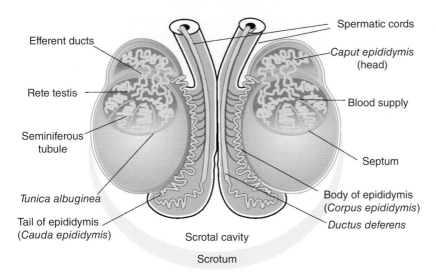

Efferent ducts

Rete testis

Seminiferous tubule

*Tunica albuginea*

Tail of epididymis
(*Cauda epididymis*)

Scrotal cavity

Scrotum

Spermatic cords

*Caput epididymis*
(head)

Blood supply

Septum

Body of epididymis
(*Corpus epididymis*)

*Ductus deferens*

**Figure 3.4** Anatomy of the adult mammalian testis. Drawing adapted from a number of sources.

Sperm released into the lumen of the seminiferous tubules pass via the rete testis through the ductuli efferentia into the caput epididymis. They traverse the epididymis over a period of 2–14 days, undergoing a number of changes in preparation for fertilization, and are then stored sequentially in the cauda, vas, seminal vesicles and ampullae prior to ejaculation. The seminal vesicles, prostate and urethral glands add glandular secretions to the sperm at the time of ejaculation. Figure 3.4 illustrates the anatomy of the adult mammalian testis.

## Spermatogenesis

In the fetal testis, primordial germ cells differentiate into spermatozoal stem cells, type A (A0 or As) spermatogonia. The process of spermatogenesis is initiated at puberty and continues throughout the reproductive life of the individual. This need for continual production requires a thriving stem cell population, major expansion of progenitor cells, morphological transformation from spermatid to sperm and the acquisition of motility. The entire process is subject to a high level of control and orchestrated organization, with complex interactions between the germ cells, testicular somatic cells, and a number of endocrine and growth factors.

Spermatogenesis can be divided into three well-defined phases, and each phase is associated with a specific type of precursor cell:

1. Proliferation (mitotic expansion, spermatocytogenesis): spermatogonia

2. Reduction division (meiotic reduction): spermatocytes
3. Differentiation (morphological transformation, spermiogenesis): spermatids.

These precursor stem cells line the basement membrane of the seminiferous tubules, have large spherical or oval nuclei, and are connected to each other via intercellular bridges to form a germ cell syncytium. They are in contact with Sertoli cells, which extend from the epithelium into the lumen of the tubules. At puberty, the spermatogonia start to proliferate by mitoses; this is followed by meiosis and a gradual reorganization of cellular components and a loss of cytoplasm.

### Spermatocytogenesis

- At intervals after puberty, stem cells in the germinal epithelium of the seminiferous tubules (type A spermatogonia) replicate their DNA and divide by mitosis.
- Each mitotic division produces two cells: another type A spermatogonium and a second cell, which enters a pool of undifferentiated spermatogonia – transient amplifying progenitor cells, Aa1, that transition without cell division into type A1 differentiating spermatogonia.
- These A1 cells undergo five synchronized cell divisions to form A2, A3, A4, Intermediate (In) and B spermatogonia, which then move into the adluminal compartment and start their differentiation by entering into meiosis.

## Meiosis

The transition from undifferentiated (A) to A1 spermatogonia represents an irreversible commitment to meiosis, and is controlled by numerous intrinsic factors and by at least one extrinsic factor: retinoic acid (RA), a metabolite of vitamin A (see Griswold, 2016 for review). In the adluminal compartment, the cells undergo two meiotic divisions to form two daughter secondary spermatocytes initially, and eventually four early spermatids. Through a series of different phases, meiosis (reduction division) converts diploid stem cells (spermatogonia) containing 46 chromosomes into haploid gametes, with 23 chromosomes. In the first phase of meiosis, type B spermatogonia (2n:2c) become primary spermatocytes (1n:2c). These cells divide again to become secondary spermatocytes (1n:1c). The cells go through this stage quickly and complete the second meiotic division. After the second meiotic division, the cells are known as spermatids. These cells must now go through a process of maturation (spermiogenesis) in order to finally emerge as mature spermatozoa (1n:1c).

## Spermiogenesis

Spermatid differentiation occurs in four stages (Figure 3.5):

1. Golgi phase
2. Cap phase
3. Acrosomal phase
4. Maturation phase.

Spermatid nuclei now contain haploid sets of chromosomes. Their autosomes continue to direct the synthesis of low levels of rRNA, mRNA and proteins as they enter into their prolonged phase of terminal differentiation, spermiogenesis. During this phase, round spermatid cells are converted into elongated sperm cells with a condensed nucleus and a flagellum. They do not divide again, either by mitosis or meiosis, but must differentiate to acquire functions that will allow them to traverse the female tract and fertilize an oocyte. This differentiation process takes approximately 2 weeks in most species and follows well-defined stages:

1. Spermatid DNA becomes highly condensed and somatic histones are replaced with protamines.
2. The acrosome, a sac containing enzymes necessary for oocyte penetration, is constructed from Golgi membranes.
3. Cytoplasmic reorganization gives rise to the midpiece, which contains mitochondria and associated control mechanisms necessary for motility.
4. The flagellar apparatus (tail) is formed, which will make the cells motile.
5. A residual body casts off excess cytoplasm.

Sperm modeling is probably regulated by the Sertoli cells, and the cells are moved to the center of the tubular lumen as spermatogenesis proceeds. The rate of progression of cells through spermatogenesis is constant and is not affected by external factors such as hormones. The timing of stored mRNA translation is a major point of control: for example, the protamine1 gene is transcribed in round spermatids, and the resulting mRNA is stored for up to 1 week before it is

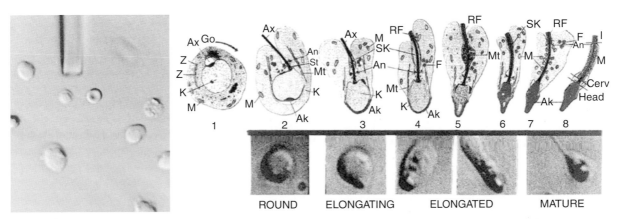

**Figure 3.5** Developing sperm. A = acrosome; An = annulus; Ax = axoneme; C = centriole; F = flowerlike structures; Fs = flagellar substructures; M = mitochondria; Mp = middle piece; Mt = manchette; Ne = neck; PP = principal piece; R = ring fibers; Sb = spindle-shaped body. Courtesy of M. Nijs and P. Vanderzwalmen, Belgium.

59

translated in elongating spermatids. Other mRNAs are stored for only hours or a few days, indicating that there must be a defined temporal program of translational control.

- Sertoli cells are connected by tight junctions and act as nurse cells during spermatogenesis.
- Tight junctions restrict the passage of substances from the blood to the lumen of the seminiferous tubules and therefore form a blood–testis barrier. This barrier protects sperm from antibodies circulating in the bloodstream.

## Molecular Features of Spermatogenesis

- The trigger that determines which spermatogonia become committed to meiosis is not known.
- DNA is transcribed from both diploid (proliferative type A [A0] spermatogonia) and haploid (committed type B [A1] spermatogonia) genomes throughout the process.
- Only type B spermatogonia undergo differentiation into spermatozoa, and the vast majority of the germ cell cytoplasm is lost during the terminal stages of differentiation, when the spermatids condense into spermatozoa.
- The reduction process that generates haploid sperm cells takes at least 65 days in humans and involves six successive stages over four consecutive spermatogenic cycles.
- Note the nomenclature relating to chromosome complement (n) and DNA copy number (c). 1c is the DNA copy number of a haploid gamete, and no gamete is ever tetraploid.

## Pathology Affecting Spermatogenesis

- A number of different pathologies can disrupt the orderly pattern of spermatogenesis, causing immature forms, especially spermatocytes to slough into the tubular lumen. Less frequently, maturation may proceed to the spermatid stage and be arrested there.
- Any lesion that causes generalized arrest of maturation, or a mixture of maturation arrest and atrophy to a stage preceding spermiogenesis, will result in azoospermia.
- The tubular epithelium is very sensitive to toxins and to ischemia; damage may result in partial, focal or total obliteration of the spermatogenic

epithelium, including the Sertoli cells, while the Leydig cells remain functionally normal.
- In cases of severe injury, the tubules may be totally destroyed and become hyalinized, or may be replaced by fibrous tissue. Since the whole tubule is destroyed, this disorder is associated with a much reduced testis size, with absence of Sertoli cells resulting in raised serum FSH.
- Focal lesions can cause oligospermia of varying severity, and patients with focal lesions may have normal levels of FSH in their serum.

## Epididymal Maturation

Mammalian spermatozoa leaving the testis are not capable of fertilizing oocytes. They gain this ability while passing down the epididymis, a process known as epididymal maturation. The epididymis is divided into different regions: the caput is the upper third, formed by efferent ductules that are lined by pseudostratified columnar ciliated epithelium (such as is found in nasal and bronchial passages; patients with upper epididymal obstruction often have associated nasal or respiratory problems, as in mucoviscidosis, Young's syndrome). The vasa efferentia tubules unite to form the single coiled tubule of the corpus, which has flatter, non-ciliated epithelium and microvilli on the luminal surface. It starts to form a muscular wall toward the cauda, where the lumen is wider, and spermatozoa can be stored prior to ejaculation.

During its journey through the different regions of the epididymis, the head of the spermatozoon acquires the ability to interact with the zona pellucida, with an increase in net negative charge. Many antigens with a demonstrable role in oocyte binding and fusion are synthesized in the testis as precursors, and then activated at some point in the epididymis either through direct biochemical modification, through changing their cellular localization or both. Examples of such antigen processing include a membrane-bound hyaluronidase, fertilin, proacrosin, 1,4-galactosyltransferase (GalTase) and putative zona ligands sp56 and p95. The terminal saccharide residues of membrane glycoproteins and lipids also undergo changes in their physical and chemical composition.

Although all the necessary morphological structures for flagellar activity are assembled during spermiogenesis, testicular spermatozoa are essentially immotile, even when washed and placed in a physiological solution. Spermatozoa from the caput epididymis begin to display motility, and by the time they reach the cauda they are capable of full progressive forward motility. Demembranation and exposure to ATP, cAMP and $Mg^{2+}$ triggers movement, which suggests that the ability to move is probably regulated at the level of the plasma membrane. Transfer of a forward motility protein and carnitine from the epididymal fluid is believed to be important for the development of sperm motility. Since the osmolality and chemical composition of the epididymal fluid vary from one segment to the next, it may be that the sperm plasma membrane is altered stepwise as it progresses down the duct, and motility is controlled by an interplay between cAMP, cytosolic $Ca^{2+}$ and pH. During maturation, the spermatozoa use up endogenous reserves of metabolic substrates, becoming dependent on exogenous sources such as fructose; at this point they shed their cytoplasmic droplet.

## DNA Packaging in Sperm

The amount of DNA in the sperm nucleus (approximately 1 m in length) has to be packaged into a volume that is typically less than 10% of the volume of a somatic cell nucleus; a different mechanism of packaging is required, as illustrated in Figure 3.6.

- Somatic cell DNA is packaged into nucleosomes by a process of primary compaction that uses histones. A 10-nm fiber is supercoiled into the 30-nm solenoid, and supercoiled again into loops (Figure 3.6A–D. These loops are the major structural form of interphase chromatin.

- During spermatogenesis, DNA is initially packaged by histones (as in Figure 3.6A–D) but following meiosis, at the secondary spermatocyte stage of spermiogenesis, histones are replaced first by transition proteins and then by protamines (Figure 3.6G). The solenoid structure is replaced by torroids (doughnut shapes), which are in turn supercoiled into torroidal loops. This highly compacted structure shuts down transcription during spermiogenesis. The loop domains shown in Figure 3.6E and J represent the chromatin state in the interphase somatic cell nucleus (Figure 3.6E) and the sperm nucleus (Figure 3.6J). Sperm appear poised for transcription.

## Gene Expression during Spermatogenesis

Gene expression during spermatogenesis can be subdivided into two distinctive phases:

1. Prior to meiosis, all stages up to and including the completion of telophase: diploid cells.
2. During spermiogenesis: late secondary spermatocytes are haploid cells, and the developmental process from this stage onwards is referred to as spermiogenesis.

Genes are expressed from both the diploid and the haploid genomes. DNA transcription is often

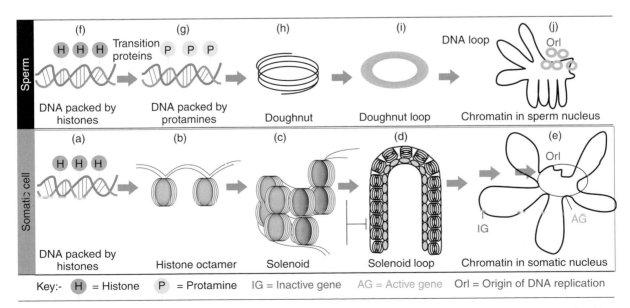

Key:-  (H) = Histone  (P) = Protamine  IG = Inactive gene  AG = Active gene  Orl = Origin of DNA replication

**Figure 3.6** DNA packaging in somatic cells and spermatozoa. See color plate section. Image adapted with permission from Ward, 1993.

coordinated with mRNA translation into its protein product (e.g., histones, X-linked lactate dehydrogenase). In spermiogenesis, however, transcription may be shut down well before the protein appears, i.e., the mRNA is translated later (e.g., PGK2, acrosin). As spermatogenesis progresses, the transcripts encoding the same protein differ in size, due to alterations in the length of the mRNA polyA tail. (A similar phenomenon occurs in oogenesis, as described later.)

### Control of Gene Expression during Spermatogenesis

- Between primitive spermatogonial and final mature spermatozoa, cellular chromatin is restructured so that certain genes are repressed, potentiated, or potentiated and transcribed.
- The gene for phosphoglycerokinase 1 (PGK1), an essential glycolytic enzyme, lies on the X chromosome, and is highly expressed, potentiated and transcribed early in spermatogenesis. As the cells progress into meiosis, the X chromosome becomes progressively inactivated, and during spermiogenesis expression of PGK1 is replaced by expression of an autosomal homologue, PGK2.
- During spermiogenesis (the haploid stages of spermatogenesis), cellular histones are replaced first by testis-specific histones and then by the transition protein TNP2 and the protamines PRM1 and PRM2. This substitution is a prerequisite for the extremely compact packaging of sperm DNA. These genes are located on chromosome 16.
- Not all histones are replaced. Human sperm retain approximately 15–20% of their chromatin in a nucleosomal configuration, and we now know that mature sperm cells retain a complex repertoire of mRNAs that may be involved in embryogenesis.

The ultimate aim of the male reproductive system is to parcel the male genetic package, a set of 23 chromosomes, into the head of a single spermatozoon, and deliver this to the female reproductive tract, in the right place at the right time. However, in order to fertilize the oocyte and initiate embryonic development, the spermatozoon must also contribute two epigenetic factors: an oocyte-activating factor and the centrosome or cell division mechanism (see Chapter 4).

## Development of the Ovary

The female genital tract develops from the mesonephros; the nephric duct and mesonephric tubules degenerate, and the oviducts and uterus evolve from the paramesonephric duct. This is a transport epithelium, which contains both ciliated and secretory cells: the ampulla develops from a secretory region. In the epiblast of early female embryos, a small number of progenitor cells come under the influence of locally secreted factors that suppress genes responsible for somatic development (e.g., Hox) and permit expression of genes that are specific for germline development, such as Stella and Blimp1 (Saitou et al., 2005). Primordial germ cells containing two X chromosomes are translocated from the genital ridge to the primordial gonad, and these are known as oogonia. The sex cords, instead of penetrating deeply into the genital ridge as in males, condense as small clusters around the PGCs, and these clusters of cells initiate the formation of primordial follicles (Figure 3.7). Cells of the cortical sex cords will form the somatic components of the follicle: granulosa, theca, endothelial cells and supporting connective tissue. Once they reach the gonadal ridge (approximately Days 25–30), the oogonia start to replicate by mitosis for a limited period. Cells from the mesonephros invade to form the ovarian medulla, forcing the germ cells toward the ovarian cortex. Whereas in male embryos spermatogonia do not start to enter meiosis until the onset of puberty, in females the oogonia start to enter into their first meiotic division around the twelfth week of gestation, at the end of the first trimester. In humans, the population of oogonia is estimated to increase from a pool of around 600 000 at 8 weeks to a maximum of 6–8 million at 16–20 weeks. At this stage they become primary oocytes and do not replicate further by mitosis. Oocytes that are not incorporated into follicles degenerate, and thus the number of oocytes is then reduced to around 1–2 million at birth, when the ovary is now populated with its full complement of oocytes.

After the oogonia enter meiosis I, they arrest in the diplotene stage of prophase I, after chromatid exchange and crossing-over (diakinesis) have taken place – the last phase of prophase I (see Chapter 1, Figure 1.13). These arrested oocytes are said to be in the dictyate (germinal vesicle) stage. The chromosomes disperse and appear as visible chromosomal threads packaged within a large nucleus, the germinal

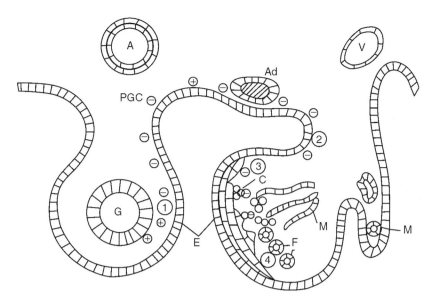

**Figure 3.7** Development of the human ovary from PGC. PGCs travel along the gut (G) mesentery (1) to the gonadal ridge (2), and after proliferation and migration become associated with cortical cords (C, 3). They begin meiosis and become enveloped within follicles (F, 4). Ad = adrenal gland; A = aorta; V = cardinal vein; E = coelomic epithelium; M = mesonephric tubules and duct. Reproduced with permission from Gosden (1995).

vesicle (GV). The first meiotic prophase stage can be seen at around 9–10 weeks, and diplotene stage chromosomes are apparent around 16 weeks, during the second trimester of pregnancy. The oocytes remain arrested at this stage until the onset of ovulatory cycles at puberty: subsequent developmental stages that lead to the resumption of meiosis are not completed unless the Graafian (antral) follicle is recruited after puberty. The process of oogenesis, from primordial germ cell to preovulatory oocyte, takes a minimum of 11 years; human oocytes complete meiosis only after fertilization.

The oogonia within the embryonic ovary are initially arranged into clusters called syncytia, which are connected by intercellular bridges. Organelles, mitochondria and other cellular factors are probably exchanged through these connections. These syncytia are programmed to break down on a large scale during fetal life, and this is followed by the formation of primordial follicles. A single layer of pregranulosa cells surrounds a single oogonium; once a complete cell layer has been formed around individual oocytes, the surrounding stromal cells secrete type IV collagen, laminin and fibronectin. These proteins form a thin basement membrane around each cluster of cells, and a discrete population of primordial follicles is formed. Each follicle has an oocyte arrested in prophase I of meiosis, surrounded by a single layer of flattened stromal pregranulosa cells that are linked to the oocyte by gap junctions and other cellular connections. The primordial follicles become localized to the peripheral region of the ovarian cortex and remain there in a quiescent state for many years (Figure 3.8a). In this pool of follicles, each will either undergo a phase of growth and development that lasts approximately 6 months, or will become atretic and die. When they resume their growth after puberty, usually only one oocyte matures and is ovulated per month for the remaining 35 or so years of the reproductive lifespan (Figure 3.8b). Oocytes must complete their growth phase and resume meiosis before they can be fertilized.

### Ovarian Reserve

Primordial follicles are the most abundant follicle type within the adult ovary, but there is a high rate of wastage. From around Day 100 of fetal life onwards, oocytes that have arrested in meiotic prophase start to undergo atresia, and this continues throughout fetal and neonatal life. This programmed elimination of germ cells may be associated with a redistribution of organelles (e.g., mitochondria) in order to provide optimal function for the remaining oocytes. Pregranulosa cells may be involved in this degenerative process. In the mouse, around 70% of oogonia are lost by apoptosis upon entry into meiosis; in humans, the population is reduced to approximately 1–2 million by birth. This pool of oocytes (the ovarian reserve) was traditionally viewed as the finite resource of oocytes that dictates the reproductive lifespan of the individual (Figure 3.9). However, this dogma has recently been challenged (Johnson et al., 2005).

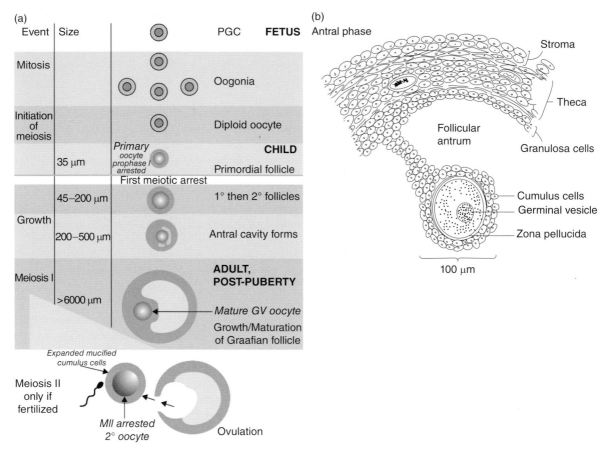

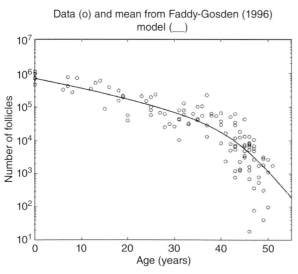

**Figure 3.8** (a) Schematic diagram of oocyte and follicular development from prenatal through to adult life. (b) Schematic diagram of preovulatory antral follicle.

**Figure 3.9** Variation in total numbers of follicles in human ovaries from neonatal age to 51 years. After Faddy & Gosden (1996).

# Follicle Development
## Formation of Primordial Follicles

In humans, the first primordial follicles can be seen during the fourth month of fetal gestation, and they begin to grow at approximately 20 weeks of fetal life, under the influence of gonadotropins. At this stage the oogonia are still active, before their arrest at the dictyate stage in prophase 1. Their pregranulosa cells enter a period of quiescence, and cell proliferation will not resume until the primordial follicle begins to grow, often months or years after it was formed. The primordial follicles are first established in the medullary region of the ovary, and they continue their development in the more peripheral parts (cortex). During the growth phase, the follicle develops morphologically, acquiring a theca interna containing steroidogenic cells, and a theca externa of connective tissue cells forming its outer layers. The basement membrane around it must either expand or be remodeled to adjust to its increasing size, and it becomes a dynamic system that nurtures the oocyte, responding to endogenous and exogenous influences via autocrine and paracrine effects. Follicular development is regulated by the oocyte itself, in combination with numerous cell interactions. A number of key molecules involved in the regulation have been identified, products of genes that are expressed specifically in oocytes: FIGalpha/FIGLA, GDF-9, BMP-6 and BMP-15, AMD, cKit, Kit ligand, etc.

Primordial follicles remain in their arrested state for up to 50 years, waiting for a signal to resume development. After puberty, a few primordial follicles become recruited to the growth phase every day, and these then go through three phases of development: primary or preantral, secondary or antral (also known as Graafian), and finally, preovulatory (Figure 3.8). As described below, the follicular cells produce growth factors and hormones, and also provide physical support, nutrients (such as pyruvate), metabolic precursors (such as amino acids and nucleotides) and other small molecules that can equilibrate between the two compartments.

## Follicular Cells

The mass of granulosa cells associated with the oocyte from the antral follicle stage until after fertilization is known as the cumulus oophorus, a complex tissue that is unique to eutherian mammals.

- Cumulus cells contribute to the intrafollicular environment of the developing oocyte, and the oocyte and its surrounding cells are in close association; electron microscopy shows gap junctions between the apposing membranes (Figure 3.10).
- In later stages of growth, the oocyte plasma membrane increases in surface area and is organized into long microvilli, presumably required for an increase in transmembrane transport. Under the control of the FIGalpha gene, the oocyte secretes a dense fibrillar material that forms a 5- to 10-μm layer around the female gamete, called the zona pellucida (Figure 3.11). At this stage, follicle cells remain in contact with the oocyte by means of long interdigitating microvilli, which gives a striated image under the light microscope: this is known as the zona radiata.

- Cumulus cells express the ganglioside GM3, which has been implicated in cell recognition, differentiation and signaling. Blocking the gap junctions interferes with transmission or action of molecules such as 2-deoxyglucose, transforming growth factor alpha (TGF-α) and mitogenic agents on the oocyte.
- In many species (but not in humans), physically removing the cumulus cells can inhibit oocyte maturation. Signaling between oocyte and cumulus occurs in both directions, and cumulus cells express growth factor receptors and the mRNA for a number of growth factors. They are also a source of prostaglandins and express angiogenic factors (e.g., vascular endothelial growth factor, VEGF) which may have a role in neovascularization of follicles and angiogenesis at the implantation site of the embryo.
- The cumulus cells become polarized during oocyte maturation and begin to secrete a hyaluronic acid extracellular matrix.

## Follicular Development after Puberty

Very small follicles have no independent blood supply; in medium-sized follicles, an anastomotic network of arterioles appears just outside the basement membrane. This network becomes more extensive as the follicle grows, and each ripe preovulatory follicle has its own rich blood supply. Changes in hormone levels during folliculogenesis affect the composition of the

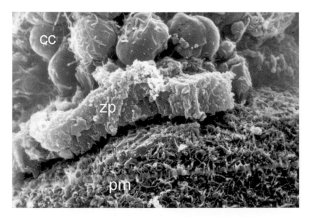

**Figure 3.10** Cumulus–cell interactions. Scanning electron micrograph of the surface of an unfertilized metaphase II human oocyte, with the zona pellucida (zp) and cumulus cells (cc) partially dissected to demonstrate the microvillar organization of the plasma membrane (pm). From Dale, 1996.

65

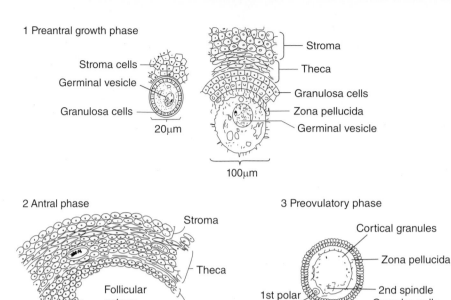

**Figure 3.11** Oogenesis in the human. Modified with permission from Johnson [2018].

follicular fluid, which is probably the source of energy substrates for the developing oocyte. The oocyte plays a fundamental role in follicle development and controls the differentiation of follicular granulosa cells. In order to acquire its necessary developmental competence, there must be communication between the oocyte and granulosa cells.

### Follicle Recruitment: From Primordial to Preantral (Primary) Follicle

In humans the number of follicles recruited into development at any given time ranges between 2 and 30, related to age. The precise mechanisms that regulate the initiation of primordial follicle growth are not well understood, and two possible mechanisms have been proposed:

(a) Growth initiation is a preprogrammed feature of the ovary: the first primordial follicles to enter the growth phase are those that contain the first oocytes to enter meiosis in the human prenatal ovary (or prenatal/early postnatal mouse ovary; Henderson and Edwards, 1968).

(b) Initiation is regulated by certain growth factors or peptides

Primordial follicles that enter the growth phase show two distinct morphological changes:

1. The oocyte increases in size.
2. Flattened pregranulosa cells become cuboidal in appearance.

However, more subtle biochemical, physiological and molecular changes occur prior to these events; e.g., increased expression of the proliferating cell nuclear antigen has been correlated with the earliest stages of follicle growth (Oktay et al., 1995). A number of other genes that are expressed exclusively in the oocyte or germline have also been identified, including growth development factor (GDF)-9, required by the granulosa cells, and Oct-4 (also known as Oct-3), a POU factor that is also expressed in pluripotential stem cells of the embryo (Rosner et al., 1990). Follicles that have started the growth phase are referred to as early primary follicles.

## Follicular Destiny

One of the most intriguing mysteries in ovarian physiology is what determines whether one follicle remains quiescent, another begins to develop but later becomes atretic, while still a third matures and ovulates.

- Over 99% of follicles are destined to die rather than ovulate; the degenerative process by which these cells are irrevocably committed to undergo cell death is termed atresia.
- Atretic oocytes show germinal vesicle breakdown, followed by fragmentation and disruption of the oocyte–cumulus complex; granulosa cells from an aspirated atretic follicle show clear signs of fragmentation.
- Despite the critical role of atresia during the recruitment of follicles for ovulation, the mechanisms underlying its onset and progression remain poorly understood. There are four degenerative stages during ovarian development which result in a massive loss of ovarian cells:

  1. During migration of primordial germ cells from the yolk sac to the genital ridge; many of these cells undergo degeneration.
  2. At the time of entry into the first meiotic stage, some germ cells undergo attrition before follicles are formed.
  3. In the later stages of development, early antral follicles either differentiate or undergo atresia.
  4. If ovulatory signals are absent, the mature follicle also may undergo degeneration.

Ovarian stimulation with FSH during ART cycles rescues follicles that were destined for atresia; therefore, most atretic follicles are evidently normal, or we would have seen more defects from children conceived by ART.

## Preantral to Antral (Secondary) Follicle

The oocyte continues to increase in size, and the granulosa cells proliferate and divide; when one to two layers of granulosa cells surround the oocyte, the follicle reaches a transitional stage. Further growth produces a secondary follicle with multiple layers of granulosa cells, and the follicles become associated with small blood vessels. This is a significant feature, since the preantral development of ovarian follicles depends upon locally acting factors and oocyte–granulosa cell communication events,

independent of the gonadotropins that are delivered via the bloodstream. In humans, the theca layer does not form until the follicle contains between three and six layers of granulosa cells.

### Antral to Preovulatory Development

Growth factors and hormones induce further follicular growth, the theca and granulosa cell layers proliferate, and the oocyte expands in size, accumulating water, ions, lipids, RNA and proteins. Follicle-stimulating hormone (FSH) is required for the formation of follicular fluid, and several pockets of this fluid, precursor spaces of the antral cavity, begin to form between the granulosa cells. The fluid is derived from the bloodstream, with added glycoproteins secreted by the granulosa cells. When five to eight layers of granulosa cells surround the oocyte, these pockets of fluid merge to form the antral cavity (follicular antrum). As the antral cavity extends, the oocyte takes up an acentric position in the follicle, and is surrounded by two or more layers of granulosa cells (Figure 3.11).

Under the influence of FSH released from the pituitary, the granulosa cells differentiate into two distinct populations:

1. The oocyte and its surrounding follicular cells form a network or syncytium, a close association that is essential for follicular growth to continue. Cumulus granulosa cells surround the oocyte; these cells are mitotically inactive and do not divide further. The innermost layers of cells become columnar, forming the corona radiata, and these cells communicate with the oocyte via gap junctions linking them with the oolemma.
2. Mural granulosa cells line the follicle wall; these cells stop dividing and also become columnar in appearance. Under the influence of FSH, they express receptors for luteinizing hormone (LH) and steroidogenic enzyme pathways become active within the cells.

Other candidates involved in granulosa cell differentiation include insulin-like growth factors IGF-I and IGF-II; the oocyte itself may also play an important role.

### Preovulatory Antral Follicles

In humans, the oocyte is 120 μm in size at the time of antral cavity formation. The oocyte is now capable of resuming meiosis, but only a limited number of oocytes proceed past the antral stage toward ovulation. Around 20 antral follicles are recruited each month from the total number available, and even fewer are selected to ovulate (this number varies between species). The remaining follicles degenerate through apoptosis and become atretic. The recruited follicles continue to grow, and (in monovular species) one follicle in the cohort is selected to become dominant. This preovulatory follicle then grows rapidly. In humans the size increases from 6.9 mm (±0.5) to a size of 18.8 mm (±0.5) over a period of 10–20 days. The follicular basement membrane must expand by approximately 400 times its original size to accommodate this follicular growth. The granulosa cell population increases from approximately 2–5 million to 50 million, and the mural granulosa cells differentiate further.

### Ovulation

1. Within a few hours of the LH surge, the follicle becomes more vascularized and swollen, and expansion of the granulosa/cumulus mass causes the follicle to form a visible bulge on the surface of the ovary. The projecting follicle wall becomes thin, forming the stigma.
2. A combination of tension and the action of a collagenase enzyme causes the follicle wall to rupture, and follicular fluid containing the cumulus–oocyte complex (COC) is released from the antral cavity.
3. The fimbriated mouth of the oviduct scrapes the sticky mass of cumulus-enclosed oocyte from the surface of the ovary; synchronized beating of cilia in the tubal wall move the COC along the oviduct. The oocyte remains viable in the oviduct for as long as 24 hours.

### Generation of the Corpus Luteum

After ovulation, the follicular basement membrane degenerates, and blood vessels populate the remaining structure of the follicle to form the corpus luteum. This structure contains large luteal cells derived from luteinized granulosa cells, and smaller luteal cells derived from the theca interna. Both populations of cells release progesterone. If pregnancy is not established, the corpus luteum remains in the ovary for 2–14 days (varying with species), and then degenerates by luteolysis.

## Oocyte Maturation and Ovulation

### Oocyte Growth

The environment in the developing follicle provides an essential niche for oocyte survival, nourishment

and development, but oocyte growth does not run strictly in parallel with follicular development (see Figure 3.8). The primordial human follicle contains a primary oocyte approximately 35 μm in size, and grows to its final size of 120 μm over a period of around 85 days. During this time, it must acquire competence and the ability to be successfully fertilized and then support early embryo development. This process of oocyte maturation involves the coordination of integrated, but independent nuclear and cytoplasmic events: the nucleus undergoes germinal vesicle breakdown, resumption of meiosis and completion of the first meiotic division. Cytoplasmic maturation requires relocation of cytoplasmic organelles and establishment of oocyte polarity, with an increase in the number of mitochondria and ribosomes. There are alterations in membrane transport systems, and the developing Golgi apparatus expands and migrates to the periphery. Organelles appear in the cytoplasm that reflect storage and export of materials: membrane-bound vesicles, multivesicular and crystalline bodies, fat droplets and glycogen granules.

During its growth phase, the oocyte prepares and stores reserves that will be needed for the first stages of fertilization and initiation of embryo development: water, lipids, carbohydrates and ions accumulate, and RNA and proteins are synthesized and stored. As the follicle moves from the primordial to the primary stage, the diameter of the oocyte also increases. Although the distribution of organelles and storage materials does not show a definite and obvious polarity, spatial patterning cannot be entirely ruled out in mammalian eggs (Gardner, 1999). A number of features can be seen during these stages:

1. The numbers of mitochondria increase to approximately $10^5$, and they become more spherical, with fewer concentrically arched cristae, indicating that they are less active.
2. Under the control of the FIG alpha gene, genes coding for the zona pellucida proteins (ZP1, ZP2, ZP3, ZP4) are expressed coordinately and specifically. The proteins that will make up the zona pellucida (ZP) are secreted, and this forms a 5- to 10-μm layer around the oocyte. At this stage, the ZP maintains communication between the oocyte and the granulosa cells; ZP3 is the primary sperm receptor.
3. Cytoplasmic organelles become far more abundant, with the notable exception of centrioles,

which disappear and are not found until after fertilization. The numbers of ribosomes multiply fourfold to around 108 in the mature oocyte.

4. Large amounts of RNA are synthesized and stored: the human oocyte has an estimated 1500 pg of total RNA, in contrast to 14 fg in the spermatozoon.

## Oocyte Polarity

Polarization represents a differential distribution of morphological, biochemical, physiological and functional parameters in the cell. The appearance of polarization may be associated with triggering the developmental program. The growing oocyte does not have a homogeneous structure; in particular, many cytoplasmic organelles become segregated to various regions of the oocyte, and this regional organization determines some of the basic properties of the embryo. In all animal oocytes, the pole where the nuclear divisions occur (forming a cleavage furrow), resulting in the formation of the polar bodies, is called the animal pole. The opposite pole (opposite to the extruded polar body) is called the vegetal pole, and often contains a high concentration of nutrient reserves. Scanning electron microscopy shows that mouse oocytes have a microvillus-free area on the plasma membrane, adjacent to the first polar body and overlying the meiotic spindle. Human oocytes show no polarity in the distribution and length of the microvilli, either in the animal or the vegetal pole. Studies with fluorescent lectins reveal no signs of polarization in membrane sugar distribution. However, Antczak and Van Blerkom (1997) found that two regulatory proteins involved in signal transduction and transcription activation (leptin and STAT3) are polarized in mouse and human oocytes and preimplantation embryos. They suggest that a subpopulation of follicle cells may be partly responsible for the polarized distribution of these proteins in the oocyte, and that they may be involved in determining its animal pole, and in the establishment of the inner cell mass and trophoblast in the preimplantation embryo. The intracellular location of mRNAs and protein translation machinery is related to cell cytoskeleton regulation. Several lines of evidence suggest that mammalian ooplasm redistributes after sperm entry during fertilization (Edwards and Beard, 1997). The meiotic spindle that begins to form just before ovulation migrates to the cortex, and its position determines the cleavage plane for extruding the first polar body.

# Storing Information

The three main classes of RNA (mRNA, tRNA and rRNA) are all involved in the synthesis of protein. The relative amounts of these three types of RNA present during oogenesis varies from species to species, in the order of 60–65% rRNA, 20–25% tRNA and 10–15% mRNA.

Whereas in species such as *Xenopus* and *Drosophila* the embryo retains the vast majority of stored mRNA until the blastula stage to direct protein synthesis later in development, mammalian oocytes contain a finite amount of stored RNA, which supports only the very early stages of preimplantation embryo development. The dictyate chromosomes in mammalian oocytes actively synthesize ribosomal and mRNA as the follicle starts to grow; there is a dramatic increase in the size of the nucleolus as RNA accumulates in the nucleus, including a significant proportion of translatable polyadenylated mRNA. Nucleosomes contain DNA packaged within chromatin, which also contains structural proteins such as histones; careful regulation of transcriptional machinery controls the expression of particular genes at specific times. When the oocyte is fully grown, transcription of new RNA stops almost completely following germinal vesicle breakdown until the time of zygotic genome activation (ZGA) when the new embryonic genome starts to direct further development. During the period prior to ZGA, the oocyte is dependent upon its pool of stored mRNA, which has been processed with elegant mechanisms that control its expression. The stability of mRNA is related to the length of its polyA tail: a long polyA tail is required for translation, but this long tail also makes the message vulnerable to degradation. There are at least two different mechanisms of mRNA adenylation in oocyte cytoplasm: the genes are transcribed with long polyA tails, but some messengers are transcribed and translated during growth, whereas others are 'masked' by deadenylation, reducing the tail to less than 40 'A' residues: this prevents their translation and also protects these messages from degradation. In later stages of maturation, the masked genes can then be activated by selective polyadenylation when their products are required. Both gene types contain a highly conserved specific sequence in their 3′ untranslatable regions (UTRs) that signals polyadenylation. The mRNA for the masked transcripts also contains a further sequence 5′ to the polyadenylation signal, known as

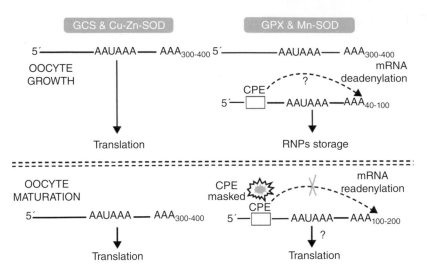

**Figure 3.12** mRNA processing during oocyte maturation. CPE = cytoplasmic polyadenylation element; RNPs = ribonucleoproteins. With thanks to Y. Ménézo.

the cytoplasmic polyadenylation element or the adenylation control element (ACE). It seems that this sequence controls the expression of stored mRNAs: ACE-containing mRNAs are masked and protected from degradation, whilst non-ACE-containing mRNAs, available for immediate translation, have long and relatively stable polyA tails (Figure 3.12). The mRNAs are also packaged in association with ribonucleoprotein (RNP) particles, and this may represent another control mechanism as part of the complex regulation of transcription and translation. Packaging with RNPs probably plays a part in controlling the access of ribosomes to regulatory elements within the mRNA.

### Oocyte Reserves

The growing oocyte contains a large amount of information that is masked, but the rest of the protein synthesizing machinery is functional. Many proteins synthesized during oogenesis are stored in the oocyte cytoplasm for later use; for example, the enzymes necessary for DNA synthesis are present in the growing oocyte and yet DNA replication is switched off. Experiments with interspecies nuclear transfer using nuclei from fibroblast cells transferred into bovine, sheep and monkey enucleated oocytes revealed that the first two cell division cycles were regulated by the oocyte cytoplasm; thereafter, the donor nucleus assumed regulatory control, but development arrested after a limited number of cleavage divisions (Fulka *et al.*, 1998). This again demonstrates that the oocyte itself has a large reserve of functional

activity, sufficient to sustain initial cell division cycles – but differentiation events in both cytoplasmic and nuclear compartments are essential for continued development.

## Stages of Oocyte Maturation

During the final stages of follicle development, mural granulosa cells increase their estrogen synthesis, and serum estrogen levels are significantly elevated. This exerts a positive feedback on the pituitary to increase its release of gonadotropins, in particular LH, resulting in the preovulatory LH surge. Binding of LH to its receptors on mural granulosa is enhanced, and this activates the pathways that promote oocyte maturation. The increased binding eventually downregulates the steroidogenic pathway that leads to estradiol synthesis, and the cells switch their steroid synthesis to the production of progesterone for the luteal phase. Under the influence of LH, the primary oocyte matures via a complex interplay between the follicular cells and the oocyte, involving numerous metabolic pathways. The final stages that lead to ovulation include:

1. *Nuclear maturation* to allow resumption of meiosis beyond arrest in prophase I. The midcycle surge of LH initiates a complex cascade of events, which will be described in detail below.

2. *Cytoplasmic maturation.* During oocyte growth, the Golgi apparatus enlarges and develops into separate units in the cortex; these export

glycoproteins to the zona pellucida and form approximately $5 \times 10^3$ cortical granules that collect at the surface of the oocyte. The cortical granules contain enzymes that are later released to modify the zona pellucida (see Chapter 4). A fine network of endoplasmic reticulum extends throughout the cytoplasm, with dense patches of membrane that become oriented closer to the periphery of the cortex, where they may be involved in calcium release for cortical granule exocytosis. An important feature of cytoplasmic maturation is the translation of mRNA species that have accumulated in a stable and dormant form during oogenesis.

3. *Cumulus expansion/mucification.* The preovulatory hormone surge leads to changes in the morphology of the cumulus granulosa cells, and they secrete hyaluronic acid into the intercellular spaces. Oocytes also produce a soluble factor that initiates production of hyaluronic acid by the cumulus granulosa cells, and the matrix thus formed transforms the granulosa cells from a tightly packed cellular mass to a more diffuse and dispersed mucified mass. The syncytial relationship between the cumulus cells and the oocyte is lost, intercellular communication via gap junctions between the cumulus cells and the oocyte is terminated, and metabolites and informational molecules can no longer pass. These events may act as the trigger for resumption of meiosis.

---

**Nuclear Maturation during Development of the Graafian Follicle**

1. In response to the preovulatory surge of gonadotropins, the concentration of cAMP within the oocyte falls.

2. Mitochondria increase in volume, are reduced in number and move to the perinuclear region, an area that requires high concentrations of ATP during the formation of the first meiotic spindle.

3. Chromatin forms a dense ring around the nucleolus; microtubular organizing centers (MTOCs) congregate as microtubules in the cytoplasm and reorganize to form a functional spindle apparatus. NB: Meiotic spindles in human oocytes do not have detectable MTOCs, and the spindle is assembled very slowly over

a period of several hours (see Chapter 1: Meiosis in Human Oocytes).

4. The chromosomes condense, the germinal vesicle membrane breaks down and the first meiotic spindle forms.

5. The spindle migrates to the animal pole of the oocyte and changes orientation.

6. The first meiotic division proceeds through metaphase I, and then to telophase I. Asymmetrical cell division gives rise to the large functional oocyte and the smaller first polar body.

7. As soon as meiosis I is complete, the oocyte enters into the second meiotic division, and this secondary oocyte arrests again at metaphase II – ready for fertilization.

8. The trigger for the resumption of the second meiotic arrest is supplied by the fertilizing spermatozoon, and meiosis is completed with the extrusion of the second polar body (in the animal kingdom only coelenterates and echinoderms have completed meiosis before sperm entry).

**Timing of events:**

| | |
|---|---|
| LH surge: 0 | GV with nucleolus |
| +15 hours | GVBD |
| +20 hours | first meiotic metaphase |
| +35 hours | second meiotic metaphase |
| +38 hours | ovulation |

---

### Nuclear Maturation: Resumption of Meiosis

Nuclear maturation specifically refers to the first resumption of meiosis, with transformation of the fully grown primary oocyte in the antral follicle into the unfertilized secondary oocyte; this process follows the preovulatory surge of FSH and LH, just prior to ovulation. The germinal vesicle membrane breaks down, and the nucleus progresses from the dictyate state of the first meiotic prophase through first meiosis to arrest again at metaphase II. Up to this stage, the primary oocyte has been maintained in meiotic arrest by a complex balance of cell cycle protein activity, intracellular levels of cAMP and other intracellular messengers. The mid-cycle surge of LH causes the level of cAMP in the oocyte to fall below this threshold level, and a cascade of events is initiated that finally leads to breakdown of the germinal vesicle (GVBD) and resumption of meiosis (see Chapter 1: Meiosis in Human Oocytes). This cascade involves intracellular ionic messengers, such as $Ca^{2+}$ and $H^+$, and a series of cell cycle complexes that have accumulated within the oocyte, including maturation-promoting factor (MPF) and cytostatic factor (CSF). The surge levels of LH shift follicular steroidogenesis from predominantly estrogen to progesterone production, and this may actively promote the resumption of meiosis by stimulating the oocyte to produce a signal that induces GVBD. The nucleus of the germinal vesicle usually contains only one nucleolus, which enlarges from 2 to almost 10 μm in diameter; this nucleolus disappears when the germinal vesicle breaks down. A rim of chromatin forms around the nucleolus in large oocytes, and this is a sign that they are capable of resuming meiosis.

## Control of Nuclear Maturation

The control of nuclear maturation involves a complex interplay between numerous metabolic pathways in both the somatic granulosa cells and the oocyte. The follicle cells are in direct physical contact with the oocyte, and they either maintain meiotic arrest or stimulate resumption of meiosis by transferring the appropriate signals. The metabolic pathways within the granulosa cells are in turn regulated by the binding of gonadotropins to their cell surface receptors. Small molecules including adenosine, uridine, hypoxanthine and their metabolites diffuse between granulosa cells and the oocyte via gap junctions. The precise mechanism for the maintenance of arrest remains to be elucidated, and two mechanisms have been proposed:

1. Adenosine stimulates oocyte adenylate cyclase via a surface receptor on the oolemma, and hypoxanthine prevents hydrolysis of cAMP: high levels of cAMP sustain meiotic arrest.
2. Adenosine could participate directly in meiotic arrest via its conversion to ATP, a substrate for adenyl cyclase within the oocyte. Purines may also participate in cell signaling via G-proteins on the oolemma and plasma membranes of the cumulus cells.

Production of active MPF in the oocyte cytoplasm mediates nuclear maturation.

1. MPF consists of two components:

    (a) A 34-kDa protein, serine/threonine kinase, that is activated by dephosphorylation; homologous to the product of the cdc2 gene in fission yeast.

    (b) Cyclin B: activated by phosphorylation, and is probably a substrate for the product of the Mos proto-oncogene.

    - MPF activity is low in GV stage oocytes and increases during GVBD.
    - MPF activity is high after the resumption of meiosis, during both metaphase I and metaphase II.

2. The action of phosphokinase A (PKA) prevents GVBD.

    (a) A decrease in intracellular cAMP reduces PKA activity, and this allows cyclin B and p34cdc2 to associate and form MPF.

    (b) p39mos then participates in the activation of MPF, possibly by cyclin B phosphorylation. Synthesis of p39mos is stimulated by progesterone, and this may be a key event in the induction of meiotic maturation.

    (c) By maintaining cyclin B in its phosphorylated (active) form, p39 may stabilize MPF and act as a CSF, thereby maintaining metaphase II arrest.

The product of the oncogene Mos is expressed early in oocyte maturation and disappears immediately after fertilization. The Mos protein has the same effects as CSF, arresting mitosis at metaphase with high p34cdc2 activity. It is thought that CSF is in part or entirely Mos, and that the second meiotic arrest is due to transcription of the Mos oncogene as the oocyte matures.

In summary, the production of a viable oocyte depends on three key processes:

1. The fully grown oocyte must recognize regulatory signals generated by follicular cells.
2. Extensive reprogramming within the oocyte must be induced; this involves activation of appropriate signal transduction mechanisms.
3. Individual molecular changes must be integrated to drive the two parallel, but distinct, processes involved in meiotic progression and the acquisition of developmental competence.

The oocyte depends on the follicular compartment for direct nutrient support and for regulatory signals. After the LH surge, new steroid, peptide and protein signals are generated, and alterations to preovulatory steroid profiles can selectively disrupt protein reprogramming and individual components of the fertilization process.

Localized short- and long-lived maternal mRNAs regulate the initial stages of development and differentiation both in the oocyte and in the early embryo. There is no doubt that the process of oocyte growth and maturation is a highly complex process, involving a three-dimensional series and sequence of regulatory elements at several different molecular levels. The final evolution of a mature oocyte which has the potential for fertilization and further development is dependent upon the correct completion and synchronization of all processes involved: although an overview is emerging, many aspects still remain to be elucidated. Thus, it is impossible to assess and gauge the consequences of manipulations during assisted reproduction practice, and it is essential to maintain an awareness of the complexity and sensitivity of this delicate and highly elegant biological system. Our in-vitro attempts to mimic nature will only succeed if they are carried out within this frame of reference (see also Chapter 11: In-Vitro Growth).

# Further Reading

### Gametogenesis

Antczak M, Van Blerkom J (1997) Oocyte influences on early development: the regulatory proteins leptin and STAT3 are polarized in mouse and human oocytes and differentially distributed within the cells of the preimplantation stage embryo. *Molecular Human Reproduction* 3: 1067–1086.

Bachvarova R (1985) Gene expression during oogenesis and oocyte development in mammals. In: Browder, LW (ed.) *Developmental Biology. A Comprehensive Synthesis, Vol. 1: Oogenesis.* Plenum, New York, pp. 453–524.

Bellve A, O'Brien D (1983) The mammalian spermatozoon: structure and temporal assembly. In: Hartmann JF (ed.) *Mechanism and Control of Animal Fertilization.* Academic Press, New York, pp. 56–140.

Braun RE (2000) Temporal control of protein synthesis during spermatogenesis. *International Journal of Andrology* 23(Suppl. 2): 92–94.

Briggs D, Miller D, Gosden R (1999) Molecular biology of female gametogenesis. In: Fauser BCJM, Rutherford AJ, Strauss JF, Van Steirteghem A (eds.) *Molecular Biology in Reproductive Medicine.* Parthenon Press, New York, pp. 251–267.

Buccione R, Schroeder AC, Eppig JJ (1990) Interactions between somatic cells and germ cells throughout mammalian oogenesis. *Biology of Reproduction* 43: 543–547.

Byskov AG, Andersen CY, Nordholm L, *et al.* (1995) Chemical structure of sterols that activate oocyte meiosis. *Nature* 374: 559–562.

Canipari R (2000) Oocyte-granulosa cell interactions. *Human Reproduction Update* 6: 279–289.

Canipari R, Epifano O, Siracusa G, Salustri A (1995) Mouse oocytes inhibit plasminogen activator production by ovarian cumulus and granulosa cells. *Developmental Biology* 167: 371–378.

Cho WK, Stern S, Biggers JD (1974) Inhibitory effect of dibutyryl cAMP on mouse oocyte maturation in vitro. *Journal of Experimental Zoology* 187: 383–386.

Choo YK, Chiba K, Tai T, Ogiso M, Hoshi M (1995) Differential distribution of gangliosides in adult rat ovary during the oestrous cycle. *Glycobiology* 5: 299–309.

Clarkson MJ, Harley VR (2002) Sex with two SOX on: SRY and SOX9 in testis development. *Trends in Endocrinology and Metabolism* 13(3): 106–111.

Dale B (1996) Fertilization. In: Greger R, Windhorst U (eds.) *Comprehensive Human Physiology.* Springer-Verlag, Heidelberg, pp. 2265–2275

Dekel N (1996) Protein phosphorylation/dephosphorylation in the meiotic cell cycle of mammalian oocytes. *Reviews of Reproduction* 1: 82–88.

Dong J, Albertini DF, Nishimori K, Kumar TR, Lu N, Matzuk MM (1996) Growth differentiation factor-9 is required during early ovarian folliculogenesis. *Nature* 383: 531–535.

Eddy EM (1998) Regulation of gene expression during spermatogenesis. *Seminars in Cell and Developmental Biology* 9: 451–457.

Edwards RG, Beard H (1997) Oocyte polarity and cell determination in early mammalian embryos. *Molecular Human Reproduction* 3: 868–905.

Elder K, Elliott T (eds.) (1998) The use of epididymal and testicular sperm in IVF. *Worldwide Conferences in Reproductive Biology 2.* Ladybrook Publications, Australia.

Epifano O, Dean J (2002) Genetic control of early folliculogenesis in mice. *Trends in Endocrinology and Metabolism* 13(4): 169–173.

Eppig JJ, O'Brien MJ (1996) Development in vitro of mouse oocytes from primordial follicles. *Biology of Reproduction* 54: 197–207.

Faddy MJ, Gosden RG (1995) A mathematical model for follicle dynamics in human ovaries. *Human Reproduction* 10: 770–775.

Faddy MJ, Gosden RG (1996) Ovary and ovulation: a model conforming the decline in follicle numbers to the age of menopause in women. *Human Reproduction* 11(7): 1484–1486.

Fulka J Jr., First N, Moor RM (1998) Nuclear and cytoplasmic determinants involved in the regulation of mammalian oocyte maturation. *Molecular Human Reproduction* 4(1): 41–49.

Gardner R (1999) Polarity in early mammalian development. *Current Opinion in Genetics and Development* 9(4): 417–421.

Gosden, R (1995) Ovulation 1: oocyte development throughout life. In: Grudzinskas JG, Yovich JL (eds.) *Gametes: The Oocyte*. Cambridge University Press, Cambridge, UK, pp. 119–149.

Gosden RG, Boland NI, Spears N, *et al.* (1993) The biology and technology of follicular oocyte development in vitro. *Reproductive Medicine Reviews* 2: 129–152.

Gosden RG, Bownes M (1995) Cellular and molecular aspects of oocyte development. In: Grudzinskas JG, Yovich JL (eds.) *Cambridge Reviews in Human Reproduction, Gametes – The Oocyte*. Cambridge University Press, Cambridge, UK, pp. 23–53.

Gougeon A (1996) Regulation of ovarian follicular development in primates: facts and hypotheses. *Endocrine Reviews* 17: 121–155.

Griswold MD (2016) Spermatogenesis: the commitment to meiosis. *Physiological Reviews* 96: 1–17.

Gurdon JB (1967) On the origin and persistence of a cytoplasmic state inducing nuclear DNA synthesis in frog's eggs. *Proceedings of the National Academy of Sciences of the USA* 58: 545–552.

Henderson SA, Edwards RG (1968) Chiasma frequency and maternal age in mammals. *Nature* 217(136): 22–28.

Hess RA (1999) Spermatogenesis, overview. In: Knobil E, Neill JD (eds.) *Encyclopedia of Reproduction*, vol. 4. Academic Press, New York, pp. 539–545.

Hillier SG, Whitelaw PF, Smyth CD (1994) Follicular oestrogen synthesis: the 'two-cell, two-gonadotrophin' model revisited. *Molecular and Cellular Endocrinology* 100: 51–54.

Hirshfield AN (1991) Development of follicles in the mammalian ovary. *International Review of Cytology* 124: 43–100.

Hutt KJ, Albertini DF (2007). An oocentric view of folliculogenesis and embryogenesis *Reproductive BioMedicine Online* 14(6): 758–764.

Johnson J, Bagley J, Skaznik-Wikiel M, *et al.* (2005) Oocyte generation in adult mammalian ovaries by putative germ cells in bone marrow and peripheral blood. *Cell* 122: 303–315.

Johnson M (2018) *Essential Reproduction*, 8th edn. Wiley-Blackwell, Oxford.

Jones R (1998) Spermiogenesis and sperm maturation in relation to development of fertilizing capacity. In: Lauria A, Gandolfi F, Enne G, Giannaroli I, *et al.* (eds.) *Gametes: Development and Function*. Serono Symposia, Rome, pp. 205–218.

Kobayashi M, Nakano R, Ooshima A (1990) Immunohistochemical localization of pituitary gonadotrophins and gonadal steroids confirms the 'two-cell, two-gonadotrophin' hypothesis of steroidogenesis in the human ovary. *Journal of Endocrinology* 126(3): 483–488.

Kramer JA, McCarrey JR, Djakiew D, Krawetz SA (1998) Differentiation: the selective potentiation of chromatin domains. *Development* 125: 4749–4755.

MacLaren A (2003) Primordial germ cells in the mouse. *Developmental Biology* 262(1): 1–15.

Masui Y (1985) Meiotic arrest in animal oocytes. In: Metz CB, Monroy A (eds.) *Biology of Fertilization*. Academic Press, New York, pp. 189–219.

Matzuk MM, Burns KH, Viveiros MM, Eppig JJ (2002) Intercellular communication in the mammalian ovary: oocytes carry the conversation. *Science* 296 (5576): 2178–2180.

McNatty KP, Fidler AE, Juengel JL, *et al.* (2000) Growth and paracrine factors regulating follicular formation and cellular function. *Molecular and Cellular Endocrinology* 163: 11–20.

Merchant-Larios H, Moreno-Mendoza N (2001) Onset of sex differentiation: dialog between genes and cells. *Archives of Medical Research* 32(6): 553–558.

Moore HDM (1996) The influence of the epididymis on human and animal sperm maturation and storage. *Human Reproduction* 11(Suppl.): 103–110.

Nurse P (1990) Universal control mechanisms resulting in the onset of M-phase. *Nature* 344: 503–508.

Oatley JM, Brinster RL (2012) The germline stem cell niche unit in mammalian testes. *Physiological Reviews* 92: 577–595.

Oktay K, Schenken RS, Nelson JF (1995) Proliferating cell nuclear antigen marks the initiation of follicular growth in the rat. *Biology of Reproduction* 53(2): 295–301.

Pereda J, Zorn T, Soto-Suazo M (2006) Migration of human and mouse primordial germ cells and colonization of the developing ovary: an ultrastructural and cytochemical study. *Microscopy Research and Technique* 69(6): 386–395.

Perez GI, Trbovich AM, Gosden RG, Tilly JL (2000) Mitochondria and the death of oocytes. *Nature* 403(6769): 500–501.

Picton HM, Briggs D, Gosden RG (1998) The molecular basis of oocyte growth and development. *Molecular and Cellular Endocrinology* 145: 27–37.

Reynard K, Driancourt MA (2000) Oocyte attrition. *Molecular and Cellular Endocrinology* 163: 101–108.

Rosner MH, Vigano MA, Ozato K, *et al.* (1990) A POU-domain transcription factor in early stem cells and germ cells of the mammalian embryo. *Nature* 345(6277): 686–692.

Sagata N (1996) Meiotic metaphase arrest in animal oocytes: its mechanisms and biological significance. *Trends in Cell Biology* 6: 22–28.

Sagata N (1997) What does Mos do in oocytes and somatic cells? *BioEssays* 19: 13–21.

Saitou M, Payer B, O'Carroll D, Ohinata Y, Surani MA (2005). Blimp1 and the emergence of the germ line during development in the mouse. *Cell Cycle* 4: 1736–1740.

Schatten H, Sun QY (2009) The role of centrosomes in mammalian fertilization and its significance for ICSI. *Molecular Human Reproduction* 15(9): 531–538.

Spears N, Boland NI, Murray AA, Gosden RG (1994) Mouse oocytes derived from in vitro grown primary ovarian follicles are fertile. *Human Reproduction* 9: 527–532.

Starz-Gaiano M, Lehmann R (2001) Moving towards the next generation. *Mechanisms of Development* 105(1–2): 5–18.

Sutovsky P, Fléchon JE, Fléchon B, *et al.* (1993) Dynamic changes of gap junctions and cytoskeleton in in vitro culture of cattle oocyte cumulus complexes. *Biology of Reproduction* 49: 1277–1287.

Swain A, Lovell-Badge R (1999) Mammalian sex determination: a molecular drama. *Genes and Development* 13(7): 755–767.

Taylor CT, Johnson PM (1996) Complement-binding proteins are strongly expressed by human preimplantation blastocysts and cumulus cells as well as gametes. *Molecular Human Reproduction* 2: 52–59.

Telfer EE (1996) The development of methods for isolation and culture of preantral follicles from bovine and porcine ovaries. *Theriogenology* 45: 101–110.

Telfer EE, McLaughlin M (2007) Natural history of the mammalian oocyte. *Reproductive BioMedicine Online* 15(3): 288–295.

Van Blerkom J, Motta P (1979) *The Cellular Basis of Mammalian Reproduction.* Urban and Schwarzenberg, Baltimore.

Ward WS (1993) Deoxyribonucleic acid loop domain tertiary structure in mammalian spermatozoa. *Biology of Reproduction* 48(6): 1193–1201.

Ward WS, Coffey DS (1991) DNA packaging and organization in mammalian spermatozoa: comparison with somatic cells. *Biology of Reproduction* 44(4): 569–574.

Wassarman PM (1996) Oogenesis. In: Adashi EY, Rock JA, Rosenwaks Z (eds.) *Reproductive Endocrinology, Surgery and Technology,* vol. 1. Lippincott-Raven Publishers, Philadelphia, pp. 341–359.

Wassarman PM, Liu C, Litscher ES (1996) Constructing the mammalian egg zona pellucida: some new pieces of an old puzzle. *Journal of Cell Science* 109: 2001–2004.

Whitaker M (1996) Control of meiotic arrest. *Reviews of Reproduction* 1: 127–135.

Yanagamachi R (1994) Mammalian fertilization. In: Knobil E, Neill J (eds.) *The Physiology of Reproduction.* Raven Press, New York, pp. 189–317.

## Sperm Chromatin Packaging and RNA Carriage

Balhorn R (1982) A model for the structure of chromatin in mammalian sperm. *Journal of Cell Biology* 93: 298–305.

Balhorn R, Gledhill BL, Wyrobek AJ (1977) Mouse sperm chromatin proteins: quantitative isolation and partial characterization. *Biochemistry* 16: 4074–4080.

Bench G, Corzett MH, DeYebra L, Oliva R, Balhorn R (1998) Protein and DNA contents in sperm from an infertile human male possessing protamine defects that vary over time. *Molecular Reproduction and Development* 50: 345–353.

Cho C, Willis WD, Goulding EH, *et al.* (2001) Haploinsufficiency of protamine-1 or -2 causes infertility in mice. *Nature Genetics* 28: 82–86.

Gardiner-Garden M, Ballesteros M, Gordon M, Tam PP (1998) Histone- and protamine-DNA association: conservation of different patterns within the beta-globin domain in human sperm. *Molecular and Cellular Biology* 18: 3350–3356.

Gatewood JM, Cook GR, Balhorn R, Bradbury EM, Schmid CW (1987) Sequence-specific packaging of DNA in human sperm chromatin. *Science* 236: 962–964.

Gatewood JM, Cook GR, Balhorn R, Schmid CW, Bradbury EM (1990) Isolation of 4 core histones from human sperm chromatin representing a minor subset of somatic histones. *Journal of Biological Chemistry* 265: 20662–20666.

Miller D (2000) Analysis and significance of messenger RNA in human ejaculated spermatozoa. *Molecular Reproduction and Development* 56: 259–264.

Miller D, Ostermeier GC (2006) Towards a better understanding of RNA carriage by ejaculate spermatozoa. *Human Reproduction Update* 12: 757–767.

Wykes SM, Krawetz SA (2003) The structural organization of sperm chromatin. *Journal of Biological Chemistry* 278: 29471–29477.

## Sex-Determining Mechanisms

Miller D (2004) Sex determination: insights from the human and animal models suggest that the mammalian Y chromosome is uniquely specialised for the male's benefit. *Journal of Men's Health and Gender* 1: 170–181.

Morais da Silva S, Hacker A, Harley V, *et al.* (1996) Sox9 expression during gonadal development implies a conserved role for the gene in testis differentiation in mammals and birds. *Nature Genetics* 14: 62–68.

Sekido R, Bar I, Narvaez V, Penny G, Lovell-Badge R (2004) SOX9 is up-regulated by the transient expression of SRY specifically in Sertoli cell precursors. *Developmental Biology* 274: 271–279.

Sekido R, Lovell-Badge R (2008) Sex determination involves synergistic action of SRY and SF1 on a specific Sox9 enhancer. *Nature* 453: 930–934.

# Gamete Interaction

Mature human gametes ready for fertilization differ in their state of nuclear maturation: the spermatozoon has completed meiosis and the oocyte is arrested at metaphase II. However, both gametes must also undergo a process of cytoplasmic maturation before they are capable of fertilization. This involves a complex series of biochemical, physiological and structural events that occur in a carefully orchestrated temporal and spatial pattern in parallel with, but independent from, nuclear maturation. Cytoplasmic and nuclear maturation are often asynchronous (Dale, 2018a): therefore, a cohort of human metaphase II oocytes collected after controlled ovarian hyperstimulation in an IVF program may appear to be similar with regards to the nuclear apparatus, but they are in fact at various stages of cytoplasmic maturation. This may partly explain the different developmental capabilities of embryos generated from a single cohort of oocytes.

Sperm–oocyte interaction is a complex process of cell–cell interaction that requires species-specific recognition and binding of the two cells. While interacting, each gamete triggers a cascade of events in its partner which changes them from arrested to developmentally competent cells. Controlled, synchronous gamete activation is essential for embryonic development; however, the biochemical and physiological processes that ultimately lead to the fusion of the male and female pronuclei are still poorly understood. In human assisted reproductive technology, although the technique of intracytoplasmic injection of spermatozoa (ICSI) essentially bypasses the initial stages of fertilization, including sperm capacitation and the interaction of the gametes, successful fertilization still requires the controlled and correct activation of both the spermatozoon and oocyte.

Mammalian fertilization is internal, and the male gametes must be introduced into the female tract at coitus. Coitus itself ranges from minutes in humans to hours in camels but is accompanied by many physiological changes. In the human, tactile and psychogenic stimuli can initiate penile erection, caused by decrease in resistance and consequently dilatation in the arteries supplying the penis, with closure of the arterio-venous shunts and venous blood valves. Vasocongestion can increase the volume of the testes by as much as 50%. Sequential contraction of the smooth muscles of the urethra and the striated muscles in the penis results in ejaculation of semen, with mixing of three different components: prostatic liquid rich in acid phosphatase, the vas deferens fraction containing spermatozoa and the seminal vesicle fraction containing fructose.

In the woman, tactile stimulation of the glans clitoris and vaginal wall leads to engorgement of the vagina and labia majora, and the vagina expands. Orgasm is accompanied by frequent vaginal contractions, with uterine contractions beginning in the fundus and spreading to the lower uterine segment. In man, rabbit, sheep, cow and cat, the semen is ejaculated into the vagina. In the pig, dog and horse, it is deposited directly into the cervix and uterus. In many species, the semen coagulates rapidly after deposition in the female tract, as a result of interaction with an enzyme of prostatic origin. The coagulation may serve to retain spermatozoa in the vagina or to protect them from the acid environment.

In the human, this coagulum forms a loose gel which is dissolved within 1 hour by progressive action of a second proenzyme, also of prostatic origin. Within minutes of coitus, spermatozoa may be detected in the cervix or uterus; 99% of the spermatozoa are lost from the vagina, but the few that enter the tract may survive for many hours in the cervical crypts of mucus. Abnormal sperm with poor motility are less able to penetrate the cervical mucus, and this may represent one means of sperm selection in natural conception. In the absence of progesterone, cervical mucus permits sperm penetration into the upper female tract, and contractions of the myometrium during the periovulatory period may assist sperm movement toward the utero-tubal junction. Kinz *et al.* (1996) suggested that there may be a mechanism that preferentially draws sperm toward the isthmus on the same side as the ovarian dominant follicle. A few thousand sperm swim through the utero-tubal junctions to reach the oviducts, where they interact with oviductal epithelium: the oviductal environment and its secretions play a critical role in the transport and interaction of both gametes. Sperm are trapped and stored in the initial part of the oviduct, which may contribute to preventing polyspermic fertilization by allowing only a few sperm to reach the ampulla at a time.

## Sperm–Oocyte Ratios: Reduction by Elimination

In the course of evolution, spermatozoal wastage has apparently been retained as a requirement for the union of one spermatozoon with one oocyte. In most animals, spermatozoa are produced in huge excess, irrespective of whether fertilization occurs externally or internally: in humans and other mammals the sperm:oocyte ratio at origin can be as high as $10^9$:1. If we examine animal sperm size and number in relation to body mass, it appears that evolutionary responses have favored sperm number rather than sperm size with increasing body size: larger animals such as elephants produce more sperm per ejaculate (corrected for body mass) than a small mammal such as a mouse. Despite large sperm numbers in mammals, behavioral adaptations are required to ensure fertilization. Mating must be synchronized, and the sperm need to be deposited in the female tract. The vast majority of spermatozoa are rapidly eliminated from the tract, and only a minute fraction successfully migrate to the site of fertilization.

In mice, the major barrier for sperm ascent is the utero-tubal junction, with spermatozoa being progressively released from the lower part of the oviductal isthmus at ovulation. In humans, the first barrier to sperm ascent is the highly folded mucus-filled cervix, where sperm are retained and released over a period of several days. In-vivo studies that counted spermatozoa in situ revealed a few hundred spermatozoa in sheep ampullae and only five in a human female ampulla (Dale & Monroy, 1981). An in-vivo study of fertilization in the mouse showed a 1:1 sperm–oocyte ratio in the ampullae – supernumerary spermatozoa were never observed.

Human in-vitro fertilization practice routinely involves inseminating cumulus-intact oocytes with a concentration of at least 100 000 spermatozoa/mL. The oocytes remain in this sperm bath for 18 hours before transfer to fresh medium to check for fertilization. However, removing oocytes from the sperm bath at various times prematurely followed by culture in sperm-free medium showed that an initial exposure of 5 minutes was sufficient for fertilization to progress (Gianaroli *et al.*, 1996). In these experiments, approximately 10 spermatozoa entered the cumulus complex, with one successfully reaching and fertilizing the oocyte. The remainder were blocked at various levels in the cumulus complex. This confirms the concept that large numbers of spermatozoa are not required for fertilization in mammals and reinforces the idea that not more than a handful of spermatozoa approach the oocyte in natural fertilization. There is evidence to show that sperm respond to chemotactic stimuli from mature oocytes and surrounding cumulus cells: progesterone acts as the principal chemoattractant, and calcium entry is an important second messenger (see Tosti & Ménézo, 2016). An olfactory receptor gene expressed in the testis may be involved in sperm chemotaxis in humans (Spehr *et al.*, 2004). Chemical modulation of the zona pellucida (ZP) by oviductal-specific glycoproteins before the oocyte encounters the spermatozoon has also been described (Coy & Aviles, 2010), and this may also be involved in fine tuning sperm–oocyte interactions in mammals.

In summary, although great quantities of spermatozoa are produced, few reach the oocyte under natural conditions. Those that do must then traverse and interact with the cumulus and coronal cells, which reduce the number of spermatozoa that can reach the oocyte to bind to and penetrate the ZP. The ZP is composed of several glycoproteins that differ between species, and this layer impedes sperm progression even further. The ZP modulates sperm binding and protects the embryo during early development, but we know little about its topographical constitution and whether sperm entry is piloted to a specific site. In many animals, including mammals, the extracellular coats of the oocyte may be removed without inhibiting fertilization, and initial gamete interactions may be bypassed by microinjecting the spermatozoon directly into the oocyte. This is a laboratory artifact, and it is often erroneously interpreted as showing redundancy of the extracellular coats. In nature, passage through these coats is a prerequisite for normal fertilization, oocyte activation and subsequent paternal nuclear decondensation.

## Polyspermy

The entry of more than one spermatozoon into a mammalian oocyte results in abnormal cleavage, and the embryo will block in development: this is known as pathological polyspermy. Images of oocytes in the laboratory with hundreds of spermatozoa attached to their surface have led to the notion that oocytes have evolved mechanisms that allow the penetration of a single spermatozoon, while repelling supernumerary spermatozoa. However, these images are a laboratory artifact. As discussed above, under natural conditions, the number of spermatozoa at the site of fertilization is extremely low compared with the numbers originally deposited in the female tract. This is regulated initially by the female reproductive tract, and then by a bottleneck created by extracellular coats of the oocyte. In order to reach the oocyte plasma membrane, the fertilizing spermatozoon must encounter and respond to a correct sequence of signals from the oocytes' extracellular coats. Those that fail to respond are halted in their progression by defective signaling and fall by the wayside. In nature, final sperm:oocyte ratios approach unity, and it would therefore appear that the achievement of monospermy has evolved via selective pressures rather than mechanisms that prevent polyspermy.

The initial stages of fertilization depend principally on two structures: the acrosome of the spermatozoon and the ZP of the oocyte. Three major events are involved in sperm–oocyte interactions:

1. The spermatozoon attaches to the ZP.
2. The spermatozoon undergoes the acrosome reaction, releasing digestive enzymes, and exposing the inner acrosomal membrane.
3. This highly fusogenic sperm membrane makes contact with the oocyte plasma membrane and the two membranes fuse together.

## Gamete Activation

Both spermatozoa and oocytes are in a quiescent state that is maintained by numerous carefully orchestrated cellular and molecular mechanisms, and their transition from arrested to developmentally competent cells is known as gamete activation. The cascades of events involved in mutual gamete activation are interconnected, with shared molecules and signaling pathways: calcium represents a key molecule for both gametes in each step of the process. Successful fertilization is dependent upon both gametes achieving full competence after the complex series of events necessary for their activation.

## Sperm Activation

Before the male gamete can initiate the steps required for successfully fertilizing an oocyte, the spermatozoon must itself be activated, a process that involves several behavioral, physiological and structural changes. Some of these changes are induced by exposure to environmental signals, and others are induced whilst the spermatozoon is interacting with the oocyte and its extracellular investments. The steps include changes in motility, capacitation, acrosome reaction, penetration of the ZP, binding to the oolemma and membrane fusion.

### Motility

Spermatozoa are maintained in the testis in a quiescent state. Metabolic suppression is regulated by physical restraint, low pH and low oxygen tension in the seminal fluid. They acquire motility during the process of epididymal maturation, but only become fully motile after ejaculation and capacitation. Sperm motility is regulated by intracellular ions and is associated with changes in the membrane potential, in particular a potassium-induced hyperpolarization (Miller *et al.*, 2015).

### Capacitation and Hyperactivation

Spermatozoa are not capable of fertilization immediately after ejaculation. They develop the capacity to fertilize (capacitate) after a period of time in the female genital tract; since epididymal maturation and capacitation are unique to mammals, this may represent an evolutionary adaptation to internal fertilization. During capacitation, the spermatozoa undergo a series of changes that give them the 'capacity' for binding to and penetrating the oocyte. These changes include an increase in membrane fluidity, cholesterol efflux, ion fluxes that alter sperm membrane potential, increased tyrosine phosphorylation of proteins, induction of hyperactive motility and the acrosome reaction.

Hyperactivation involves a change in flagellar beating, with an increase in the amplitude of flagellar bend; this may provide a force that helps in the release of spermatozoa from the oviductal epithelium and enhances the sperm's ability to navigate toward the oocyte. Hyperactivation may also help the sperm to penetrate the ZP.

Capacitation is a transitory state: the time required for capacitation varies from species to species and ranges from less than 1 hour in the mouse to 1–4 hours in the human. Only 10% of the available population are capacitated at any one time: capacitated spermatozoa are continuously replaced from the stored pool, ensuring that fertile spermatozoa are available over the period of several hours when ovulation may occur (Forman & Fissore, 2015).

Two changes take place: the epididymal and seminal plasma proteins coating the spermatozoa are removed, followed by an alteration in the glycoproteins of the sperm plasma membranes (an antigen on the plasma membrane of the mouse spermatozoon, laid down during epididymal maturation, cannot be removed by repeated washing, but disappears, or is masked during capacitation). The events are regulated by the activation of intracellular signaling pathways, involving cAMP, protein kinase A, receptor tyrosine kinases and non-receptor tyrosine kinases. A number of different molecules regulate these pathways, including calcium, bicarbonate, reactive oxygen species, GABA, progesterone, angiotensin and cytokines. Phosphorylation of sperm proteins is an important part of capacitation, and this has been shown to be associated with the change in the pattern of sperm motility described above, hyperactive motility, recognizable by an increase in lateral head displacement. There is also some evidence that spermatozoa can translate some mRNA species during capacitation (Gur and Breitbart, 2006).

In the human, capacitation in vivo probably starts while the spermatozoa are passing through the cervix. Many enzymes and factors from the female tract have been implicated in causing capacitation, such as aryl-sulfatase, fucosidase and taurine. The factors involved are not species specific, and capacitation may be induced in vitro in the absence of any signals from the female tract. Follicular fluid can also promote capacitation in vitro. A low molecular weight motility factor found in follicular fluid, ovary, uterus and oviduct may increase sperm metabolism (and hence motility) by lowering ATP and increasing cyclic AMP levels within the sperm. Table 4.1 demonstrates the duration of fertility and motility of mammalian spermatozoa within the oviduct, together with the fertilizable life of oocytes.

Chemically defined media with appropriate concentrations of electrolytes, metabolic energy sources and a protein source (serum albumin) will also induce the acrosome reaction in a population of washed sperm. The removal or redistribution of glycoproteins on the sperm cell surface during capacitation exposes receptor sites that can respond to oocyte signals, leading to the acrosome reaction.

**Table 4.1** Survival parameters of mammalian gametes in vitro

| | Time required for capacitation (h) | Duration of sperm motility (h) | Duration of sperm fertility (h) | Fertilizable life of oocytes (h) |
|---|---|---|---|---|
| Mouse | <1 | 13 | 6 | 15 |
| Sheep | 1–5 | 48 | 30–48 | 12–15 |
| Rat | 2–3 | 17 | 14 | 12 |
| Hamster | 2–4 | – | – | 9–12 |
| Pig | 3–6 | 50 | 24–48 | 10 |
| Rabbit | 5 | 43–50 | 28–36 | 6–8 |
| Rhesus monkey | 5–6 | – | – | 23 |
| Man | 5–6 | 48–60 | 24–48 | 6–24 |
| Dog | – | 268 | 134 | 24 |

Reproduced with permission from Gwatkin (1974).

- Capacitation is temperature dependent and only occurs at 37–39°C.
- Sperm surface components are removed or altered during capacitation.
- In vitro, the acrosome reaction cannot occur until capacitation is complete.

## Acrosome Reaction (AR)

The acrosome is a membrane-bound cap that covers the anterior portion of the sperm head; it contains a large array of hydrolytic enzymes including hyaluronidase, acrosin, proacrosin, phosphatase, arylsulfatase, collagenase, phospholipase C and β-galactosidase. The acrosome originates in the Golgi system of the early spermatid, in a series of concentrically arranged membranes around an aggregation of small vesicles. One of the vesicles increases in size and fills with particulate material, and the vesicle grows by fusion of several smaller vesicles. When the future acrosomal vesicle reaches a certain size, it migrates toward the nucleus. The nucleus then starts to elongate, the vesicle loses much of its fluid content and its membrane wraps around the front of the nucleus to form the typical acrosome.

When the capacitated spermatozoon attaches to the ZP, the permeability of the sperm plasma membrane is altered, causing a transient change in the concentration of several intracellular ions. This triggers the acrosome reaction, which is the final prerequisite step in the activation of the spermatozoon before gamete fusion is possible. The reaction consists of three stages:

1. The outer acrosomal membrane fuses with the overlying sperm head plasma membrane, allowing the contents to be released; this can be monitored in vitro using a fluorescent tag in the acrosome reaction to ionophore challenge (ARIC) test.
2. The acrosomal granule breaks down, releasing lysins. These enzymes 'dissolve' a pathway through the ZP.
3. When the sperm head plasma membrane contacts the oocyte plasma membrane, the two membranes fuse.

It appears that some of the sperm that may reach the zona are not triggered into the acrosome reaction, and are not able to penetrate the egg. In order for sperm to attach, a specific molecular fit may be required to induce the acrosome reaction. In the human, the membranes start to fuse near the border between the acrosomal cap and its equatorial segment. Once the correct trigger signals have been received, the acrosome reaction is relatively rapid, taking 2–15 minutes in vitro. Gametes collected from the ampullae of mammals after mating show that free-swimming spermatozoa have unreacted acrosomes, and those within the cumulus mass have either reacted acrosomes or are in the process of reacting. The majority of spermatozoa attached to the surface of the ZP surface have reacted acrosomes.

The acrosome reaction only occurs in the presence of $Ca^{2+}$: it may be induced artificially by adding Ca ionophore A23187, a chemical that carries $Ca^{2+}$ across cell membranes to the sperm cytoplasm (Figure 4.1), or simply by increasing the external concentration of $Ca^{2+}$. An artificially high pH of about 9–9.5 will also induce the AR. It appears that the physiological events leading to the AR parallel those leading to activation of the oocyte, including changes in the ion permeability of the plasma membrane, alterations in the intracellular level of free $Ca^{2+}$ and an alkalinization of the cytoplasm. The influx of calcium triggers the fusion of the acrosomal membranes and the exocytosis of the acrosomal

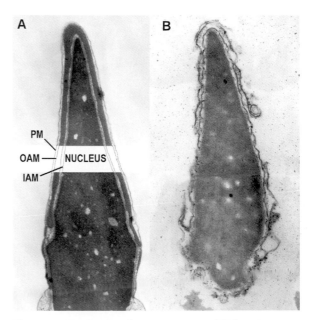

**Figure 4.1** Transmission electron microscope (TEM) section through a human spermatozoon showing the plasma membrane (PM) and outer (OAM) and inner (IAM) acrosomal membranes. To the right is a TEM of a human spermatozoon after exposure to the calcium ionophore A23187 has triggered the acrosome reaction.

contents. The sequence of events leading to exocytosis may involve several second messenger pathways, including:

- Changes in intracellular calcium
- Activation of cAMP and phosphokinase A pathways
- Phospholipase C generating InsP3 and diacylgycerol (DAG)
- Phospholipase D generating phosphatidic acid
- Activation of phospholipase A2 generating arachidonic acid.

Completion of the acrosome reaction does not necessarily ensure successful fertilization in vitro; enormous variability can be found in a population of spermatozoa surrounding the cumulus mass. Some will acrosome react too soon, others too late: in some the trigger stimulus will be inadequate, perhaps in others the transduction mechanism will fail at some point. The cumulus mass is composed of both cellular and acellular components, and the acellular matrix is made up of proteins and carbohydrates, including hyaluronic acid. As described earlier, in vivo, very few spermatozoa reach the site of fertilization: therefore, the idea that large populations of spermatozoa surrounding the oocyte mass dissolve the cumulus matrix, as observed during IVF, is probably incorrect in vivo. Fertilization occurs before the dispersion of the cumulus mass, and in vivo the sperm:oocyte ratio is probably close to 1:1.

## Oocyte Activation

### The Zona Pellucida

The ZP is secreted by the growing oocyte, a glycoprotein sheet several micrometers thick that provides a protective coat for the oocyte and developing embryo. If we accept the concept that polyspermy prevention is a laboratory artifact, it probably serves mainly as a protective coat for the developing embryo. Electron microscopy shows the outer surface to have a latticed appearance, consisting of 70% protein, 20% hexose, 3% sialic acid and 2% sulfate. In the mouse oocyte, the zona contains three glycoproteins, ZP1, ZP2 and ZP3, with apparent molecular weights of 200 000, 120 000 and 83 000, respectively; each is heavily glycosylated. Filaments of ZP2 and ZP3 polymers are crosslinked noncovalently, and ZP1 dimers create bridges between them to form a matrix (Wassarman *et al.*, 1996). In the mouse, ZP2 is distributed throughout

the thickness of the zona, and ZP3 binds to primary receptors on capacitated spermatozoa, inducing a cascade of events that lead to the acrosome reaction. Sperm receptors for ZP2, in contrast, are located on the inner acrosomal membrane and therefore are unmasked only after the AR has taken place. Following the AR, ZP2 binds the sperm to the zona, and the sperm penetrate the ZP to fuse with the oocyte plasma membrane. The zona in many species, including humans, contains a fourth zona protein, ZP4, which is absent in mice.

The ZP gene family has an ancient phylogeny, and the coding sequences of the murine and human ZP genes are 74% identical. All ZP proteins contain a structural element, the ZP domain (ZPD), composed of 260 amino acids, and this structural element is also found in many other proteins with different functions, including receptors and intracellular signaling related to differentiation and morphogenesis. There are 10 ZPD proteins in nematodes, more than 20 in flies and over 100 in birds.

Synthesis of these glycoproteins is regulated in a temporal sequence during oogenesis. In mammals and amphibians, ZP genes are transcribed exclusively by oocytes and/or follicle cells. ZP2 is expressed at low levels in resting oocytes, but ZP1 and ZP3 are expressed only in growing oocytes. In fish and birds, the ZP proteins are synthesized in the ovary and/or the liver. ZP3, an 83-kDa glycoprotein, appears to be the primary adhesion molecule. The bioactive component within ZP3 is thought to be related to its carbohydrate composition, with the terminal sugar residue being either a terminal alpha-linked galactose or a terminal N-acetylglucosamine. Other studies have suggested that ZP1 may also be involved in primary adhesion events in the rabbit and the human. ZP2 and ZP3 are the two major subunits of the ZP; the N-terminal region of ZP2 may regulate sperm recognition in mouse and human oocytes. When sperm bind to ZP3, they undergo the acrosome reaction.

Studies carried out using human ZP have revealed that ZP2 is modified by cleavage, similar to the mouse model. Sperm penetration through the zona is inhibited after fertilization. After sperm penetration, the zona undergoes modifications consistent with its role as a protective device. However, unlike the mouse, the ZP can still bind spermatozoa and induce the AR. Thus, fertilization does not abolish ZP bioactivity. This difference may be linked to the presence of

ZP4 – the precise events that describe the role of the zona proteins in gamete interaction require further study in humans (Lefièvre et al., 2004; Conner et al., 2005; Patrat et al., 2006; Tanphaichitr et al., 2015; Tosti & Ménézo, 2016).

## Cytoplasmic Maturation

During stages of oogenesis, the oocyte has accumulated reserves of proteins and mRNAs that allow it to remain quiescent, in a state of developmental arrest that is characterized by blocks at both nuclear and cytoplasmic levels. Arrest during the first meiotic prophase is characterized by the germinal vesicle; following germinal vesicle breakdown, meiosis is again arrested, and this block is removed by the fertilizing spermatozoon (Table 4.2). Two types of protein kinase in the cytoplasm maintain the second meiotic arrest: maturation promoting factor (MPF) and cytostatic factor (CSF). Oocytes acquire competence for successful fertilization and the ability to sustain early development via cytoplasmic maturation, a process that may be considered a parallel to sperm capacitation. Several milestones in development must be reached before an oocyte is capable of being fertilized correctly (see Tosti & Ménézo, 2016 for review and Figure 4.2 for overview):

1. MPF is expressed at a high level.

   - Core components of MPF = CSF and cyclin-dependent kinase1(Cdk1/Cdk2).
   - CSF maintains the anaphase-promoting complex/cyclosome (APC/C) inactive, via a signaling cascade involving early mitotic inhibitors, Emi2/Erp1.

2. High levels of other factors are present within the oocyte, including c-mos, mitogen-activated protein kinase (MAPK) and active p34cdc2.

3. Progression to the MII stage of meiosis. The first polar body must be extruded into the perivitelline space, between the oolemma and ZP.

4. Virtually all transcription ceases by the time of germinal vesicle breakdown (GBVD). The expression of genes beyond this stage switches to translation of stored mRNA.

These points are summarized in Table 4.2 and Figure 4.2.

The first event of activation in oocytes of most species is an increase in ionic permeability of the plasma membrane. In the human, the spermatozoon induces an outward current in the oocyte plasma membrane by activating calcium-gated potassium channels. In vitro, the activation competence of oocytes is continually changing, and is not a stable, prolonged feature of ovulated eggs; therefore, timing is critical in the handling of in-vitro manipulations.

# Sperm–oocyte Fusion

The process of membrane fusion between gametes is temperature, pH and $Ca^{2+}$ dependent, and the two membranes must be in close approximation. Fusion appears to be mediated or facilitated by membrane-associated proteins, but terminal saccharides of glycoproteins are not directly involved in the process.

**Table 4.2** Expression of factors during late stages of oogenesis in preparation for fertilization

| | G2 → M phase | | | | | |
| --- | --- | --- | --- | --- | --- | --- |
| | First meiotic block | | | Second meiotic block | | |
| | Germinal vesicle | Germinal vesicle breakdown | Metaphase I | First polar body | Metaphase II | Post fertilization |
| Phos p34cdc2 | ++ | − | − | − | − | ++ |
| Active p34cdc2 | − | ++ | ++ | ++ | ++ | − |
| MPF | · | ++ | ++ | − | ++ | − |
| c-mos | + | + | ++ | ++ | ++ | − |
| MAPK | − | ++ | ++ | ++ | ++ | − |
| cAMP | ++ | − | − | − | − | − |

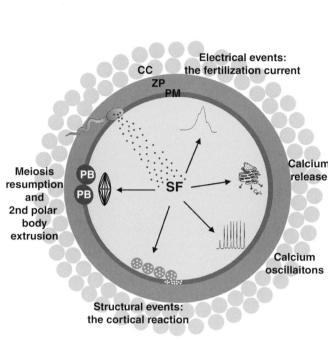

| EVENT | COMPONENTS INVOLVED |
|---|---|
| Sperm factor release | PLC ζ/γ <br> PAWP <br> PIP2 |
| Fertilization current | fertilization channels <br> sodium/calcium currents <br> calcium-activated potassium channels <br> calcium-activated chloride channels |
| Calcium release and oscillations | calcium ions <br> calcium stores <br> STIM/ORAI/SERCA <br> IP3/cADPr/NAADP <br> TPCs |
| Structural modifications | CG <br> calcium <br> SFE1/SFE9/proteoliaisin/rendezvin <br> PKC <br> SNAREs <br> α-SNAP/ NSF <br> ovastacin |
| Meiosis resumption | MPF/MAPKZP2 <br> cyclin B <br> PKC/CAMKII/calcineurin <br> EMI2/ERP <br> Mos <br> Cdk1/Cdc2 <br> zinc <br> mRNA polyadenylation |

**Figure 4.2** Sperm-induced oocyte activation. Left panel: image representing events occurring during sperm-induced oocyte activation: upon release of the sperm factor (SF), electrical modification of oocyte plasma membrane properties generates an outward (in mammals) or inward ion current (non-mammals). Release of calcium from the intracellular stores generates calcium oscillations. Physical changes of the oocyte occur by release of CG contents, and finally meiosis is resumed, allowing completion of the cell cycle, extrusion of the polar body and triggering of zygote formation. Right panel: table reporting the event and the components involved. PLCζ = phospholipase C; PAWP = postacrosomal sheath WW domain-binding protein; PIP2 = phosphatidylinositol (4,5)-bisphosphate; IP3 = inositol 1,4,5-trisphosphate; cADPr = cyclic adenosine diphosphoribose; NAADP = nicotinic acid adenine dinucleotide phosphate; TPCs = two-pore channels; SFE1, SFE9 = structural matrix proteins; PKC = protein kinase C; SNAP = N-ethylmaleimide-sensitive factor attachment protein alpha; NSF = N-ethylmaleimide sensitive factor; MPF = maturation-promoting factor; MAPK = mitogen-activated protein kinase; CAMKII = calcium calmodulin-dependent protein kinase; EMI/ERP = early mitotic inhibitors; Mos = serine/threonine kinase; Cdk1 = cyclin-dependent kinase; CG = cortical granule; SF = sperm factor. Reproduced with permission from Tosti & Ménézo (2016).

During penetration of the zona, the spermatozoon loses its acrosomal contents, and only the inner acrosomal membrane is in direct contact with the zona. In eutherian mammals, the post-acrosomal region of the sperm head plasma membrane only attains fusibility after the acrosome reaction; this area apparently fuses with the oocyte plasma membrane, and the two membranes become continuous (Figure 4.3).

The surface of the oocyte membrane is organized into evenly spaced short microvilli that seem to facilitate gamete fusion; these microvilli have a low radius of curvature which may help to overcome opposing electrostatic charges. In mouse and hamster, the area overlying the metaphase spindle is microvillus-free, and spermatozoa are not able to, or are less likely to, fuse with this area. The human oocyte, however, has

(a)

(b)

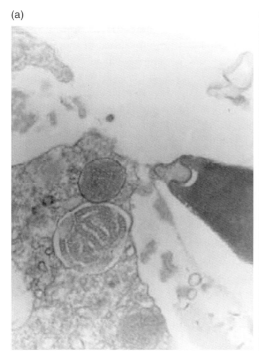

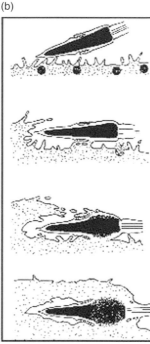

**Figure 4.3** (a) Transmission electron micrograph showing the point of sperm–oocyte fusion in the sea urchin. Sperm factor must flow through this cytoplasmic bridge of 0.1 mm diameter. The large granule (1 mm) below the spermatozoon is a cortical granule. (b) Stages in sperm–oocyte fusion in the mammal. Modified with permission from Yanagimachi (1994).

microvilli present over the entire surface, with no obvious polarity at this stage. There may, however, be 'hotspots' for sperm entry into the oocyte; this is an area that requires further research.

## The Oocyte Plasma Membrane

Lipids in the plasma membrane are organized asymmetrically into 'rafts,' domains of 10–200 nm, which make up to 20% of the surface area of somatic cells. They are thought to be platforms for membrane trafficking, signal transduction and viral entry, containing regions of high cholesterol, sphingomyelin and gangliosides, and are enriched in phospholipids with saturated fatty acyl chains. Caveolin, a major raft component, serves as a scaffolding to embed and inactivate many proteins and enzymes. Lipid rafts are less fluid than the rest of the plasma membrane and display lateral movement in response to physiological stimuli. In mouse, sea urchin and amphibians, fertilization may be inhibited by methyl-beta-cyclodextrin (MBCD), which disrupts rafts by dispersing important raft proteins, such as CD9, and inhibits Src kinase activation and the completion of meiosis. In mouse oocytes, MBCD disrupts both planar and caveolar rafts, which are thought to be the sites of mammalian sperm–egg binding and fusion. Phosphatidic acid

(PA) may be responsible for stabilizing rafts. Other lipids may also affect rafts and membrane fusion, for example production of ceramide during fertilization may lead to clustered rafts and an increase in raft diameter. Cortical microfilaments are important in raft biology, and PA is a major regulator of cytoskeletal fibers.

Several lipids seem to have roles in membrane fusion events at fertilization, including the acrosome reaction, gamete fusion and cortical exocytosis, regulating receptors and releasing intracellular calcium. In *Xenopus* oocytes, phosphatidic acid can activate Src tyrosine kinase or phospholipase C during fertilization, leading to an increase in intracellular calcium. Lipases such as phospholipase D, C and A2, sphingomyelinase, lipin 1 and autotaxin are involved in generating lipid second messengers at fertilization.

In the human oocyte, lipid raft microdomains are enriched in the ganglioside GM1 and the tetraspanin protein CD9. GM1 is involved in a variety of processes such as virus docking, signal transduction and protein binding, while CD9 seems to be the most important membrane component involved in sperm penetration in mammals. Sperm penetration into the human oocyte appears to be dependent on the density and organization of GM1 microdomains at the site

85

where the sperm arrives – these can be considered docking sites. Sperm bind at these GM1 microdomains, but do not penetrate. The lipid rafts with CD9, distinct to those with GM1, may be sites for stable binding. GM1 organization and the stability of these plasma membrane rafts depend on underlying mitochondrial activity and efficiency.

---

### Izumo1 and Juno

A great deal of research has been directed toward identifying the molecules on the oocyte surface and sperm acrosomal membrane that are responsible for gamete fusion. *Izumo 1* (named after a Japanese marriage shrine) is a mouse spermatozoal transmembrane protein that interacts with *Juno* (after the Roman goddess of fertility and marriage), a receptor found on the surface of the unfertilized oocyte. Juno is a member of the Folr4 folate receptor family, and is anchored to glycophosphatidylinositol (GPI). Juno has thus far been identified on mouse, opossum, pig and human oocytes. Juno is rapidly lost from the oocyte surface after fertilization; Juno–Izumo1 interaction appears to be a necessary adhesion step for gametes, rather than a membrane fusion event. Fusion probably requires other membrane proteins, perhaps such as EEF-1(Eukaryotic Elongation Factor 1) and myomaker (Wassarman, 2014). The strength of sperm binding may be increased by local clustering of Juno on the oocyte membrane, organized by the tetraspanin CD9. This protein has a clear role in sperm–oocyte fusion in its own right, but the corresponding sperm ligand is unknown. Members of the CRISP (cysteine-rich secretory proteins) family are also known to participate in the process of capacitation and mammalian sperm–ZP interactions.

---

Lipid rafts may concentrate signaling proteins at the site of gamete interaction to promote adhesion and fusion. Plasma membrane fusion of the two gametes leading to cell–cell continuity is the last step in the interaction of gametes and leads to oocyte activation and the formation of the zygote. Although the mechanism is still not clear, lipid rafts and associated transmembrane proteins Izumo 1, Juno and CD9 play a fundamental role (Wassarman, 2014).

The sperm plasma membrane remains fused with the oocyte plasma membrane and indicates the point of 'entry.' Sperm motility is required for penetration, but not for gamete fusion; the fertilizing spermatozoon continues flagellar movement for around 20 seconds after attachment to the oocyte surface.

In small mammals sperm–oocyte fusion is quite advanced after 3 minutes, the entire incorporation of the sperm head takes 15 minutes, and pronucleus formation takes about 60 minutes. In some mammals (e.g., the Chinese hamster) the tail is not incorporated, while in others it is incorporated by the progressive fusion of the oocyte and spermatozoal plasma membranes. After incorporation, the midpiece mitochondria and axial filament of the tail appear to disintegrate. Immediately after fusion, the sperm plasma membrane remains localized to the point of entry, integrated into the oocyte plasma membrane, but by the time that the pronuclei have formed, sperm surface antigen has spread all over the surface of the zygote.

## The Cortical Reaction

### Cortical Contractions

In mammals, the calcium wave at fertilization triggers contraction of the acto-myosin cytoskeleton, which induces rhythmic movement in the cortical cytoplasm. Sperm entry causes a change in the shape of the oocyte: a fertilization cone is formed, and the zygote flattens along the axis that bisects the fertilization cone. In mouse, sperm-induced cytoplasmic movements are synchronous with pulsations seen in the fertilization cone, and last for 4 hours, until the pronuclei are formed. These pulsations are actin-dependent, and are associated with intracellular calcium waves. It may be postulated that calcium activates kinases such as protein kinase C or $Ca^{2+}$/calmodulin-dependent kinase 11, which are known to regulate the cytoskeleton.

### Cortical Granules

Cortical granules (CG) are spherical membrane-bound organelles containing enzymes and mucopolysaccharides that lie peripherally in the oocyte (Figure 4.4). They contain enzymes and mucopolysaccharides, and are synthesized in the early stages of oocyte growth. The exact timing is species-specific: in rat and mouse, they first appear in the unilaminar follicle, while in humans, monkeys and the hamster they first appear in multi-layered follicles. Small vesicles are formed from the Golgi membranes, and these migrate to the subcortical area and coalesce to form mature cortical granules. Cortical granules continue to be produced up to the time of ovulation.

In all animals, including the sea urchin, granule migration depends on cytoskeletal elements. The

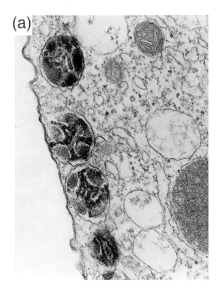
(a)

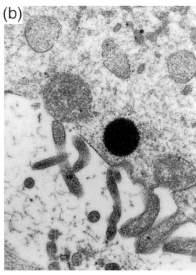
(b)

**Figure 4.4** Transmission electron micrographs of the surface of unfertilized oocytes of the sea urchin (a) and human (b), showing the cortical granules.

family of Rab proteins, the largest family of mono-meric small GTPases, is a major effector. These proteins function as molecular switches between active (GTP-bound) and inactive (GDP-bound) conformations. During their active state they cooperate with downstream 'effector' proteins, which are involved in different cellular activities such as vesicle formation, motility and the movement of vesicles and organelles along cytoskeletal elements. In mouse oocytes the cortical granules translocate along the actin network regulated by Rab27a, which is a marker for cortical granules. Two pathways are involved: myosin Va transports the granules along the actin, and granules then attach to Rab11a vesicles that move to the plasma membrane (Holubcova *et al.*, 2013).

In the majority of mammals, including the human, granules are evenly distributed throughout the cortex. However, in mouse and hamster oocytes the surface area around the animal pole, the site of the meiotic spindle, is devoid of granules: up to 24% of the surface area around this site is free of cortical granules. In mouse oocytes the number of cortical granules decreases from 7400 to 4100 after extrusion of the polar bodies, suggesting that some may be exocytosed in this area before fertilization, this may prevent sperm penetration in the area overlying the female meiotic plate. Prefertilization release of cortical granules in some mammals may serve to condition the ZP for subsequent interaction with the spermatozoa.

Two classes of proteins, v and t SNARES (soluble NSF attachment protein receptors), have been shown to play a role in cortical granule docking and exocytosis. Alpha-SNAP (N-ethylmaleimide-sensitive factor attachment protein alpha) and NSF (N-ethylmaleimide sensitive factor) are also implicated in the mouse cortical reaction.

Two populations of cortical granules can be distinguished in mammalian oocytes, based on their electron density: one has an electron dense core, the other has fluffy or granular contents. These might reflect different stages in granule maturity, different types of granules or different stages of exocytosis. They contain between 4 and 14 proteins, which are glycosylated with complex carbohydrates. Those identified so far include:

- Several proteinases, including a trypsin-like molecule, tissue-type plasminogen activator (tPA), a serine proteinase and ZP2 proteinase, which converts ZP2 (120 kDa) to ZP2f (90 kDa).
- An ovoperoxidase, involved in catalyzing the cross-linking of tyrosines in the ZP to harden it.
- Calreticulin, a chaperone protein responsible for glycoproteins.
- N-acetylglucosaminidase, a glucosidase, p32 and p75, which have all been recognized in mouse cortical granules by specific antibodies, although their roles are not clear.
- Ovastacin, a protein of the metalloproteinase family, similar to hatching enzyme.

Immediately after sperm penetration, cortical granules fuse with the oocyte plasma membrane and release their contents into the perivitelline space by exocytosis – this cortical reaction is the first morphological indication of oocyte activation. The cortical reaction elicits the zona reaction (zona hardening), changing the characteristics of the ZP, and at the same time the egg plasma membrane becomes a mosaic of cortical granule membrane and original plasma membrane. In mammalian oocytes the change is dramatic and rapid, and does not require any new protein synthesis within the cell, but seems to be related to metabolic de-repression of the oocyte. The resulting transient increase in surface area due to CG/oolemma fusion facilitates the necessary increase in metabolic turnover required by the activated oocyte. In the mouse, the action of proteinases or glycosidases results in hydrolysis of ZP3 receptors, which changes the role of the ZP from sperm receptor to protective coat.

The early embryo is a compact mass of cells that are continually dividing, and the embryo is continually changing shape. Such movement would be hindered if the cells were attached to a rigid structure, and the fluid-filled perivitelline space (PVS) acts as a flexible boundary that allows movement, while the hardened zona provides a protective structure. The PVS may also serve as a microenvironment, buffering the embryo from changes in its external environment. The hardened ZP keeps the dividing blastomeres of the embryo in close contact and protects them from

potential microbial invasion. The embryo remains in this protective zona coat until hatching, just prior to implantation.

After penetrating the zona and oolemma, the naked sperm nucleus enters the oocyte cortex, moves laterally, rotates approximately 180 degrees and during the next 10 minutes starts to develop into the male pronucleus. The mitochondria and tail of the spermatozoon also enter the cytoplasm but later degenerate.

## Release from Meiotic Arrest

The final phase of oocyte activation is resumption and completion of meiosis, leading to extrusion of the polar body and zygote cleavage. The universal messenger that triggers reinitiation of meiosis in oocytes at fertilization is an increase in intracellular $Ca^{2+}$ released from intracellular stores in periodic waves or transients (Figure 4.5).

A variety of physical and chemical stimuli can parthenogenetically cause calcium to be released in a similar fashion, but the kinetics of these calcium transients are different, and they do not sustain development. There are two hypotheses as to how the spermatozoon triggers intracellular $Ca^{2+}$ release:

## The G-protein Hypothesis

This model for oocyte activation was extrapolated from the events known about calcium response to hormones in somatic cells. Hormone-receptor

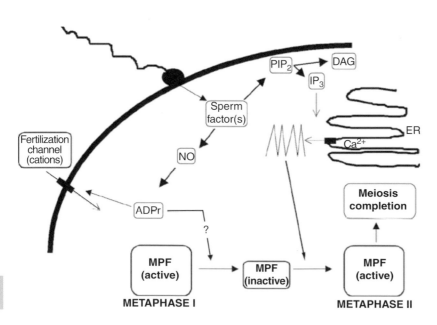

**Figure 4.5** Schematic showing the likely mechanisms involved in oocyte activation after being triggered by the fertilizing sperm. IP3 = inositol 1,4,5-trisphosphate; NO = nitric oxide; DAG = diacylglycerol; PIP2 = phosphatidylinositol-4,5-bisphosphate; cADPr = cyclic adenosine diphosphoribose; MPF = maturation-promoting factor. From Dale et al. (1999).

binding on the outer surface of the plasma membrane signals through a G-protein in the plasma membrane; this signal triggers the activation of phospholipase C, leading to the formation of inositol 1,4,5-trisphosphate ($IP_3$) and hence calcium release. This model of oocyte activation suggests that the sperm behaves as an 'honorary hormone': the attachment of sperm to a sperm receptor triggers $IP_3$ formation through a G-protein linked to this receptor.

## The Soluble Sperm Factor Hypothesis

The sperm factor hypothesis, proposed by Dale and colleagues in the early 1980s, suggests that intracellular calcium release is triggered by a diffusible messenger(s)in the cytoplasm of the spermatozoon, which enters the oocyte cytoplasm after sperm–oocyte fusion. The first direct evidence for a soluble sperm factor was shown by microinjecting the soluble components from spermatozoa into sea urchin and ascidian oocytes. Several activation events were triggered, including cortical granule exocytosis and gating of plasma membrane currents. The same conclusion was reached when the experiment was repeated in mammals. The soluble sperm factor hypothesis gained further support with the advent of ICSI in the 1990s, where the events of oocyte activation, including calcium release, occur even when the surface membrane events are bypassed.

Soluble extracts of spermatozoa can activate oocytes from different phyla as well as different species: mammalian oocytes can be partially activated by microinjecting sea urchin spermatozoa into the cytoplasm. Thus, sperm factors do not appear to be species specific, nor indeed phylum specific. Sperm extracts can also trigger calcium oscillations in somatic cells, suggesting that they may be common calcium-releasing agents rather than sperm-specific molecules. It is possible that both soluble sperm factor and membrane transduction mechanisms interact to trigger oocyte activation. Spermatozoa contain many calcium-releasing molecules, including adenosine diphosphate ribose (ADPr), $IP_3$, nicotinamide nucleotide metabolites, calcium ions and relatively large proteins. Recently, phospholipase C zeta 1, identified in mammalian and human sperm, has been shown to trigger calcium release and lead to oocyte activation. Mammals, together with sea urchins and ascidians, belong to the deuterostome group of animals that show remarkable similarities in gamete physiology.

Since changes in plasma membrane conductance, calcium ion release and MPF inactivation are common to all these oocytes at fertilization, the sperm-borne trigger might also be expected to be common. It remains to be seen if phospholipase C zeta 1 is found in the spermatozoa of these other deuterostomes and indeed if this lipase triggers other activation events in the mammalian oocyte such as the ADPr/NO pathway (Dale *et al.*, 2010, Dale, 2018b).

---

**Intracellular Calcium Release**

The pattern of calcium release at fertilization varies from species to species. There are three categories of calcium release mechanisms in oocytes, related to the type of receptor on the intracellular calcium store:

1. Inositol 1,4,5-trisphosphate ($IP_3$)-induced calcium release (IICR). $IP_3$ is produced by the action of phospholipase C on plasma membrane lipid phosphatidylinositol bisphosphate, and IICR is triggered by the binding of $IP_3$ to its receptor on the endoplasmic reticulum.

2. Calcium-induced calcium release (CICR). CICR is triggered by opening the ryanodine receptor on an intracellular store but can also be triggered in a mechanism involving the $IP_3$ receptor. This can also be triggered by calcium itself and appears to be modulated by cyclic ADP ribose. Cyclic ADP ribose is, in turn, produced by metabolism of nicotinamide adenine diphosphate ($NAD^+$) by ADP ribosyl cyclase or $NAD^+$ glycohydrolase.

3. $NAADP^+$-induced calcium release. Other calcium-releasing second messengers have been identified, including cATP ribose and $NAADP^+$. Since $NAD^+$, NADH, $NADP^+$ and NADPH can be metabolized to calcium-releasing second messengers in sea urchin microsomes, it is possible that other calcium-releasing second messengers may be discovered in the nicotinamide nucleotide family.

In mammalian oocytes there is a large increase in the sensitivity to CICR at fertilization, together with a series of repetitive calcium spikes. This again suggests that both CICR and IICR are activated at fertilization.

---

## Centrosomes and Centrioles

The centrosome provides the 'division center' for the new zygote, forming the basis for the mitotic spindle that guides the chromosomes through its process of duplication and division. In studies on sea urchins and roundworms at the turn of the century, Boveri at the Stazione Zoologica in Naples showed that the male gamete provided this 'division center' for the zygote, and predicted that the structure is a cyclical reproducing organ of the cell. The centrosome is paternal in origin, contributed by the sperm: two notable exceptions to this are the mouse and hamster, where it is apparently maternal in origin, lending support to the observation that these rodents are poor model systems for human fertilization. In frogs, however, although the centrosome is contributed by the sperm, it lacks tubulin, which is needed for microtubule nucleation. Tubulin is provided by the oocyte cytoplasm, and therefore the functional frog centrosome is a mosaic of paternal and maternal components.

In somatic cells the centrosome is composed of two structures known as centrioles (Figure 4.6), which are made up of nine triplets of microtubules arranged in a pinwheel shape. These centrioles are placed at right angles to each other and are surrounded by dense pericentriolar material. During interphase, the centrosome divides to form the poles of the mitotic spindle; after division, this segregates with the chromosomes to each of the daughter cells. In contrast, during oogenesis the centrosome degenerates after meiosis, leaving the oocyte without a 'division center'; this is then contributed by the sperm during fertilization. The sperm centrosome has a functional proximal centriole, close to the nucleus, and a degenerate distal centriole.

After the sperm enters the oocyte, a small 'aster' of microtubules grows out from the centriole, and this aster directs the migration of the sperm pronucleus to the center of the oocyte to make contact with the decondensing maternal pronucleus. This initiates the migration of the maternal pronucleus toward the forming male pronucleus. Microtubules extend from a point in between the now juxtaposed male and female pronuclei, and the centrioles duplicate and migrate to opposite poles during mitotic prophase to set up the first mitotic spindle of the zygote. The zygotic centrosome duplicates and then splits apart during interphase.

Although the centrioles are the main organelles associated with cell division, it is now thought that the pericentriolar material may be principally responsible for organizing the microtubules. In cases of polyspermy, when the oocyte is fertilized by more than one sperm, human oocytes develop multiple asters, each associated with a sperm.

Parthenogenetically activated cattle and human oocytes can organize their microtubules without sperm entry, but this takes place later, and less completely than it does after sperm entry. Defective centrosome function can result in fertilization failure – microtubules are present in the second meiotic spindle of unfertilized oocytes that are arrested in metaphase. During parthenogenesis, where there is no sperm to contribute a centrosome, there is no aster of nucleated microtubules, and the microtubules are found in the cytoplasm throughout the oocyte. In this

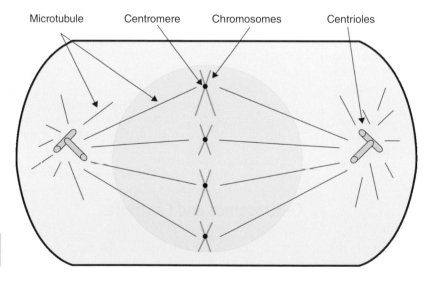

Microtubule    Centromere    Chromosomes    Centrioles

**Figure 4.6** Schematic representation of the spindle apparatus, showing centrioles, microtubules and chromosomes with centromeres.

case, the female centrosome becomes functional, duplicating and forming the mitotic spindle poles.

Six hours post-insemination, a small microtubule sperm aster extends from the sperm centrosome, and the activated egg extrudes the second polar body.

## Pronucleus Formation

During spermatogenesis, gene expression is repressed, DNA replication ceases and sperm chromatin is tightly packed into a nuclear envelope that lacks pores. The mammalian sperm nucleus is packed with proteins that contain highly charged basic amino acids (protamines) that condense the DNA and repress transcription. Extensive disulfide linking in the protamines makes the sperm head rigid, a property that is necessary for penetration of the zona. Protamine cross-linking in the human spermatozoon is regulated by $Zn^{2+}$ present in prostatic gland secretions. When the sperm nucleus enters the oocyte cytoplasm, the process is reversed, with changes in morphology and biochemical processes. The sperm nuclear membrane breaks down, and under the influence of factors in the oocyte cytoplasm, the highly condensed chromatin starts to swell and become dispersed, so that filaments of chromatin are released into the cytoplasm. The factors that cause decondensation are apparently not species-specific, since human sperm can decondense when microinjected into an amphibian oocyte; a reduced form of glutathione is probably responsible for facilitating the process, by reducing disulfide bonds in sperm nuclear protamines.

The mammalian oocyte is at the metaphase II stage at the time of sperm entry; the sperm nuclear envelope dissolves and chromatin starts to decondense while the oocyte transits from metaphase II to telophase II. During telophase II, the sperm chromatin completes its decondensation as the female pronucleus develops. Sperm protamines are replaced by histones, and the male and female pronuclear envelopes then develop synchronously. However, research suggests that paternal histones delivered to the egg are retained in the male pronucleus and contribute to zygotic chromatin (van der Heijdn et al., 2008). Between 4 and 7 hours after fusion, a new nuclear membrane forms around the decondensed male and female chromatin, creating pronuclei that contain the two sets of haploid chromosomes. Oocyte cytoplasm contains factors that are necessary for the development of the male pronucleus; these factors are again not species-specific, since human spermatozoa can develop into normal pronuclei in hamster oocytes and form a normal chromosome complement. In hamster oocytes, a maximum of five pronuclei will decondense at any time, indicating that the factors may be present in limited quantities.

Bovine sperm tagged with a mitochondrion-specific vital dye have been used to follow sperm incorporation and the conversion of sperm-derived components within the bovine zygote. The zygotes were then fixed at various times after fertilization for immunochemistry and ultrastructural studies. These experiments showed that complete incorporation of the sperm can be inhibited by the microfilament disrupter cytochalasin B, and therefore this process depends upon the integrity of oocyte microfilaments. After sperm incorporation, the mitochondria were displaced from the sperm midpiece, and the sperm centriole was exposed to egg cytoplasm. The microtubule-based sperm aster then formed, initiating union of male and female pronuclei. The disassembly of the sperm tail occurred as a series of precisely orchestrated events, involving the destruction and transformation of particular sperm structures into zygotic and embryonic components.

## Nucleolar Precursor Bodies and Nucleoli

When the two pronuclei are formed in the zygote, they contain structures known as nucleolar precursor bodies (NPBs); the number and pattern displayed by their arrangement became popular as criteria for evaluating the embryonic potential of individual zygotes (Tesarik and Greco, 1999; Scott et al., 2000). Spermatozoal nucleoli are destroyed during spermatogenesis (Schulz and Leblond, 1990), and oocyte nucleolar material is required for the reassembly of nucleoli in both female and male pronuclei (Ogushi et al., 2008).

Tesarik and colleagues (1986, 1988) described the mechanism of NPB and nucleolar formation in human embryos, a scheme that differs from the process that takes place during the differentiation of adult somatic cells. In somatic cells, nucleoli are periodically reconstituted during mitotic telophase, with first a dense fibrillar component and then a granular component appearing around specific loci on chromosomes bearing rRNA genes, usually located at or close to a secondary constriction. In contrast, rDNA of the mammalian zygote and embryo appears to be incapable of starting transcription and thus triggering the nucleogenetic process unless it is associated with nuclear precursors.

The sequence of events described by Tesarik and colleagues for human embryos involves four stages:

1. Transcriptionally inactive rDNA has not yet penetrated into the homogeneous nuclear precursor (pre-nucleoli).
2. rDNA penetrates into the heterogeneous nuclear precursor and turns on the synthesis of pre-rRNA, whose processing is still inactive.
3. Processing of pre-rRNA is progressively activated in compact fibro-granular nucleoli.
4. Active pre-rRNA synthesis and processing occur in reticulated nucleoli.

This scheme, however, did not include information about the paternal or maternal origin of the components. The oocyte nucleolus is derived from material that is present in the germinal vesicle, and its content may change during the process of oocyte maturation. It is composed of approximately 700 proteins, with roles in many cellular processes, including cell cycle regulation and apoptosis. Ogushi *et al.* (2008) conducted a series of experiments leading to the conclusion that the nucleoli of both male and female pronuclei are maternal in origin, derived exclusively from maternal nucleolar remnants retained at the time of GVBD. Microsurgical removal of murine and pig oocyte nucleoli during prophase I indicated that the nucleoli did not contain the factors necessary for oocyte maturation. However, after fertilization of mature oocytes without nucleoli, no nucleoli were then visible in the resulting zygote pronuclei, and these zygotes could not complete development to blastocyst stage. Transfer of GVs to recipient cytoplasts indicated that material(s) within the mature oocyte GV, showing a ring of condensed chromatin around the nucleolus just prior to GVBD, is essential for full-term development. Although the oocyte nucleolus is clearly involved, the factors have not been identified, and may include precursor molecules required for the assembly of fully functional nucleoli at a later stage in the development of the embryo.

Lefèvre (2008) described and summarized these experiments: 'The nucleoli of the two pronuclei are exclusively of maternal origin, and the oocyte nucleolar material is essential for the reassembly of nucleoli in both male and female pronuclei.'

## Syngamy

After the male and female pronuclei are formed, they gradually migrate over a period of a few hours to the center of the oocyte, until they are adjacent to each other. During this period DNA is synthesized, in preparation for the first mitotic division. The process of migration has been studied extensively in the sea urchin and the mouse. In the mouse, fluorescein conjugated probes for cytoskeletal elements show a thickened area of microfilaments below the cortex of the polar body region. In addition to the spindle microtubules there are 16 cytoplasmic microtubule-organizing centers (MTOCs) or foci, and each centrosomal focus organizes an aster. These foci condense on the surface of the envelope just before the pronuclear membranes disintegrate. The mitotic metaphase spindle then forms, which involves duplication of the proximal centriole contributed by the sperm centrosome to form a pair of polar centrioles, and the chromosomes are aligned along the spindle equator. The plane of cell division is mediated by astral microtubules that extend from the mitotic spindle to the plasma membrane. Between 18 and 24 hours after gamete fusion, the two sets of chromosomes come together in syngamy (Figure 4.7), a cleavage furrow forms as soon as the first mitotic anaphase and telophase are completed, and the zygote becomes a two-cell embryo. Surprisingly, the male and female chromosomes do not mix immediately, but remain separate throughout the first cleavage division. The dynamic process of spindle assembly during this first cleavage division was examined using inverted light-sheet microscopy to produce three-dimensional images of live mouse zygotes. Differential labeling of maternal and paternal chromosomes, together with fluorescent-labeling of MTOCs, showed that two bipolar spindles form in the zygote: the male and female chromosomes each assemble their own machinery for chromosome separation (Reichmann *et al.*, 2018). The two spindles align their poles during anaphase, but keep the male and female genomes apart until they align in parallel before segregating the genomes during the first cleavage division. Further analysis suggested that each of the two spindles around the parental genomes functions independently before the chromosomes congress, and then segregate during first anaphase. The two spindles must be closely aligned prior to anaphase: if they are not correctly aligned in parallel, the chromosomes can be segregated in different

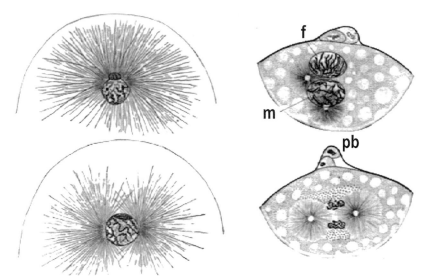

**Figure 4.7** A drawing showing (left) the fusion of male and female pronuclei to form the zygote nucleus as in sea urchins. In the majority of animals (and usually in mammals) the pronuclear membranes break down without fusing, allowing the chromosomes to interact in the cytoplasm (frames on the right). pb = polar body. Reproduced from Wilson (1900).

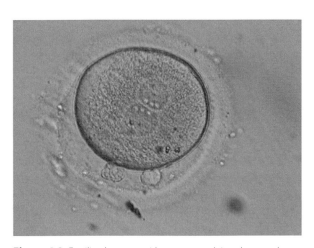

**Figure 4.8** Fertilized oocyte with two pronuclei and two polar bodies clearly visible; nucleolar precursor bodies are aligned in the pronuclei.

directions, leading to blastomeres with more than one nucleus per cell. Zygotes in which the two spindles were aligned parallel to each other before anaphase divided into two blastomeres with single nuclei. This mechanism might provide a basis for the frequent observation of multinucleated blastomeres after human IVF procedures.

## 'The Sun in the Egg'

The union of egg and sperm haploid genomes to form the genome of a new diploid organism is a moment of fundamental biological significance.

Leopold Auerbach of Breslau, Germany (1828–1897) described two protoplasmic vacuoles in a newly fertilized egg, as well as a radiating figure between them. In 1876, Oscar Hertwig identified these vacuoles as the male and female pronuclei (Figures 4.7 and 4.8), and he observed their fusion. When the two nuclei merged together in syngamy, he described the figure as follows:

> Es entsteht so vollstandig das Bild einer Sonner im Ei.
> It arises to completion like a sun within the egg.

In an analysis of Hertwig's paper, Paul Weindling (1991) proposed, 'This vivid image conveyed the discovery of the moment at which a new life was formed. The metaphor expressed awareness that the force of natural powers was greater than the sum of two cells.'

## Further Reading

### Books and Reviews

Auerbach L (1874) *Organologische Studien*. Breslau.

Boveri T (1902) Über mehrpolige Mitosen als Mittel zur Analyse des Zellkerns. *Verhandlungen der physicalisch-medizinischen Gesselschaft zu Würzburg N.F.* 35: 67–90.

Coy P, Aviles M (2010) What controls polyspermy in mammals: the oviduct or the oocyte? *Biological Reviews* 85: 593–605.

Dale B (1983a) *Fertilization in Animals*. Edward Arnold, London.

Dale B (2018b) *Fertilization: The Beginning of Life*. Cambridge University Press, Cambridge, UK.

Dale B (2018) Polyspermy. In: Skinner M (ed.) *Encyclopedia of Reproduction*, 2nd edn. Elsevier, New York, pp. 309–313.

Edwards RG (1982) *Conception in the Human Female.* Academic Press, New York.

Fleming TA, Johnson MH (1988) From egg to epithelium. *Annual Review of Cell Biology* 4: 459–485.

Forman H, Fissore R (2015) Fertilization in mammals. In: Plant TM, Zelezni AJ (eds.) *Knobil and Neill's Physiology of Reproduction*, 4th edn. Elsevier, New York, pp. 149–196.

Gwatkin R (1974) *Fertilization Mechanisms in Man and Mammals.* Plenum Press, New York.

Lauria A, Gandolfi E, Enne G, Gianaroli L (eds.) (1998) *Gametes: Development and Function*. Serono Symposia, Rome.

Nuccitelli R, Cherr G, Clark A (1989) *Mechanisms of Egg Activation.* Plenum Press, New York.

Schatten G (1994) The centrosome and its mode of inheritance: the reduction of the centrosome during gametogenesis and its restoration during fertilization. *Developmental Biology* 165(2): 299–335.

Tosti E, Boni R (2004) Electrical events during gamete maturation and fertilization in animals and humans. *Human Reproduction Update* 10(1): 53-65.

Tosti E, Ménézo Y (2016) Gamete activation: basic knowledge and clinical applications. *Human Reproduction Update* 22(4): 420–439.

Wilson EB (1900) *The Cell in Development and Inheritance.* Macmillan, London.

Yanagimachi R (1981) Mechanisms of fertilization in mammals. In: Mastroianni L, Biggers JD (eds.) *Fertilization and Embryonic Development in Vitro.* Plenum Press, New York, pp. 81–182.

Yanagimachi R (1994) Mammalian fertilization. In: Knobil E, Neill J (eds.) *The Physiology of Reproduction.* Raven Press, New York, pp. 189–317.

## Publications

Breitbart H, Spungin B (1997) The biochemistry of the acrosome reaction. *Molecular Human Reproduction* 3(3): 195–202.

Cappell SD, Mark KG, Garbett D, Pack LR, Rape M, Meyer T (2018) Emi1 switches from being a substrate to an inhibitor of APC/C$^{Cdh1}$ to start the cell cycle. *Nature* 558: 313–317.

Cohen-Dayag A, Tur-Kaspa I, Dor J, Mashiach S, Eisenbach M (1995) Sperm capacitation in humans is transient and correlates with chemotactic responsiveness to follicular factors. *Proceedings of the National Academy of Sciences* 92: 11039–11043.

Collas P (1998) Cytoplasmic control of nuclear assembly. *Reproduction, Fertility, and Development* 10: 581–592.

Collas P, Poccia D (1998) Remodeling the sperm nucleus into a male pronucleus at fertilization. *Theriogenology* 49(1): 67–81.

Conner SJ, Lefièvre L, Hughes DC, Barratt CL (2005) Cracking the egg: increased complexity in the zona pellucida. *Human Reproduction* 20: 1148–1152.

Dale B (2016) Achieving monospermy or preventing polyspermy? *Research and Reports in Biology* 7: 47–57.

Dale B, DeFelice LJ (1990) Soluble sperm factors, electrical events and egg activation. In: Dale B (ed.) *Mechanism of Fertilization: Plants to Humans.* NATO ASI cell biology ser H 45. Springer, Berlin, pp. 475–487.

Dale B, DeFelice LJ (2011) Polyspermy prevention: facts and artifacts. *Journal of Assisted Reproduction and Genetics* 28: 199–207.

Dale B, Di Matteo L, Marino M, Russo G, Wilding M (1999) Soluble sperm activating factor. In: Ganon C (ed.) *The Male Gamete: from Basic Knowledge to Clinical Applications.* Cache River Press, Vienna, IL, pp. 291–302.

Dale B, Marino M, Wilding M (1998) Soluble sperm factor, factors or receptors. *Molecular Human Reproduction* 5: 1–4.

Dale B, Monroy A (1981) How is polyspermy prevented? *Gamete Research* 4: 151–169.

Dale B, Tosti E, Iaccarino M (1995) Is the plasma membrane of the human oocyte reorganized following fertilisation and early cleavage? *Zygote* 3(1): 31–36.

Dale B, Wilding M, Coppola G, Tosti E (2010) How do spermatozoa activate oocytes. *Reproductive BioMedicine Online* 21: 1–3.

Davidson EH (1990) How embryos work: a comparative view of diverse modes of cell fate specification. *Development* 108: 365–389.

Eisenbach M, Ralt D (1992) Precontact mammalian sperm-egg communication and role in fertilization. *American Journal of Physiology* 262: 1095–1101.

Foltz KR, Lennarz WJ (1993) The molecular basis of sea urchin gamete interactions at the egg plasma membrane. *Developmental Biology* 158: 46–61.

Gianaroli L, Magli C, Ferraretti A, *et al.* (1996) Reducing the time of sperm-oocyte interaction in human IVF improves the implantation rate. *Human Reproduction* 11: 166–171.

Gianaroli L, Tosti E, Magli C, Ferrarreti A, Dale B (1994) The fertilization current in the human oocyte. *Molecular Reproduction and Development* 38: 209–214.

Gupta SK (2015) Role of zona pellucida glycoproteins during fertilization in humans. *Journal of Reproductive Immunology* 108: 90–97.

Gur Y, Breitbart H (2006) Mammalian sperm translate nuclear-encoded proteins by mitochondrial-type ribosomes. *Genes and Development* 20(4): 411–416.

Hertwig O (1876) Beiträge zur Kenntniss der Bildung, Befruchtung und Theilung des thierischen Eies. *Morphologische Jahrbuch* 1: 347–434.

Hewitson L, Simerley C, Schatten G (1999) ICSI: Unravelling the mysteries. *Nature Medicine* 5(4): 431–433.

Holubcova Z, Howard G, Schuh M (2013) Vesicles modulate an actin network for asymmetric spindle positioning. *Nature Cell Biology* 15: 937–947.

Holy J, Schatten G (1991) Spindle pole centrosomes of sea urchin embryos are partially composed of material recruited from maternal stores. *Developmental Biology* 147: 343–353.

Jaffe L (1980) Calcium explosions as triggers of development. *Annals of the New York Academy of Sciences* 339: 86–101.

Kinz G, Beil D, Deininger H, Wildt L, Leyendecker G (1996) The dynamics of rapid sperm transport through the female genital tract: evidence from vaginal sonography of uterine peristalsis and hysterosalpingoscintigraphy. *Human Reproduction* 11(3): 627–632.

Lanzafame F, Chapman M, Guglielmino A, Gearon CM, Forman RG (1994) Pharmacological stimulation of sperm motility. *Human Reproduction* 9(2): 192–194.

Lefèvre B (2008) The nucleolus of the maternal gamete is essential for life. *Bioassays* 30: 613–616.

Lefièvre L, Conner SJ, Salpekar A, *et al.* (2004) Four zona pellucida glycoproteins are expressed in the human. *Human Reproduction* 19: 1580–1586.

Lennarz WJ (1994) Fertilization in sea urchins: how many different molecules are involved in gamete interaction and fusion? *Zygote* 2(1): 1–4.

Maro B, Gueth-Hallonet C, Aghion J, Antony C (1991) Cell polarity and microtubule organization during mouse early embryogenesis. *Development Supplement* 10: 17–25.

Miller MR, Mansell SA, Meyers SA, Lishko PV (2015) Flagellar ion channels of sperm: similarities and differences between species. *Cell Calcium* 58: 105–113.

Myles DG (1992) Molecular mechanism of sperm-egg membrane binding and fusion in mammals. *Developmental Biology* 158: 35–45.

Nasr-Esfahani MH, Razavi S, Mardani M, Shirazi R, Javanmardi S (2007) Effects of failed oocyte activation and sperm protamine deficiency on fertilization post-ICSI. *Reproductive BioMedicine Online* 14(4): 422–429.

Ogushi S, Palmieri C, Fulka H, *et al.* (2008) The maternal nucleolus is essential for early embryonic development in mammals. *Science* 319: 613–616.

Patrat C, Auer J, Fauque P, *et al.* (2006) Zona pellucida from fertilised human oocytes induces a voltage-dependent calcium influx and the acrosome reaction in spermatozoa, but cannot be penetrated by sperm. *BMC Developmental Biology* 6: 59.

Ralt D, Goldenberg M, Fetterolf P, *et al.* (1991) Sperm attraction to a follicular factor(s) correlates with human egg fertilizability. *Proceedings of the National Academy of Sciences of the USA* 88: 2840–2844.

Reichmann J, Nijmeijer B, Hossein MJ (2018) Dual spindle formation in zygotes keeps parental genomes apart in early mammalian embryos. *Science* 361(6398): 189–193.

Sakkas D, Ramalingam M, Garrido N, Barratt CLR (2015) Sperm selection in natural conception: what can we learn from Mother Nature to improve assisted reproduction outcomes? *Human Reproduction Update* 21(6): 711–726.

Santella L, Alikani M, Talansky B, Cohen J, Dale B (1992) Is the human oocyte plasma membrane polarized? *Human Reproduction* 7: 999–1003.

Santella L, Dale B (2015). Assisted yes, but where do we draw the line? *Reproductive BioMedicine Online* 31: 476–478.

Schatten G, Simerly C, Schatten H (1991) Maternal inheritance of centrosomes in mammals; studies on parthenogenesis and polyspermy in mice. *Proceedings of the National Academy of Sciences of the USA* 88(15): 6785–6789.

Schulz MC, Leblond CP (1990) Nucleolar structure and synthetic activity during meiotic prophase and spermiogenesis in the rat. *American Journal of Anatomy* 189: 1–10.

Scott L, Alvero R, Leondires M, *et al.* (2000) The morphology of human pronuclear embryos is positively related to blastocyst development and implantation. *Human Reproduction* 15: 2394–2403.

Shapiro S (1987) The existential decision of a sperm. *Cell* 49: 293–294.

Simerly C, Wu G, Zoran S, *et al.* (1995) The paternal inheritance of the centrosome, the cell's microtubule-organising center, in humans and the implications of infertility. *Nature Medicine* 1: 47–53.

Spehr M, Schwane K, Riffell JA, *et al.* (2004) Particulate adenylate cyclase plays a key role in human sperm olfactory receptor-mediated chemotaxis. *Journal of Biological Chemistry* 279: 40194–40203.

Suarez SS, Pacey AA (2006) Sperm transport in the female reproductive tract. *Human Reproduction Update* 12(1): 23–27.

Sutovsky P, Navara CS, Schatten G (1996) Fate of the sperm mitochondria, and the incorporation, conversion, and disassembly of the sperm tail structures during bovine fertilization. *Biology of Reproduction* 55: 1195–1205.

Tanphaichitr N, Kongmanas K, Kruevaisayawan H, *et al.* (2015) Remodeling of the plasma membrane in preparation for sperm-egg recognition: roles of acrosomal proteins. *Asian Journal of Andrology* 17: 574–582.

Tesarik J, Greco E (1999) The probability of abnormal preimplantation development can be predicted by a single static observation on pronuclear stage morphology. *Human Reproduction* 14: 1318–1323.

Tesarik J, Kopecny V (1989a) Developmental control of the human male pronucleus by ooplasmic factors. *Human Reproduction* 4: 962–968.

Tesarik J, Kopecny V (1989b) Nucleic acid synthesis and development of human male pronucleus. *Journal of Reproduction and Fertility* 86: 549–558.

Tesarik J, Kopecny V (1989c) Development of human male pronucleus: ultrastructure and timing. *Gamete Research* 24: 135–149.

Tesarik J, Kopecny V, Plachot M, Mandelbaum J (1988) Early morphological signs of embryonic genome expression in human preimplantation development as revealed by quantitative electron microscopy. *Developmental Biology* 128: 15–20.

Tesarik J, Kopecny V, Plachot M, Mandelbaum J, Da Lage C, Fléchon J-E (1986) Nucleologenesis in the human embryo developing in vitro: ultrastructural and autoradiographic analysis. *Developmental Biology* 115: 193–203.

Tesarik I, Sousa M, Testart J (1994) Human oocyte activation after intracytoplasmic sperm injection. *Human Reproduction* 9: 511–514.

Tosti E (1994) Sperm activation in species with external fertilization. *Zygote* 2(4): 359–361.

van der Heijdn GW, Ramos L, Baart EB, *et al.* (2008) Sperm derived histones contribute to zygotic chromatin in humans. *BMC Developmental Biology* 8: 34.

Ward CR, Kopf GS (1993) Molecular events mediating sperm activation. *Developmental Biology* 158: 9–34.

Wassarman PM (1990) Profile of a mammalian sperm receptor. *Development* 108: 1–17.

Wassarman P (2014) Sperm protein finds its mate. *Nature* 508: 466–467.

Wassarman PM, Florman HM, Greve IM (1985) Receptor-mediated sperm-egg interactions in mammals. In: Metz CB, Monroy A (eds.) *Fertilization*, vol. 2. Academic Press, New York, pp. 341–360.

Wassarman PM, Liu C, Litscher ES (1996) Constructing the mammalian egg zona pellucida: some new pieces of an old puzzle. *Journal of Cell Science* 109: 2001–2004.

Weindling PJ (1991) *Darwinism and Social Darwinism in Imperial Germany: The Contribution of the Cell Biologist Oscar Hertwig (1849–1922)*. G. Fischer Verlag, Stuttgart, p. 71.

Zumoffen CM, Massa E, Caille AM, Munuce MJ, Ghersevich SA (2015) Effects of lactoferrin, a protein present in the female reproductive tract, on parameters of human sperm capacitation and gamete interaction. *Andrology* 3: 1068–1075.

# First Stages of Development

## Preimplantation Development

After completing fertilization with fusion of the pronuclei during syngamy, the zygote now has a diploid complement of chromosomes, undergoes its first mitotic division and then continues to divide by mitosis into a number of smaller cells known as blastomeres. In humans, the first few cleavage divisions take place in the oviduct, before the embryo reaches its site of implantation in the uterus (Figure 5.1).

In contrast to oogenesis, where the cell undergoes a period of growth without replication or division, early embryo cleavage involves intense DNA replication and cell division in the absence of growth; the overall size of the embryo does not change as a result of the early cleavage divisions. As cleavage progresses, the embryo polarizes, and differences arise between the blastomeres; this process of differentiation may be regulated by unequal distributions of cytoplasmic components previously laid down in the

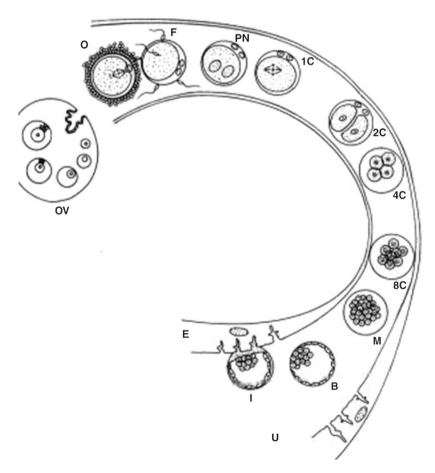

**Figure 5.1** Development of the mammalian embryo. The oocytes released from the ovary (OV) enter the ampulla where they are fertilized (F) and then are transported along the fallopian tube, cleaving to generate the morula stage (M). The blastocyst(B) expands, hatches and then implants (I) in the endometrium (E) of the uterus (U). From Sathananthan *et al.* (1993), with permission.

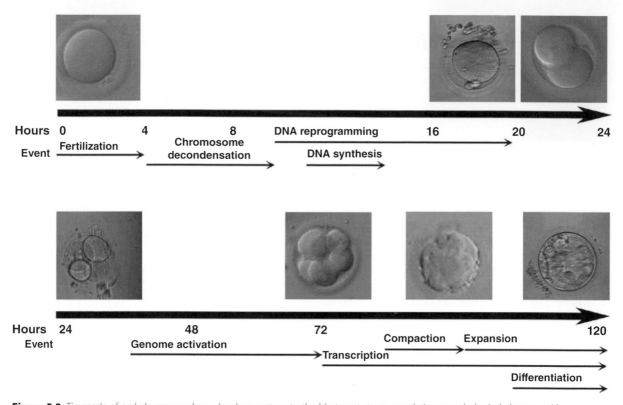

Hours  0          4         8    DNA reprogramming     16      20      24

Event  Fertilization       Chromosome           decondensation      DNA synthesis

Hours  24          48        72      Compaction   Expansion     120

Event         Genome activation        Transcription                  Differentiation

**Figure 5.2** Timescale of early human embryo development up to the blastocyst stage, correlating morphological changes with developmental events. Time is in hours.

oocyte during oogenesis, or by changes occurring in the blastomeres as a result of new embryonic gene transcription during development (Figure 5.2). Each blastomere nucleus will be subjected to a different cytoplasmic environment, which, in turn, may differentially influence activity of the genome. As a result, after the onset of zygote gene activation and subsequent differentiation, eventually the blastomeres set off on their own specific program of development. Maternal mRNA encoding developmental information is essential in early differentiation and has been found to persist during specific patterns of gene expression until gastrulation in some species; embryos in some bats and marsupials can remain in a state of diapause (dormancy) within the uterine cavity for many months. In mammals, maternal mRNA rapidly disappears after the major activation of the genome, i.e., at the two-cell stage in the mouse, four- to six-cell in humans, and eight-cell in sheep and cattle. Localized short- and long-lived maternal mRNAs probably regulate the initial stages of differentiation; there is some evidence to suggest that stores of maternal RNA in the oocytes of older women may be depleted, perhaps due to dysfunction or disruption of the mechanisms that control its storage.

## Genome Activation

As described in Chapter 3, the developing oocyte accumulates reserves of mRNA, proteins, organelles, etc. These maternal transcripts and proteins are required to support and direct early development, and are progressively degraded as the new embryonic genome is increasingly transcribed. In vitro, the early embryo shows very little metabolic activity during its first few cleavage divisions. Stored maternal mRNA directs the first two cleavage divisions, and then activation of the new embryonic genome provides novel transcripts and reprograms the pattern of gene expression to direct further development. After the long period of gene suppression in both gametes, the new embryonic cell cycle must be precisely timed and regulated, with a correct timing of DNA synthesis during S-phase. The cycle during which the zygote genome is activated is always the longest cell cycle of preimplantation development: any delay at this time may cause the level of mRNA to fall below a critical threshold, and without appropriate zygotic genome activation (ZGA), the mammalian embryo fails to develop further. This critical transition takes place during the four-to eight-cell stage in humans, and maternal mRNA rapidly disappears whilst the zygote genome gradually increases its expression. However, the transition is not absolute; maternal transcripts are degraded at different rates, and the stability of the maternally encoded proteins vary, so that some maternal information may still contribute to embryonic development after the embryonic genome is activated. A small amount of maternal message is needed almost up until the blastocyst stage; therefore, previous failures at any stage of oocyte development, maturation and handling can affect development even after ZGA. Gene expression involves conformational changes in nucleosome organization (like uncoiling a spring), regulated by interactions among DNA methylation, histone acetylation and messenger RNA polyadenylation patterns. Activation of the embryonic genome follows a series of progressive steps; the timing and coordination of gene expression can be regulated at the level of maternal mRNA translation. The newly formed embryonic genome undergoes extensive epigenetic modifications that result in a program of gene expression that is highly regulated. Any disruption during these initial steps can have a far-reaching impact on embryo development.

1. Maternal RNA transcripts are depleted, and new embryonic mRNA is transcribed. The replacement of maternal transcripts by those of the zygote occurs at different rates for different genes; this may be due to the relative importance of different transcripts for immediate developmental events, or because the protein products differ in their stability, or both. The expression of approximately 1800 mRNAs is modulated during the first 3 days of development; the majority are downregulated or destroyed, a small number are upregulated on days 1 and 2, and a large group of mRNAs become increasingly abundant on Day 3 (Dobson et al., 2004); there may represent preferentially stable mRNAs in the pool of maternal mRNA that is being degraded.

2. There is a qualitative shift in protein synthesis and in post-translational modification.

3. A functional nucleosomal structure develops, the nuclear organizing region (NOR).

Establishing the precise timing of genome activation is related to the sensitivity of methods available for its detection; new protein synthesis activity has been detected at different stages in different species:

| Rabbit | 1–2 cells |
|---|---|
| Mouse | 2 cells |
| Cow | 4–8 cells |
| Human | 4 cells |
| Sheep | 8–16 cells |
| Drosophila | 4000 cells |
| Xenopus | 5000 cells |

Recent transcriptome analysis has shown that gene expression during ZGA is carefully orchestrated: genes involved in transcription and RNA metabolism are highly expressed (Hamatani et al., 2004; Wang et al., 2004; Zeng & Schultz, 2004), and most of the newly synthesized ZGA transcripts are quickly translated (Flach et al., 1982). Epigenetic chromatin remodeling has been proposed as the main mechanism regulating the ZGA: epigenetic marks involve post-translational modifications of nucleosomal histones (methylation, acetylation, phosphorylation and ubiquitination), DNA methylation and non-histone proteins that bind to chromatin.

There is evidence to suggest that a minor degree of transcriptional activity does take place prior to the major activation of the genome, with a period of minor gene activation from the paternal pronucleus in the one-cell embryo, followed by a period of gene activation in the two-cell embryo when maternal mRNA and zygotic gene transcripts are handled differently, so that transcription and translation of nascent transcripts is delayed (Wiekowski et al., 1991; Nothias et al., 1995; Schultz, 2002). In human preimplantation embryos, reverse transcriptase-polymerase chain reaction (RT-PCR) detected early transcripts for two paternal Y chromosome genes, ZFY and SRY. ZFY transcripts were detected at the pronucleate stage, 20–24 hours after in-vitro insemination, and at intermediate stages up to the blastocyst stage. SRY transcripts were also detected at two-cell to blastocyst stages (Ao et al., 1994).

In 1938, the Carnegie Institution of Washington funded a 7-year study with the aim of finding and characterizing early embryos recovered from fertile married women undergoing therapeutic hysterectomy. Over a period of 15 years, Arthur Hertig and John Rock examined excised fallopian tubes and uteri, allowing them to describe 34 embryos aged up to 17 days post-fertilization: the earliest were at the two-cell stage, and the latest were undergoing gastrulation (Hertig *et al.*, 1954, 1956). Their analyses led them to make several key observations about the dynamics of fertilization and early embryo development, as well as providing insight into rates of embryo loss after natural conception.

Cleavage increases the number of nuclei, which amplifies the number of templates that will facilitate the production of specialized proteins needed for the later processes of compaction and differentiation to the blastocyst stage. As mentioned above, changes in chromatin structure, rather than changes in the activity of the transcriptional apparatus, may underlie the timing and basis for ZGA. Transcription factors must be available that can bind to the DNA, and a functional physical structure, the NOR develops, producing conformational changes in the DNA structure that will allow the binding of promoters and enhancers of transcription. In the mouse and rabbit, there is a general chromatin-mediated repression of promoter activity. Repression factors are inherited by the maternal pronucleus from the oocyte, but are absent in the paternal pronucleus; they become available sometime during the transition from a late one-cell to a two-cell embryo (Henery *et al.*, 1995). This means that paternally inherited genes are exposed to a different environment in fertilized eggs than are maternally inherited genes, a situation that could contribute to genomic imprinting.

The formation of the NOR is related to the nuclear:cytoplasmic ratio. A titratable factor in the cytoplasm, possibly related to cdc25, may be diluted with the increase in nuclear:cytoplasmic ratio, driving maturation promoting factor (MPF) and a kinase cascade that triggers mitosis. The gradual depletion of cdc25 causes a pause in cleavage, which allows time for the NOR to develop, and mitosis induces a general repression of promoters prior to initiation of zygotic gene expression. Enhancers then specifically release this repression. A biological clock may delay transcription until both paternal and maternal genomes are replicated; they must then be remodeled from a postmeiotic state to one in which transcription is repressed by chromatin structure. The chromatin structure must have a configuration that allows specific transcription enhancers to relieve/reverse repression at appropriate times during development. Differential hyperacetylation of histone H4 (particularly on DNA in the male pronucleus) has been implicated in the remodeling of maternal and paternal chromatin, and depletion of maternally derived histones has also been suggested as one of the mechanisms involved in ZGA (Adenot *et al.*, 1997).

Chromatin-mediated repression of promoter activity prior to ZGA is similar to that observed during *Xenopus* embryogenesis; this mechanism ensures that genes are not expressed until the appropriate time in development. When the time is right, positive factors such as enhancers can begin their activity. The mechanism by which enhancers communicate with promoters seems to change during development and may depend upon the presence of specific co-activators. In the mouse, ZGA occurs during the second cell division cycle (two-cell stage) and seems to be regulated by a 'zygotic clock' that measures the time following fertilization rather than progression through the first cell cycle. There is evidence that circadian clock genes may be involved in programming an appropriate timing, so that development is synchronized with endocrine and other local factors to ensure successful implantation. In support of this concept, expression of circadian clock genes has been found in the reproductive tract and conceptus of the mouse during the first 4 days of pregnancy (Johnson *et al.*, 2002). It may be that in vivo, mammalian ZGA is a time-dependent mechanism that must interact in synchrony with the cell cycle and other physiological events.

In human embryos, the major wave of genome activation occurs on Day 3, independent of cell number: embryos that arrest with fewer than eight cells still show evidence of ZGA (Dobson *et al.*, 2004). This corresponds to the first wave of ZGA in mice, at 26–29 hours post fertilization (Vassena *et al.*, 2011). Further changes in morphology, i.e., compaction and cavitation, also depend on timing of development, rather than cell number – irrespective of lysis or fragmentation of one or more blastomeres. Inherited maternal/paternal factors have a significant influence on zygote development, including those that mediate RNA metabolism/translation and cytokinesis as well as ploidy and epigenetic factors. During further development, the embryo's morphology, physiology and metabolism are shaped by an interplay between its genotype and its response to environmental factors. The human embryo is exquisitely sensitive to environmental signals and shows a high degree of plasticity by modulating its metabolism, gene expression and rate of cell division. This developmental plasticity, with effects on gene methylation and expression, has the potential to influence later health and well-being in postnatal life (Bateson *et al.*, 2004; Rosenbloom, 2018).

## Imprinting

During oogenesis and spermatogenesis, the maternal and paternal chromosomes are packaged in a manner that affects subsequent transcription of some of the genes during development. The DNA sequence that specifies the parental genes is not altered, but the way in which it is chemically modified and packaged in chromatin affects the expression of the genes. Because the genetic code itself remains the same, this modification is referred to as an epigenetic change, and the phenomenon is known as imprinting. The pattern of epigenetic change is parentally specific, i.e., the genes affected (imprinted) in oocytes differ from those imprinted in sperm – there is differential expression of the two parental alleles of a gene. In terms of function, this means that although the oocyte and the sperm each contribute a complete set of genes, each set on its own is not competent to direct a complete program of development; a fully functional genome requires the combination of both paternal and maternal genes. The process of genomic imprinting is established during gametogenesis, and the nucleus of the zygote has an imprint memory that is retained by the embryo into both prenatal and postnatal life. Imprinting is highly regulated during preimplantation development; the topic is thus highly significant and relevant to in-vitro manipulations and culture, and will be discussed in detail in Chapter 15.

## Compaction

The first event that determines the directed development of previously undifferentiated blastomeres is compaction. During the first few cleavage divisions to reach the four- to eight-cell stage, individual blastomeres can be clearly seen in the developing embryo. At about the third cleavage division there is

a significant increase in RNA and protein synthesis, a marked change in the patterns of phospholipid synthesis, and the embryo undergoes compaction to form a morula. During this transition as the embryo is compacting, it must also make fundamental decisions regarding cell position, polarity and fate. The process is calcium-dependent, and requires prior transcription of the zygote genome. With compaction, the blastomeres flatten against each other and begin to form junctions between them, so that the boundaries between blastomeres can no longer be distinguished. The cells of the compacted embryo become highly polarized and tightly associated, with redistribution of surface microvilli and other plasma membrane components.

Coordination of these complex developmental processes requires communication between the cells; two types of intercellular junction have been described:

1. Structural tight junctions and desmosomes anchor the cells together and form an impermeable epithelial barrier between cells. Tight junctions are composed of several integral and peripheral proteins, including occludin and cingulin (ZO-1).
2. Low-resistance junctions such as gap junctions allow the flow of electrical current and the direct transfer of small molecules, including metabolites and second messengers (cAMP) between blastomeres.

Compaction has been extensively studied in the mouse: the distribution of dense microvillar and amicrovillar regions indicates surface polarity, and the distribution of endocytotic vesicles and actin filaments, as well as the location of the cell nucleus, demonstrates polarity in the cytoplasm. In the mouse, isolated blastomeres that are decompacted experimentally maintain their polarity, and compaction does not require either a prior round of DNA replication or protein synthesis (Kidder and McLachlin, 1985). Therefore, the four-cell embryo probably contains some of the proteins required for compaction. Although the factors that trigger the timing of its onset are not known, experimental evidence suggests that this may be regulated by post-translational modification of specific proteins such as E-cadherin. E-cadherin protein (uvomorulin) is expressed in the oocyte, and during all stages of preimplantation development. It is uniformly distributed on the surface of blastomeres and accumulates in the regions of intercellular contact during compaction. E-cadherin phosphorylation can be observed in the mouse eight-cell embryo. Culturing embryos in calcium-free medium inhibits E-cadherin phosphorylation and prevents compaction, but the situation is complex, and precise mechanisms behind the molecular basis for compaction and its timing remain unclear.

In human embryos, tight junctions begin to appear on Day 3, at the 6- to 10-cell stage, heralding the onset of compaction. The surface morphology of human oocytes and embryos has been studied with scanning electron microscopy (Santella *et al.*, 1992; Dale *et al.*, 1995; Nikas *et al.*, 1996), and this showed that unfertilized oocytes 1 day after insemination were evenly and densely covered with long microvilli. The length and density of microvilli appeared to decrease in fertilized oocytes, and a further decrease was observed in Day 2 and Day 3 embryos with 2–12 cells. There was no evidence of surface polarity until Day 4, when it was evident in the majority of embryos with 10 or more cells. The microvilli appeared dense again with a polarized distribution over the free surface of the compacted blastomeres.

In the mouse, gap junctions are expressed at the eight-cell stage, and their de novo assembly during compaction is a time-dependent event. Inhibition of DNA synthesis during the third and fourth cell cycles has no effect on the establishment of gap junctional coupling during compaction (Valdimarsson and Kidder, 1995), but a delay of 10 hours in DNA synthesis during the second cell cycle results in the failure of gap junctional coupling at the time of compaction.

In human embryos, gap junctions are not apparently well developed until the early blastocyst stage, when intercellular communication is clearly seen between inner cell mass (ICM) cells (Figures 5.3 and 5.4; Dale *et al.*, 1991).

Following compaction, the developing embryo is described as a morula, seen in the human normally 4 days after fertilization. The embryo now shows a significant increase and change of pattern in RNA, protein and phospholipid synthesis, and this results in a process of differentiation so that cells are now allocated to an ICM, with outer cells forming an epithelial layer of trophectoderm. Whereas early

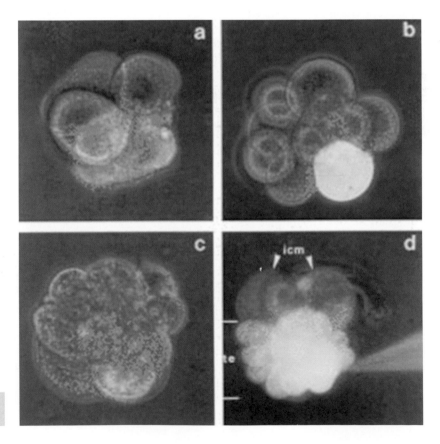

**Figure 5.3** Functional expression of gap junctions in the early human embryo shown by micro injection of the low molecular weight tracer lucifer yellow. There is no dye spread in four cells (a), ten cells (b) or morula (c). However, transfer occurs in the blastocyst stage (d). icm = inner cell mass. Reproduced with permission from Dale *et al.* (1991).

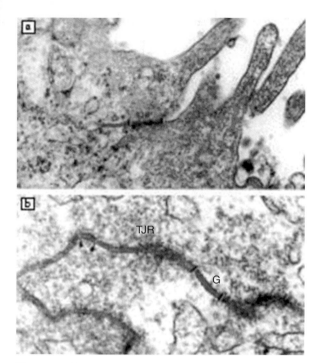

**Figure 5.4** Transmission electron micrographs showing tight junctions (TJR) and gap junctions (G) in the human morula. (a) is a section at the apical level between two polar cells at a magnification of ×75 500; (b) shows a typical section between a polar and an apolar cell at ×158 000. Arrowheads show sites of tight membrane contact. Reproduced with permission from Gualtieri *et al.* (1992).

blastomeres are totipotent (as evidenced by experimental embryo splitting and chimera formation), at compaction the cells polarize radially, and differential division across this axis creates different populations of cells, with unequal distributions of organelles:

1. Outer polar cells with surface microvilli and redistribution of other plasma membrane components are restricted to the free outer surface of the embryo, and these cells form the trophectoderm.

2. Inner apolar cells with tight junctions containing basal nuclei, which will form the ICM.

These morphological transitions are thought to be brought about by differential gene expression with corresponding protein expression profiles, but these have not yet been clearly defined at the molecular level. Experimental interference with adhesion between cells during compaction shows that this process is important in determining cell lineages. ICM cells preferentially communicate with each other and not with trophectoderm cells via gap junctions, whereas trophectoderm cells communicate with each other and

not with ICM cells. The ratio of trophectoderm to ICM cells can be influenced by culture conditions in vitro, and this might have implications for further embryonic/fetal development.

## Cavitation

Between the 16- and 32-cell stage, a second morphological change occurs, known as cavitation. The trophectoderm is the first cell to differentiate after ZGA, and these polarized blastomeres compact to construct functional complexes of junctions and systems that can then transport ions and water to fill the blastocoelic cavity with fluid. Activation of $Na^+$, $K^+$ ATP-ase systems in the trophectoderm cells results in energy-dependent active transport of sodium pumped into the central area of the embryo, followed by osmotically driven passive movement of water to form a fluid-filled cavity, the blastocoele. The movement of other ions such as chloride and bicarbonate also contributes to blastocoele formation. Immuno-histochemistry shows that the trophectoderm cells are sitting on a basement membrane, and tight junctions form a continuous belt between trophectoderm cells, preventing leakage of small ions in the blastocoelic fluid.

Blastocoele formation and expansion is critical for further development, as it is essential for further differentiation of the ICM. This is now bathed in a specific fluid medium, which may contain factors and proteins that will influence cell proliferation and differentiation. The position of cells within the ICM in relation to the fluid cavity might also contribute to the differentiation of the outer cells into primitive endodermal cells.

Apoptosis can be seen at the blastocyst stage, localized to the ICM: this may represent a mechanism for the elimination of inappropriate or defective cells.

The trophectoderm cells will eventually form the placenta and extraembryonic tissue. Myxoploidy of trophectoderm cells is a common feature in all animal species, regardless of their implantation mechanisms; mouse and cow, which differ completely in their mechanism of implantation, show this feature, with chromosome complements of 2n, 4n, 8n in their trophectoderm cells. However, in humans it could possibly be considered as the initiation of syncytio-trophoblast formation. The regulation of this process, and apparent lack of division in these cells, remains a mystery – but it seems to be related to the appearance of giant cells in the trophectoderm, suggesting that regulation of the nuclear/cytoplasmic ratio is involved. It is interesting to note that there is a counterpart of 'giant cells' in the uterus around the time of implantation. A retroviral syncytin envelope gene with cell–cell fusion activity has been identified in mammalian syncytiotrophoblast, and is postulated to be responsible for syncytiotrophoblast formation (Heidmann *et al.*, 2009).

## Blastocyst Expansion and Hatching

The embryo is enclosed in the zona pellucida during these early stages of development, keeping the cells together prior to compaction and acting as a protective barrier. If the ICM divides at this early stage, monozygotic (identical) twins may develop.

In humans, the early blastocyst (Day 4/5) initially shows no increase in size, and a cavity representing <30% of its volume is visible. It subsequently expands over the next 1 or 2 days (Day 5/6) by active accumulation of fluid in the central blastocoelic cavity, which expands to form 70% of the embryo volume. Blastocyst expansion is driven by the trophectoderm, as described above.

Time-lapse imaging reveals that expansion is a dynamic process, with pulses of oscillating contraction/blastocoel collapse/recovery at intervals of 2 to 4 hours (Huang *et al.*, 2016). Variations between different embryos can be seen, particularly at later

times during the periods of expansion. The data further suggest that periodicity and amplitude of oscillations may be modulated by the zona pellucida: embryo-specific variations in expansion kinetics may reflect variations in the zona. Rates of blastocyst expansion were found to correlate with viability/implantation, with stronger contractions related to impaired zona hatching, i.e., inadequate recovery from blastocoel contraction may jeopardize hatching and subsequent implantation. Blastocyst expansion could thus represent an in-vitro 'stress test' of embryo viability, confirming that this feature is a useful tool in selection of embryos for transfer (see Chapter 11).

Before the blastocyst can start the process of implantation, it must free itself from the protective zona pellucida, which becomes visibly thinner as the late blastocyst expands; in vitro, initiation of the hatching process can be seen as trophectoderm cells 'escaping' from the zona pellucida (Figure 5.5). Hatching is completed within a few hours, and the freed blastocyst is separated from its empty zona (see also Chapter 11, Figure 11.8).

## Cell Fate and Cell Lineages

The fate of each blastomere is influenced by mechanisms that achieve a balance between pluripotency and differentiation; the expression of lineage-specific genes differs between different species. At the earliest stages of development, the transcriptional machinery

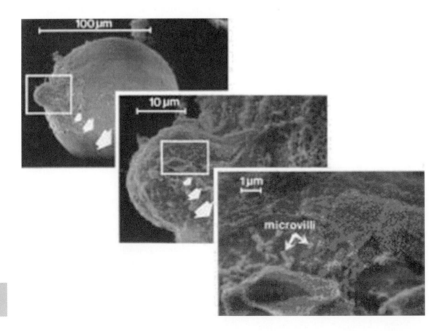

**Figure 5.5** Scanning electron micrograph of a hatching human embryo. The microvilli on the surface of the trophectoderm cells are bared owing to internal pressure in the blastocoel and dissolution of the zona pellucida.

that will direct differentiation is not switched on, and transcription is under the control of specific transcriptional regulators, regulatory RNAs and chromatin remodeling machinery, which are in turn influenced by epigenetic marks, cell positional history, cell polarity and orientation of division. As discussed in Chapter 3, the mammalian oocyte has evidence of polarity, and this has been confirmed in human oocytes. Maternal factors are subsequently important in establishing polarities, regulating cleavage planes and in allocating specific blastomeres to their eventual fate. By the morula stage, cell fate decisions have been made, and an axis is established with embryonic (ICM) and abembryonic (trophectoderm) poles. Cells positioned on the inside of the morula retain pluripotency, and those on the outside develop into extraembryonic trophectoderm which will support the development of the embryo in the uterus and influence embryonic patterning before gastrulation via signaling mechanisms. The generation of inside cells requires outer cells to divide in an orientation such that one daughter cell is directed inwards during the 8- to 16-cell and 16- to 32-cell stages; these divisions are known as differentiative, in contrast to conservative divisions in which both daughter cells remain on the outside. Because inside and outside cells will follow different fates, differentiative divisions probably distribute cell fate-determining factors asymmetrically between the daughters. Several molecules that influence polarization have been identified: the $Ca^{2+}$-dependent E-cadherin molecule is implicated in generating blastomere polarity, localized geographically at division together with the actin microfilament stabilizing protein ezrin. Homologues of PAR (partitioning defective proteins) also influence the regulation of cell polarization and the control of asymmetric cell divisions via positioning effects on the spindle. The transcription factor Cdx2 is required for the commitment of outer cells to the trophoblast (see Chapter 7).

The molecular basis for the generation and stabilization of polarity in development is not fully understood, but evidence is accumulating to suggest that cell fate may be determined as early as the four-cell stage in human embryos: mRNAs specific for a trophectoderm lineage (beta-hCG) were identified in a single blastomere of a four-cell embryo, and not at the two-cell stage; a single putative trophectodermal precursor appears to emerge during the second cleavage division (Hansis *et al.*, 2002; Edwards and Hansis,

2005). In mouse embryos, lineage tracing experiments using fluorescent tracers and optional sectioning indicate that differences in developmental properties of individual blastomeres may be determined at the two-cell stage (Piotrowska *et al.*, 2001; Piotrowska-Nitsche *et al.*, 2005). These experiments showed that the first cell to divide to the four-cell stage contributed preferentially to the embryonic cell lineage, whereas the later-dividing blastomere contributed to the abembryonic (trophectoderm) lineage. By the blastocyst stage, the position of cells within regions of the blastocyst has an influence on their subsequent fate in postimplantation development (Gardner, 2001, 2007).

Although transcription in human blastomeres has been found to be similar up to the precompaction eight-cell stage, it is possible that they are already programmed to express lineage-associated genes (Galan *et al.*, 2010; Wong *et al.*, 2010). Single-cell RNA sequencing and analysis of protein distribution in human and mouse embryos from the zygote to the eight-cell stage revealed transcriptional programs that are conserved between the species, as well as some that are specific to human embryos (Blakeley *et al.* 2015). In a further study, CRISPR-Cas9 genome editing that targeted the OCT 4 gene (*POU5F1*) in mouse and human zygotes revealed that the loss of OCT 4 affects human and mouse embryos differently: the targeted human embryos initiated blastocyst formation, but the ICM formed poorly, and the embryos subsequently collapsed. The mutation downregulated both extraembryonic trophectoderm genes (*CDX2*) and those that regulate the pluripotent epiblast, including *NANOG*. OCT4-targeted mouse embryos continued to blastocyst development and maintained their expression of genes such as *NANOG* (Fogarty *et al.*, 2017). These studies suggest that OCT4 has a different function in humans than in mice and is required earlier in human blastocyst development: its expression can be detected during cleavage and morula stages.

The ICM is a transitory state, and before the blastocyst implants into the uterine wall, its cells diverge into either early epiblast (E) or hypoblast/primitive endoderm (PE, see Chapter 6). The mechanisms of segregation have been extensively studied in the mouse, and Roode *et al.* (2012) observed that human embryos segregate PE by mechanisms that differ from those identified in mouse, rat and cow embryos, suggesting that the specification of cell lineages is different in different species. Glinsky *et al.* (2018)

identified multilineage precursor cells emerging in human embryos at the morula stage on Day 4 that were sustained up to Day 7 of development. These cells were described as having a Multilineage-Markers-Expression phenotype (MLME cells); they suggest that lineage specification thus begins prior to the ICM stage, and that MLME cells congregate in the ICM, where they continue differentiation into more specialized cell types.

It is important to recognize that each step in the creation of a blastocyst is dependent upon the previous step, with new avenues for interaction between the cell populations leading to ever-increasing complexity of the embryo. In vitro, manipulations and culture environment have the potential for disrupting the highly sophisticated and carefully orchestrated events necessary for normal development and implantation.

## Preimplantation Development in Mouse and Human Embryos

Although mouse and human embryos appear similar in morphology during their early post-fertilization development, key molecular differences in gene expression patterns and in developmental timing have been identified (Niakan & Eggan, 2013). The centrosome structure is contributed by the oocyte in the mouse, and by the sperm cell in humans. The pattern of DNA methylation and X-inactivation also differs between the two species (Fulka *et al.* 2004). Human embryos are far more susceptible to genetic instability than are mouse embryos, and numerous studies have revealed significant differences in cell cycle regulation, control of apoptosis and cytokine expression. Some of the established differences are summarized in Table 5.1 and Figure 5.6.

## Causes of Early Embryo Arrest

Cleaved embryos do frequently arrest their development in culture, and a great deal of research has been carried out in animal systems to elucidate possible causes and mechanisms. Studies conducted over the past 15 years continue to reveal that cultured embryos show significant changes in their patterns of gene expression. These changes affect not only survival during the preimplantation period but may also affect the ability of the embryo to implant and continue through normal fetal development. They may also have an impact on post-partum health and susceptibility to disease in later life. Understanding the mechanisms and signaling pathways involved in the embryo's response to culture environments is of paramount importance in minimizing potential hazards to normal human preimplantation development in vitro. Differences observed in gene expression patterns between cultured and in-vivo-derived embryos may be due to changes in gene transcription, or to changes in mechanisms that cells use to regulate mRNA stability and half-life.

The longest cell division cycle during development is that during which genome activation takes place, when maternal transcripts are degraded and massive synthesis of embryonic transcripts is initiated. Maternal reserves are normally sufficient until transcription begins, but epigenetic effects of defective sperm can lead to accumulation of delays, with resulting arrested development. Antisperm antibodies can have deleterious effects at this stage, by immunoneutralization of proteins that signal division (CS-1) or regulation (Oct-3). After genome activation, the next critical stage is morula/blastocyst transition. Complex remodeling takes place, and poor sperm quality can compromise this transition (see Ménézo and Janny, 1997).

Embryonic arrest is frequently a result of events surrounding maturation but can be a result of any metabolic problem. In bovine and pig oocytes, insufficient glutathione inhibits decondensation of the sperm head and polar body formation, and genetic factors regulate the speed of preimplantation development. Genetic factors implicate enzyme deficiencies or dysfunctional regulation, which may have deleterious effects. In domestic animals, as in humans, there is an age-related maternal effect. Maternal age has an effect on embryo quality, especially on blastocyst formation – this may be related to an ATPase-dependent $Na^+/K^+$ pump mechanism, or to a poor stock of mRNA, poor transcriptional and/or post-transcriptional regulation or accelerated turnover of mRNA.

In clinical IVF, detection of two pronuclei is regarded as evidence that normal fertilization has taken place, and the formation of a normal mitotic spindle following fertilization is critical in order to ensure correct chromosomal alignment. Mistakes at this stage can be lethal, resulting in chromosomal disorders such as aneuploidy. In some cases a first cleavage division takes place when no pronuclei have

**Table 5.1** Comparison of human and mouse preimplantation development

| Parameter | Human | Mouse |
| --- | --- | --- |
| Average cell cycle time | 13–16 hrs | 10 hrs |
| Average embryo diameter | 140 μm (Volume = 8× that of mouse) | 70 μm |
| Zygotic gene expression | 4–8 cell stage, D3 | 2-cell stage, D1–2 |
| Waves of transcription | MII – 4c, maternal genes only 8c-blastocyst: maternal genes downregulated, zygotic genes upregulated | 2-cell: genes required for transcription & RNA processing 4–8 cell: genes involved in morphology & function |
| Compaction | 8–16 cell stage, D4 | Late 8-cell stage, D3 |
| Cavitation | From 35 cells, D4 to early D5 | From 32 cells, D3.25 |
| Blastocyst formation | 108–136 hrs; 64–100 cells, late D5 128–256 cells, early to late D6 >256 cells | 84–96 hrs; <64 cells D3.5 >64 cells D3.75 to D4.25 ~164 cells |
| Oct4 expression | 7-8c, D3; required for blastocyst formation Persistently expressed in TE, downregulated in a subset of PE cells, restricted to ICM on D6 | 4c, D2; downregulated in TE by D4.5, not required for blastocyst formation |
| GATA2 & 3 expression | Trophoblast of late blastocysts | Cleavage stage in all cells, then restricted to outer trophoblast in late blastocysts |
| Segregation of epiblast/hypoblast from ICM | D7; not dependent on FGF signaling | D4.5; dependent on FGF signaling, involves NANOG and Gata6 |
| Epiblast morphology | Flattened bilaminar disc | Cup-like egg cylinder |
| Implantation | Between D6 and D8 TE cells form invasive cytotrophoblast (CT) cells; CT cells proliferate & differentiate in placental villi: Multinucleated syncytial cells Extravillous trophoblast cells that invade uterine decidua | Day 4–4.5 Minimal early invasion; TE cells form early proliferative cells adjacent to the epiblast Polyploid trophoblast giant cells are budded off through endoreduplication, giving rise to extraembryonic ectoderm |
| Stem cell doubling time | 30–35 hrs | 12–15 hrs |
| Maintenance of stem cell lines | Does not require LIF | LIF-dependent |

been detected during the previous 24–28 hours, a phenomenon that has been described as 'silent fertilization.' The first cell division tends to be asymmetrical, and the embryos arrest during cleavage. Van Blerkom *et al.* (2004) undertook a multi-year study of oocytes and embryos in which silent fertilization was suspected, using scanning laser confocal fluorescence microscopy to study chromosomal and microtubular structures. They were able to visualize maternally and paternally derived spindles in embryos that had

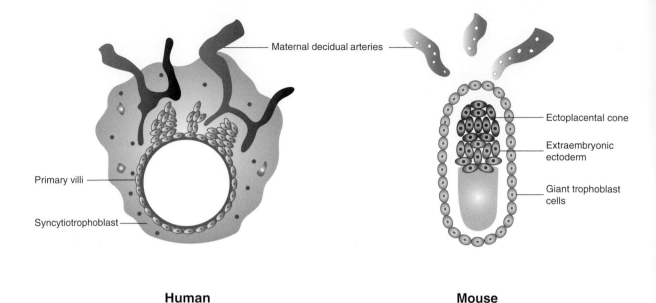

**Human**    **Mouse**

**Figure 5.6** Comparison of human and mouse peri-implantation development. Left panel: early human postimplantation development, with syncytiotrophoblast and primary villi. Right: early mouse postimplantation development, with extraembryonic ectoderm and ectoplacental cone. Reproduced with permission from Baines & Renaud (2017), with thanks to Alejandra Ontiveros.

shown no sign of pronuclear evolution after multiple, closely spaced inspections at the 1-cell stage, with maternal and paternal spindles well separated. The authors suggest that the evolution of such embryos may have an unusual pattern of chromosomal segregation, leading to micro- or multinucleation. The mechanisms involved in silent fertilization could be due to defects in normal calcium signaling, inadequate cytoplasmic maturity or delayed release of sperm-derived factors that also modulate calcium signaling.

Fluorescent in-situ hybridization (FISH) analysis of cleaved human embryos has confirmed that chromosomal aberrations are found in a significant proportion of embryos which develop with regular cleavage and morphology; this undoubtedly contributes to the high wastage of embryos in human IVF.

## Paternal Factors

Sperm quality may have an influence on embryogenesis and implantation potential. Increasing paternal age is thought to have an influence on fertility, possibly through increased nondisjunction in the sperm. Damage during spermatogenesis may be induced by reactive oxygen species and defective oxidative phosphorylation, or via inherited dysfunctional mitochondrial DNA. Fertilization by a sperm that is diploid, with incomplete decondensation and DNA activation or inadequate chromatin packaging, may cause aneuploidy or lack of genome competence in the embryo. The quality of condensation and packaging of sperm DNA are important factors for the initiation of human embryo development, even after ICSI. The centrosome, involved in microtubular organization, is the first epigenetic contribution of the sperm, and correct and harmonious microtubule arrangement is necessary for chromosome segregation and pronuclear migration. An abnormal sperm carrying an imperfect centrosome can disrupt mitosis, provoking problems at the beginning of embryogenesis with the formation of fragments, abnormal chromosome distribution and early cleavage arrest. Up to 25% of apparently unfertilized eggs may show signs of having initiated fertilization, but then have anomalies that prevent cell division. In bulls, there is a positive correlation between sperm aster formation at the time of fertilization and the bull's fertility. In the human, paternal Y-linked genes are transcribed as early as the zygote stage, and compromised paternal genetic material could be transcribed at even this early stage, causing fertilization failure or embryonic arrest. Finally, as discussed in Chapter 3, spermatozoa lacking in or with defective oocyte activating factor may only partially activate oocytes and lead to abortive development.

## Metabolic Requirements of the Early Mammalian Embryo in Vitro

Maternal oocyte reserves that are stored during the maturation process must be capable of supporting metabolism in the early embryo prior to ZGA. Genes coding for all of the required enzymes must be expressed with correct timing and in the appropriate equilibrium. There must also be an effective mechanism for repairing damaged DNA in the oocyte and sperm; an estimated 1.5 to 2 million repair operations are performed during the first cell cycle, and these are dependent upon adequate maternal reserves of mRNA, proteins, organelles, etc.

When the oocyte is fertilized and starts the process of transcription, the new embryo must maintain equilibrium between many different parameters:

1. The endogenous pool of metabolites, largely the result of final stages of oocyte maturation
2. Metabolic turnover of RNA messengers and proteins
3. Active uptake of sugars, amino acids and nucleic acid precursors
4. Passive transport, especially of lipids
5. Incorporation of proteins such as albumin, which can bind lipids, peptides and catecholamines.

Although maternal reserves play an important role, the environment of the embryo is also critical. Culture media rarely reflect in-vivo conditions: the efficacy of transport systems into the oocyte and early embryo must be taken into account. Culture conditions have a direct impact on transcription and translation; embryonic metabolism may be depressed, protein turnover accelerated and mitochondrial function may be impaired. Suboptimal culture conditions have been shown to decrease cell numbers and jeopardize embryo viability.

ATP as an energy source is a basic requirement, and mammalian cells can generate ATP either by aerobic oxidation of substrates to carbon dioxide and water, or by anaerobic glycolysis of glucose to lactic acid. Under in-vitro conditions, oocytes and embryos generate ATP by aerobic oxidative metabolism of pyruvate, lactate, amino acids and possibly lipids. These metabolites have been shown to be important prior to genomic activation; pyruvate can

also remove toxic ammonium ions via transamination to alanine.

## Pentose Phosphate Pathway, NADPH and Glutathione

An important feature of early embryo metabolism is linked to the activation process that is induced by sperm entry, which increases glycolysis and glucose uptake through transporters. These may provide energy by generating ATP, but upregulation of the pentose phosphate pathway (PPP) at the time of pronuclear formation is a more significant metabolic parameter during this period. The PPP generates ribose 5-phosphate, a nucleotide precursor for subsequent DNA synthesis and replication. Upregulation of glucose metabolism via the PPP requires a fully grown pronucleus; the activity of the PPP influences the onset of the first S-phase in both male and female pronuclei, and continues to influence embryo development up to the blastocyst stage. The PPP also generates NADPH, which is involved in the majority of anabolic pathways: 1 mole of glucose 6-phosphate generates 1 mole of ribose 5-phosphate plus 2 moles of NADPH. NADPH further allows methionine to be recycled from homocysteine, with the formation of folic acid via methylene tetrahydrofolate reductase (MTHFR) (see Chapter 1: The 1-Carbon Cycle). This pathway influences imprinting processes in the oocyte, and is also involved in thymidine synthesis (5-methyl-uracyl, see section Vitamins). NADPH is also required to reduce oxidized glutathione (GSSG). The synthesis of glutathione from cysteine is energy consuming (ATP), and therefore recycling of GSSG is important, reducing energy consumption and decreasing the need for available cysteine.

Glutathione is necessary for sperm head swelling, and the impact of glutathione mobilization on further embryonic development is immediate: an increase in the rate of blastocyst formation is observed, with increased cell number per blastocyst formed. This is probably due to the universal role of glutathione in protection against oxidative stress.

## Glucose

Sugar metabolism is complex; active transport of hexoses has been shown in mouse embryos, and glucose and lactate are necessary for mouse embryo development in vitro. Hexoses are essential for

109

energy generation during preimplantation development: 1 mole of glucose generates from 30 to 36 moles of ATP. However, the equilibrium between sugars and other metabolic compounds is of paramount importance. It has been suggested that glucose is toxic during in-vitro culture before genomic activation and that glucose and phosphate together may inhibit early embryo development. The mechanisms proposed include induction of glycolysis at the expense of substrate oxidation, through disrupted mitochondrial function. High levels of glucose can lead to excessive free radical formation, but the toxic effect is dependent upon the overall composition of the media; in some systems the negative effect of glucose may be counterbalanced by the presence of a correct amino acid balance, i.e., the presence of sulfur amino acids and derivatives that neutralize reactive oxygen species (ROS). Amino acids and EDTA suppress glycolysis through different combinations, and act in combination to further suppress glycolysis. After genome activation, glucose becomes a key metabolite, required for lipid, amino acid and nucleic acid synthesis. It is also essential for blastocyst hatching.

## Lipids

Lipids are essential for very early stages of development: meiotic resumption and oocyte competence depend on lipid beta-oxidation, and lipids are then required immediately after fertilization. Three times more ATP can be generated from one chain of fatty acid (palmitate) than from one molecule of glucose. Mitochondria are involved in the metabolism of lipids, and this requires the presence of carnitine as a catalyst. Lipids can be synthesized (through C-2 condensation reactions), accumulated from the surrounding medium or carried with albumin. Cholesterol synthesis is possible, but slow: there is a rate-limiting step at the level of hMG (3-hydroxy-3-methyl-glutaryl) CoA reductase. If synthesis of cholesterol is experimentally inhibited by chetosterol, the embryos arrest and die.

## Electrolytes

The correct balance of electrolytes is always an essential basis for biochemical processes that lead to energy production and cAMP-based regulatory mechanisms. $K^+$ and $HCO_3$ are involved in sperm capacitation, and intracellular regulation is a vital aspect of correct homeostasis. $HCO_3$ has a particular role in activation, via an increase in sperm cAMP levels. The carbon from $HCO_3$ can be incorporated during anabolic processes in the embryo. Iron and copper cations appear to arrest embryo development, encouraging free radical formation; therefore, EDTA (or penicillamine) in early stage culture media is beneficial as a chelating agent (but not in fertilization medium, as it chelates calcium, which is essential for sperm motility, capacitation and the acrosome reaction). EDTA is also a free radical scavenger. A suggestion that EDTA might be deleterious after genome activation and should be removed in the second phase of culture has been shown to be invalid.

## Amino Acids

Amino acids are important regulators of embryo development. The concept of 'essential and non-essential' amino acids is not valid for preimplantation development, as their role is unlikely to be equivalent to their definition as 'essential' in terms of nutrition for the entire individual. In vivo, genital tract secretions contain all of the amino acids; these are essential for translation of stored polyadenylated mRNAs for new protein synthesis during the first 3 days after fertilization. The ratio between different amino acids appears to be more important than their actual concentration in culture media, as they compete with each other for membrane transport systems; an imbalance between amino acid concentrations reflects their capacity for active transport into the embryo, as well as their ability to act as organic osmolytes. Differing affinities for transport mechanisms mean that disequilibrium in the external milieu will be reflected in anomalies of the endogenous pool, with potentially deleterious effects on protein synthesis. Active transport mechanisms have been confirmed by the finding that amino acids are found at a higher concentration inside embryos than in the surrounding medium. Sulfur amino acids play a particularly important role, in that methionine, via $S$-adenosylmethionine, is used for transmethylation reactions involving proteins, phospholipids and nucleic acids, and is probably involved in imprinting through this process. The balance between methionine and other amino acids is crucial: methionine has a very high affinity for transporters, and its presence in excess may prevent uptake of other amino acids, creating an imbalance in the endogenous pool.

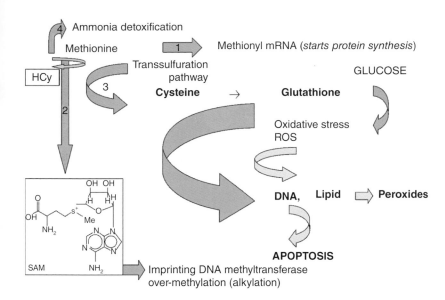

**Figure 5.7** Methionine utilization in the preimplantation embryo. HCy = homocysteine; ROS = reactive oxygen species. With thanks to Y. Ménézo.

Methylation of nucleic acids is known to modulate gene expression and to participate in the mechanism of genomic imprinting (Figure 5.7, see Chapter 1). S-amino acids also participate in protecting the embryo from free oxygen radicals: cysteine is a precursor for the synthesis of hypotaurine and taurine, and taurine can neutralize toxic aldehyde by-products of peroxidative reactions. Cysteine is a precursor of cysteamine and glutathione, and redox coupling between these amino acids helps the embryo to maintain its redox potential and prevent damage from peroxidative reactions. Homocysteine competes for the same transporter as methionine for entry into the embryo and thus inhibits methylation; the pathway that recycles homocysteine to methionine via the CBS (cystathionine beta synthase pathway) is poorly expressed or nonexistent in the human oocyte (Benkhalifa *et al.*, 2010). Ultimately, the initiation of all protein synthesis requires methionyl tRNA, and the availability of cysteine and methionine is therefore crucial during early embryogenesis. A shortage of these compounds, linked to either maternal age or transporter deficiency, is detrimental.

Glutamine is also an important source of carbon and energy; in vitro it may be deaminated into glutamic acid, but it is also converted to pyroglutamic acid (or pyrollidone carboxylic acid, PCA), which cannot be used for anabolism. However, glutamine is only weakly degraded in slightly alkaline conditions, corresponding to culture media. Introducing Gly-glutamine and Ala-glutamine into culture media to prevent degradation does not help, as they are converted to Gly-PCA and Ala-PCA.

Glycine is an energy source, as it can be deaminated immediately to form glycollate and glyoxylate (C-2 metabolites), and also acts as a precursor for peptides, proteins and nucleic acids. It is a chelating agent for toxic divalent cations, has an in-vitro osmoregulatory role and is implicated in the regulation of intracellular pH of the embryo.

Deamination reactions are an important part of the biochemical and metabolic processes, and free ammonia is immediately recycled by efficient enzyme systems present in the oviduct (Figure 5.8). In vitro, in the presence of incubator carbon dioxide, free ammonia forms carbonate and ammonium bicarbonate, both unstable compounds. If the embryo cultures are 'open,' without oil, ammonia is liberated and eliminated by the carbon dioxide atmosphere. However, within microdrops under oil, ammonia can accumulate, which is toxic to the embryo; Gardner and Lane (1993) demonstrated severe teratogenic effects in mouse embryos.

## Nucleotides

At a very early stage, embryos can synthesize purine and pyrimidine bases, precursors of RNA and DNA; these are required for DNA repair processes, which are very important during this period of

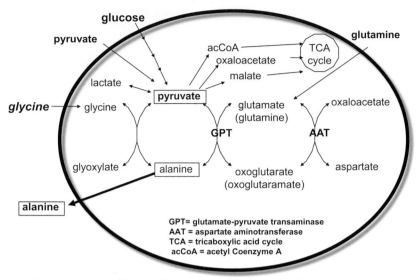

→→ Nitrogen recycling in the mammalian preimplantation embryo

**Figure 5.8** Nitrogen recycling in the mammalian preimplantation embryo (with thanks to Y. Ménézo). acCoA = acetyl coenzyme A; TCA cycle = tricarboxylic acid cycle.

development (Ménézo *et al.*, 2010, 2013). Following DNA damage caused by ROS, the oxidized deoxynucleoside triphosphate pool is a significant contributor to genetic instability. These oxidized bases must be removed in order to avoid their reintroduction into DNA. The nucleotide pool sanitization enzymes are the first defense against mutagenesis, and the human oocyte is well equipped with NUDT (nucleoside diphosphate linked moiety X), the major enzyme involved. However, there is a requirement for ATP, CTP and TTP. For example, GTP must replace oxidized G (8-oxoguanosine, the most common DNA decay linked to ROS) in DNA. These bases can also be actively transported from the surroundings; the embryo probably uses this mechanism, as uptake is generally less energy consuming than full synthesis. There is an exponential increase in the accumulation of these precursors during the transition from morula to blastocyst as the number of cells increases.

## Vitamins

It is difficult to measure vitamin uptake, but indirectly it is clear that folic acid and vitamin B12, necessary for methylation processes, are mandatory cofactors. Thymine is also known as 5-methyluracil, a pyrimidine nucleobase: inhibition of this methylation process by methotrexate leads to thymidine starvation and developmental arrest (O'Neill, 1998). Other vitamins such as vitamin C and vitamin E may act as redox regulators.

## Growth Factors

The potential role of growth factors in culture media remains open. Numerous growth factors are present in the oviduct and uterus, and they clearly play a role in vivo. Co-culture systems demonstrated a positive effect of growth factors on cell number, embryo quality and freeze–thaw tolerance. However, this positive aspect represents the balanced interaction of several growth factors, such as leukemia inhibitory factor (LIF), growth hormone (GH) and mitogenic colony-stimulating factor, rather than the action of a single one. Some may slow down, and several may accelerate embryonic development: the addition of a single growth factor in vitro remains questionable at this point.

## Further Reading

### Books and Reviews

Balinsky BI (1965) *An Introduction to Embryology*. Saunders, London.

Cummins JM, Jequier AM, Kan R (1994) Molecular biology of human male infertility: links with ageing, mitochondrial genetics, and oxidative stress? *Molecular Reproduction and Development* 37: 345–362.

Dekel N (1996) Protein phosphorylation/ dephosphorylation in the meiotic cell cycle of mammalian oocytes. *Reviews of Reproduction* 1: 82–88.

Eddy EM (1998) Regulation of gene expression during spermatogenesis. *Seminars in Cell and Developmental Biology* 19: 451–457.

Eppig JJ (2001) Oocyte control of ovarian follicular development and function in mammals. *Reproduction* 122: 829–838.

Gilchrist RB, Lane M, Thompson JG (2008) Oocyte-secreted factors: regulators of cumulus cell function and oocyte quality. *Human Reproduction Update* 14(2): 159–177.

Jurisicova A, Acton BM (2004) Deadly decisions: the roles of genes regulating programmed cell death in human preimplantation embryo development. *Reproduction* 128(3): 281–291.

Kane MT, Morgan PM, Coonan C (1997) Peptide growth factors and preimplantation development. *Human Reproduction Update* 3: 137–157.

Kola I, Trounson A (1989) *Dispermic Human Fertilization: Violation of Expected Cell Behaviour*. Academic Press, San Diego.

Masui Y (2001) From oocyte maturation to the in vitro cell cycle: the history of discoveries of Maturation Promoting Factor (MPF) and Cytostatic Factor (CSF). *Differentiation* 69: 1–17.

Ménézo Y, Dale B, Cohen M (2010) DNA damage and repair in human oocytes and embryos: a review. *Zygote* 18(4): 357–365.

Reik W, Dean W, Walter J (2001) Epigenetic reprogramming in mammalian development (Review). *Science* 293: 1089–1093.

Sathananthan AH, Ng SC, Bongo A, Trounson A, Ratnam S (1993) *Visual Atlas of Early Human Development of Assisted Reproduction Technology*. Singapore University Press, Singapore.

Schultz RM (2002) The molecular foundations of the maternal to zygotic transition in the preimplantation embryo. *Human Reproduction Update* 8(4): 323–331.

Tosti E (2006) Calcium ion currents mediating oocyte maturation events (Review). *Reproductive Biology and Endocrinology* 4: 26–35.

Van den Bergh M, Ebner T, Elder K (2012) *Atlas of Oocytes, Zygotes and Embryos in Reproductive Medicine*. Cambridge University Press, Cambridge, UK.

## Publications

Adams JM, Cory S (1998) The Bcl-2 protein family: arbiters of cell survival. *Science* 281: 1322–1326.

Adenot PG, Mercier Y, Renard JP, Thompson EM (1997) Differential H4 acetylation of paternal and maternal chromatin precedes DNA replication and differential transcriptional activity in pronuclei of 1-cell mouse embryos. *Development* 124(22): 4615–4625.

Alikani M (2007) The origins and consequences of fragmentation in mammalian oocytes and embryos. In: Elder K, Cohen J (eds.) *Human Preimplantation Embryo Selection*. Taylor-Francis, London, pp. 51–78.

Alikani M, Cohen J, Tomkin G, *et al.* (1999) Human embryo fragmentation in vitro and its implications for pregnancy and implantation. *Fertility and Sterility* 71: 836–842.

Antczak M, Van Blerkom J (1997) Oocyte influences on early development: the regulatory proteins leptin and STAT3 are polarized in mouse and human oocytes and differentially distributed within the cells of the preimplantation stage embryo. *Molecular Human Reproduction* 3: 1067–1086.

Ao A, Erickson RP, Winston RML, Handyside AH (1994) Transcription of paternal Y-linked genes in the human zygote as early as the pronucleate stage. *Zygote* 2: 281–287.

Bachvarova R (1992) A maternal tail of poly(A): the long and short of it. *Cell* 69: 895–897.

Baines KJ, Renaud SJ (2017) Transcription factors that regulate trophoblast development and function. *Progress in Molecular Biology Translational Science* 145: 39–88.

Barritt J, Brenner CA, Cohen J, Matt DW (1999) Mitochondrial DNA rearrangements in oocytes and embryos. *Molecular Human Reproduction* 5(10): 927–933.

Bateson P, Barker D, Clutton-Brock T, *et al.* (2004) Developmental plasticity and human health. *Nature* 430(6998): 419–421.

Benkhalifa M, Montjean D, Cohen-Bacrie P, Ménézo Y (2010) Imprinting: RNA expression for homocysteine recycling in the human oocyte. *Fertility and Sterility* 93(5): 1585–1590.

Blakeley P, Fogarty NME, del Valle I, *et al.* (2015) Defining the three cell lineages of the human blastocyst by single-cell RNA-seq. *Development* 142: 3151–3165.

Bonnerot C, Vernet M, Grimber G, Brioand P, Nicolas JF (1993) Transcriptional selectivity in early mouse embryos: a qualitative study. *Bioessays* 15(8): 531–538.

Bouniol-Baly C, Nguyen E, Besombes D, Debey P (1997) Dynamic organization of DNA replication in one cell mouse embryos: relationship to transcriptional activation. *Experimental Cell Research* 236: 201–211.

Braude P, Bolton V, Moore S (1988) Human gene expression first occurs between the four- and eight-cell stages of preimplantation development. *Nature* 332: 459–461.

Brenner C, Wolny YM, Adler RR, Cohen J (1999) Alternative splicing of the telomerase catalytic submit in human oocytes and embryos. *Molecular Human Reproduction* 5(9): 845–850.

Brenner CA, Wolny YM, Barritt JA, *et al.* (1998) Mitochondrial DNA deletion in human oocytes and embryos. *Molecular Human Reproduction* 4(9): 887–892.

Brison DR, Schulz RM (1997) Apoptosis during mouse blastocyst formation: evidence for a role for survival factors including transforming growth factor alpha. *Biology of Reproduction* 56: 1088–1096.

Brison DR, Schulz RM (1998) Increased incidence of apoptosis in TGF-alpha deficient mouse blastocysts. *Biology of Reproduction* 59: 136–144.

Calarco PG (1995) Polarization of mitochondria in the unfertilized mouse oocyte. *Developmental Genetics* 16: 36–43.

Chen C, Sathanantan AH (1986) Early penetration of human sperm through the vestments of human eggs in vitro. *Archives of Andrology* 16: 183–197.

Cho WK, Stern S, Biggers JD (1974) Inhibitory effect of dibutyryl cAMP on mouse oocyte maturation in vitro. *Journal of Experimental Zoology* 187: 383–386.

Clayton L, McConnell JM, Johnson MH (1995) Control of the surface expression of uvomorulin after activation of mouse oocytes. *Zygote* 3(2): 177–189.

Conaghan J, Handyside AH, Winston RM, Leese HJ (1993) Effects of pyruvate and glucose on the development of human preimplantation embryos in vitro. *Journal of Reproduction and Fertility* 99(1): 87–95.

Coticchio G, Fleming S (1998) Inhibition of phosphoinositide metabolism or chelation of intracellular calcium blocks FSH-induced but not spontaneous meiotic resumption in mouse oocytes. *Developmental Biology* 203: 201–209.

Dale B, Gualtieri R, Talevi R, *et al.* (1991) Intercellular communication in the early human embryo. *Molecular Reproduction and Development* 29: 22–28.

Dale B, Marino M, Wilding M (1998) Sperm-induced calcium oscillations: soluble factor, factors or receptors? *Molecular Human Reproduction* 5: 1–4.

Dale B, Tosti E, Iaccarino M (1995) Is the plasma membrane of the human oocyte re-organized following fertilization and early cleavage? *Zygote* 3: 31–37.

Delhanty JDA, Harper JC, Ao A, Handyside AH, Winston RML (1997) Multicolour FISH detects frequent chromosomal mosaicism and chaotic division in normal preimplantation embryos from fertile patients. *Human Genetics* 99: 755–760.

De Sousa PA, Caveney A, Westhusin ME, Watson AJ (1998) Temporal patterns of embryonic gene expression and their dependence on oogenetic factors. *Theriogenology* 49: 115–128.

Dobson AT, Raja R, Abeyta MJ, *et al* (2004) The unique transcriptome through day 3 of human preimplantation development. *Human Molecular Genetics* 13(14): 1461–1470.

Dominko T, First N (1997) Timing of meiotic progression in bovine oocytes and its effect on early embryo development. *Molecular Reproduction and Development* 47: 456–467.

Dulcibella T (1996) The cortical reaction and development of activation competence in mammalian oocytes. *Human Reproduction Update* 2(1): 29–42.

Edwards RG, Beard H (1997) Oocyte polarity and cell determination in early mammalian embryos. *Molecular Human Reproduction* 3: 868–905.

Edwards RG, Hansis C (2005) Initial differentiation of blastomeres in 4-cell human embryos and its significance for early embryogenesis and implantation. *Reproductive BioMedicine Online* 11(2): 206–218.

Eichenlaub-Ritter U (2002) Manipulation of the oocyte: possible damage to the spindle apparatus. *Reproductive BioMedicine Online* 5: 117–124.

Eppig JJ, Chesnel F, Hirao Y, *et al.* (1997) Oocyte control of granulosa cell development: how and why. *Human Reproduction* 12(11 Suppl.): 127–132.

Flach G, Johnsom MH, Braude PR, Taylor RAS, Bolton VN (1982) The transition from maternal to embryonic control in the 2-cell mouse embryo. *The EMBO Journal* 1(6): 681–686.

Fogarty NME, McCarthy A, Snijders KE, *et al.* (2017) Genome editing reveals a role for OCT4 in human embryogenesis. *Nature* 550: 67–73.

Fulka J Jr., First NL, Moor RM (1998) Nuclear and cytoplasmic determinants involved in the regulation of mammalian oocyte maturation. *Molecular Human Reproduction* 4: 41–49.

Fulka H, Mrazek M, Tepla O, Fulka J (2004) DNA methylation pattern in human zygotes and developing embryos. *Reproduction* 128: 703–708.

Gabdoulline R, Kaisers W, Gaspar A, *et al.* (2015) Differences in the early development of human and mouse embryonic stem cells. *PLoS One* 10(10): e0140803.

Galan A, Montaner DD, Poo M, *et al.* (2010) Functional genomics of 5- to 8-cell stage human embryos by blastomere single-cell cDNA analysis. *PLoS One* 5: e13615.

Gardner DK (1998) Changes in requirements and utilization of nutrients during mammalian preimplantation embryo development and their significance in embryo culture. *Theriogenology* 49: 83–102.

Gardner DK, Lane M (1993) Amino acids and ammonium regulate mouse embryo development in culture. *Biology of Reproduction* 48(2): 377–385.

Gardner RL (2001) Specification of embryonic axes begins before cleavage in normal mouse development. *Development* 128(6): 839–847.

Gardner RL (2007) The axis of polarity of the mouse blastocyst is specified before blastulation and independently of the zona pellucida. *Human Reproduction* 22: 798–806.

Glabowski W, Kurzawa R, Wisniewska B, *et al.* (2005) Growth factors effects on preimplantation development of mouse embryos exposed to tumour necrosis factor alpha. *Reproductive Biology* 5(1): 83–99.

Glinsky G, Durruthy J, Wossidlo M *et al.* (2018) Single cell expression analysis of primate-specific retroviruses-derived HPAT lincRNAs in viable human blastocysts identifies embryonic cells co-expressing genetic markers of multiple lineages. *Heliyon* 4(2018): e00667.

Gopichandran N, Leese HJ (2003) Metabolic characterisation of the bovine blastocyst, inner cell mass, trophectoderm and blastocoel fluid. *Reproduction* 126: 299–308.

Grammont G, Irvine KD (2002) Organiser activity of the polar cells during Drosophila oogenesis. *Development* 129: 5131–5140.

Gregory L (1998) Ovarian markers of implantation potential in assisted reproduction. *Human Reproduction* 13(Suppl. 4): 117–132.

Grobstein C (1988) Biological characteristics of the preembryo. *Annals of the New York Academy of Sciences* 541: 346–348.

Gualtieri R, Santella L, Dale B (1992) Tight junctions and cavitation in the human pre-embryo. *Molecular Reproduction and Development* 32: 81–87.

Guyader-Joly C, Khatchadourian C, Ménézo Y (1996) Comparative glucose and fructose incorporation and conversion by in vitro produced bovine embryos. *Zygote* 4: 85–91.

Hales BF, Barton TS, Robaire B (2005) Impact of paternal exposure to chemotherapy on offspring in the rat. *Journal of the National Cancer Institute Monograph* 34: 28–31.

Hales BF, Robaire B (2001) Paternal exposure to drugs and environmental chemicals: effects on progeny outcome. *Journal of Andrology* 22(6): 927–936.

Hamatani T, Carter MG, Sharov AA, Ko MS (2004) Dynamics of global gene expression changes during mouse preimplantation development. *Developmental Cell* 6(1): 117–131.

Hamberger L, Nilsson L, Sjögren A (1998) Microscopic imaging techniques: practical aspects. *Human Reproduction* 13: Abstract book 1: 15, L.

Hansis C, Grifo JA, Tang Y, Krey LC (2002) Assessment of beta-HCG, beta-LH mRNA and ploidy in individual human blastomeres. *Reproductive BioMedicine Online* 5(2): 156–161.

Hardy K (1999) Apoptosis in the human embryo. *Reviews of Reproduction* 4: 125–134.

Harper JC, Delhanty JDA (2008) Preimplantation genetic diagnosis. In: Rodeck CH, Whittle MJ (eds.) *Fetal Medicine: Basic Science and Clinical Practice*, 2nd edn. Churchill Livingstone, Edinburgh, pp. 323–330.

Heidmann O, Vernochet C, Dupressoir A, Heidmann T (2009) Identification of an endogenous retroviral envelope gene with fusogenic activity and placenta-specific expression in the rabbit: a new 'syncytin' in a third order of mammals. *Retrovirology* 6: 107.

Heikinheimo O, Gibbons W (1998) The molecular mechanisms of oocyte maturation and early embryonic development are unveiling new insights into reproductive medicine. *Molecular Human Reproduction* 4(8): 745–756.

Henery CC, Miranda M, Wiekowski M, Wilmut I, DePamphilis ML (1995) Repression of gene expression at the beginning of mouse development. *Developmental Biology* 169(2): 448–460.

Henkel R, Miller C, Miska H, Gips H, Schill WB (1993) Early embryology: determination of the acrosome reaction in human spermatozoa is predictive of fertilization in vitro. *Human Reproduction* 8(12): 2128–2132.

Hertig AT, Rock J, Adams EC (1956) A description of 34 human ova within the first 17 days of development. *American Journal of Anatomy* 98(3): 435–493.

Hertig A, Rock J, Adams E, Mulligan W (1954) On the preimplantation stages of the human ovum: a description of four normal and four abnormal specimens ranging from the second to the fifth day of development. *Contributions to Embryology of the Carnegie Institution of Washington* 35: 119–220.

Hewitson LC, Simerly CR, Dominko T, Schatten G (2000) Cellular and molecular events after in vitro fertilization and intracytoplasmic sperm injection. *Theriogenology* 53: 95–104.

Hewitson LC, Simerly C, Schatten G (1997) Inheritance defects of the sperm centrosome in humans and its possible role in male infertility. *International Journal of Andrology* 20(Suppl. 3): 35–43.

Hewitson LC, Simerly CR, Tengowski MW, *et al.* (1996) Microtubule and chromatin configuration during Rhesus intracytoplasmic sperm injection: successes and failures. *Biology of Reproduction* 55: 271–280.

Houghton FD (2005) Role of gap junctions during early embryo development. *Reproduction* 129: 129–131.

Houghton FD (2006) Energy metabolism of the inner cell mass and trophectoderm of the mouse blastocyst. *Differentiation* 74: 11–18.

Huang TTF, Chinn K, Kosasa T, *et al.* (2016) Morphokinetics of human blastocyst expansion in vitro. *Reproductive BioMedicine Online* 33: 659–667.

Huarte J, Stutz A, O'Connell ML, *et al.* (1992) Transient translational silencing by reversible mRNA deadenylation. *Cell* 69: 1021–1030.

Ivanov PL, Wadhams MJ, Roby RK, *et al.* (1996) Mitochondrial DNA sequence heteroplasmy in the Grand Duke of Russia Georgij Romanov establishes the authenticity of the remains of Tsar Nicholas II. *Nature Genetics* 12: 417–420.

Janny L, Ménézo YJR (1994) Evidence for a strong paternal effect on human preimplantation embryo development and blastocyst formation. *Molecular Reproduction and Development* 38: 36–42.

Jansen S, Esmaeilpour T, Pantaleon M, Kaye PL (2006) Glucose affects monocarboxylate cotransporter (MCT) 1 expression during mouse preimplantation development. *Reproduction and Fertility* 131: 469–479.

Jennings MO, Owen RC, Keefe DD, Kim ED (2017) Management and counseling of the male with advanced paternal age. *Fertility and Sterility* 107(2): 324–328.

Johnson MH (2002) Time and development. *Reproductive BioMedicine Online* 4(Suppl. 1): 39–45.

Johnson MH, Day ML (2000) Egg timers: how is developmental time measured in the early vertebrate embryo? *Bioessays* 22: 57–63.

Johnson MH, Lim A, Fenando D, Day ML (2002) Circadian clockwork genes are expressed in the reproductive tract and conceptus of the early pregnant mouse. *Reproductive BioMedicine Online* 4(12): 140–145.

Kaneda H, Hayashi J, Takahama S, *et al.* (1995) Elimination of paternal mitochondrial DNA in intraspecific crosses during early mouse embryogenesis. *Proceedings of the National Academy of Sciences of the USA* 92: 4542–4546.

Katari S, Turan N, Bibikova M, *et al.* (2009) DNA methylation and gene expression differences in children conceived in vitro or in vivo. *Human Molecular Genetics* 18(20): 3769–3778.

Kawamura K, Fukuda J, Shimizu Y, Kodama H, Tanaka T (2005) Survivin contributes to the anti-apoptotic activities of transforming growth factor alpha in mouse blastocysts through phosphatidylinositol 3′-kinase pathway. *Biology and Reproduction* 73: 1094–1101.

Kidder GM, McLachlin JR (1985) Timing of transcription and protein synthesis underlying morphogenesis in preimplantation mouse embryos. *Developmental Biology* 112: 265–275.

Krakauer DC, Mira A (1999) Mitochondria and germ cell death. *Nature* 400: 125–126.

Lane M, Gardner DK (1997) Nonessential amino acids and glutamine decrease the time of the first three cleavage divisions and increase compaction of mouse zygotes in vitro. *Journal of Assisted Reproduction and Genetics* 14(7): 398–403.

Lane M, Gardner DK (2000) Lactate regulates pyruvate uptake and metabolism in the preimplantation mouse embryo. *Biology and Reproduction* 62: 16–22.

Lee L, Miyano T, Moor RM (2000) Localisation of phosphorylated MAP kinase during the transition from meiosis I to meiosis II in pig oocytes. *Zygote* 8: 119–125.

Lefièvre L, Conner SJ, Salpekar A, *et al.* (2004) Four zona pellucida glycoproteins are expressed in the human. *Human Reproduction* 19(7): 1580–1586.

Levy R, Elder K, Ménézo Y (2004) Cytoplasmic transfer in oocytes: biochemical aspects. *Human Reproduction Update* 10(3): 241–250.

Lightman A, Kol S, Wayner V, *et al.* (1997) The presence of a sponsoring embryo in a batch of poor quality thawed embryos significantly increases pregnancy and implantation rate. *Fertility and Sterility* 67(4): 711–716.

Lin YC, Chang SY, Lan KC, *et al.* (2003) Human oocyte maturity in vivo determines the outcome of blastocyst development in vitro. *Journal of Assisted Reproduction and Genetics* 20(12): 506–512.

Lo H (1996) The role of gap junction membrane channels in development. *Journal of Bioenergetics and Biomembranes* 8(4): 399–409.

Majumder S, DePamphilis ML (1994) Requirements for DNA transcription and replication at the beginning of mouse development. *Journal of Cell Biochemistry* 55(1): 59–68.

Marangos P, FitzHarris G, Carroll J (2003) $Ca^{2+}$ oscillations at fertilization in mammals are regulated by the formation of pronuclei. *Development* 130: 1461–1472.

Maro B, Gueth-Hallonet C, Aghion J, Antony C (1991) Cell polarity and microtubule organization during mouse early embryogenesis. *Development, Supplement* 1: 17–25.

Mattioli M, Barboni B (2000) Signal transduction mechanism for LH in the cumulus oocyte complex. *Molecular and Cellular Endocrinology* 161: 19–23.

Memili E, Dominko T, First N (1998) Onset of transcription in bovine oocytes and embryos. *Molecular Reproduction and Development* 51: 36–41.

Memili E, First NL (1999) Control of gene expression at the onset of bovine embryonic development. *Biology of Reproduction* 61: 1198–1207.

Ménézo Y, Janny L (1997) Influence of paternal factors in early embryogenesis. In: Barratt C, De Jonge C, Mortimer D, Parinaud J (eds.) *Genetics of Human Male Infertility*. EDK, Paris, pp. 246–257.

Ménézo Y, Lichtblau I, Elder K (2013). New insights into human embryo metabolism in vitro and in vivo. *Journal of Assisted Reproduction and Genetics* 30(3): 293–303.

Mio Y (2006) Morphological analysis of human embryonic development using time-lapse cinematography. *Journal of Mammalian Ova Research* 23(1): 27–35.

Munné S, Alikani M, Tomkin G, Grifo J, Cohen J (1995) Embryo morphology, developmental rates, and maternal age are correlated with chromosome abnormalities. *Fertility and Sterility* 64: 382–391.

Nargund G, Bourne T, Doyle P, *et al.* (1996) Associations between ultrasound indices of follicular blood flow, oocyte recovery and preimplantation embryo quality. *Human Reproduction* 11(1): 109–113.

Niakan KK, Eggan K (2013) Analysis of human embryos from zygote to blastocyst reveals distinct gene expression patterns relative to the mouse. *Developmental Biology* 375: 54–64.

Niemann H, Wrenzycki C (1999) Alterations of expression of developmentally important genes in preimplantation bovine embryos by in vitro culture condition: implications for subsequent development. *Theriogenology* 53: 21–34.

Nikas G, Ao A, Winston RM, Handyside AH (1996) Compaction and surface polarity in the human embryo in vitro. *Biology of Reproduction* 55: 32–37.

Nikas G, Paraschos T, Psychoyos A, Handyside AH (1994) The zona reaction in human oocytes as seen with scanning electron microscopy. *Human Reproduction* 9(11): 2135–2138.

Nothias JY, Majumder S, Kaneko KJ, DePamphilis ML (1995) Regulation of gene expression at the beginning of mammalian development. *Journal of Biological Chemistry* 270: 22077–22080.

Nothias JY, Miranda M, De Pamphilis ML (1996) Uncoupling of transcription and translation during zygotic gene activation in the mouse. *EMBO Journal* 14: 5715–5725.

O'Neill C (1998) Role of autocrine mediators in the regulation of embryo viability: lessons from animal models. *Journal of Assisted Reproduction and Genetics* 15(8): 460–465.

Orsi NM, Leese HJ (2004) Ammonium exposure and pyruvate affect the amino acid metabolism of bovine blastocysts in vitro. *Reproduction* 127: 131–140.

Payne D, Flaherty SP, Barry MF, Matthews CD (1997) Preliminary observations on polar body extrusion and pronuclear formation in human oocytes using time-lapse video cinematography. *Human Reproduction* 12(3): 532–541.

Payne D, Flaherty SP, Newble CD, Swann NJ, Wang XJ, Matthews CD (1994) The influence of sperm morphology and the acrosome reaction on fertilization. *Human Reproduction* 9: 1281–1288.

Pfeffer PL (2018) Building principles for constructing a mammalian blastocyst embryo. *Biology* 7: pii: E41. DOI: 10.3390/biology7030041

Picton HM, Briggs D, Gosden RG (1998) The molecular basis of oocyte growth and development. *Molecular and Cellular Endocrinology* 145: 27–37.

Piotrowska K, Wianny F, Pedersen RA, Zernicka-Goetz M (2001) Blastomeres arising from the first cleavage division have distinguishable fates in normal mouse development. *Development* 128: 3739–3748.

Piotrowska-Nitsche K, Perea-Gomez A, Haraguchi S, *et al.* (2005) Four-cell stage mouse blastomeres have different developmental properties. *Development* 132: 479–490.

Piotrowska-Nitsche K, Zernicka-Goetz M (2005) Spatial arrangement of individual 4-cell stage blastomeres and the order in which they are generated correlate with blastocyst pattern in the mouse embryo. *Mechanisms of Development* 122: 487–500.

Posillico J, and The Metabolomics Study Group for Assisted Reproductive Technologies (2007) Selection of viable embryos and gametes by rapid, noninvasive metabolomic profiling of oxidative stress biomarkers. In: Elder K, Cohen J (eds.) *Human Preimplantation Embryo Evaluation and Selection*. Taylor-Francis, London, pp. 245–262.

Puissant F, Van Rysselberge M, Barlow P, *et al.* (1987) Embryo scoring as a prognostic tool in IVF treatment. *Human Reproduction* 2: 705–708.

Robaire B, Hales BF (2003) Mechanisms of action of cyclophosphamide as a male-mediated developmental toxicant. *Advances in Experimental Medicine and Biology* 518: 169–180.

Roode M, Blair K, Snell P, Elder K, *et al.* (2012) Human hypoblast formation is not dependent on FGF signaling. *Developmental Biology* 361: 358–363.

Rosebloom T (2018) Developmental plasticity and its relevance to assisted human reproduction. *Human Reproduction* 33(4): 546–552.

Rossant J (2004) Lineage development and polar asymmetries in the peri-implantation mouse blastocyst. *Seminars in Cell and Developmental Biology* 15(5): 573–581.

Sakkas D, Urner F, Bizzaro D, *et al.* (1998) Sperm nuclear DNA damage and altered chromatin structure: effect on fertilization and embryo development. *Human Reproduction* 13(Suppl. 4): 11–19.

Santella L, Alikani M, Talansky BE, Cohen J, Dale B (1992) Is the human oocyte plasma membrane polarized? *Human Reproduction* 7: 999–1003.

Sapienza C, Peterson AC, Rossant J, Balling R (1987) Degree of methylation of transgenes is dependent on gamete of origin. *Nature* 328(6127): 251–254.

Sathanathan AH, Chen C (1986) Sperm-oocyte membrane fusion in the human during monospermic fertilization. *Gamete Research* 15: 177–186.

Sathananthan AH, Ng SC, Trounson AO, Ratnam SS, Bongso TA (1990) Human sperm-oocyte fusion. In: Dale B (ed.) *Mechanism of Fertilization: Plants to Humans.* NATO ASI Series, Vol. h45. Springer-Verlag, Berlin, pp. 329–350.

Schatten G (1994) The centrosome and its mode of inheritance: the reduction of the centrosome during gametogenesis and its restoration during fertilization. *Developmental Biology* 165(2): 299–335.

Schatten G (1999) Fertilization. In: Fauser BCJM (ed.) *Molecular Biology in Reproductive Medicine.* Parthenon Publishing, London, pp. 297–311.

Schatten G, Simerly C, Schatten H (1991) Maternal inheritance of centrosomes in mammals; studies on parthenogenesis and polyspermy in mice. *Proceedings of the National Academy of Sciences of the USA* 88(15): 6785–6789.

Schultz RM (1995) Role of chromatin structure in zygotic gene activation in the mammalian embryo. *Seminars in Cell Biology* 6(4): 201–208.

Schultz RM (1999) Preimplantation embryo development. In: Fauser BCJM (ed.) *Molecular Biology in Reproductive Medicine.* Parthenon Publishing, London, pp. 313–331.

Shabazi MN, Jedrusik A, Vuoristo S *et al.* (2016). Self-organisation of the human embryo in the absence of maternal tissues. *Nature Cell Biology* 18(6): 700–708.

Simerly C, Navara CS (2007) The sperm centriole: its effect on the developing embryo. In: Elder K, Cohen J (eds.) *Human Preimplantation Embryo Evaluation and Selection.* Taylor&Francis, London, pp. 337–354.

Simerly C, Wu G, Zoran S, *et al.* (1995) The paternal inheritance of the centrosome, the cell's microtubule-organising center, in humans and the implications for infertility. *Nature Medicine* 1: 47–53.

Spanos S, Becker DL, Winston RM, Hardy K (2000) Anti-apoptotic action of insulin-like growth factor-1 during human preimplantation embryo development. *Biology and Reproduction* 63: 1413–1420.

Stein P, Worrad DM, Belyaev ND, Turner BM, Schultz RM (1997) Stage-dependent redistributions of acetylated histones in nuclei of the early preimplantation mouse embryo. *Molecular Reproduction and Development* 47(4): 421–429.

Steuerwald N (2007) Gene expression analysis in the human oocyte and embryo. In: Elder K, Cohen J (eds.) *Human Preimplantation Embryo Evaluation and Selection.* Taylor&Francis, London, pp. 263–272.

Sun QY (2003) Cellular and molecular mechanisms leading to cortical reaction and polyspermy block in mammalian eggs. *Microscopy Research and Technique* 61(4): 342–348.

Surani MA, Barton SC, Norris ML (1986) Nuclear transplantation in the mouse: heritable differences between parental genomes after activation of the embryonic genome. *Cell* 45(1): 127–136.

Temeles GL, Ram PT, Rothstein JL, Schulz RM (1994) Expression patterns of novel genes during mouse preimplantation embryogenesis. *Molecular Reproduction and Development* 37: 121–129.

Tesarik J, Greco E (1999) The probability of abnormal preimplantation development can be predicted by a single static observation on pronuclear stage morphology. *Human Reproduction* 14: 1318–1323.

Tesarik J, Kopecny V (1989a) Developmental control of the human male pronucleus by ooplasmic factors. *Human Reproduction* 4: 962–968.

Tesarik J, Kopecny V (1989b) Nucleic acid synthesis and development of human male pronucleus. *Journal of Reproduction and Fertility* 86: 549–558.

Tesarik J, Kopecny V (1989c) Development of human male pronucleus: ultrastructure and timing. *Gamete Research* 24: 135–149.

Tesarik J, Kopecny V, Plachot M, Mandelbaum J (1988) Early morphological signs of embryonic genome expression in human preimplantation development as revealed by quantitative electron microscopy. *Developmental Biology* 128: 15–20.

Torres-Padilla ME, Zernicka-Goetz M (2006) Role of TIF1α as a modulator of embryonic transcription in the mouse zygote. *Journal of Cell Biology* 174(3): 329–338.

Valdimarsson G, Kidder GM (1995) Temporal control of gap junction assembly in preimplantation mouse embryos. *Journal of Cell Science* 108 (Pt 4): 1715–1722.

Vassena R, Boué S, González-Roca E, *et al.* (2011) Waves of early transcriptional activation and pluripotency program initiation during human preimplantation development. *Development* 138(17): 3699–3709.

Van Blerkom J, Davis P, Alexander S (2004) Occurrence of maternal and paternal spindles in unfertilized human oocytes: possible relationship to nucleation defects after silent fertilization. *Reproductive BioMedicine Online* 8(4): 454–459.

Wang QT, Piotrowska K, Ciemerych MA, *et al.* (2004) A genome-wide study of gene activity reveals developmental signaling pathways in the preimplantation mouse embryo. *Developmental Cell* 6(1): 133–144.

Warner CM, Cao W, Exley GE *et al.* (1998) Genetic regulation of egg and embryo survival. *Human Reproduction* 13(Suppl. 3): 178–190.

Wassarman P (1987) The biology and chemistry of fertilization. *Science* 235: 553–560.

Wassarman P (1990) Profile of a mammalian sperm receptor. *Development* 108: 1–17.

Wassarman PM, Florman HM, Greve IM (1985) Receptor-mediated sperm–egg interactions in mammals. In: Metz CB, Monroy A (eds.) *Fertilization*, Vol. 2. Academic Press, New York, pp. 341–360.

Wiekowski M, Miranda M, DePamphilis ML (1991) Regulation of gene expression in preimplantation mouse embryos: effects of the zygotic clock and the first mitosis on promoter and enhancer activities. *Developmental Biology* 147(2): 403–414.

Wolffe AP (1998) Packaging principle: how DNA methylation and histone acetylation control the transcriptional activity of chromatin. *Journal of Experimental Zoology* 282: 239–244.

Wong C, Loewke K, Bossert N, *et al.* (2010) Non-invasive imaging of human embryos before embryonic genome activation predicts development to the blastocyst stage. *Nature Biotechnology* 28: 1115–1121.

Woodward BJ, Lenton EA, MacNeil S (1993) Requirement of preimplantation human embryos for extracellular calmodulin for development. *Human Reproduction* 8(2): 272–276.

Worrad DM, Turner BM, Schultz RM (1995) Temporally restricted spatial localization of acetylated isoforms of histone H4 and RNA polymerase II in the 2-cell mouse embryo. *Development* 121(9): 2949–2959.

Xu Y, Zhang JJ, Grifo JA, Krey LC (2005) DNA methylation patterns in human tripronucleate zygotes. *Molecular Human Reproduction* 11(3): 167–171.

Zeng F, Schultz R (2005) RNA transcript profiling during zygotic gene activation in the preimplantation mouse embryo. *Developmental Biology* 283: 40–57.

# Implantation and Early Stages of Fetal Development

## Implantation

During the transition from morula to blastocyst the embryo enters the uterus, where it is sustained by oxygen and a rich supply of metabolic substrates in uterine secretions. The subsequent sequence of events that lead to implantation is a crucial milestone in mammalian embryo development. Carefully orchestrated programs are set into action, which establish diverse cell lines, specify cell fate and major remodeling that will generate the embryo and its extraembryonic tissues: during gastrulation, the three primary germ layers that lead to body formation are formed. The critical conditions that are created in this early stage will pave the way to a successful pregnancy.

At the site of implantation the trophectoderm cells produce proteolytic enzymes that digest a passage through the zona pellucida, as the blastocyst 'hatches' free of the zona. The uterine environment may also contain proteolytic enzymes, but very little is known about the molecular basis for hatching. The exposed cell layers of the hatched blastocyst make firm physical contact and implantation starts. The process of implantation (Figure 6.1), leading to the successful establishment of a pregnancy, must be carefully coordinated in time and in place. The embryo and the uterus, both highly complex structures, must interact correctly and at the appropriate time in order for a pregnancy to be established; a multitude of different factors can influence their respective unique developmental characteristics. Implantation is initiated via a molecular dialogue between the 'free' hatched blastocyst and the endometrium, which allows the embryo to attach to the endometrial epithelium (decidua). The blastocyst trophectoderm secretes hCG, which provides direct signaling to the epithelial cells of the endometrium; hCG is detectable in maternal circulation within 3 days of embryo attachment to the endometrial epithelium – i.e., 9–12 days post ovulation. Trophectoderm cells from the blastocyst migrate between the epithelial cells, displace them and penetrate up to the basement membrane. The process of implantation can be divided into three stages: apposition, adhesion and invasion; the three phases must occur during a period when the uterine endometrium is maximally receptive, a period that is known as the 'implantation window.'

## Apposition: The Embryo/Endometrial Dialogue

The embryo enters the uterus 3 or 4 days after ovulation, and hatches from the zona pellucida as an expanded blastocyst on Day 5–6, so that the hatched blastocyst is 'apposed' to the uterine endometrium. Apposition is facilitated by the transient appearance of specialized epithelial cellular membrane protrusions or 'pinopodes,' which surround the pits in endometrial glands and actively reabsorb the uterine secretory phase fluid. Their appearance is progesterone-dependent, they are present for only 2–3 days (between Days 5 and 7 post ovulation), and they are a morphological marker of the opening of the implantation window (Nikas et al., 1995).

The uterine epithelium is coated with a network of glycoproteins (glycocalyx), which acts as a physical barrier to cell–cell interaction. The uterus is not receptive at this stage: the thick mucin coat, long microvilli and negative charge on the cellular surface membranes prevent blastocyst attachment. The embryo must first overcome this 'glycocalyx barrier,' which contains mucins expressed by endometrial cells, via localized (i.e., embryo driven) enzymatic cleavage of the extracellular glycoproteins, or via binding of receptors expressed by the embryo and subsequent cleavage of the mucins. During the receptive stage, the microvilli on the apical surface of the uterine epithelial cells shorten and MUC1 expression decreases in the immediate vicinity of the blastocyst. In response to estrogen, expression of maternal factors such as LIF is increased, which

(a)

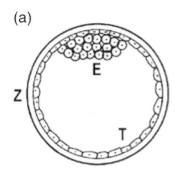

(b)

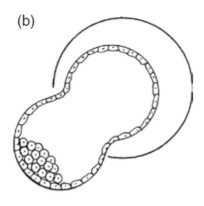

**Figure 6.1** Detailed anatomy of implantation in the mammal
(a) Expanded blastocyst showing the flat layer of trophectoderm cells (T) which will become part of the extraembryonic tissue and the inner cell mass (E) from which the embryo derives. (b) Diagram shows hatching, probably due in part to the production of a proteolytic-like enzyme by some of the trophectoderm cells. (c) Invasion of the epithelium (Ep) of the endometrium (En).
St = syncytiotrophoblast. Z = zona pellucida.

(c)

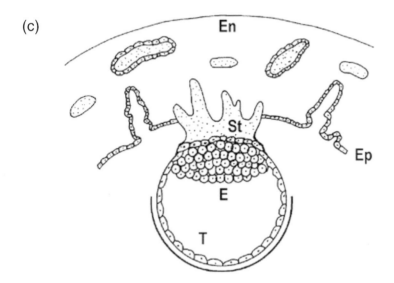

promotes endometrial receptivity to blastocyst attachment. Under these conditions, the progesterone-primed uterine wall increases expression of epidermal growth factor (EGF) and heparin-binding EGF-like growth factor (HB-EGF). EGF and HB-EGF bind EGF receptors and heparin sulfate proteoglycans on the trophoblast surface, which induces receptor phosphorylation and a second messenger cascade by the trophoblast; the blastocyst then hatches from the zona pellucida. When apposition is achieved, the adhesion molecules have access to each other, and the embryonic cytotrophoblast cells of the trophectoderm become attached to the endometrial cells.

## Adhesion

The embryo is thought to attach (adhere) to the endometrium on Day 6–7 post ovulation, mediated by the polar trophectoderm, the trophoblast cells immediately next to the inner cell mass. Once the embryo and endometrial adhesion molecules have free access to each other, the embryonic trophoblast cells attach to the endometrial epithelial cells: an erosive syncytium of trophoblast cells (syncytiotrophoblast) spreads from the polar trophectoderm into the basal decidua (Figure 6.2a). Several families of adhesion molecules are thought to be involved to a greater or lesser degree in human embryo attachment, including the integrins, tastin/trophinin complexes, heparan sulfate proteoglycans, cadherins, lectin/glycan interactions and glycan/glycan interactions. The integrin family is one of the key adhesion factors involved in human implantation. Experimental evidence has shown that hCG upregulates the integrin avb3, and interleukins IL-1α and IL-1β from the embryo are also involved. Human

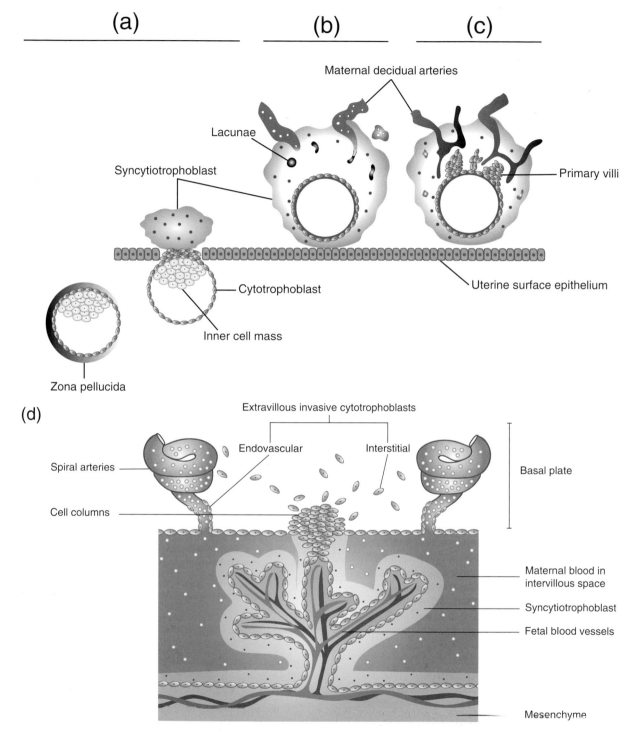

**Figure 6.2** (a) Preimplantation and peri-implantation blastocyst, showing both polar and mural trophectoderm, and the emergence of the primitive syncytiotrophoblast from the polar trophectoderm. (b and c) Postimplantation trophoblast development. Note the development of lacunae in the syncytiotrophoblast and the emergence of the primary villi (b). (d) Anatomy of the definitive placenta, showing both the villous trophoblast organized into chorionic villi and the extravillous cytotrophoblast cells organized into trophoblast cell columns. Adapted with permission from Baines & Renaud (2017), with thanks to Alejandra Ontiveros.

oocytes, early embryos and blastocysts express integrins, and they are also widely expressed by the glandular epithelium. Some are synthesized at a constant rate ($\alpha2$, $\alpha3$, $\alpha6$, $\beta1$, $\beta4$, $\beta5$), whereas others vary during stages of the cell cycle ($\alpha1$, $\alpha9$, $\alpha v$, $\beta3$, $\beta6$). The $\alpha v$ family of integrins are most likely to be involved in attachment; they bind fibronectin, osteopontin, vitronectin and other components of the extracellular matrix.

---

### What Is Trophoblast?

**(From Lee *et al.*, 2016.)**

Differentiation of the implanting blastocyst trophectoderm (TE) into subpopulations of trophoblast cells is a key early event in establishing a pregnancy. During the first trimester of gestation, trophoblast cells proliferate rapidly in the developing placenta, and any dysfunction at this stage will have an impact on obstetric outcome. Trophoblast cells differentiate in two main pathways: villous (VCT) and extravillous (EVT) cytotrophoblast. Whereas most somatic cells are human leukocyte antigen (HLA) class I positive and express HLA-A, HLA-B, HLA-C and HLA-E, human first trimester trophoblast cells never express HLA-A and HLA-B, and are the only cells that normally express HLA-G.

1. VCTs fuse to form an overlying syncytiotrophoblast (ST); these cells are HLA class I null.
2. EVTs form multinucleated placental bed giant cells deep in the decidua and myometrium; they express HLA-C, HLA-E and HLA-G.

## Invasion

Pre-villous trophoblast starts to differentiate between Days 7 and 12, and endometrial transformation (stromal decidualization) is underway by Day 12 post ovulation (Duc-Goiran *et al.*, 1999). Cytotrophoblasts of the embryonic trophectoderm are mononuclear undifferentiated stem cells that are precursors of all trophoblast forms. These differentiate into subsets via a complex process of gene repression to prevent their self-renewal and induction of genes that promote new biochemical functions (see Baines & Renaud, 2017 for review).

1. Junctional trophoblast cells from the polar trophectoderm mediate the attachment of the placenta to the uterus.

2. Invasive intermediate trophoblasts migrate into the uterine tissue.
3. Villous syncytiotrophoblast makes the majority of the placental hormones, including hCG, and regulates nutrient exchange between maternal and fetal blood.

Mononuclear trophoblast cells fuse to form a mitotically inactive syncytiotrophoblast with small chambers (lacunae) that connect together and fill with maternal blood from eroded decidual blood vessels. This invasion of the uterine decidua establishes an interface between fetus and mother, so that nutrients and waste products can be transferred. It also fulfills a mechanical function by stabilizing the placental tissue within the uterus. Cytotrophoblast cells proliferate rapidly to form large finger-like villous projections that penetrate the syncytiotrophoblast (VCT). At their tips, the villi continue as columns of cytotrophoblast cells that make contact with the endometrium and extend laterally, fusing with neighbors to form the cytotrophoblast shell. The shell represents the maternal–fetal interface, anchoring the conceptus to the endometrium. A subpopulation of trophoblast, the extravillous trophoblast (EVT), arises from the outer surface. These cells migrate into the wall of the uterus and play a critical role in remodeling the uterine spiral arteries that ultimately supply the placenta. These villi initially radiate out from the entire conceptus, and then regress gradually, apart from those adjacent to the decidua basalis, where the placenta will develop (Figure 6.2b).

EVTs invade the endometrium and upper layers of the myometrium and remodel the extracellular matrix in order to selectively permeate uterine spiral arteries. The colonized blood vessels are then modified to yield widened, low-resistance channels that can carry an increased maternal blood flow to the placenta. The mother must protect herself from these invasive trophoblasts migrating toward the uterine spiral arteries, and the endometrial stroma transforms itself into a dense cellular matrix known as the decidua, which will form the maternal part of the placenta. During decidualization, the spindle-shaped stromal fibroblasts enlarge and differentiate into plump secretory decidual cells, creating a tough extracellular matrix that is rich in fibronectin and laminin. This transformation occurs under the influence of progesterone.

The reaction is initially localized to cells surrounding the spiral arteries, but subsequently spreads to neighboring cells. The majority of cells of the decidua express leukocyte antigens. The largest single population of white blood cells in the endometrium are natural killer large granular lymphocytes (or natural killer [NK] cells), with smaller numbers of macrophages and T cells also present. The abundance of NK cells increases dramatically between ovulation and implantation, influenced by steroid hormones (King *et al.*, 1998). The decidua forms a physical barrier to invasive cell penetration and also generates a local cytokine milieu that promotes trophoblast attachment.

The first signs of the decidualization reaction can be seen as early as Day 23 of the normal menstrual cycle (10 days after the peak of the luteinizing hormone surge), when the spiral arteries of the endometrium first become prominent. Over the next few days, the effect of progesterone causes the stromal cells surrounding the spiral arteries to transform and differentiate into predecidual cells. This progressive decidualization of the endometrial stroma prepares the uterine lining for the presence of the invasive trophoblasts, but simultaneously closes the door to implantation. At this stage the embryo first becomes visible to the maternal immune system.

The invasion stage requires a very delicate balancing of conflicting biological needs between the early fetus and the mother, with a complex regulation of adhesion molecule expression, coordinated in time and in space. The invading cells use collagenases, and also express plasminogen activator inhibitor type 1, suggesting that the plasminogen activator system may also be involved. They lose integrins associated with basement membrane interactions (possibly laminin), and gain integrins that can interact with fibronectin and type I collagen. The outer layer trophoblast cells fuse to form a multinucleated syncytiotrophoblast layer that covers the columns of invading cells. This layer proliferates rapidly and forms numerous processes, the chorionic villi (the chorion is the layer that surrounds the embryo and extraembryonic membranes). Cyclic AMP and its analogs, and more recently hCG itself, have been shown to direct cytotrophoblast differentiation toward a syncytiotrophoblast phenotype that actively secretes the placental hormones.

At the point where chorionic villi make contact with external extracellular matrix (decidual stromal, ECM), another population of trophoblasts proliferates from the cytotrophoblast layer to form the junctional trophoblast. The junctional trophoblasts make a unique fibronectin, trophouteronectin (TUN), which appears to mediate the attachment of the placenta to the uterus. Transforming growth factor-β (TGF-β) and, more recently, leukemia inhibitory factor (LIF) have been shown to downregulate hCG synthesis and upregulate TUN secretion. These cells also make urokinase-type plasminogen activator and type 1 plasminogen activator inhibitor (PAI-1). Experiments using in-vitro model systems showed that phorbol esters increase trophoblast invasiveness and upregulate PAI-1 in cultured trophoblasts. Uterine prostaglandins (PGF2 and PGE2) are regulated by steroids and are involved in regulating the formation of the decidua.

## The Implantation Window

The existence of a transient implantation window has been well documented for rodent species. In these species, the window is maternally directed, and the receptive state is sustained for less than 24 hours. In the human, the window appears to be approximately 5 days long (Day 6 to Day 10 post ovulation in the normalized 28-day menstrual cycle), and the opening of the receptive phase is not as clearly defined as its termination. In the mouse, hatched blastocysts readily attach and spread in an integrin-dependent process on any surface that includes ligands found in the stroma during pregnancy (fibronectin, collagen, laminins, vitronectin, thrombospondin, etc.) as well as on artificial substrates like Matrigel. However, during human embryo implantation, trophoblast is penetrated through the epithelium, and the process is likely to be more strongly regulated by complex and multifactorial interactions between embryo and endometrium.

## Summary

Successful implantation requires both a synchronous development and a synchronized interaction between blastocyst and endometrium. Direct signaling from the embryo to the endometrium upregulates molecules such as the integrins, and this signaling promotes blastocyst adhesion. The blastocyst initially derives nourishment from uterine secretions, but in order to continue growing the conceptus must develop its own vascular system and, as a first step, induces a highly specialized reaction in the uterine stroma that initiates sprouting and growth of capillaries – the primary decidual reaction. The decidualized stromal cells make pericellular fibronectin. There is a dramatic transformation of endometrial stromal cells and a massive leukocyte infiltration by NK cells and macrophages. Maternal hormones influence the communication between the embryo and the endometrium, via effects on cytokines, adhesion molecules, prostaglandins, metalloproteases and their inhibitors, and angiogenic growth factors.

The molecular mechanisms behind this complex and sophisticated process have been studied using animal models, and knockout (KO) mouse studies have positively identified genes for receptivity (LIF, HMX3), responses to embryo (Cox2) and decidualization (IL-11R). Other factors identified as having a role include immune response gene (IRG1), progesterone receptor knock-out (PRKO), estrogen receptor knock-out (ERKO), homeobox protein A10 (Hoxa10), IHH (Indian Hedgehog gene) and immune regulating hormone 1 (IIRH1). Estrogen and progesterone receptors and the signaling pathways that interact with them are clearly important, including the IGF-I and EGF family and prostaglandins. Research in humans continues, now using endometrial organoid culture and microarray technology to look at gene expression in order to identify those factors that determine a receptive endometrium, with the hope of elucidating mechanisms that may enhance successful implantation after ART (Sherwin *et al.*, 2007; Simon *et al.*, 2009; Turco *et al.*, 2017).

---

**Steroid Hormones and Implantation**

**Estrogen** acts during the proliferative phase of the menstrual cycle to promote the development of the endometrium, and it opens the window of receptivity via several mechanisms:

- Causes loss of surface negative charge, shortening of microvilli and thinning of the mucin coat with changes in its molecular composition
- Stimulates the synthesis of at least 12–14 endometrial polypeptides, as well as estrogen and progesterone receptors
- Acts on luminal epithelial cells to make them responsive or sensitive to a blastocyst signal, promoting trophectoderm attachment to the luminal cells

- Stimulates the release of glandular epithelial secretions that include cytokines, and this activates the implantation process.

**Progesterone** is secreted by the corpus luteum after ovulation, and stimulates the secretory activity of the uterus:

- Produces intense edema in the stroma
- Increases blood vessel volume threefold
- Stimulates the formation of pinopodes and primes the decidua.

Steroids regulate the action of **uterine growth factors** which are synthesized at various stages of the menstrual cycle: IGF-I and IGF-II, EGF, HB-EGF, FGF, β-FGF, α-FGF, TGF-β1, PDGF-β.

# Early Placental Development

The definitive placenta has two anatomically distinct compartments that provide specialized functions. In general, cells that are near the embryo promote exchange between maternal and fetal blood, and trophoblast cells developing next to the basal decidua interact with the stroma to facilitate blood flow to the placenta. In humans, the maternal–fetal exchange surface is organized into tree-like structures, the chorionic villi. These are made up of an outer lining of trophoblast cells (chorion) and an inner core of vascularized mesoderm, which originates from the allantois: the placenta is therefore known as chorioallantoic. The blood vessels that form within the core connect with the fetal circulation via the umbilical vessels; the chorionic villi are bathed in maternal blood, and nutrients are transported into the villous core, where they can enter the fetal circulation.

Maintaining an ongoing pregnancy after implantation depends upon successful placental development, and any defects in the process can lead to a spectrum of disorders that may present at different times: miscarriage, pre-eclampsia, fetal growth restriction, stillbirth, preterm rupture of membranes and premature delivery.

After implantation, the endometrial glands are highly active, and secretions from these glands, 'uterine milk,' deliver nutrients into the placenta until 10 weeks of pregnancy. These secretions contain cytokines, transport proteins and growth factors that stimulate trophoblastic cell proliferation. The glands usually regress over the first trimester, but still communicate with the intervillous space for at least 10 weeks. In animal models, signals from the conceptus increase 'uterine milk' protein production, i.e., there is a signaling dialogue between the trophoblast and the endometrial glands in early pregnancy, which determines healthy placental development. Any defects or deficiency in this dialogue may result in fertility problems or recurrent miscarriage.

### Natural Killer (NK) Cells

- Lymphocytes in circulating peripheral blood that have the ability to kill target cells are known as peripheral blood natural killer cells (pbNK cells); they have the intrinsic ability to kill some leukemic cell lines in vitro and are an important component of the immune system. Through cytotoxicity and cytokine secretion, they act as a first line of defense against viruses and in controlling the early spread of tumors.
- Immune cells with a similar phenotype represent around 30% of stromal cells in late secretory endometrium and are found in the lining of the uterus at implantation as well as during development of the placenta in the first trimester of pregnancy. These cells were given the name 'uterine killer cells' (uNK cells): this is a misnomer, as they have very poor 'killer' functions, and instead are thought to have an important role in regulating trophoblast invasion and placentation, playing an important part in building a healthy placenta before the period of accelerated fetal growth. Their origin is unclear, but they are thought to arise from immature progenitor cells in the circulation that migrate into the uterine mucosa and develop there.
- The name 'uterine killer cells' led to a myth that uNK cells can kill the embryo and may be involved in failed IVF and recurrent miscarriage; however, they are never in contact with the embryo, but only with placental trophoblast cells, and there is no evidence that they can kill trophoblast cells under natural conditions.
- uNK and pbNK cells are quite distinct, with different types of receptors regulating their function: any parameter used to test NK cell function in a peripheral blood sample cannot reflect the function of uNK cells. Despite the widespread use of NK cell testing and immunotherapy as a means of enhancing pregnancy outcome in IVF, there is no scientific rationale or evidence that justifies strategies aiming to target or modulate uNK cell function (Moffett & Shreeve, 2015).

At 6 weeks of gestation, early trophoblastic villi cover the entire gestational sac, merging at their tips to form the cytotrophoblastic shell that forms a boundary with the endometrium at the interface between maternal and fetal tissues. Trophoblast cells from the cytotrophoblast shell migrate down the lumina of spiral arteries, effectively plugging them during the first trimester. Seventy percent of miscarriages show an incomplete shell, and this is associated with abnormal early onset of maternal arterial blood flow. Mesenchyme from the extraembryonic somatic mesoderm eventually fills the trophoblastic villi, and blood vessels form which then connect the maternal to the fetal circulation via the umbilical cord.

## Early Postimplantation Embryogenesis

Most of our knowledge about early postimplantation development was gained from studies in chick, mouse and other mammalian species. Fixed and stained human embryos after pregnancy loss at different stages of gestation provided information about the early human postimplantation period. The Carnegie Collection of Human Development at the National Institute of Child and Human Development in Washington DC has made a collection of several thousand serial microscopic cross-sections, which are available for study (O'Rahilly and Müller, 1987). Human embryos have been classified into 23 developmental stages based on a number of morphological features, known as the Carnegie stages. These stages represent a series of events that occur during development, with overlap between the different stages. From 1994 onwards the Visible Embryo Project (www.visembryo.com) used computer technology to reconstruct accurate three-dimensional images of human development. A digital image database of serially sectioned human embryos from the Carnegie Collection is available online as The Heirloom Collection, supported by the National Library of Medicine in the USA.

More recently, Shabazi et al. (2016) developed an in-vitro system to culture human embryos in the absence of maternal tissues from early cleavage or blastocyst stages through to postimplantation stages up to day 12–13, and compared their observations with the Carnegie series. Using immunostaining for lineage-specific markers, they identified the series of events that occur after implantation: segregation of epiblast and hypoblast progenitors (Day 7); epiblast polarization and formation of the proamniotic cavity (Day 8–10); differentiation of the trophoblast into cytotrophoblast and syncytiotrophoblast (Day 8–10); formation of the prospective amniotic ectoderm and yolk sac and bilaminar disc (Day 11). By extending the studies using human pluripotent stem cells, they showed that embryonic cell lineages reorganize via cellular polarization, leading to cavity formation. Unexpectedly, the human embryos were able to self-organize autonomously, without the participation of maternal tissue.

The brief overview presented below describing early embryo development is based upon the Carnegie Collection of beautiful color three-dimensional reconstructions and animations, which can be viewed at: http://virtualhumanembryo.lsuhsc.edu/.

## 7–12 Days Post Ovulation

Once the blastocyst has hatched and trophoblast cells have started the process of implantation, the cells of the inner cell mass start to reorganize into distinct layers, each layer destined for a different developmental fate. Cellular morphology changes, and there is active movement of individual cells and groups of cells, setting up new relationships between them. In the human embryo, the first 14–18 days of development are concerned mainly with the differentiation of various extraembryonic tissues, and after this time separate tissues can begin to be identified.

## 13–15 Days Post Ovulation (Second Week of Development)

Cells of the inner cell mass separate into two different sheets of cells to form a bilaminar embryonic disc (Figure 6.3):

Dorsal germinal layer = epiblast

Ventral germinal layer = hypoblast.

The flatter hypoblast cells lie on top of the epiblast and will form the yolk sac; the epiblast contains the cells of the future embryo.

The two layers of the embryonic disc divide the blastocyst into two chambers, the amnion and the yolk sac (Figure 6.5); outside the embryo, the extraembryonic spaces (chorionic, amniotic, yolk sac) continue to develop, the endometrium is being converted into the decidua and early placentation has begun. The amnion fills with fluid that cushions the developing fetus; the yolk sac contributes to the formation of the extraembryonic membranes, chorion and amnion. It is also the site of early blood cell formation, and part of the yolk sac becomes incorporated into the gut later in development. The cells of the trophoblast form another chamber, the extraembryonic coelom, around the amnion, yolk sac and developing embryo; this will later become the chorionic sac and placenta.

## 13–15 Days Post Ovulation (End of Second Week of Development)

Embryonic epiblast cells move along the surface, begin to pile up near the center to form a node

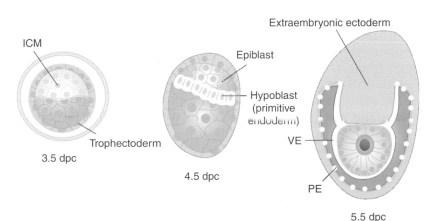

**Figure 6.3** Peri-implantation development. Diagram of mouse blastocyst showing epiblast layer. ICM = inner cell mass; VE = visceral endoderm; dpc = days post conception. With thanks to Cindy Lu and Elizabeth Robertson.

ICM

Extraembryonic ectoderm

Epiblast

Hypoblast (primitive endoderm)

Trophectoderm

VE

PE

3.5 dpc

4.5 dpc

5.5 dpc

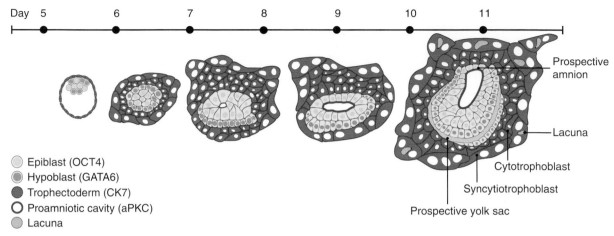

Day 5 6 7 8 9 10 11

Prospective amnion

Lacuna

Cytotrophoblast

Syncytiotrophoblast

Prospective yolk sac

- Epiblast (OCT4)
- Hypoblast (GATA6)
- Trophectoderm (CK7)
- Proamniotic cavity (aPKC)
- Lacuna

**Figure 6.4** Schematic model of human embryo morphogenesis during peri-implantation and early implantation. (See color plate section) Day 7: segregation of epiblast and hypoblast progenitors; Day 8–10: polarization and formation of the proamniotic cavity in the epiblast; Day 8–10: differentiation of the trophectoderm (TE) into cytotrophoblast and syncytiotrophoblast cells; Day 10–11: formation of the prospective amniotic epithelium, the prospective yolk sac and the bilaminar disc. Adapted with permission from Shabazi *et al.* (2016), with thanks to Alejandra Ontiveros.

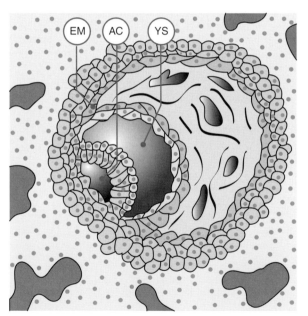

EM AC YS

**Figure 6.5** Diagrammatic representation of human embryo transverse section on approximately Day 14 post ovulation, indicating extraembryonic mesoblast (EM), amniotic cavity (AC) and yolk sac (YS, also known as umbilical vesicle).

and then move internally to create a furrowed cell mass, the primitive streak (Figure 6.6a). This is a visible feature showing that cells are migrating, and the furrow begins to extend toward the cranial

(head) end of the bilaminar disc (Figure 6.6b). Cells near the advancing edge of the streak begin to pull apart slightly to form an open pit, and cells bordering this pit then migrate between the epiblast and hypoblast to create a new layer, the mesoderm. Cells from the epiblast also displace the hypoblast, creating the endoderm. The cells that remain on the surface will form ectoderm, and this formation of a now trilaminar disc is known as gastrulation. During gastrulation, cells from the mesoderm form the notochord, which will define the primitive axis of the embryo and establish cranio-caudal orientation and bilateral symmetry of the fully developed body. The three layers of cells form the primary germ cells that will evolve into the specialized cells, tissues and organs of the body:

*Endoderm* (inner layer): forms the lining of the primitive digestive tract and its associated glandular structures, as well as portions of the liver, pancreas, trachea and lungs.

*Mesoderm* (middle layer): initially forms a loose aggregate of cells, the mesenchyme; this then organizes into regions that evolve into the vertebral column, skeletal muscle, ribs, skull and the dermis of the skin. Mesenchymal cells also form tubular structures: urogenital system, heart, blood

(a)    Actual Size 0.2mm

(b)    Actual Size 0.4mm

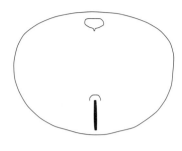 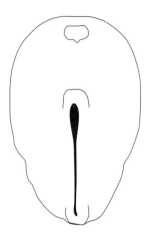

**Figure 6.6** Third week of fetal development, dorsal views; dates are approximate, stages overlap. (a) 13 days post ovulation, Carnegie Stage 6; primitive streak and node (bottom) and prechordal plate (top). (b) 16 days post ovulation, Carnegie Stage 7; neurolation. (c) 17–19 days post ovulation, Carnegie Stage 8; primitive pit, notochordal and neurenteric canals. (d) 19–21 days post ovulation, Carnegie Stage 9; appearance of somites. Illustrations drawn by Luke Ebbutt-James, Cambridge, UK.

(c)    Actual Size 1.0 - 1.5mm

(d)    Actual Size 1.5 - 2.5mm

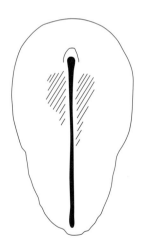 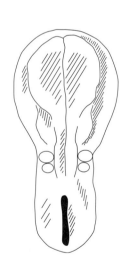

vessels, and the lining of the pericardial, pleural and peritoneal cavities.

*Ectoderm* (outer layer): develops into skin epidermis, brain and spinal cord. Sensory receptors for vision, hearing and smell, as well as the future autonomic nervous system and adrenal medulla, also develop from ectoderm.

## 17–19 Days (Third Week of Development)

After gastrulation, the mesoderm starts to segment into mesenchymal tissue somites, and the notochord induces rapid growth in the ectoderm. Over the next 2–3 days, the ectodermal layer thickens to form a neural plate, which folds to form a neural groove (Figure 6.6c): the nervous system is one of the first

129

organs to develop. During this process of neurolation, the ectoderm will subdivide into neural tissue and epithelial tissue lineages (pigmented cells of the epidermis, adrenal medullary cells, skeletal and connective tissues of the head). Somites continue to form in the mesoderm, the neural groove fuses dorsally to form a tube at the level of the fourth somite, and closes. The cranial end of the neural plate is wider, enclosing the region that will form the brain. The spinal cord will form at the caudal end, which is narrower (the notochord is eventually replaced by the vertebral column).

## 19–21 Days (End of Third Week of Development)

Rapid cellular growth elongates the embryo and expands the yolk sac. Primordial germ cells can be identified at the root of the allantois. A head fold rises on either side of the primitive streak, and endocardial cells begin to fuse and form two endocardial tubes which will develop into the heart. Pairs of mesodermal somites can be seen on either side of the neural groove (Figure 6.6d), appearing first in the caudal region. The neural folds rise and fuse along the length of the neural tube (Figure 6.7a), along with budding somites that close the neural tube (like a zipper). The neural tube begins to close in the middle of the embryo (cervical area), and then extends in both cranial and caudal directions. Failure of the neural tube to close correctly at this stage can lead to anomalies such as spina bifida (caudal) or anencephaly (cranial). Masses of cells detach themselves from the side of the neural plate and form the neural crest, precursor cells of numerous differentiated cells of the nervous and glandular systems. The heart tube becomes S-shaped, with the beginning of cardiac muscle contraction. Secondary blood vessels appear in the chorion/placenta, and hematopoietic cells appear in the yolk sac.

## 23-27 Days (Fourth Week)

A primitive S-shaped tubal heart begins to beat, and the developing neural tube curves the embryo into a C-shape (Figure 6.7b). The forebrain is closed when 20 somites are present, eyes and ears begin to form, and pharyngeal arches are present. Valves and septa begin to appear in the heart, and a blood circulatory system continues to develop.

### Genes Significant in Early Development

- Homeobox genes are a highly conserved family of transcription factors that switch on cascades of other genes that are involved in the regulation of embryonic development of virtually all multicellular animals.
- Wnt genes encode short-range secreted proteins that are involved in cell adhesion and cell–cell signaling.
- Cellular adhesion molecules such as the integrins are important for cellular recognition and binding that influence cell migration. Laminin and fibronectin are also involved in cell migration.
- The fate of a migrating cell is apparently determined largely by its final destination. RhoB and Slug proteins, which promote cell migration, are present at the gastrulation stage, and the loss of N-cadherin helps to initiate the migration of neural crest cells.
- Hedgehog genes encode signaling molecules that are involved in patterning processes; this family of genes is named after a *Drosophila* gene whose loss of function produced an embryo covered with pointed denticles, like a hedgehog. Three homologous genes have been found in mammals: Sonic hedgehog, Shh (named after the Sega Genesis video game), Desert hedgehog, Dhh and Indian hedgehog, Ihh.
- Shh is secreted by the notochord and has numerous critical roles in development, involved in the patterning of many systems, including the brain and spinal cord, as well as in establishing left–right axis patterning. Differentiation pathways appear to be influenced by different levels of Shh, in combination with other paracrine factors, including Wnt and FGF.
- The Shh transcription pathway controls cell division in adult stem cells and has been linked to the formation of some cancerous tumors.

## 28-35 Days (Fifth Week)

Somites organize themselves into myotomes, the groups of tissues that will develop into the musculoskeletal structure of the body wall, and rudiments of the ribs and limbs begin to appear (Figure 6.7c and d). Sclerotomes give rise to the axial skeleton, myotomes to striated muscle, and dermatomes to subcutaneous

(a)    Actual Size 1.5 – 3.0mm

(b)    Actual Size 3.0 – 5.0mm

**Figure 6.7** Fourth week of fetal development, dorsal views; dates are approximate, stages overlap. (a) 21–23 days post ovulation, Carnegie Stage 10; neural folds/heart folds begin to fuse. (b) 25–27 days post ovulation, Carnegie Stage 12; upper limb buds appear. (c) 26–30 days post ovulation, Carnegie Stage 13; pharyngeal arches and upper limb buds visible. (d) 31–35 days post ovulation, Carnegie Stage 14; esophagus forming, lens vesicle opens to the surface and optic cup develops, upper limb buds elongate and taper. Illustrations drawn by Luke Ebbutt-James, Cambridge, UK.

(c)    Actual Size 4.0 – 6.0mm

(d)    Actual Size 5.0 – 7.0mm

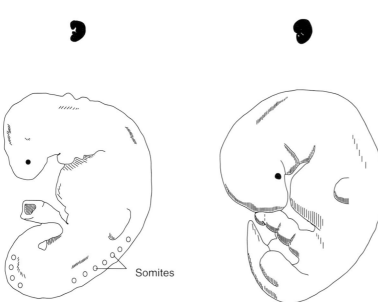

Somites

tissue and skin. Arches that form the face and neck can be seen under the enlarging forebrain. The digestive epithelial layer begins to differentiate into the future locations of the liver, lung, stomach and pancreas.

## 35-42 Days (Sixth Week)

By Day 35 (fifth week of development = 6 weeks from last menstrual period), when clinical pregnancy after IVF can be confirmed by ultrasound visualization of gestational sac and fetal heartbeat (Figure 6.8),

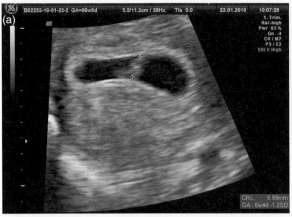

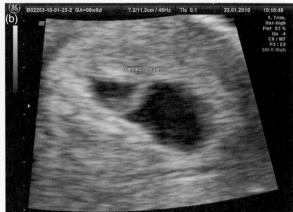

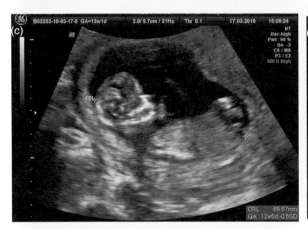

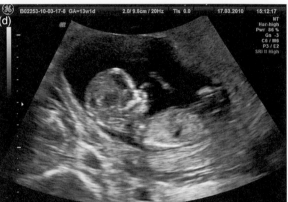

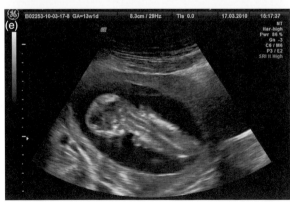

**Figure 6.8** Ultrasound scans of early pregnancy. Six-week scan, showing crown–rump length (crl) = 6.89 mm, = 6 weeks + 4 days. (b) Another view of (a), illustrating fetal pole. (c) Twelve-week scan, crl = 65.57 mm, = 12 weeks + 6 days. (d) Thirteen-week scan, clear view of head and body. (e) Another view of (d), showing the vertebral column. Images courtesy of Baby Premier, division of Specialist Medical Imaging Ltd.

the three primary germ layers have expanded and undergone a dramatic process of differentiation and transformation, to form a clearly recognizable fetus. The beating heart has chambers, and all limbs and body systems are under development. Medial thickening of the coelomic epithelium represents the formation of primordial gonads. The size of the fetus is now approximately 7.0–9.0 mm, and it will continue to grow at a rate of around 1 mm per day during the first trimester. By the beginning of the second trimester, the basic brain structure is complete, and genitalia begin to show signs of gender characteristics.

## Ultrasound Confirmation of Clinical Pregnancy

1. **Gestational sac**: can be seen at around 4 weeks' gestation but may not be visible until the end of the fifth week. It is characteristic of early pregnancy, but does not correspond to anatomical features of the embryo. Gestational sacs are also found in ectopic pregnancies.
2. **Yolk sac**: visible during the fifth week, and grows to be no larger than 6 mm. Larger yolk sacs usually indicate an abnormal pregnancy; yolk sacs that are misshapen, are 'floating' within the gestational sac and contain echogenic (instead of sonolucent) material are ominous findings for the pregnancy.
3. **Fetal heartbeat (FH)**: using transvaginal ultrasound, fetal cardiac activity can sometimes be seen along the edge of the yolk sac before a fetal cell mass is identifiable. In normal pregnancies, the fetal heartbeat may not be seen until the fetal pole is around 4 mm in size. Failure to identify a FH in a fetus >4 mm in size is an ominous sign.
4. **Fetal pole**: the fetus in its somite stage, first visible separation from the yolk sac by transvaginal scan (TVS) just after 6 weeks' gestation (Day 35 post ovulation).
5. **Crown–rump length (CRL)**: single most accurate measure of gestational age up to 12 weeks' gestation.

## Pregnancy Failures

1. **Miscarriage**: spontaneous abortion prior to 20 weeks' gestation.
2. **Biochemical pregnancy**: early pregnancy loss, prior to 6 weeks from last menstrual period.
3. **Blighted ovum**: anembryonic gestation. Sac appears normal on TVS, but an embryo never develops; probably due to early embryonic death with continued trophoblast development.
4. **Missed abortion**: nonviable intrauterine pregnancy that has not yet aborted. TVS shows gestational sac with no FH; can be due to a blighted ovum, or early demise of an embryo after detection of FH. The cervical os is closed.
5. **Threatened abortion**: vaginal bleeding and/or abdominal/pelvic pain during early pregnancy; the cervical os is closed, and no tissue has been passed. FH is still present on TVS.
6. **Inevitable abortion**: vaginal bleeding, usually with abdominal pain and cramps. FH is absent, cervical os is open, but no tissue has been passed. Usually progresses to complete abortion.
7. **Incomplete abortion**: Heavy vaginal bleeding, with tissue having been passed, but some remaining in utero.
8. **Complete abortion**: bleeding, abdominal pain; all products of conception have been passed; empty uterus must be confirmed by TVS.
9. **Recurrent abortion**: history of more than three spontaneous abortions.

## Ectopic Pregnancy

- A hatched blastocyst can sometimes implant in sites outside the uterus, most commonly in the fallopian tube. Other sites include the utero-cervical isthmus (cervical pregnancy) and the utero-tubal junction; more rarely, implantation can take place in the ovary, or in the peritoneal or abdominal cavity.
- Occasionally two embryos will implant at different sites: one in each tube (bilateral tubal pregnancy) or one in the uterus and one at an ectopic site (heterotopic pregnancy).
- An embryo can continue to grow at an ectopic site for several weeks, with signs and symptoms of early pregnancy in the mother. If undetected, ectopic pregnancy can result in a life-threatening crisis due to tubal rupture or erosion into a blood vessel.

# Further Reading

### Implantation

Baines KJ, Renaud SJ (2017) Transcription factors that regulate trophoblast development and function. In: Huckle WR (ed.) *Progress in Molecular Biology and Translational Science*, vol. 145. Academic Press, Burlington, MA pp. 39–88.

Bourgain C, Devroey P (2007) Histologic and functional aspects of the endometrium in the implantatory phase. *Gynecologic and Obstetric Investigation* 64(3): 131–133.

Campbell S, Swan HR, Seif MW, Kimber SJ, Aplin JD (1995) Cell adhesion molecules on the oocyte and preimplantation human embryo. *Molecular Human Reproduction* 1(4): 171–178.

Cheon YP, Xu X, Bagchi MK, Bagchi IC (2003) IRG1 is a novel target of progesterone receptor and plays a critical role during implantation in the mouse. *Endocrinology* 144(12): 5623–5630.

Duc-Goiran P, Mignot TM, Bourgeois C, Ferré F (1999) Embryo-maternal interactions at the implantation site: a delicate equilibrium (Review). *European Journal of Obstetrics, Gynecology, and Reproductive Biology* 83(1): 85–100.

Grewal S, Carver JG, Ridley AJ, Mardon HJ (2008) Implantation of the human embryo requires Rac1 dependent endometrial stromal migration. *Proceedings of the National Academy of Sciences USA* 105: 16189–16194.

Hempstock J, Cindrova-Davies T, Jauniaux E, Burton G (2004) Endometrial glands as a source of nutrients, growth factors and cytokines during the first trimester of human pregnancy: a morphological and immunohistochemical study. *Reproductive Biology and Endocrinology* 2: 58. DOI:10.1186/1477-7827-2-58.

Horcajadas JA, Pellicer A, Simón C (2007) Wide genomic analysis of human endometrial receptivity: new times, new opportunities. *Human Reproduction Update* 13(1): 77–86.

King A, Burrows T, Verma S, Hiby S, Loke YW (1998) Human uterine lymphocytes. *Human Reproduction Update* 4(5): 480–485.

Kliman HJ (2000) The story of decidualization, menstruation, and trophoblast invasion. *American Journal of Pathology* 157: 1759–1768.

Lee CQE, Gardner L, Turco M, Zhao N, *et al.* (2016) What is trophoblast? A combination of criteria define human first trimester trophoblast. *Stem Cell Reports* 6: 257–272.

Lee K, Jeong J, Kwak I, *et al.* (2006) Indian hedgehog is a major mediator of progesterone signaling in the mouse uterus. *Nature Genetics* 38: 1204–1209.

Mardon H, Grewal S (2007) Experimental models for investigating implantation of the human embryo. *Seminars in Reproductive Medicine* 25: 410–417.

Moffett A, Shreeve N (2015) First do no harm: uterine natural killer (NK) cells in assisted reproduction. *Human Reproduction* 30(7): 1519–1525.

Nikas G, Drakakis P, Loutradis D, *et al.* (1995) Uterine pinopodes as markers of the 'nidation window' in cycling women receiving exogenous oestradiol and progesterone. *Human Reproduction* 10(5): 1208–1213.

Parr MB, Parr EL (1964) Uterine luminal epithelium: protrusions mediate endocytosis, not apocrine secretion, in the rat. *Biology of Reproduction* 11(2): 220–233.

Psychoyos A (1986) Uterine receptivity for nidation. *Annals of the New York Academy of Sciences* 476: 36–42.

Psychoyos A, Nikas G, Gravanis A (1995) The role of prostaglandins in blastocyst implantation. *Human Reproduction* 10(Suppl. 2): 30–42.

Sherwin JR, Sharkey AM, Cameo P, *et al.* (2007) Identification of novel genes regulated by hCG in baboon endometrium. *Endocrinology* 148: 618–626.

Simon C, Gimeno MJ, Mercader A, *et al.* (1997) Embryonic regulation of integrins in endometrial epithelial cells. *Journal of Clinical Endocrinology and Metabolism* 82: 2607–2616.

Simon L, Spiewak KA, Ekman GC, *et al.* (2009) Stromal progesterone receptors mediate induction of IHH in uterine epithelium. *Endocrinology* 150: 3871–3876.

Turco M, Gardner L, Hughes J, *et al.* (2017) Long-term, hormone-responsive organoid cultures of human endometrium in a chemically defined medium. *Nature Cell Biology* 19(5): 568–577.

Wang H, Dey SK (2006) Roadmap to embryo implantation. *Nature Reviews Genetics* 7: 185–199.

Wilcox AJ, Baird DD, Dunson D, McChesney R, Weinberg CR (2001) Natural limits of pregnancy testing in relation to the expected menstrual period. *Journal of the American Medical Association* 286(14): 1759–1761. Erratum in: *JAMA* 2002; 287(2): 192.

Wilcox AJ, Baird DD, Weinberg CR (1999) Time of implantation of the conceptus and loss of pregnancy. *New England Journal of Medicine* 340(23): 1796–1799.

## Embryogenesis

www.visembryo.com

http://embryology.med.unsw.edu.au/

Deglincerti A, Croft GF, Pietila LN, Zernicka-Goetz M, Siggia ED, Brivanlou AH (2016) Self-organization of the in vitro attached human embryo. *Nature* 533: 251–254.

Dorus S, Anderson JR, Vallender EJ, *et al.* (2006) Sonic Hedgehog, a key development gene, experienced intensified molecular evolution in primates. *Human Molecular Genetics* 15(13): 2031–2037.

Gilbert SF (2000) *Developmental Biology*. Sinauer Associates, Sunderland, MA.

Herzog W, Zeng X, Lele Z, *et al.* (2003) Adenohypophysis formation in the zebrafish and its dependence on sonic hedgehog. *Developmental Biology* 254: 1.

O'Rahilly RF, Müller F (1987) *Developmental Stages in Human Embryos*. Carnegie Institution of Washington, Washington, DC.

Shabazi MN, Jedrusik A, Vuoristo S *et al.* (2016) Self-organization of the human embryo in the absence of maternal tissues. *Nature Cell Biology* 18(6): 700–708.

# Stem Cell Biology

## Stem Cells and Stem Cell Lines

Every cell in an individual has a unique chromosome complement, with 20 000–25 000 genes coded into a DNA sequence of 3 billion base pairs, packed into 23 pairs of chromosomes: a total of 46 chromosomes in each diploid human cell. All of these cells have the same genetic information, copied during mitotic divisions by replicating the DNA during each cell cycle. The pattern of gene activity in each cell (gene expression/transcription) dictates its function and fate, enabling different cells to differentiate and carry out distinct functions.

After an oocyte has been fertilized, the one-cell zygote is **totipotent**, with the potential to give rise to a complete organism, including both embryonic and extraembryonic cells. As cell division proceeds, blastomeres lose the potential to give rise to an entire organism, and by the time that a fully expanded blastocyst has formed, three types of morphologically and molecularly distinct cells have emerged: **trophectoderm** cells surround an inner cell mass, which contains **epiblast** progenitor cells and **primitive endoderm** cells. The embryo itself is derived exclusively from epiblast progenitor cells; trophectoderm cells will form fetal components of the placenta, and primitive endoderm will form the yolk sac, which is derived from extraembryonic endoderm. Continued development of the embryo requires the support of all of these extraembryonic cell types.

Epiblast progenitor cells of the blastocyst inner cell mass are considered to be **pluripotent**, as they have the potential to give rise to the three primary germ layers that will form all of the tissues of the fetus: mesoderm, endoderm and ectoderm. Significantly, these progenitor cells do not have the potential to give rise to a whole organism without the supporting extraembryonic cells. Following implantation, the pluripotent embryonic cells become committed to more specialized cells that increasingly lose their potential to contribute to all three germ layers. **Multipotent** cells have been identified in the developing embryo and in the adult, which have the potential to continually give rise to the same cell (**self-renew**) and also have the potential to give rise to other cells with a more specialized function. Hematopoietic stem cells are multipotent cells that replenish all blood cells by dividing to form two types of cell: one daughter cell maintains a stem cell population, and the second daughter cell has the potential to continue to alter its pattern of gene expression and differentiate. The daughter cells that become more specialized with each cell division go through distinct populations of **transit amplifying cells**, proliferative cells that retain their self-renewal property until they reach the end of their production line and are terminally differentiated. Other types of stem cell, such as neural stem cells, are **oligopotent**, giving rise to diverse but restricted populations of specific self-renewing subtypes. **Unipotent** cells, such as spermatogonial stem cells, are self-renewing cells that have the potential to give rise to a single lineage, spermatogonia. Figure 7.1 illustrates a hierarchy of stem cell potential.

Two properties are unique to all types of stem cell:

1. They have the capacity for long-term self-renewal.
2. They have the potential to give rise to cells other than themselves.

A **stem cell line** is a population of cells that has been grown and maintained in vitro. When maintained under appropriate conditions, these cells continue to grow in tissue culture for very long periods of time.

## Mammalian Stem Cell Lines

Following the derivation and culture of human embryonic stem cell lines in the late 1990s (Thomson *et al.*, 1998), debate and controversy escalated

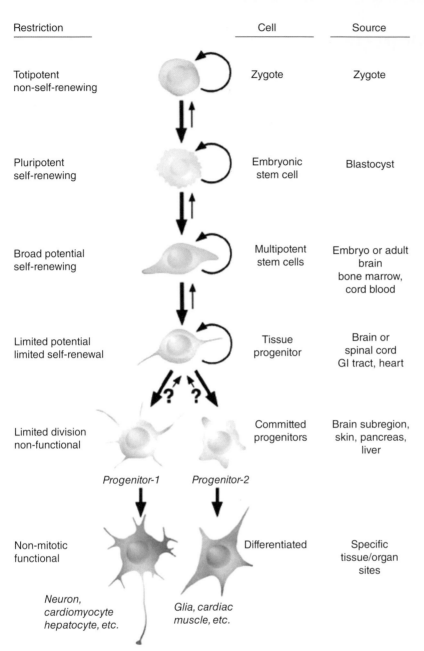

| Restriction | Cell | Source |
|---|---|---|
| Totipotent non-self-renewing | Zygote | Zygote |
| Pluripotent self-renewing | Embryonic stem cell | Blastocyst |
| Broad potential self-renewing | Multipotent stem cells | Embryo or adult brain bone marrow, cord blood |
| Limited potential limited self-renewal | Tissue progenitor | Brain or spinal cord GI tract, heart |
| Limited division non-functional | Committed progenitors | Brain subregion, skin, pancreas, liver |
| Non-mitotic functional | Differentiated | Specific tissue/organ sites |

*Progenitor-1*  *Progenitor-2*

*Neuron, cardiomyocyte hepatocyte, etc.*  *Glia, cardiac muscle, etc.*

**Figure 7.1** Potential pathways for stem cell development. Adapted from Gage (2000), with permission from AAAS.

surrounding the use of surplus human embryos donated for research. Despite the controversial ethico-legal perspectives, in many countries throughout the world IVF clinics have embryos that are either unsuitable for treatment or are surplus to the patient's requirements. Given the opportunity for appropriate counseling and informed consent, many patients choose to make a contribution to science by donating surplus embryos for research rather than allowing them to perish (Franklin *et al.*, 2008). There is no doubt that embryos donated for stem cell research represent a very valuable resource for scientific investigation, with the potential to make a significant contribution to our understanding of early developmental processes and the molecular pathology of disease. Stem cell biology has become an integral part of ART; the principles and the science underpinning this new area of developmental and regenerative biology should be viewed within the perspective and frame of reference of the first stages of postimplantation development, as presented in the brief synopsis in Chapter 6.

# Human Embryonic Stem Cells (hESCs)

Human embryonic stem cells are derived from the in-vitro expansion of epiblast progenitors within the inner cell mass of a preimplantation blastocyst. hESCs are capable of indefinite self-renewal, and maintain the potential to differentiate into cell types from the three embryonic germ layers (pluripotency). Because they remain pluripotent when maintained in vitro, they provide an ideal resource for investigating and studying the pathways that lead to the establishment of cells that might be relevant to clinical treatment, such as dopamine-producing neurons and insulin-producing cells of the pancreas.

The goal of hESC research is to elucidate the pathways that direct differentiation in vitro, with the aim of providing functional and therapeutically relevant cells. These cells can be used to investigate mechanisms of disease progression, and for research into drugs that might inhibit or reverse pathological processes. hESCs also provide an insight into aspects of early embryonic development that are otherwise inaccessible to research, due to ethical and practical considerations; they can be used as a tool to investigate how cells can be manipulated to regenerate damaged or diseased cells in the human body. Lastly, hESC-differentiated cells may eventually prove to be useful in cell transplantation approaches for the treatment of disease (see Trounson & DeWitt [2016] and Chen *et al.* [2014], for reviews).

Several strategies have been applied to promote the differentiation or selection of therapeutically relevant cell types, including the addition of growth factors or cytokines, as well as other ways of manipulating gene expression. One major hurdle to this approach is that the process of directing the differentiation of hESCs into functionally relevant specialized cells is very inefficient, and their intrinsic potential can allow them to switch from pluripotency toward uncontrolled differentiation during expansion in culture. This inefficiency may be the result of heterogeneity within a starting stem cell population, in addition to the lack of information about the developmental events that promote the emergence of specialized cells in vivo – differentiation into a particular lineage is a highly complex process, controlled by a multitude of overlapping parameters. The constraints of in-vitro culture conditions also hinder the ability to mimic in-vivo events.

The large-scale availability of treatments involving pluripotent stem cells will require further research to elucidate the fine details of the growth and stability of the cells, as well as a secure and thorough regulatory pathway to ensure their safety.

**Tissue stem cells** in fetal or adult tissue can supply cells to parts of the body that require a continuous supply of regenerative cells. Tissue stem cells include blood and intestinal stem cells; these are partially committed cells that can function to regenerate their respective adult tissues as required. They commonly reside in a microenvironment (niche) in a quiescent state where they are provided with signals and support that promote the maintenance of self-renewal. Stem cells exit the niche as they undergo cellular commitment/differentiation.

# Multipotent Stem Cells

- All blood cell types are continuously replaced from a store of hematopoietic stem cells (HSCs) in the bone marrow.
- The lining of the gut (gut epithelium) has intestinal stem cells in the small intestine that produce four different cell lineages (Paneth, goblet, absorptive columnar, enteroendocrine).
- Epidermal stem cells in the skin and hair follicle can regenerate damaged epithelium.
- Skeletal muscle stem cells (satellite cells) are quiescent cells that can also give rise to committed progeny such as myofibers in response to injury or disease.

# Oligopotent Stem Cells

- Neural stem cells are restricted self-renewing subtypes that give rise to three lineages: neurons, oligodendrocytes, astrocytes.

# Unipotent Stem Cells

- Spermatogonial stem cells give rise to spermatogonia.

**HSCs in Treatment**

- Leukemias, lymphomas and other blood disorders have been successfully treated with bone marrow transplants since the 1960s. The donor tissue must be human leukocyte antigen (HLA) matched to that of the recipient, or the cells will be rejected by the recipient's immune system.
- During the past decade, IVF in combination with preimplantation genetic diagnosis (PGD) has been used to select embryos that are HLA matched to a sibling who has a blood disorder. Cord blood isolated from the baby ('savior sibling') at the time of delivery is then prepared to provide a supply of HSCs for transplant to the sibling.
- It had been suggested that HSCs may have 'plasticity,' i.e., the ability to engraft in other locations and then transdifferentiate to cell types appropriate to their new location. However, so far this concept is unsubstantiated, and there is no evidence that blood-forming stem cells can serve as a significant source of regenerative cells in the repair of nonblood tissues.

## Differentiation

Cells can be distinguished from one another by their patterns of gene expression, which includes expression of both protein coding and noncoding RNAs, the secretion of proteins, their response to extracellular signals and the distribution of epigenetic chromatin modification. Changes to any or all of these processes can influence the differentiation of stem cells. For example, hESCs express the transcription factors OCT4, NANOG and SOX2 and require extracellular signals such as fibroblast growth factor (FGF) and Activin/Nodal to maintain self-renewal. Changes in the levels and balance between FGF and Activin/Nodal can influence the maintenance and differentiation of hESCs: in the presence of too much Activin/Nodal they resemble endoderm cells, and too little Activin/Nodal will cause differentiation into ectoderm cells. The mechanisms involved in the maintenance of hESCs is poorly elucidated, but is likely to involve cell signaling pathways that function at different levels, with multiple feedback controls and intercellular gene regulation:

1. Gene expression: transcription factors are proteins that function to promote or repress gene expression at the DNA level. For example, OCT4 is thought to maintain hESCs by binding to genomic regulatory regions to promote the expression of pluripotency-associated genes and repress the expression of genes associated with differentiation.

2. Extracellular signals: small proteins that are produced and secreted (cytokines) by a stem cell niche can contribute to the maintenance of self-renewal. These proteins are often required to maintain stem cells in culture, such as the addition of cytokines FGF and epidermal growth factor (EGF) to neural stem cells grown in vitro.

3. Chromatin modifications: DNA is packaged with histones to form nucleosomes. Post-translational modification of histone tails forms a code that can determine states of gene expression that are heritable, modifying gene expression by influencing the access of transcription factors to genomic regulatory regions.

4. Physical context: the presence of extracellular matrix and physical contact with other cells can influence the maintenance and differentiation potential of stem cells.

**Tissue Stem Cells in Treatment**

**From Trounson & DeWitt (2016).**

- Mesenchymal stem cells (MSCs) from bone marrow, placenta, umbilical cord and adipose tissue are being used in clinical trials for bone repair, joint and lower back pain, and graft versus host disease (GvHD).
- MSCs have been applied as therapy for myocardial infarction, cartilage repair, diabetes, and pulmonary, neurological and liver disease.
- Neural stem cells from adult and fetal tissues are being studied for diseases of the eye, spinal cord injury and neurodegenerative disorders such as Parkinson's disease and amyotrophic lateral sclerosis.
- Limbal stem cells of the cornea have been approved for autologous therapies and as allogeneic transplants involving donor cells.
- Gene therapy strategies are being studied as a means of DNA-editing hematopoietic stem cells in order to replace a mutated gene with a normal copy to cure single-gene diseases such as thalassemia, sickle cell disease, adrenoleukodystrophy and severe combined immunodeficiency.

**Potential Therapeutic Applications for ESCs**

1. Platform for drug discovery: hESCs can be differentiated into clinically relevant cells from individuals that harbor disease-associated gene expression. For example, hESCs have been established from individuals with amyotrophic lateral sclerosis, and these hESCs were differentiated to motor neurons, the cells that are damaged in these patients. These hES-differentiated cells can be used to screen for small molecules (drugs) that might inhibit the progression of the disease and be effective in patient treatment.

2. Exogenous: transplantation of stem cells that have been differentiated in vitro toward a particular cell lineage, e.g., neuronal stem cells for neurodegenerative diseases that involve death or dysfunction of just one, or a few, cell types, such as dopaminergic neurons to treat Parkinson's disease, insulin-producing beta-cells to treat diabetes, etc. This approach has at least two significant considerations:

   - in-vitro stem cell differentiation must be completely controlled, as there may be a possibility of malignant transformation
   - transplant rejection unless the cells are immune matched.

3. Autologous: the patient's own stem cells are manipulated in vitro to induce/repress gene expression and returned to the specific site that requires healing/treatment.

4. Endogenous stem cell renewal: the patient's own stem cells are manipulated to renew themselves in situ; this requires:

   - identification of stem cells in different parts of the body
   - interpretation of how they interact with their niche/microenvironment.

# Evolution of Stem Cell Research

The derivation of human ESCs in 1998 ignited an explosion of interest in stem cell biology and its therapeutic potential, and research in the field evolved very rapidly over the subsequent decade. In the words of the French philosopher Auguste Comte (1798–1857) 'To understand science, it is necessary to know its history,' and this is particularly true of stem cell science, where each significant achievement has been based upon the findings of prior decades of research. Successful derivation of human ESCs was based on research using murine ESCs, and this required information that was gained from previous stem cell models using mouse and human embryonal carcinoma cell lines. Similarly, the recent elucidation of discrete factors that can induce somatic cells into forming pluripotent stem cells (iPSCs) depended on studies in mouse and human embryonic stem cells. There is no doubt that novel trends will continue to emerge, and in order to fully comprehend the potential and the possible directions that lie in the future of stem cell research, it is important to be aware of the milestones that have marked its evolution so far.

# Early Culture Systems

During the early 1960s, Robert Edwards recognized the extraordinary potential of stem cell biology, and in collaboration with Robin Cole and John Paul in Glasgow, he isolated stem cells from the inner cell mass (ICM) of rabbit blastocysts. They cultured zona-free rabbit ICM on collagen surfaces, sometimes with HeLa feeder layers, and established cell colonies that showed differentiation to muscle, blood islands, neurons and complex groups of differentiating cells (Figure 7.2). Four immortal cell lines (two epithelioid and two fibroblastic) that survived more than 200 generations of subculture were established and cryopreserved. All cell lines remained diploid for several generations (Cole *et al.*, 1965, 1966; Edwards, 2008).

In further studies by Richard Gardner (1968), ICM cells isolated from mice with marker (coat color) genes were injected directly into the blastocoelic cavity of recipient mice, forming chimeras which showed that the grafted cells had colonized several different tissues; this indicated that the injected ICM cells were multipotent. After human blastocysts first became available through IVF, Edwards and his team attempted to prepare human ESCs in vitro (Fishel *et al.*, 1984), but this early work had to be abandoned due to ethico-legal problems surrounding the use of human embryos for research.

# Embryonal Carcinoma (EC) and Embryonal Germ (EG) Cell Lines

In the early 1970s, stem cell lines that could be propagated in vitro were derived from murine teratocarcinomas (Kahn and Ephrussi, 1970); these cell lines were capable of unlimited self-renewal and

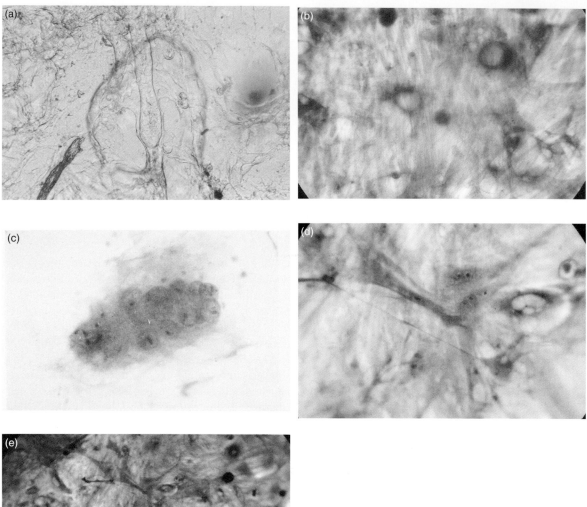

**Figure 7.2** Cell colonies derived from intact zona-free rabbit blastocysts after 20 days in culture (Cole *et al.*, 1966). (a) Cell masses derived from a zona-free rabbit blastocyst. (b) Muscle differentiating after continued culture. (c) A single blood island that developed among cell outgrowths from rabbit ICM. (d) A group of neurons in the same outgrowths. (e) A complex group of differentiating cells in which muscle cells are mixed with various types of differentiating cells – a pathologist discerned several cell types in this mass of cells. Reprinted with permission from Edwards (2008).

multilineage differentiation. Mouse EC cells express antigens and proteins that are similar to cells present in the ICM, which led to the concept that EC cells are an in-vitro counterpart of the pluripotent cells present in the ICM (Martin, 1981); this provided the intellectual framework for working toward derivation of both mouse and human embryonic stem (ES) cells. Human EC lines were established in 1977 (Hogan *et al.*, 1977), and these proved to differ from mouse EC lines, both

in expression of surface markers, and in their in-vitro properties. Unlike mouse EC lines, the human cells are highly aneuploid and have a limited ability to differentiate into a wider range of somatic cell types. Nonetheless, these human cell lines provided a useful model in which to study cell differentiation (Andrews *et al.*, 1984b; Thompson *et al.*, 1984; Pera *et al.*, 1989). Both mouse and human EC culture systems enabled numerous improvements in technique and methodology, as well as initiating studies on factors that are involved in the control of differentiation in vitro.

Stem cell lines derived from mouse testicular teratomas (EG cells) were found to contribute to a variety of tissues in chimeras, including germ cells (Stevens, 1967); this provided a practical way to introduce modifications to the mouse germline (Bradley et al., 1984). Pluripotent EG cells were successfully derived directly from primordial germ cells in vitro in 1992 (Matsui et al., 1992; Resnick et al., 1992).

## Mouse Embryonic Stem Cells

Using culture conditions that had been used for mouse EC cells (inactivated fibroblast feeder layers and serum), the first mouse ES cell lines were derived from the ICM of mouse blastocysts (Evans and Kaufman, 1981; Martin, 1981). It was subsequently found that the efficiency of mouse ES cell derivation is strongly influenced by genetic background and that different culture conditions were required for strains that were initially thought to be nonpermissive. Further experiments revealed that mouse ES cells could be sustained by conditioned medium harvested from feeder layers, in the absence of the feeder cells themselves. Fractionation of conditioned medium led to the identification of leukemia inhibitory factor (LIF) as one of the cytokines that sustains mouse ES cells (Smith et al., 1988; Williams et al., 1988). LIF activates the transcription factor Stat3, which inhibits differentiation and promotes viability. Further investigation of the signaling pathways showed that the proliferative effect of LIF requires a finely tuned balance between positive and negative effectors/factors. If serum is removed from the medium, mouse ES cells can be maintained in an undifferentiated state by adding LIF in combination with bone morphogenetic protein (BMP), a member of the TGF-alpha superfamily (Ying et al., 2003).

The subsequent two decades of research using murine ESCs led to numerous advances in culture system techniques and technology, and the identification of several types of in-vitro differentiated cells (including neural tissue) introduced the therapeutic potential and hope of eventual therapies to treat degenerative diseases – neurodegenerative disease in particular. The murine ES model contributed enormously to many different aspects of developmental biology: a large collection of genes, factors, markers

and signaling pathways involved in differentiation have now been identified, providing clues toward achieving directed differentiation of these pluripotent cells in vitro (Yu et al., 2007).

## Human Embryonic Stem Cells

A considerable delay (17 years) ensued between the derivation of mouse ES cells in 1981 and the first establishment of human ES cell lines in 1998. This was due to at least two factors:

1. Suboptimal media and conditions for human embryo culture meant that human blastocysts were rarely available (especially for research purposes). Media optimized for extended culture were introduced during the mid-1990s, and blastocyst culture then became a more practical reality.
2. Initial culture systems for hESC derivation were based on those that were successful in the mouse, and it eventually became apparent that there are significant species-specific differences between mouse and human ES cells.

Isolation of ICMs from human blastocysts was reported in 1994 (Bongso et al., 1994), but they were cultured in conditions that allowed derivation of mouse ES cells, and this resulted only in differentiation of the human cells instead of their derivation into stable pluripotent cell lines. In the mid-1990s, ES cell lines were derived from two nonhuman primates: the rhesus monkey and the common marmoset (Thomson et al., 1995, 1996). Using experience gained from these primate models, in 1998 Thompson and his colleagues then reported the isolation of pluripotent stem cell lines derived from human blastocyst ICM cultured on inactivated mouse feeder layers. These cell lines expressed markers for pluripotency and could be maintained undifferentiated in long-term culture. The cultured cells also maintained the potential to form derivatives from all three germ layers when injected into severe combined immunodeficiency (SCID) mice. Media containing LIF and its related cytokines, required for mouse ESCs, failed to support human or nonhuman primate ES cells (Thomson et al., 1998; Dahéron et al., 2004; Humphrey et al., 2004); the fact that fibroblast feeder layers supported both mouse and human ES cells was apparently a fortunate coincidence.

Reubinoff et al. (2000) then reported directed differentiation of hESCs, producing three neural cell lines (astrocytes, dendrocytes, mature neurons) from an early neural progenitor stem cell in spontaneously differentiating cultures. A huge expansion in research activity followed this initial report, and over the next few years panels of markers associated with pluripotency and with stages of differentiation were identified. Research continues into elucidating pathways of differentiation and identifying factors that sustain hESCs in culture, as well as active factors that decay with de-differentiation, or change during re-differentiation. The body of published literature surrounding hESCs is now vast; by manipulating culture conditions, spontaneous differentiation to numerous different cell types has been observed, including beating heart cells (Mummery *et al.*, 2002), insulin-secreting cells, hepatocytes, cartilage, etc. Protocols are now available for directing at least partial differentiation of hESCs toward numerous different fates: early endoderm, hepatic cells, pancreatic cells, cardiomyocytes, endothelial cells, osteogenic cells, hematopoietic cells, lymphocytes, myeloid cells, etc. (see Sullivan *et al.*, 2007). hESC lines have also been genetically modified, with fluorescent reporter genes introduced into key gene loci that can be traced during in-vitro differentiation in order to identify subsets of cells along developmental pathways (Davis *et al.*, 2008a; Hatzistavrou *et al.*, 2009).

---

**Somatic Cell Nuclear Transfer: Cloning**

See (Figure 7.3).

1. **Therapeutic cloning**: the nucleus of an adult somatic (differentiated) cell is reprogrammed by insertion into an enucleated donor oocyte. The oocyte is then activated by electrofusion to stimulate cleavage, grown in culture to the blastocyst stage, and the ICM of this blastocyst used for stem cell derivation. The resulting stem cell lines are immunologically identical (HLA matched) to the somatic cell that was reprogrammed and could theoretically be used for potential therapies without transplant rejection. The technique has been successful in nonhuman primates (rhesus macaque), although with very low efficiency: two primate ESC lines were derived from the use of 304 oocytes (Byrne *et al.*, 2007). A report that several patient-specific stem cell lines had been established in Korea subsequently proved to be based on data that was fabricated, and the papers were withdrawn (Hwang *et al.*, 2004, 2005). In view of the extreme difficulty in obtaining donor oocytes, and the inefficiency of the technique so far, it may be that pursuing research with iPS cells is a better strategy than therapeutic cloning.

2. **Reproductive cloning**: somatic cell nuclear transfer (SCNT) is carried out as for therapeutic cloning, but the resulting embryo is transferred to the uterus. Dolly, the much-celebrated sheep, was the first example of successful mammalian reproductive cloning, demonstrating that a differentiated adult cell could be reprogrammed to generate an entire organism (Wilmut *et al.*, 1997). This success confirmed John Gurdon's remarkable discoveries during the 1950s, when he was able to produce tadpoles after somatic cell nuclear transfer into *Xenopus laevis* eggs (Gurdon, 1962). The technique has been used in a variety of large and small animals, including cows, goats, mice, pigs, cats, rabbits and a gaur. However, reproductive cloning is both expensive and highly inefficient; more than 90% of cloning attempts fail, and imprinting defects have been identified in cloned animals, with abnormalities of immune function and growth and numerous other disorders. Experiments with cloned mice indicate that approximately 4% of their genes function abnormally, due to imprinting defects.

# Epiblast Stem Cells (EpiSCs)

As described in Chapter 6, one of the first stages of postimplantation development is the separation of the ICM into two lineages, the hypoblast and the pluripotent epiblast.

Pluripotency can be considered as two states: newly segregated epiblast cells contain 'naïve' or ground state pluripotency, and following implantation these respond to signals from the extraembryonic tissues to become primed for differentiation. The two types of cells are characterized by expression of core pluripotency factors Oct4, Sox3 and Nanog, but they differ in their expression of other genes and their culture requirements.

Experiments with mouse embryos established that the epiblast in the late blastocyst is functionally and molecularly distinct from blastomeres, and from the ICM (Nichols and Smith, 2009). A strategically important milestone was reached in 2007, with the isolation of primed pluripotent stem cell lines derived from postimplantation (E5.5 to E6) mouse and rat epiblast (Brons *et al.*, 2007; Tesar *et al.*, 2007).

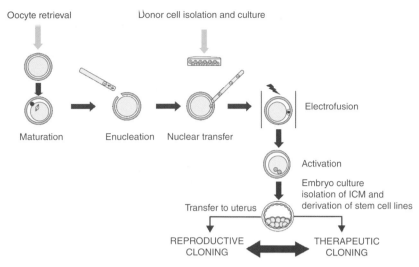

Oocyte retrieval

Donor cell isolation and culture

Maturation    Enucleation    Nuclear transfer

Electrofusion

Activation

Embryo culture
isolation of ICM and
derivation of stem cell lines

Transfer to uterus

REPRODUCTIVE
CLONING

THERAPEUTIC
CLONING

**Figure 7.3** Transfer of a diploid somatic cell nucleus into an enucleated metaphase II oocyte followed by activation by electrofusion leads to the creation of an embryo that has the chromosome complement of the somatic cell. A resulting blastocyst stage embryo can be transferred to a recipient uterus and allowed to develop to term into an animal with characteristics of the transferred somatic nucleus (reproductive cloning), or inner cell mass cells may be used to generate stem cell lines that are genetically matched to the donor of the somatic cell (therapeutic cloning).

Intriguingly, these EpiSCs differ significantly from mouse ESCs, but have key features in common with human cells. The two factors required for mouse ESC derivation (LIF and/or BMP4) have no effect on epiblast cell isolation, a similar situation to human ESC derivation. Instead, the signaling factors that are important for human ESCs (FGF and Activin/Nodal) are apparently critical for EpiSC derivation. The pattern of gene expression by EpiSCs differs from that of mouse ESCs, but they do retain the ability to proliferate indefinitely, as well as the potential for multilineage differentiation. Mouse ES cells can be induced to become EpiSCs, and the reverse transition has also been observed (Bao *et al.*, 2009). It is possible that the unique properties that hESCs have in common with EpiSCs could reflect a different origin that had not previously been recognized in hESCs; i.e., they may represent a later stage of development (postimplantation epiblast) than mouse ES cells. Activin/Nodal signaling seems to have an evolutionarily conserved role in the maintenance of pluripotency. This also reinforces the significant species-specific differences in genetic and signaling pathways for lineage specification between humans and rodents. Several key TGF-ß signaling pathways were found to be enriched and differentially expressed in the human EPI and TE, and inhibiting this pathway downregulated Nanog expression in human, but not in mouse EPI cells – TGF-ß signaling is required for the development of pluripotent

EPI in human blastocysts (Roode *et al.*, 2012). The differences between species in expression of early lineage-specific genes have significant implications for developmental control and stem cell derivation.

## Induced Pluripotent Cell Lines (IPSCs/PiPSCs)

The concept of reversing the programming of differentiated tissues to pluripotent states was introduced with the first somatic cell nuclear transfer (SCNT) experiments by John Gurdon during the late 1950s, using *Xenopus* oocytes (Gurdon, 1962). Several decades later, the birth of 'Dolly the Sheep' provided the first confirmation in mammals that a differentiated somatic cell could be converted to a totipotent state by inserting its nucleus into an enucleated oocyte. Dolly was born at the Roslin Institute in Edinburgh on July 5, 1996. The somatic cell nucleus was taken from a mammary gland cell and transferred into an unfertilized ovine oocyte that was then stimulated to divide by electrical pulse activation; the hybrid cell developed to blastocyst stage and was transferred to a recipient surrogate mother. Dolly died on February 14, 2003 from a progressive lung disease, 5 months before her 7th birthday.

With accumulated information regarding pluripotency in ESC, pinpointing key genes that might be used to reprogram somatic cells became a major research goal. Panels of genes that are enriched in ESC populations and thought to be involved in maintenance of

143

pluripotency were screened, with the target of identifying factors that have the ability to reprogram somatic mouse cells into proliferation. From a panel of 24 target genes, four factors were found that together induced a transformation of mouse fibroblasts into cells that closely resemble mouse ES cells: OCT4, SOX2, c-Myc and Klf4 (Takahashi and Yamanaka, 2006). The experiments were conducted by using retroviruses to insert key pluripotency genes into the fibroblasts; the cells that resulted had properties analogous to ESCs in culture and also formed teratomas when injected into mice. The same technique was subsequently applied to successfully reprogram human fibroblasts into hES-like cells (Takahashi *et al.*, 2007a; Lowry *et al.*, 2008). A further independent study using human cells screened a panel of 14 genes that are enriched in hESCs and succeeded in reprogramming human fibroblasts with the introduction of genes for OCT4, SOX2, NANOG and LIN28 (Yu *et al.*, 2007). Human iPS cells satisfy all the original criteria proposed for characterization of hESCs: morphology is similar, they express typical hESC surface antigens and genes, differentiate into multiple lineages in vitro, and when injected into SCID mice they form teratomas containing cells derived from all three primary germ layers. Since this initial report, numerous combinations of somatic cell type and cocktails of factors have been studied and continue to be investigated: some cell types can be reprogrammed more efficiently than others, and different types of cell respond to different expression levels and combinations of factors. The number of factors investigated continues to grow, and the original four now only head a list of related proteins that seem to enhance the efficiency of transformation in some cells (Heng *et al.*, 2010). Efforts to elucidate the mechanisms by which such a limited number of transcription factors can erase and reprogram a differentiated state continue: the DNA-binding sites of OCT4, SOX2 and NANOG have been studied, and it seems that these three factors can also activate or repress the expression of many other genes, including transcription factors that are important during early stages of development (Boyer *et al.*, 2005).

## Factors Used to Induce Pluripotency

### OCT4
- POU domain transcription factor.
- Expression restricted to pluripotent cells of the embryo.
- Expressed in undifferentiated ES, EC and EG cells.
- Essential for formation of the ICM.
- In the absence of OCT4, all cells in the embryo become trophectoderm.
  - Deletion in ES cells causes differentiation into trophectoderm.
  - Overexpression causes differentiation to endoderm/mesoderm.

### SOX2
- High mobility group (HMG) box transcription factor.
- Expressed in ICM and trophectoderm.
- Required for development of the embryonic lineage.
- Also required for proliferation of extraembryonic ectoderm.
- Interacts specifically with OCT4 to influence expression of target genes.
- SOX2 controls OCT4 expression, and they perpetuate their own expression when they are co-expressed.

### c-Myc
- Transcription factor that activates expression of a large number of genes through binding on enhancer box sequences (E-boxes).
- Has a direct role in DNA replication, can drive cell proliferation by upregulating cyclins/downregulating p21.
- Also has roles in cell growth, apoptosis, differentiation, stem cell renewal.
- Proto-oncogene: upregulated in many types of cancers.

### Klf4: A Member of the Krüppel-like Family of Transcription Factors
- Can act as a transcriptional activator or repressor, depending on promoter context and interaction with other transcription factors.

### NANOG
- Homeodomain transcription factor.
- Expression is tightly associated with pluripotency.
  - Essential for early development and for reprogramming.
  - Required for development of the epiblast.

### LIN28: Marker of Undifferentiated HESCs
- Encodes a cytoplasmic mRNA-binding protein that binds to and enhances the translation of IGF2 mRNA.

### Protein-Induced Pluripotent Stem Cell Lines (piPSCs)

In further attempts to overcome the problem of viral vectors, modified versions of the protein products themselves have also been used. Stable iPSCs from human fibroblasts were generated by using a cell-penetrating peptide to deliver the four proteins OCT4, SOX2, Klf4 and c-Myc (Zhou *et al.*, 2009; Cho *et al.*, 2010). The cells produced by this DNA-vector free, direct protein transduction method have been called 'protein-induced pluripotent stem cells,' piPSCs. Experiments have been carried out using recombinant proteins, as well as proteins derived from cell fractions. Since the first discovery that somatic cells could be induced into pluripotency, methods and protocols have been refined, and a great deal of research is now focused toward practical application of the technology in defining pathophysiology of disease and potential drug discovery for treatment of human disease (Negoro *et al.*, 2017). Pioneering studies have demonstrated that iPSCs derived from cells carrying monogenic disorders can mimic disease phenotypes in vitro when differentiated into cell types that are characteristic of the disease, providing a unique in-vitro human model that can be used for drug screening or further research (see Hamazaki *et al.*, 2017 for review).

## Germline Stem Cells and Implications for In-vitro Gametogenesis

### Spermatogonial Stem Cells (SSC)

As described in Chapter 3, primordial germ cells differentiate into type A (A0) spermatogonia in the fetal testis, and spermatogonia in the seminiferous tubules differentiate into mature sperm after puberty. Type A spermatogonia in the basal compartment of the tubules divide by mitosis to form two cells, another parent type A cell and a second (type B) diploid cell that is irreversibly committed to entering meiosis in order to start the journey toward mature haploid sperm cell production. Spermatogenesis continues throughout the life of a normal adult male, producing millions of sperm each day. The relatively small population of self-renewing type A spermatogonia are known as spermatogonial stem cells (SSCs), and these adult tissue stem cells are essential for male fertility, balancing self-renewal with differentiating divisions for continuous sperm production. hSSCs are unipotent stem cells; despite stages

of amplification and differentiation, they ultimately produce only one cell type: mature sperm.

Their active proliferation makes them highly susceptible to damage by chemotherapy and radiation, and therefore patients undergoing treatment for cancer may become temporarily or permanently infertile. Semen and/or testicular biopsy cryopreservation have long been offered to men prior to initiation of gonadotoxic treatment; this option is not possible for prepubertal boys, who have not yet started spermatogenesis. The potential of using SSCs as a means of preserving a patient's fertility remains an active focus for research directed toward understanding:

1. How SSCs keep their germline identity, and their paternal-specific pattern of epigenetic imprinting
2. The testicular niche and the intercellular communications that balance self-renewal with differentiation in order to allow lifelong gametogenesis.

In 1994, Brinster and colleagues described transplantation of SSCs from fertile donor mice to the testes of infertile recipients; the recipient mice initiated donor-derived spermatogenesis and produced functional sperm (Brinster *et al.*, 1994). Since that time, experimental SSC transplantation has been used to restore fertility, with resulting embryos or offspring, in mice, rats, goats, sheep and monkeys (Gassei & Orwig, 2016). Based upon these experiments, many centers are now cryopreserving testicular tissue or cells from prepubertal boys before they start cancer treatment, in the hope that SSC-based therapies will be available in the future. Experimental strategies under investigation to achieve in-vivo or in-vitro spermatogenesis include testicular tissue grafting, testicular tissue organ culture, SSC culture and transplantation, and iPSCs.

### Testicular Tissue Grafting

Successful homotropic and heterotropic testicular tissue grafting has been reported in rodent models, with the birth of pups after production of spermatozoa capable of ICSI fertilization. Experimental xenografting of human testicular tissue in nude mice has thus far shown poor graft survival and massive germ cell loss (Del Vento *et al.*, 2018), and although useful as an experimental model, the risk of zoonosis and epigenetic modification rules this strategy out for clinical use. Homotropic (intratesticular) grafting has the advantage that testicular tissue is transferred to its natural environment with the cells required to support spermatogenesis, the germ cell niche. Although prepubertal testicular tissue has been cryobanked in many centers over the last decade, successful clinical application by transplanting the tissue graft to restore fertility has not yet been reported. Further studies are needed to confirm the reproductive potential of spermatogonia that survive after cryopreservation, and to explore the biology of human spermatogenesis to discover whether techniques that have been successful in animal systems are likely to succeed with human tissue. Transplantation techniques will also need to be refined, with the aim of preserving the integrity of the germ cell niche that regulates self-renewal and differentiation. In the case of cancer patients, residual malignant cells may be present, and therefore this strategy may only be used for patients in whom there is no risk of malignant contamination.

### Testicular Organ Culture and Three-Dimensional Cell Culture

Principles of tissue engineering have been used to achieve in-vitro spermatogenesis, aiming to provide an environment that mimics the natural extracellular environment with synthetic or biologically derived matrices in organ or three-dimensional culture. For organ culture, intact testicular tissue is layered on an agar slab suspended in medium; for three-dimensional culture, SSCs are first dissociated from their somatic cells and then suspended in a soft agar culture system, containing 50% agar. Somatic cells are included in both systems, in order to mimic the in-vivo situation and try to promote communication between the cellular compartments. Newborn mouse organ culture systems have maintained pieces of intact testicular tissue in culture, with complete spermatogenesis after 3–6 weeks of culture and production of haploid round spermatids and sperm capable of fertilization after ICSI. Although the method has not yet been reported as successful using human tissue, the mouse model may provide increased insight into the factors that drive SSC self-renewal and differentiation.

### SSC Culture and Transplantation

Experimental animal systems suggest that only 5–10% of transplanted SSCs will form spermatogenic colonies in the recipient; the extent of spermatogenesis depends upon the number of transplanted cells. Mouse and rat SSCs obtained from prepubertal testes can be maintained in culture, retaining their biological potential for fertility restoration (de Rooij, 2017), but long-term cultures have not been established for non-rodent species (Takashima & Shinohara, 2018). These experimental systems have provided very useful models to investigate the basic biology and potential manipulation of SSCs in detail, as well as providing a model to study prepubertal testicular physiology. The number of SSCs that will be required to generate spermatogenesis in humans is not known, but it is likely that the cells must first be isolated from the testicular biopsy and propagated in vitro before autotransplantation. Although human SSC culture has been reported using a variety of different methods, the population of spermatogonia are heterogeneous with respect to self-renewal/differentiation capacity, hSSCs quickly lose germ cell identity in culture and no in-vitro culture system has been independently replicated by another group. Animal experiments have revealed that there are numerous issues yet to be resolved; in particular, epigenetic programming and stability must not be compromised, and the potential risk of reintroducing residual malignant cells must also be considered.

Detailed studies of SSCs have largely been limited to model systems, the mouse in particular. However, the Cairns laboratory based at the University of Utah carried out an elegant study in humans using stem cells isolated from adult male testicular biopsies (Guo *et al.*, 2017). The group used multiple tools for genome analysis, including single-cell RNA sequencing to establish gene expression profiles and outline the stages that sperm stem cells undergo during normal development. Their results revealed that the process is much more complex in humans than had been previously understood. Four distinct cellular phases of maturation were outlined, as stem cells progressed from a quiescent to a proliferative state, and then to a phase of differentiation as the cells matured to become sperm. These data provide an important framework for further studies that can help toward understanding pathologies that lead to infertility and cancer in men.

### Induced Pluripotent Germline Stem Cells (iPSCs)

In cases where no germ cells are available in the testis or biopsy, a suggested alternative approach is to induce pluripotency or transdifferentiation of patients' somatic cells in order to derive sperm cells in vitro. However, the molecular mechanisms underlying human germ cell development are poorly understood, and this technology is still in very early stages of development. Experimental mouse models have generated haploid male gametes, but some of the offspring died prematurely (Hayashi *et al.*, 2012). Studies using human somatic cells indicate that germ cells can be derived from human iPSCs, but most of the cells remained at early stages of differentiation, and it is likely that many characteristics of normal germ cells may not be reproduced in hiPSCs, particularly in terms of epigenetic status – hiPSCs are reported to maintain some epigenetic marks of the donor cell used for reprogramming (Kim *et al.*, 2011).

## Ovarian Stem Cells (OSCs)

Oocytes begin their development in early embryonic life, when a small number of progenitor cells (primordial germ cells) in the epiblast start their journey toward the primitive ovary, where they continue to multiply as oogonia (see Chapter 3: Development of the Ovary). 'Lower' species that depend on high rates of continuous oocyte formation (invertebrates and fish/amphibians) maintain the capacity to generate germline stem cells in adult life, and model organisms such as the fly (*Drosophila melanogaster*), nematode (*Caenorhabditis elegans*) and fish (*Oryzias latipes*, Medaka) have provided valuable insight regarding the molecular mechanisms involved in OSC development and renewal.

The potential existence of OSCs in mammals was studied and analyzed in detail in the 1950s, and Zuckermann (1951) laid the foundation for the dogma that the postnatal mammalian ovary does not contain renewable OSCs. The hypothesis suggested that there is a strict prenatal period for mammalian oogenesis, with the process completed before or shortly after birth, depending on the species. This theory was confirmed by many subsequent studies over the next five decades, and the principle that OSCs do not persist in adult ovaries was widely accepted: it is clear that the pool of ovarian follicles declines with age (Faddy *et al.*, 1992; Faddy & Gosden, 2007). However, in 2004, the Tilly laboratory in Boston described OSCs in adult mouse ovaries that were capable of restoring follicles lost by atresia and ovulation (Johnson *et al.*, 2004). The following year, the same group published experiments demonstrating that the OSCs were derived from bone marrow and were able to 'seed' the ovaries on demand via circulation in the

bloodstream (Johnson *et al.*, 2005a, 2005b). The suggestion that OSCs capable of producing functional oocytes could be isolated has a major potential impact on fertility preservation options, as well as treatment of patients who are infertile due to primary ovarian insufficiency. Furthermore, the pathways that direct oocyte differentiation are not well understood either in vivo or in vitro, and OSCs may provide a valuable model for investigating normal human germ cell differentiation, the interaction with somatic cells and extracellular signals. The regenerative potential of the mammalian ovary has therefore become an area of immense interest – as well as huge debate and controversy (see Gosden 2013 and Grieve *et al.*, 2015 for reviews).

Equivocal areas in the debate include techniques used to identify specific markers and gene expression profiles, cues for differentiation and physiological interactions within their candidate niche, as well as final proof of a real physiological role (see Albertini & Gleicher, 2015). Using techniques based on expression of germ and stem cell markers combined with magnetic or fluorescent cell sorting, putative OSCs have been isolated from adult mouse, rat and bovine ovaries, as well as from human ovaries (White *et al.*, 2012; Dunlop *et al.*, 2014). Populations of OSCs established in culture continue to express specific cell markers, and in a rodent model the cells have generated follicles capable of producing healthy offspring after introducing them into a somatic ovarian environment (Hayashi *et al.*, 2012). However, many technical questions remain unanswered, and some of the studies have not been independently replicated. Although there is some evidence that putative human OSCs can form oocyte-like structures in a xenotransplant model, there are no data relating to a possible contribution to the primordial follicle pool, or to a potential physiological role during later stages of follicle development. Identifying a stem cell in the ovary is not equivalent to possible regeneration of follicles and production of oocytes with a competent and functional physiological role. The conditions under which they are isolated/characterized/cultured require further characterization and optimization, as well as their epigenetic status, crucial for normal development.

## Summary

In terms of a future role in assisted reproduction, the birth of a new baby depends critically upon the fertilization of a healthy oocyte by a healthy mature sperm. The evolution of both mature gametes depends upon stringent control of many molecular and cellular processes that are not yet fully understood during in-vivo gametogenesis. All stages of both sperm and oocyte development must be carefully evaluated and controlled, to ensure normal meiotic competence and correct epigenetic imprinting (Handel *et al.*, 2014). Fundamental and stringent translational and preclinical studies of safety and feasibility will be an important requirement before in-vitro gametogenesis may become a reality in clinical practice.

---

**Derivation of Research Stem Cell Lines from Blastocyst ICM**

See Figure 7.4a and b.

Protocol based on Sullivan *et al.* (2007); all animal-based products must be avoided if lines are being derived for potential therapeutic use.

1. Prepare feeder layers: seed mitotically inactivated fibroblasts onto gelatinized four-well culture plates at a density of approximately 50 000 cells/cm$^3$. Mouse embryonic fibroblasts (MEFs) are commonly used, inactivated either with mitomycin C or by gamma-irradiation (human fibroblast cells can also be used, isolated from a variety of sources including newborn foreskin, but for research purposes, derivation on MEFs has practical advantages and thus far appears to be more efficient).
2. Remove/dissolve the zona pellucida: different methods include the use of pronase, acid Tyrode's solution or allowing the blastocyst to hatch completely in culture.
3. Remove the trophectoderm layer, by complement-mediated lysis (immunosurgery), or by manual dissection.
4. Plate the isolated ICM clump onto a well-developed, confluent feeder layer, and incubate in human ES derivation medium, undisturbed, for 48 hours.
5. After several days, outgrowths of cells from the ICM will appear. hESCs grow in flat two-dimensional clumps and have prominent nucleoli; these can be isolated and subcultured into fresh culture dishes. The explants should not be allowed to become over-confluent and crowd the dish, or they will begin to differentiate.
6. If the subcultured cells continue to proliferate without signs of differentiation, they are a 'putative ES line,' and require extensive characterization to confirm.
7. Batches of cells can be cryopreserved at intervals during subculture.

## hESC Culture Systems

The first human ESCs were derived using inactivated mouse fibroblasts as feeder layers. The efficiency of derivation/propagation has since been greatly improved, and culture conditions that minimize the risk of xenobiotic hazard in cells, reagents and media supplements have been established. The use of feeder layers has been largely replaced by semi- or fully defined matrices such as Matrigel, recombinant proteins or synthetic polymers (Kropp *et al.*, 2016). Basic fibroblast growth factor and members of the TGF-beta superfamily are important in regulating self-renewal, and it has become apparent that maintaining the undifferentiated state involves extensive cross-talk between the intracellular signaling pathways activated by factors such as FGF, TGF-β and BMP (Rao and Zandstra, 2005). In 2005, Vallier *et al.* reported successful prolonged culture of hESCs in a chemically defined medium containing activin A (INHBA)/nodal (NODAL) and FGF2; cells cultured in this medium maintained their fundamental characteristics of pluripotency (Vallier et al., 2005). Other members of the TGF-β superfamily (BMP11/GDF11 and myostatin/GDF8) have also been identified that promote self-renewal in feeder-free and serum-free conditions (Hannan *et al.*, 2009).

Current research is now directed toward understanding the signaling pathways involved in regulating the environment of the human embryo and human pluripotent epiblast cells. Analysis of transcriptome and protein expression patterns in human embryos donated for research is contributing to the identification of components required to establish a minimal chemically defined culture medium that will support hESC growth/self-renewal in vitro in conditions that more closely match the in-vivo environment (K. Niakan, personal communication).

Derivation and propagation of hESCs require a significant commitment of time and resources. Establishing a culture of hESCs takes from 3 to 6 weeks, and the cultures need daily attention once established. With the appropriate level of skill and attention, they can be

(a)

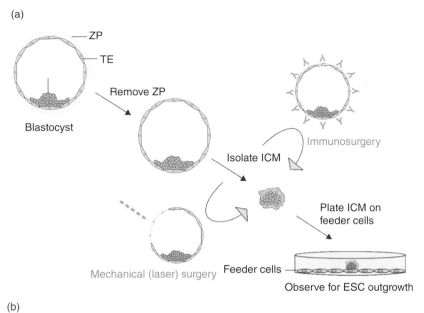

(b)

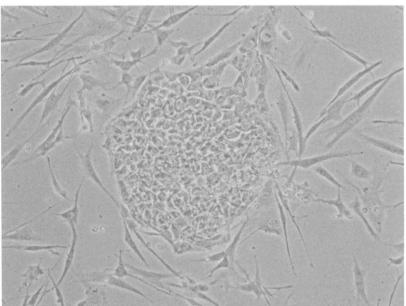

**Figure 7.4** (a) Cartoon outlining derivation of a stem cell line from a blastocyst inner cell mass (ICM) (with thanks to Alice Chen). ZP = zona pellucida; TE = trophectoderm; ESC = embryonic stem cell. (b) Phase-contrast image of a human stem cell colony, on a background of inactivated mouse fibroblasts (with thanks to Dr. Kathy Niakan).

kept in continuous culture for years, with aliquots cryopreserved during subculture. It has become clear that there is probably no standard culture method or medium that is optimal for all lines and all purposes (see under 'Books' in Further Reading).

Human ES cells have been derived not only from blastocyst ICM, but also from later stage blastocysts, morulae (Stojkovic *et al.*, 2004), single blastomeres (Klimanskaya *et al.*, 2007) and from parthenogenetic embryos (Mai *et al.*, 2007; Revazova *et al.*, 2007). It is not yet known whether the pluripotent cell lines derived from these sources have any consistent developmental differences or whether they have an equivalent potential.

## Characterization of ESC Lines

1. The cells should have the ability to be propagated in long-term culture, without visible signs of transformation.
2. Cryopreserved aliquots of cells should maintain the ability to continue propagation after freeze-thawing.
3. Identify cell surface markers characteristic of ESCs: the glycolipids SSEA3 and SSEA4, and keratan sulfate antigens Tra-1-60 and Tra-1-81.
4. Identify protein markers of pluripotency: Oct4, Nanog, Sox2.
5. Analyze chromosomal karyotype.
6. If feeder layers are removed, they should round up and clump into embryoid bodies containing undirected differentiated cell types from the three germ layers.
7. Injection of the ESCs into an immunosuppressed (SCID) mouse should result in teratoma formation. More sophisticated molecular biology tools are now being used in order to identify specific transcriptional profiles, combining immunotranscriptional and polysome translation state analyses to identify a large number of genes and cell surface markers (Kolle *et al.*, 2009).

## ESC Markers of Pluripotency

'Pluripotency' in hESCs may not be an all-or-nothing state: hESC cultures are in fact heterogeneous (Hough *et al.*, 2009). Analyzing transcripts of single hESCs for lineage-specific transcription factors revealed that there is a gradient and a hierarchy of pluripotency gene expression, with many cells coexpressing both pluripotency and lineage-specific genes. It may be that only a small fraction of the hESC culture population lies at the top of the developmental hierarchy, and that pluripotent stem cell populations may simultaneously express both stem cell and lineage-specific genes. Transcription factor networks that control pluripotency are dependent on upstream extrinsic signaling pathways, and cells along the continuum of differentiation show a progressively decreasing potential for self-renewal, with decreased expression of stem cell surface markers and pluripotency genes. The spatial organization of hESC cultures also influences the fate of individual cells, and engineering the microenvironment (niche) can be used to direct the rate and direction of differentiation by regulating the balance between inducing and inhibiting factors in the signaling pathways (Peerani *et al.*, 2007).

## Stem Cell Banking and Registries

Several thousand human embryonic stem cell lines have now been established in countries throughout the world, including several lines carrying gene defects for inherited genetic disease, derived from embryos identified as abnormal in PGD cycles. Research is accelerating via new and sophisticated molecular biology tools for gene sequencing, microarrays to map gene expression in single cells, cytokine and cDNA libraries, etc.

This fast-moving and multidisciplinary research is of critical importance to medical science, and there is a crucial need for collaboration and free exchange of information. Initiatives to facilitate collaboration and establish bench marks and good practice models have been set up (see Andrews *et al.*, 2005; Franklin *et al.*, 2008), and stem cell registries have been developed in order to collect, organize and disseminate information about specific cell lines (see Borstlap *et al.*, 2010 for review of stem cell registries). In May 2004, the world's first Stem Cell Bank was opened in the UK (www.nibsc.org/ukstemcellbank/), established in order to provide a repository for human stem cell lines of all types, and to supply well-characterized cell lines for use in basic research. The Bank has a catalog of characterized stem cell lines that have been deposited by research groups in several different countries, and details of lines that are being characterized, or are due for release, can also be found on their website. Applications to access the Bank's stem cell lines must be first approved by a UK Medical Research Council Stem Cell Steering Committee who will review the research proposal and the credentials of the research team.

In March 2009, in response to a new Executive Order from President Obama, the National Institutes of Health (NIH) in the USA published a registry of cell lines, and guidelines to establish policy and procedures for NIH-funded stem cell research: https://stemcells.nih.gov/research/registry.htm/; http://stemcells.nih.gov/policy/2009-guidelines.htm.

A global registry for human pluripotent stem cell lines supported by the European Commission was established in 2007 as an open, free access platform to coordinate research collaborations and cooperation, and promote comparable quality standards: The Human Pluripotent Stem Cell Registry, https://hpscreg.eu.

Stem cell biology is now arguably the most powerful tool available for the advancement of medical science. The possibility of studying cell fate transitions, controlling proliferation and directing differentiation by manipulating core sets of transcription factors adds a new dimension to the fields of regenerative medicine, degenerative disease and the uncontrolled proliferation of cancerous disease. Culture systems and selected populations of stem cells can be used to screen drugs and new approaches to treatment. Understanding the regulation of self-renewal at the molecular level will lead to improved systems for hESC derivation and propagation, and also has the potential to yield further insight into aspects of development that might increase the efficiency of clinical IVF. Human embryonic stem cells undergoing differentiation in culture also give us information about a period that has not previously been accessible for research, the first stages of early postimplantation human development, which are described in Chapter 6.

## Further Reading

### Website Information

Human Tissue Authority: www.hta.gov.uk
www.hta.gov.uk/policies/regulating-human-embryonic-stem-cell-lines-human-application
International Society for Stem Cell Research: www.isscr.org/about-stem-cells
University of Wisconsin News: https://news.wisc.edu/stem-cells-how-we-got-here-where-were-going/
Nature Reviews: www.nature.com/reviews/focus/stemcells/index.html

### Books and Reviews

Andrews PW (2002) From teratocarcinomas to embryonic stem cells. *Philosophical Transactions of the Royal Society of London, Series B* 357: 405–417.

Chen JC, Zhou L, Pan S-y (2014) A brief review of recent advances in stem cell biology. *Neural Regeneration Research* 9(7): 684–687.

Edwards RG (2004) Stem cells today. *Reproductive BioMedicine Online* 8(3): 275–306.

Edwards RG (2008) From embryonic stem cells to blastema and MRL mice, *Reproductive BioMedicine Online* 16(3): 425–461.

Fang F, Li Z, Zhao Q, *et al.* (2018) Human induced pluripotent stem cells and male infertility: an overview of current progress and perspectives. *Human Reproduction* 33(2): 188–195.

Freshney RI, Stacey GN, Auerbach JA (2007) *Culture of Human Stem Cells.* Wiley-Liss, Chichester, UK.

Gurdon JB, Byrne JA (2003) The first half-century of nuclear transplantation. *Proceedings of the National Academy of Sciences of the USA* 100(14): 8048–8052.

Hamazaki T, El Rouby N, Fredette NC, *et al.* (2017) Concise review: induced pluripotent stem cell research in the era of precision medicine. *Stem Cells* 35(3): 545–550.

Sell S (ed.) (2004) *Stem Cells Handbook.* Humana Press, New York.

Simon C, Pellicer A (2009) *Stem Cells in Human Reproduction: Basic Science and Therapeutic Potential.* Informa Healthcare, London.

Sullivan S, Cowan CA, Eggan K (2007) *Human Embryonic Stem Cells: The Practical Handbook.* Wiley, Chichester.

Tilly JL, Rueda BR (2008) Minireview: Stem cell contribution to ovarian development, function, and disease. *Endocrinology* 149: 4307–5211.

Trounson A, DeWitt ND (2016) Pluripotent stem cells progressing to the clinic. *Nature Reviews Molecular Cell Biology* 17: 194–200.

### Publications

Albertini DF, Gleicher N (2015) A detour in the quest for oogonial stem cells: methods matter. *Nature Medicine* 21: 1126–1127.

Andrews PW, Banting G, Damjanov I, Arnaud D, Avner P (1984a) Three monoclonal antibodies defining distinct differentiation antigens associated with different high molecular weight polypeptides on the surface of human embryonal carcinoma cells. *Hybridoma* 3: 347–361.

Andrews PW, Benvenisty N, McKay R, *et al.* (2005) The International Stem Cell Initiative: toward benchmarks for human embryonic stem cell research. *Nature Biotechnology* 23(7): 795–797.

Andrews PW, Damjanov I, Simon D, *et al.* (1984b) Pluripotent embryonal carcinoma clones derived from the human teratocarcinoma cell line Tera-2. *Laboratory Investigation* 50: 147–162.

Andrews PW, Goodfellow PN, Shevinsky LH, Bronson DL, Knowles BB (1982) Cell-surface antigens of a clonal human embryonal carcinoma cell line: morphological and antigenic differentiation in culture. *International Journal of Cancer* 29: 523–531.

Avilion AA, Nicolis SK, Pevny LH, *et al.* (2003) Multipotent cell lineages in early mouse development depend on SOX2 function. *Genes and Development* 17: 126–140.

Bao S, Tang F, Li X, *et al.* (2009) Epigenetic reversion of post-implantation epiblast to pluripotent embryonic stem cells. *Nature* 461: 1292–1295.

Beattie GM, Lopez AD, Bucay N, *et al.* (2005) Activin A maintains pluripotency of human embryonic stem cells in the absence of feeder layers. *Stem Cells* 23: 489–495.

Bendall SC, Stewart MH, Menendez P, *et al.* (2007) IGF and FGF cooperatively establish the regulatory stem cell niche of pluripotent human cells in vitro. *Nature* 448: 1015–1021.

Bongso A, Fong CY, Ng SC, Ratnam S (1994) Isolation and culture of inner cell mass cells from human blastocysts. *Human Reproduction* 9: 2110–2117.

Borstlap J, Luong MX, Rooke HM, *et al.* (2010) International stem cell registries. *In Vitro Cellular and Developmental Biology Animal* 46(3–4): 242–246.

Boyer LA, Lee TI, Cole MF, *et al.* (2005) Core transcriptional regulatory circuitry in human embryonic stem cells. *Cell* 122(6): 947–956.

Bradley A, Evans M, Kaufman MH, Robertson E (1984) Formation of germ-line chimaeras from embryo-derived teratocarcinoma cell lines. *Nature* 309: 255–256.

Brandenberger R, Wei H, Zhang S, *et al.* (2004) Transcriptome characterization elucidates signaling networks that control human ES cell growth and differentiation. *Nature Biotechnology* 22: 707–716.

Brinster RL, Zimmermann JW (1994) Spermatogenesis following male germ-cell transplantation. *Proceedings of the National Academy of Sciences USA* 91: 11298–11302.

Brons IG, Smithers LE, Trotter MW, *et al.* (2007) Derivation of pluripotent epiblast stem cells from mammalian embryos. *Nature* 448(7150): 191–195.

Byrne JA (2008) Generation of isogenic pluripotent stem cells. *Human Molecular Genetics* 17(R1): R37–41.

Byrne JA, Pedersen DA, Clepper LL, *et al.* (2007) Producing primate embryonic stem cells by somatic cell nuclear transfer. *Nature* 450(7169): 497–502.

Chambers I, Silva J, Colby D, *et al.* (2007) Nanog safeguards pluripotency and mediates germline development. *Nature* 450: 1230–1234.

Cho JH, Lee C-S, Kwon Y-W, *et al.* (2010) Induction of pluripotent stem cells from adult somatic cells by protein-based reprogramming without genetic manipulation. *Blood* 116(3): 386–395.

Cole RJ, Edwards RG, Paul J (1965) Cytodifferentiation in cell colonies and cell strains derived from cleaving ova and blastocysts of the rabbit. *Experimental Cell Research* 37: 501–504.

Cole RJ, Edwards RG, Paul J (1966) Cytodifferentiation and embryogenesis in cell colonies and tissue cultures derived from ova and blastocysts of the rabbit. *Developmental Biology* 13: 285–307.

Dahéron L, Opitz SL, Zaehres H, *et al.* (2004) LIF/STAT3 signalling fails to maintain self-renewal of human embryonic stem cells. *Stem Cells* 22(5): 770–778.

Davis RP, Costa M, Grandela C, *et al.* (2008a) A protocol for removal of antibiotic resistance cassettes from human embryonic stem cells genetically modified by homologous recombination or transgenesis. *Nature Protocols* 3: 1550–1558.

Davis RP, Ng ES, Costa M, *et al.* (2008b) Targeting a GFP reporter gene to the MIXL1 locus of human embryonic stem cells identifies human primitive streak-like cells and enables isolation of primitive hematopoietic precursors. *Blood* 111: 1876–1884.

Del Vento F, Vermeulen M, de Michele F, *et al.* (2018) Tissue engineering to improve immature testicular tissue and cell transplantation outcomes: one step closer to fertility restoration for prepubertal boys exposed to gonadotoxic treatments. *International Journal of Molecular Science* 19: 286–310.

de Rooij DG (2017) The nature and dynamics of spermatogonial stem cells. *Development* 144(17): 3022–3030.

Dietrich JE, Hiragi T (2007) Stochastic patterning in the mouse pre-implantation embryo. *Development* 134(23): 4219–4231.

Dunlop CE, Bayne RA, McLaughlin M, Telfer EE, Anderson RA (2014) Isolation, purification and culture of oogonial stem cells from adult human and bovine ovarian cortex. *Lancet* 383: S48.

Evans M, Kaufman MH (1981) Establishment in culture of stem cells from mouse embryos *Nature* 292: 154–156.

Faddy MJ, Gosden RG (2007) Numbers of ovarian follicles and testing germline renewal in the postnatal ovary: facts and fallacies. *Cell Cycle* 6(15): 1951-1952.

Faddy MJ, Gosden RG, Gougeon A, Richardson SJ, Nelson JF (1992) Accelerated disappearance of ovarian follicles in mid-life; implications for forecasting menopause. *Human Reproduction* 7: 1342–1346.

Gage FH (2000) Mammalian neural stem cells. *Science* 287(5457): 1433–1438.

Gassei K, Orwig KE (2016) Experimental methods to preserve male fertility and treat male infertility. *Fertility and Sterility* 105(2): 256–266.

Fishel S, Edwards RG, Evans CJ (1984) Human chorionic gonadotrophin secreted by preimplantation embryos. *Science* 223: 816–818.

Franklin SB, Hunt C, Cornwell G, *et al.* (2008) hESCCO: development of good practice models for hES cell derivation. *Regenerative Medicine* 3(1): 105–116.

Gardner Rl (1968) Mouse chimaeras obtained by the injection of cells into the blastocyst. *Nature* 220: 596–597.

Gosden RG (2013) Programmes and prospects for ovotechnology. *Reproductive BioMedicine Online* 27: 702–709.

Grieve KM, McLaughlin M, Dunlop CE, Telfer EE, Anderson RA (2015) The controversial existence and functional potential of oogonial stem cells. *Maturitas* 82: 278–281.

Guo G, Yang J, Nichols J, *et al.* (2009) Klf4 reverts developmentally programmed restriction of ground state pluripotency. *Development* 136(7): 1063–1069.

Guo J, Grow EJ, Yi C, *et al.* (2017) Transcription, signaling and metabolic transitions during human spermatogonial stem cell differentiation. *Cell Stem Cell* 21(4): 533–546. DOI:10.1016/j.stem.2017.09.003.

Gurdon JB (1962) The developmental capacity of nuclei taken from intestinal epithelial cells of feeding tadpoles. *Journal of Embryology and Experimental Morphology* 10: 622–640.

Gurdon JB (1968) Transplanted nuclei and cell differentiation. *Scientific American* 219(6): 24–35.

Gurdon JB, Colman A (1999) The future of cloning. *Nature* 402: 743–746.

Handel MA, Eppig JJ, Schimenti JC (2014) Applying "gold standards" to in vitro-derived germ cells. *Cell* 157: 1257–1261.

Hannah C, Hennebold J (2014) Ovarian germline stem cells: an unlimited source of oocytes? *Fertility and Sterility* 101(1): 20–30.

Hannan NR, Jamshidi P, Pera MF, Wolvetang EJ (2009) BMP-11 and myostatin support undifferentiated growth of human embryonic stem cells in feeder-free cultures. *Cloning Stem Cells* 11(3): 427–435.

Hatzistavrou T, Micallef SJ, Ng ES, *et al.* (2009) ErythRED, a hESC line enabling identification of erythroid cells. *Nature Methods* 6(9): 659–662.

Hayashi K, Ogushi S, Kurimoto K, Shimamoto S, Ohta H, Saitou M (2012) Offspring from oocytes derived from in vitro primordial germ cell-like cells in mice. *Science* 338: 971–975.

Heng BC, Richards M, Ge Z, Shu Y (2010) Induced adult stem (iAS) cells and induced transit amplifying progenitor (iTAP) cells – a possible alternative to induced pluripotent stem (iPS) cells? *Journal of Tissue Engineering and Regenerative Medicine* 4(2):159–162.

Hogan B, Fellows M, Avner P, Jacob F (1977) Isolation of a human teratoma cell line which expresses F9 antigen. *Nature* 270: 515–518.

Hough SR, Laslett AL, Grimmond SB, Kolle G, Pera MF (2009) A continuum of cell states spans pluripotency and lineage commitment in human embryonic stem cells. *PLoS One* 4(11): e7708.

Humphrey RK, Beattie GM, Lopez AD, *et al.* (2004) Maintenance of pluripotency in human embryonic stem cells is STAT3 independent. *Stem Cells* 22(4): 522–530.

Hwang W-S, Roh SI, Lee BC, *et al.* (2005) Patient-specific embryonic stem cells derived from human SCNT blastocysts. *Science* 308: 1777–1783.

Hwang W-S, Ryu YJ, Park JH, *et al.* (2004) Evidence of a pluripotent human embryonic stem cell line derived from a cloned blastocyst. *Science* 303: 1669–1674.

Illmensee K (2002) Biotechnology in reproductive medicine. *Differentiation* 69(4–5): 167–173.

Johnson J, Bagley J, Skaznik-Wikiel M, *et al.* (2005a) Oocyte generation in adult mammalian ovaries by putative germ cells in bone marrow and peripheral blood. *Cell* 122: 303–315.

Johnson J, Canning J, Kaneko T, Pru JK, Tilly JL (2004) Germline stem cells and follicular renewal in the postnatal mammalian ovary. *Nature* 428: 145–150.

Johnson J, Skaznik-Wikiel M, Lee HJ, Niikura Y, Tilly JC, Tilly JL (2005b) Setting the record straight on data supporting postnatal oogenesis in female mammals. *Cell Cycle* 4: 1469–1575.

Kahn BW, Ephrussi B (1970) Developmental potentialities of clonal in vitro cultures of mouse testicular teratoma. *Journal of the National Cancer Institute* 44: 1015–1029.

Kaji K, Norrby K, Paca A, *et al.* (2009) Virus-free induction of pluripotency and subsequent excision of reprogramming factors. *Nature* 458(7239): 771–775.

Kim J, Lengner CJ, Kirak O, *et al.* (2011) Reprogramming of postnatal neurons into induced pluripotent stem cells by defined factors. *Stem Cells* 29(6): 992–1000.

Klimanskaya I, Chung Y, Becker S, Lu SJ, Lanza R (2007) Derivation of human embryonic stem cells from single blastomeres. *Nature Protocols* 2(8): 1964–1972.

Kolle G, Ho SHM, Zhou Q, *et al.* (2009) Identification of human embryonic stem cell surface markers by combined membrane-polysome translation state array analysis and immunotranscriptional profiling. *Stem Cells* 27(10): 2446–2456.

Kropp C, Masai D, Zweigerdt R (2016) Progress and challenges in large-scale expansion of human pluripotent stem cells. *Process Biochemistry* http://dx.doi.org/10.1016/j.procbio.2016.09.032

Laslett AL, Grimmond S, Gardiner B, *et al.* (2007b) Transcriptional analysis of early lineage commitment in human embryonic stem cells. *BMC Developmental Biology* 7: 12.

Laslett AL, Lin A, Pera MF (2007c) Characterization and differentiation of human embryonic stem cells. In: Masters JR, Palsson BO, Thomson JA, *et al.* (eds.) *Embryonic Stem Cells*. Springer, the Netherlands, pp. 27–40.

Lowry WE, Richter L, Yachecko R, *et al.* (2008) Generation of human induced pluripotent stem cells from dermal fibroblasts. *Proceedings of the National Academy of Sciences of the USA* 105(8): 2883–2888.

Mai Q, Yu Y, Li T, *et al.* (2007) Derivation of human embryonic stem cell lines from parthenogenetic blastocysts. *Cell Research* 17(12): 1008–1019.

Martin GR (1981) Isolation of a pluripotent cell line from early mouse embryos cultured in medium conditioned by teratocarcinoma stem cells. *Proceedings of the National Academy of Sciences of the USA* 78: 7634–7638.

Matsui Y, Zsebo K, Hogan BL (1992) Derivation of pluripotential embryonic stem cells from murine primordial germ cells in culture. *Cell* 70: 841–847.

Mullor JL, Sánchez P, Altaba AR (2003) Pathways and consequences: Hedgehog signaling in human disease. *Trends in Cell Biology* 12(12): 562–569.

Mummery C, Ward D, van den Brink CE, *et al.* (2002) Cardiomyocyte differentiation of mouse and human embryonic stem cells. *Journal of Anatomy* 200: 233–242.

Negoro T, Okura H, Matsuyama A (2017) Induced pluripotent stem cells: global research trends. *BioResearch Open Access* 6.1. DOI: 10.1089/biores.2017.0013

Ng ES, Davis R, Stanley EG, Elefanty AG (2008) A protocol describing the use of a recombinant protein-based, animal product free medium (APEL) for human embryonic stem cell differentiation as spin embryoid bodies. *Nature Protocols* 3: 768–776.

Nichols J, Smith A (2009) Naive and primed pluripotent states. *Cell Stem Cell* 4: 487–492.

Nichols J, Zevnik B, Anastassiadis K, *et al.* (1998) Formation of pluripotent stem cells in the mammalian embryo depends on the POU transcription factor Oct-4. *Cell* 95: 379–391.

Niwa H, Miyazaki J, Smith AG (2000) Quantitative expression of Oct-3/4 defines differentiation, dedifferentiation or self-renewal of ES cells. *Nature Genetics* 24: 372–376.

O'Brien C, Lambshead J, Chy H, Zhou Q, Wang Y-C (2012) Analysis and purification techniques for human pluripotent stem cells. In: Peterson S, Loring JG (eds.) *Human Stem Cell Manual: A Laboratory Guide,* 2nd edn. Academic Press.

Pedersen R (2005) Developments in human embryonic stem cells. *Reproductive BioMedicine Online* 10(Suppl. 1): 60–62.

Peerani R, Rao BM, Bauwens C, *et al.* (2007) Niche-mediated control of human embryonic stem cell self-renewal and differentiation. *EMBO Journal* 26(22): 4744–4755.

Pera MF, Cooper S, Mills J, Parrington JM (1989) Isolation and characterization of a multipotent clone of human embryonal carcinoma-cells. *Differentiation* 42: 10–23.

Picton HM, Wyns C, Anderson RA, *et al.* (2015) A European perspective on testicular tissue cryopreservation for fertility preservation in prepubertal and adolescent boys. *Human Reproduction* 30(11): 2643–2675.

Pierce GB (1974) Neoplasms, differentiations and mutations. *American Journal of Pathology* 77(1): 103–118.

Rao BM, Zandstra PW (2005) Culture development for human embryonic stem cell propagation: molecular aspects and challenges. *Current Opinion in Biotechnology* 16(5): 568–576.

Resnick JL, Bixler LS, Cheng L, Donovan PJ (1992) Long-term proliferation of mouse primordial germ cells in culture. *Nature* 359: 550–551.

Reubinoff BE, Pera MF, Fong C-Y, Trounson A, Bongso A (2000) Embryonic stem cell lines from human blastocysts: somatic differentiation in vitro. *Nature Biotechnology* 18: 299–404.

Revazova ES, Turovets NA, Kochetkova OD, *et al.* (2007) Patient-specific stem cell lines derived from human parthenogenetic blastocysts. *Cloning Stem Cells* 9(3): 432–449.

Roode M, Blair K, Snell P, *et al.* (2012) Human hypoblast formation is not dependent on FGF signaling. *Developmental Biology* 361: 358–363.

Seifinejad A, Tabebordbar M, Baharvand H, Boyer LA, Hosseini Salekdeh G (2010) Progress and promise towards safe induced pluripotent stem cells for therapy. *Stem Cell Review* 6(2): 297–306.

Sermon CKD, Simon C, Braude P, *et al.* (2009) Creation of a registry for human embryonic stem cells carrying an inherited defect: joint collaboration between ESHRE and hESCreg. *Human Reproduction* 24(7): 1556–1560.

Silva J, Nichols J, Theunissen TW, *et al.* (2009) Nanog is the gateway to the pluripotent ground state. *Cell* 138: 722–737.

Smith AG, Heath JK, Donaldson DD, *et al.* (1988) Inhibition of pluripotential embryonic stem cell differentiation by purified polypeptides. *Nature* 336 (6200): 688–690.

Stevens LC (1967) Origin of testicular teratomas from primordial germ cells in mice. *Journal of the National Cancer Institute* 38(4): 549–552.

Stevens LC (1970) The development of transplantable teratocarcinomas from intratesticular grafts of pre- and postimplantation mouse embryos. *Developmental Biology* 21: 364–382.

Stojkovic M, Lako M, Stojkovic P, *et al.* (2004) Derivation of human embryonic stem cells from day-8 blastocysts recovered after three-step in vitro culture. *Stem Cells* 22: 790–797.

Strelchenko N, Verlinsky O, Kukharenko V, Verlinsky Y (2004) Morula-derived human embryonic stem cells. *Reproductive BioMedicine Online* 9: 623–629.

Takahashi K, Okita K, Nakagawa M, Yamanaka S (2007a) Induction of pluripotent stem cells from fibroblast cultures. *Nature Protocols* 2(12): 3081–3089.

Takahashi K, Tanabe K, Ohnuki M, *et al.* (2007b) Induction of pluripotent stem cells from adult human fibroblasts by defined factors. *Cell* 131(5): 861–872.

Takahashi K, Yamanaka S (2006) Induction of pluripotent stem cells from mouse embryonic and adult fibroblast cultures by defined factors. *Cell* 126(4): 663–676.

Takashima S, Shinohara T (2018) Culture and transplantation of spermatogonial stem cells. *Stem Cell Research* 29: 46–55.

Telfer EE, Albertini DF (2012) The quest for human ovarian stem cells. *Nature Medicine* 18(3): 353–354.

Telfer EE, Gosden RG, Byskov AG, *et al.* (2005) On regenerating the ovary and generating controversy. *Cell* 122: 821–982.

Tesar PJ, Chenoweth JG, Brook FA, *et al.* (2007) New cell lines from mouse epiblast share defining features with human embryonic stem cells. *Nature* 448: 196–199.

Thomson JA, Itskovitz-Eldor J, Shapiro SS, *et al.* (1998) Embryonic stem cell lines derived from human blastocysts. *Science* 282: 1145–1147.

Thomson JA, Kalishman J, Golos TG, *et al.* (1995) Isolation of a primate embryonic stem cell line. *Proceedings of the National Academy of Sciences of the USA* 92: 7844–7848.

Thomson JA, Kalishman J, Golos TG, *et al.* (1996) Pluripotent cell lines derived from common marmoset (*Callithrix jacchus*) blastocysts. *Biology of Reproduction* 55: 688–690.

Thompson S, Stern PL, Webb M, *et al.* (1984) Cloned human teratoma cells differentiate into neuron-like cells and other cell types in retinoic acid. *Journal of Cell Science* 72: 37–64.

Trounson A (2002) Human embryonic stem cells: mother of all cell and tissue types. Proceedings of Serono Symposia International Conference: "Robert G Edwards at 75". *Reproductive BioMedicine Online* 4(Suppl. 1): 58–63.

Trounson A, McDonald C (2015) Stem cell therapies in clinical trials: progress and challenges. *Cell Stem Cell* 17: 11–22.

Vallier L, Alexander M, Pedersen RA (2005) Activin/Nodal and FGF pathways cooperate to maintain pluripotency of human embryonic stem cells. *Journal of Cell Science* 118: 4495–4509.

White YA, Woods DC, Takai Y, Ishihara O, Seki H, Tilly JL (2012) Oocyte formation by mitotically active germ cells purified from ovaries of reproductive age women. *Nature Medicine* 18: 413–421.

Williams RL, Hilton DJ, Pease S, *et al.* (1988) Myeloid leukaemia inhibitory factor maintains the developmental potential of embryonic stem cells. *Nature* 336(6200): 684–687.

Wilmut I, Schnieke AE, McWhir J, Kind AJ, Campbell KH (1997) Viable offspring derived from fetal and adult mammalian cells. *Nature* 385: 810–813.

Wolf DP, Mitalipov S, Norgren RB Jr. (2001) Nuclear transfer technology in mammalian cloning. *Archives of Medical Research* 32(6): 609–613.

Woltjen K, Michael IP, Mohseni P, *et al.* (2009) piggyBac transposition reprograms fibroblasts to induced pluripotent stem cells. *Nature* 458(7239): 766–770.

Woods DC, Tilly JL (2013) Isolation, characterization and propagation of mitotically active germ cells from adult mouse and human ovaries. *Nature Protocols* 8: 966–988.

Ying QL, Nichols J, Chambers I, Smith A (2003) BMP induction of Id proteins suppresses differentiation and sustains embryonic stem cell self-renewal in collaboration with STAT3. *Cell* 115(3): 281–292.

Yu J, Vodyanik MA, Smuga-Otto K, *et al.* (2007) Induced pluripotent stem cell lines derived from human somatic cells. *Science* 318(5858): 1917–1920.

Zhou H, Ding S (2010) Evolution of induced pluripotent stem cell technology. *Current Opinions in Hematology* 17(4): 276–280.

Zhou H, Wu S, Duan L, Ding S (2009) Generation of induced pluripotent stem cells using recombinant proteins. *Cell Stem Cell* 4(5): 381–384.

Zou K, Yuan Z, Yang Z, *et al.* (2009) Production of offspring from a germline stem cell line from neonatal ovaries. *Nature Cell Biology* 11: 631–636.

Zuckerman S (1951) The number of oocytes in the mature ovary. *Recent Progress in Hormone Research* 6: 63–108

# The Clinical In-Vitro Fertilization Laboratory

## Introduction

In the armory of medical technology available for alleviation of disease and quality of life enhancement, there is nothing to match the unique contribution of assisted reproductive technology (ART). There is no other life experience that matches the birth of a baby in significance and importance. The responsibility of nurturing and watching children grow and develop alters the appreciation of life and health, with a resulting long-term impact upon individuals, families and, ultimately, society. Thus, the combination of oocyte and sperm to create an embryo with the potential to develop into a unique individual cannot be regarded lightly, as merely another form of invasive medical technology, but must be treated with the respect and responsibility merited by the most fundamental areas of human life.

Successful assisted reproduction involves the careful coordination of both a medical and a scientific approach for each couple undertaking a treatment cycle, with close collaboration between doctors, scientists, nurses and counselors. Only meticulous attention to detail at every step of each patient's treatment can optimize their chance of delivering a healthy baby. Appropriate patient selection, ovarian stimulation, monitoring and timing of oocyte retrieval should provide the IVF laboratory with viable gametes capable of producing healthy embryos. It is the responsibility of the IVF laboratory to ensure a stable, nontoxic, pathogen-free environment with optimum parameters for oocyte fertilization and embryo development. The first part of this book reveals the complexity of variables involved in assuring successful fertilization and embryo development, together with the fascinating and elegant systems of control that have been elucidated at the molecular level. An increased understanding of basic pathophysiology of disease has revealed that events very early in development may have an impact on health,

predisposing children to health risks. Preimplantation embryos are regularly exposed to potential environmental stress during in-vitro manipulations, and this has the capacity to impact later development via epigenetic alterations of the genome prior to establishment of the first cell lineages.

It is essential for the clinical biologist to be aware that the control mechanisms involved in human IVF are complex, and exquisitely sensitive to even apparently minor changes in the environment of gametes and embryos. Temperature and pH are of crucial importance, and many other factors can potentially affect cells at the molecular level. Multiple variables are involved, and the basic science of each step must be carefully controlled, while allowing for individual variation between patients and between treatment cycles. New technologies and strategies continue to be introduced that can influence the risks associated with in-vitro culture; the success of any new innovations in technique and technology can only be gauged by comparison with a standard of efficient and reproducible established procedures. The IVF laboratory therefore has a duty and responsibility to ensure that all of the components and elements involved are strictly controlled and regulated via an effective system of quality management, with all procedures carried out by its most valuable and critical asset: a team of highly trained and responsible professional personnel (Guo 2015; Elder *et al.*, 2015; also see Chapter 9).

## Setting Up a Laboratory: Design, Equipment and Facilities

The design of an IVF laboratory should provide a distraction- and risk-free environment in which uninterrupted concentrated attention can be comfortably and safely dedicated to each manipulation, with sensible and logical planning of workstations that are practical and easy to clean. Priority must be given to minimizing the potential for introducing infection or contamination from any source, and therefore the tissue culture area must provide aseptic facilities for safe manipulation of gametes and embryos, allowing for the highest standards of sterile technique; floors, surfaces and components must be easy to clean on a daily basis. The space should be designated as a restricted access area, with facilities for changing into clean operating theater dress and shoes before entry.

---

**The Assisted Conception Treatment Cycle**

- Consultation: history, examination, investigations, counseling, consent(s)
- Drug scheduling regimen: GnRH agonist pituitary downregulation or oral contraceptive pill to schedule withdrawal bleed
- Baseline assessment at start of treatment cycle
- Gonadotropin stimulation
- Follicular phase monitoring, ultrasound/endocrinology
- Induction of ovulation
- Oocyte retrieval (OCR)
- In-vitro fertilization/ICSI
- Embryo transfer
- Supernumerary embryo cryopreservation
- Luteal phase support
- Day 15–18 pregnancy test
- Ultrasound assessment to confirm gestational sac/fetal heartbeat

---

## Laboratory Space Layout

The range of treatment types to be offered, the number of cycles per year and the manner in which the cycles will be managed all dictate the appropriate layout design and the equipment and supplies required. Four separate areas of work should be equipped according to need, arranged and set up to accommodate the flow of work according to the sequence of procedures in an IVF cycle:

1. Andrology: semen assessment and sperm preparation; surgical sperm retrieval
2. Embryology: oocyte retrieval, fertilization, embryo culture and transfer
3. Cryopreservation: sperm, oocytes, embryos, ovarian and testicular tissue
4. Micromanipulation: ICSI, assisted hatching, biopsy procedures.

Careful consideration should be given to the physical maneuvers involved, ensuring ease and safety of movement between areas to minimize the possibility of accidents. Bench height, adjustable chairs, microscope eye height and efficient use of space and surfaces all contribute to a working environment that minimizes distraction and fatigue. The location of storage areas and equipment such as incubators and centrifuges should be logically planned for efficiency and safety within each working area; the use of mobile laboratory components allows flexibility to meet changing requirements. Many IVF laboratories are now designed with curved joins between walls, floors and ceilings to ensure that no dust settles. For optimal cleanliness on reaching the entrance of the laboratory, two-stage entrance/exits can be incorporated into the changing room areas, so that outdoor clothing is removed at the external section, and scrubs/protective clothing donned at the second stage. Hand-washing facilities must be available in the changing area; sinks should be avoided in culture area, as they can act as a source of microbial contamination.

## Light Exposure during ART Procedures

In the course of normal physiology, gametes and embryos exist in a dark environment, and therefore exposure to light is not a 'natural' situation. The potential of introducing metabolic stress through light exposure was taken into consideration during the first trials of human IVF in Oldham and Cambridge: dissecting microscopes were fitted with green filters, background lighting in the laboratory was kept low, and during the time of the embryo transfer procedure the lights were extinguished in the operating theater until the embryo transfer catheter had been safely handed over to the physician. Increasingly sophisticated technology in IVF has added the use of more powerful microscopy, with high-intensity light sources. Some spectra of light are known to be associated with generation of reactive oxygen species (ROS), and further data has accumulated about the harmful effects of ROS in IVF. The effects of light exposure in IVF procedures has been studied in detail, with the following conclusions and suggested guidelines (see Pomeroy & Reed, 2015 for review):

- Certain wavelengths of light are potentially harmful in ART, and the extent of the damage is related to the duration of exposure, wavelength and intensity. Wavelengths <300 nm UV are absorbed by plastic; near UV-wavelengths of 300–400 nm are associated with increased apoptosis in mouse blastocysts.

- Although ambient light is not a significant hazard, cool fluorescent light, as commonly used in laboratories, produces a higher level of ROS and apoptosis in mouse and hamster zygotes than does warm fluorescent light or sunlight (Takenaka *et al.*, 2007).
- Embryology laboratories should not be located in areas where direct sunlight might cause damage.
- Biological safety cabinet hood lights, ambient lights, headlamps and microscope lamps should be chosen and used with care and attention.
- Ninety-five percent of radiation exposure is from microscopes, and the use of green bypass filters may be prudent when viewing gametes and embryos under the microscope.

## Laboratory Equipment

Equipment should be selected based on its suitability for the intended purpose, capacity for the intended workload, ease of use and maintenance, availability of service and repair contracts to quality standards, and validation of evidence regarding its correct function. All equipment used in clinical treatments must be of the highest standard available, validated for the intended use, safety checked and properly calibrated, regularly cleaned and maintained. Temperature and gas levels must be strictly monitored and recorded.

Service contracts should be set up with reliable companies, who must provide calibration certificates for the machines used to service and calibrate equipment in the IVF laboratory. Provision must be made for emergency call-out, with alarms fitted to all vital equipment and back-up machines held in reserve. Essential equipment that requires contracts for service and calibration includes:

- Incubators
- Air filtration equipment
- Flow cabinets
- Microscopes
- Heated surfaces/microscope stages
- ICSI/micromanipulation workstation
- Centrifuges
- Refrigerators and freezers
- Embryo/oocyte freezing machines
- Osmometers
- Liquid nitrogen storage dewars
- Electronic witnessing system
- Ultrapure water system.

A camera and monitor system that can display and record images is also recommended as part of the basic laboratory set up, for teaching, assessment and record keeping.

### Incubators

Carefully calibrated and accurately monitored $CO_2$ incubators that are capable of controlling multiple environmental variables (gas, temperature, humidity) are critical to successful IVF: probably the laboratory's most important piece of equipment, since embryo development is compromised by environmental fluctuations. The choice of 'best' incubator varies between laboratories, depending on workflow, total cycle volume and timeframe of when the cycles are performed. Results can vary between incubators in the same laboratory, and optimal function can only be maintained by strict quality control and correct management that considers the daily patient caseload. Patient samples should be distributed to avoid overuse of any particular incubator, as repeated opening/closing jeopardizes the stability of the culture environment.

The choice of a humidified or nonhumidified incubator depends upon the type of tissue culture system used: whereas humidity is required for standard four-well 'open' culture, the use of an equilibrated humidified overlay of clinical grade mineral oil allows the use of incubators without humidity, although this may depend upon the number of days of continuous culture. Dry incubators carry less risk of fungal contamination, are easier to clean and may benefit from the use of thermocouple $CO_2$ sensors, which are not sensitive to humidity.

Traditional stand-alone incubators can accommodate culture dishes for many different patients in a secure, well-insulated environment. Newer models deliver a range of gas concentrations, with $CO_2$ concentrations of 5–6% and variable $N_2$ levels to reduce oxygen concentrations from ambient 21% to as low as 5% (Meintjes *et al.*, 2009). The larger models may incorporate a water-jacket or air-jacket in the door for additional insulation, and may or may not include an internal fan for air circulation. They can be run dry or at 95% relative humidity when water is added to the tray at the bottom of the chamber. A water-jacket not only helps to maintain a consistent temperature under normal circumstances, but also in the event of a power failure. However, the units are heavy, tend to have higher power consumption and have the accompanying risk of adding a source of potential contamination. Air-jacketed incubators warm up quickly, but do not retain heat for long periods without power; they have the benefit of being compatible with heat-sterilizing decontamination methods. Inner gas-tight split doors are essential in order to minimize recovery time after door opening, and $CO_2$ levels must be regularly (preferably continuously) monitored using an infrared $CO_2$ sensor. A single large incubator should not be used to house more than 12 cases at a time.

Smaller benchtop models are portable and therefore more flexible, with pre-mixed gas and sealed gas-tight chambers so that the dishes for each patient can be isolated. These mini-incubators heat the culture dish by direct contact with a warmed surface and are less prone to variation in temperature and pH. Their use excludes the use of laboratory air in the gas mix, and they do not need constant $CO_2$ calibration with external monitoring devices. However, it is extremely important to find a reliable source for the gas mixture, both in the accuracy of the percentages of each gas and in their purity. In addition, the culture system will lose heat rapidly if power is interrupted. In that respect, all incubators should have a back-up battery or generator to protect the power supply in case of power failure.

Large incubators can also be used to equilibrate tubes and bottles of media; this is not possible when only mini-incubators are used, so that HEPES-buffered media might be required for the majority of preparatory procedures. Large incubators also have the advantage of allowing independent probes to be installed, with failure alarms that can operate remotely. Some also have fitted HEPA-volatile organic compound (VOC) filters.

Incubators must be regularly monitored, and readings of the LED display checked and calibrated against independent recordings of temperature and pH monitored by probes placed in a standard 'test' culture system. Temperature stability can be monitored with 24-hour thermocouple readings as part of the standard maintenance schedule. There should be a schedule to ensure regular dismantling and cleaning, and a yearly inspection and general servicing by the supplier is recommended. Repeated opening and closing of the incubator affects the stability of the tissue culture environment, and the use of an accessory small bench-top mini-incubator during oocyte retrievals and manipulations helps to minimize disturbance of the larger incubators. Excessive opening/closing can also be avoided by using 'holding' incubators for transient procedures such as dish equilibration, sperm preparation methods and brief culture of thawed embryos prior to same day transfer

Irrespective of the type used, in all stand-alone incubators the dishes must be removed from the controlled environment for each stage of manipulation, exposing gametes or embryos to suboptimal temperatures and changes in pH due to reduced $CO_2$ concentration. A number of newer incubators are now available that overcome this problem by incorporating a microscope and imaging system for continuous monitoring of embryo development using time-lapse photography of individual embryos.

Choice of incubator is a critical decision for every IVF laboratory; a distinct advantage of any specific type of incubator has not been clearly demonstrated in terms of human embryo development or clinical outcomes, and selection must be individualized for every laboratory situation. A mix of incubator types helps in covering multiple scenarios, and maintains different options for their use, including implementing new technologies as these evolve. Practical issues such as cost, space, low-$O_2$ capability, gas recovery times and ease of quality management and maintenance will always be important considerations (see Swain, 2014 and Elder et al., 2015 for detailed reviews).

## Electronic Witnessing Systems

Sample mismatch, where patients are not correctly linked with their own specimens or treatments, is a catastrophic event in an IVF laboratory, with serious consequences both for patients and staff. Critical points where mismatching of gametes and embryos is most likely to occur include initial gamete collection, mixing of gametes by IVF or ICSI, transfer of gametes or embryos between tubes or dishes, freeze–thaw procedures, and intrauterine insemination or embryo transfer procedures. Adverse events involving sample misidentification invariably receive wide media attention, and have led to the implementation of specific double-checking safety protocols: double-checking of IVF clinical and laboratory protocols is now mandatory. After incidents reported in 2002, the

UK regulatory authority (Human Fertilization and Embryology Authority, HFEA) introduced double-witnessing as a requirement in 2006. Double-checking protocols can be difficult to implement because of staffing implications, and are still subject to human error: an embryologist who is continuously distracted by the demands of double-witnessing is vulnerable to errors due to attention lapse/omitting key steps. Electronic witnessing systems have been developed in order to provide safer mechanisms to prevent mix-ups at every stage in the ART procedure. Systems are now available that provide electronic identity checking/witnessing, using either barcode readers or radio frequency identification (RFID), and their use is rapidly extending to fertility clinics worldwide. RFID systems use labels that are attached to all labware, allowing sperm and oocytes to be tracked throughout the IVF process. This technology reduces the chance of human error and helps to ensure that the resulting embryo is transferred to the correct patient. Automated witnessing systems can also be incorporated into the incubator imaging system, recording bar codes of dishes while monitoring embryo development. The data can be transmitted to a computer for continuous monitoring either on site or remotely.

Electronic witnessing systems have the advantage that they can be programmed to include traceability for all the media and batches of consumables used for a specific case. They also provide information on who performs specific procedures and the time that it takes for completion, which is very useful for audit purposes. However, the systems can also breed a new generation of errors: it is essential that full risk assessments to evaluate operation in a specific laboratory and validation checks are performed before introducing e-witnessing, rather than just accepting that an electronic system will work efficiently.

## Ambient Air Quality

The quality of ambient air is a factor that may impact successful embryo development; strict management of the laboratory environment to eliminate potential contamination can contribute toward optimizing IVF outcomes (see Morbeck, 2015 and Elder et al., 2015 for reviews).

The specific air quality requirements for IVF laboratories in terms of airborne particulates vary by country/region. Air cleanliness is classified according to the number and size of particles within a sample of air, measured in particles per cubic foot or cubic meter of air.

Laboratory air quality should be maintained by use of positive air pressure relative to adjacent areas; the airflow pressures in clean areas should be continuously monitored and frequently recorded. Adjacent rooms with different clean area classification should have a pressure differential of 10–15 pascals, with the highest pressure in the most critical areas. High-efficiency particulate air (HEPA) filters that remove particles smaller than 0.3 μm and filters to remove volatile organic compounds, which can adversely affect the health of human gametes and embryos, can also be used (Cohen et al., 1997; Cutting et al., 2004). Filters must be regularly inspected and changed to ensure that their efficiency is not reduced.

The environment in a clean room is produced by incorporating parallel streams of HEPA-filtered air (laminar flow) that blow across the room to expel any dust and particles in the airflow by the shortest route, moving at a uniform velocity of 0.3–0.45 meters per second. The air velocity over critical areas must be at a sufficiently high level to sweep particles away from the area and ensure that particles do not thermally migrate from the laminar flow. At least 20 changes of air per hour are usually required for clean rooms classified as Grade B, C and D (see Table 8.1).

The airflow can either be vertical downflow (entering via filters in the roof, exiting through vents in the floor) or horizontal crossflow (entering through filters in one sidewall and exhausted above the floor in the sidewall opposite and/or recirculated via a bank of filters).

The US Federal Standard 209E defines air quality based upon the maximum allowable number of particles 0.5 μm and larger per cubic foot of air: Class 1, 100, 1000, 10 000 and 100 000. The lower the number, the cleaner the air. The ISO classifications are defined as ISO Class 1, 2, 3,4, etc. through to Class 9. The cleanest, ultrapure air is Class 1. Guidelines suggested by regulatory and legislative authorities for IVF laboratories are based on those for Good Manufacturing Procedures (GMP), which define four grades of clean area (A–D) for aseptic handling and processing of products that are to be used in clinical treatment (Tables 8.1a and 8.1b). Each area has recommendations regarding required facilities, environmental and physical monitoring of viable and nonviable particles, and personnel attire.

**Table 8.1a** Comparison of air classification systems

| WHO GMP | US 209E | US Customary | ISO/TC (209) ISO 14644 | EEC GMP |
|---------|---------|--------------|------------------------|---------|
| Grade A | M 3.5 | Class 100 | ISO 5 | Grade A |
| Grade B | M 3.5 | Class 100 | ISO 5 | Grade B |
| Grade C | M 5.5 | Class 10 000 | ISO 7 | Grade C |
| Grade D | M 6.5 | Class 100 000 | ISO 8 | Grade D |

**Table 8.1b** Classification of clean areas in terms of airborne particles

| | At rest | | In operation | |
|---|---|---|---|---|
| | Maximum permitted number of particles/m$^3$ | | | |
| Grade | 0.5–5.0 μm | >5 μm | 0.5–5.0 μm | >5 μm |
| A | 3500 | 0 | 3500 | 0 |
| B | 3500 | 0 | 350 000 | 2000 |
| C | 350 000 | 2000 | 3 500 000 | 20 000 |
| D | 3 500 000 | 20 000 | Not defined | Not defined |

- Grade A (equivalent to Class 100 [US Federal Standard 209E], ISO 5 [ISO 14644–1]) is the most stringent, to be used for high-risk operations that require complete asepsis, carried out within laminar flow biological safety cabinets (BSC).
- Grade B (equivalent to Class 100, ISO 5) provides the background environment for a Grade A zone, e.g., clean room in which the BSC is housed.
- Grade C (equivalent to Class 10 000, ISO 7) is a clean area for carrying out preparatory stages in manufacture of aseptically prepared products, e.g., preparation of solutions to be filtered.

Personnel entering all grades of clean area must maintain high standards of hygiene and cleanliness at all times, and should not enter clean areas in circumstances that might introduce microbiological hazards, i.e., when ill or with open wounds. Changing and washing procedures must be defined and adhered to, with no outdoor clothing introduced into clean areas. Wearing of watches, jewelry and cosmetics is discouraged. Changing rooms for outdoor clothing should lead into a Grade D area (not B or C). Protective clothing for the different areas is defined:

- Grade D: protective clothing and shoes, hair, beard, mustache covered.
- Grade C: single or two-piece suit with high neck, wrists covered, shoes/overshoes, hair

beard mustache covered; non-shedding materials.
- Grade A and B: headgear, beard and mustache covered, masks, gloves, non-shedding materials, and clothing should retain particles shed by operators.
- Grade D (equivalent to Class 100 000, ISO 8) is a clean area for carrying out less critical stages in manufacture of aseptically prepared products, such as handling of components after washing.

The Tissue and Cells Directive issued by the European Union (Directive 2003/94/EC) stipulates that where human cells and tissue are exposed to the environment during processing, the air quality should be Grade A with the background environment at least equivalent to Grade D, unless a less stringent air quality may be justified and documented as achieving the quality and safety required for the type of tissue and cells, process and human application concerned. Since there is no documented evidence of disease transmission in ART treatment that can be attributed to air quality in the laboratory, the European Society for Human Reproduction and Embryology (ESHRE) suggests that less stringent air quality is justified for ART (de los Santos *et al.*, 2016).

The regulatory authority in the UK (Human Fertilisation and Embryology Authority, HFEA) recommends that all work in the IVF laboratory be carried out in Class II flow cabinets delivering Grade C quality air to ensure safe handling of gametes and embryos, with the background environment as close as possible to Grade D (www.hfea.gov.uk).

Cell culture $CO_2$ incubators equipped with a HEPA filter airflow system can continuously filter the entire chamber volume every 60 seconds, providing Class 100/Grade B air quality within 5 minutes of closing the incubator door. These incubators may also incorporate a sterilization cycle (Steri-Cycle™) and can be supplied with an additional ceramic filter that excludes volatile low molecular weight organic and inorganic molecules, collectively known as volatile organic compounds (VOCs). Some air purification systems also incorporate UV filters.

## Volatile Organic Compounds

The importance of ambient air and the possible consequences of chemical air contamination have been repeatedly reviewed (Morbeck, 2015; Elder *et al.*, 2015). Whereas most organisms and species are protected to some extent from hazards in their ambient environment through their immune, digestive and epithelial systems, oocytes and embryos in vitro have no such protection, and their active and passive absorption mechanisms are largely indiscriminate. IVF laboratories set up in buildings within polluted areas, or close to airports or industrial manufacturing sites, may be subject to serious chemical air contamination, which may be reflected by inadequate pregnancy and live birth rates. Large traditional incubators obtain their ambient air directly from the laboratory room; gas mixtures are supplied in gas bottles, which may be contaminated with organic compounds or metallic contaminants. Pressurized rooms using HEPA filtration are used by many IVF laboratories, with standards applied to pharmaceutical clean rooms; however, HEPA filtration cannot effectively retain gaseous low molecular weight organic and inorganic molecules.

The four most common air pollutants are:

1. Volatile organic compounds: in urban and dense suburban areas, VOCs are produced by industry and by vehicle and heating exhausts, as well as by a variety of cleaning procedures. Instruments such as microscopes, television monitors or furniture (as a result of manufacturing processes) may also produce VOCs; perfumes, after-shave and other highly scented aerosols are also potential sources,

and all theater and laboratory staff should be discouraged from their use.

2. Small inorganic molecules such as $N_2O$, $SO_2$ and CO.

3. Substances derived from building materials, such as aldehydes from flooring adhesives, substituted benzenes, phenol and n-decane released from vinyl floor tiles; flooring adhesives have been found to be particularly aggressive in arresting embryo development. Newly painted surfaces frequently present a hazard, as many paints contain substances that are highly toxic in the IVF laboratory; laboratory renovations and painting should always be planned during a period when treatment cycles are not being performed.

4. Other polluting compounds which may be released by pesticides or by aerosols containing butane or iso-butane as a propellant. Liquids such as floor waxes may contain heavy metals, which have a drastic effect on embryo implantation potential.

Detailed studies of chemical air contamination in all areas of an IVF laboratory have revealed that there are dynamic interactive processes between air-handling systems, spaces, tools, disposable materials and other items unique to the laboratory. Anesthetic gases, refrigerants, cleaning agents, hydrocarbons and aromatic compounds may be detected, and some of these can accumulate specifically in incubators. Water-soluble and lipid-soluble solid phases such as those in incubators can interact: whereas some contaminants may be absorbed by culture media, this may be counteracted by providing a larger sink such as a humidification pan in the incubator. Mineral oil may act as a sink for other components. Unfiltered outside air may be cleaner than HEPA-filtered laboratory air or air obtained from incubators, due to accumulation of VOCs derived from adjacent spaces or specific laboratory products, including sterile Petri dishes. Standards for supplies of compressed gases are based upon criteria that are not designed for cultured and unprotected cells, with no perspective of the specific clean air needs of IVF. New incubators can have VOC concentrations more than 100-fold higher than used incubators from the same manufacturer; allowing the emission of gases from new laboratory products is crucial. Systems that can clean the air and reduce VOCs can be installed into existing air conditioning systems.

VOCs can be measured in the laboratory using sensitive hand-held monitors that use photoionization monitors to screen equipment and consumables and pinpoint sources of VOCs. Active filtration units with activated carbon filters and oxidizing material can be placed inside cell culture incubators or in the laboratory spaces themselves (Cohen *et al.*, 1997; Boone *et al.*, 1999). As always, prevention is the best strategy, and efforts should be made to eliminate potential sources such as alcohol disinfectants and anesthetic gases – as well as perfumes/after-shave lotions – from the laboratory.

## Biological Safety Cabinets

A biological safety cabinet or BSC is an enclosed workspace that provides protection either to workers, the products being handled or both. BSCs provide protection from infectious disease agents, by sterilizing the air that is exposed to these agents. The air may be sterilized by UV light, heat or passage through a HEPA filter that removes particles larger than 0.3 μm in diameter. BSCs are designated by class, based on the degree of hazard containment and the type of protection they provide. In order to ensure maximum effectiveness, certain specifications must be met:

(a) Whenever possible, a 30-cm clearance should be provided behind and on each side of the cabinet, to ensure effective air return to the laboratory. This also allows easy access for maintenance.

(b) The cabinet should have 30- to 35-cm clearance above it, for exhaust filter changes.

(c) The operational integrity of a new BSC should be validated by certification before it is put into service, or after it has been repaired or relocated.

(d) All containers and equipment should be surface decontaminated and removed from the cabinet when the work is completed. The work surface, cabinet sides and back, and interior of the glass should be wiped down at the end of each day. (70% ethanol and Fertisafe™ are effective disinfectants).

(e) The cabinet should be allowed to run for 5 minutes after materials are brought in or removed.

### BSC Classes

**Class I** (Figure 8.1a) – provides personnel and environmental protection, but no product protection. Cabinets have an open front, negative pressure and are ventilated. Nonsterile room air enters and circulates through the cabinet. The environment is protected by filtering exhaust air through a 0.3-μm HEPA filter. The inward airflow protects personnel as long as a minimum velocity of 75 linear feet per minute (lfpm) is maintained through the front opening. This type of cabinet is useful to enclose equipment or procedures that have a potential to generate aerosols (centrifuges, homogenizing tissues, cage dumping), and can be used for work involving microbiological agents of moderate to high risk.

**Class II** – incorporates both charcoal and HEPA filters to ensure an environment that is close to sterile. It provides product, personnel and environment protection, using a stream of unidirectional air moving at a steady velocity along parallel lines ('laminar flow'). The laminar flow, together with HEPA filtration, captures and removes airborne contaminants and provides a particulate-free work environment. Airflow is drawn around the operator into the front grille of the cabinet, providing personnel protection. A downward flow of HEPA-filtered air minimizes the chance of cross-contamination along the work surface. Exhaust air is HEPA filtered to protect the environment, and may be recirculated back into the laboratory (Type A, Figure 8.1b) or ducted out of the building (Type B).

Class II cabinets provide a microbe-free environment for cell culture and are recommended for manipulations in an IVF laboratory. They can be modified to accommodate microscopes, centrifuges or other equipment, but the modification should be tested and certified to ensure that the basic systems operate properly after modification. No material should be placed on front or rear grille openings, and laboratory doors should be kept closed during use to ensure adequate airflow within the cabinet. The laminar flow of air can have a significant cooling effect on culture dishes; some laboratories choose to switch off the flow of air at appropriate times when it is safe to do so.

**Class III** – is used for routine anaerobe work and is designed for work with high-risk organisms in maximum containment facilities. This cabinet provides maximum protection to the environment and the worker. It is completely enclosed with negative pressure, plus access for passage of materials through a dunk tank or double-door pass through box that can be decontaminated between uses. Air coming into and going out of the cabinet is HEPA filtered, and

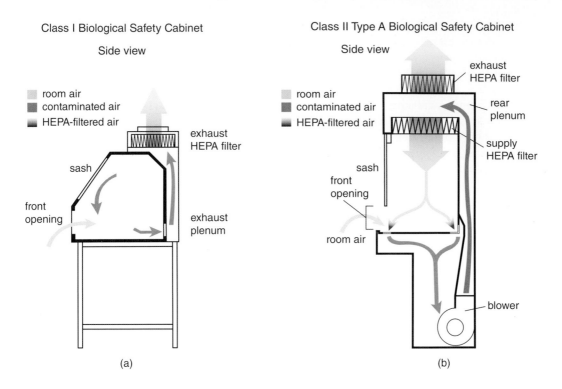

Class I Biological Safety Cabinet

Side view

Class II Type A Biological Safety Cabinet

Side view

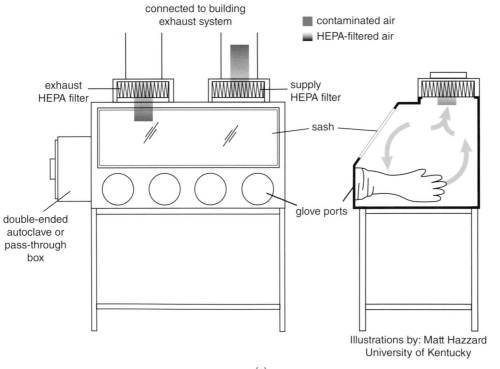

Class III Biological Safety Cabinet

Illustrations by: Matt Hazzard
University of Kentucky

**Figure 8.1 (a, b, c)** Schematic diagrams of airflow in biological safety cabinets. Reproduced with permission from Elder *et al.* (2004).

exhaust air passes through two HEPA filters or a HEPA filter and an air incinerator before discharge to the outdoors. Infectious material within the cabinet is handled with rubber gloves that are attached and sealed to ports in the cabinet (Figure 8.1c).

**Horizontal laminar flow 'clean bench'** – provides only product protection, and is not a BSC. HEPA-filtered air is discharged across the work surface toward the user. These can be used for clean activities but should never be used when handling cell cultures or infectious materials.

**Vertical laminar flow 'clean bench'** – is also not a BSC, but is useful in hospital pharmacies for preparation of intravenous drugs. Although they generally have a sash, the air is usually discharged into the room under the sash.

## Water Quality

Although the majority of media required for an IVF laboratory are now commercially available, if any solutions are to be prepared 'in house,' a reliable source of ultrapure water is a critical factor. A pure water source is also required for washing and rinsing nondisposable equipment. Weimer *et al.*, (1998a) carried out a complete analysis of impurities that can be found in water: this universal solvent provides a medium for most biological and chemical reactions, and is more susceptible to contamination by other substances than any other common solvent. Both surface and ground water are contaminated with a wide range of substances, including fertilizers, pesticides, herbicides, detergents, industrial waste effluent and waste solvents, with seasonal fluctuations in temperature and precipitation affecting the levels of contamination. Four categories of contaminants are present: inorganics (dissolved cationic and anionic species), organics, particles and microorganisms such as bacteria, algae, mold and fungi. Chlorine, chloramines, polyionic substrates, ozone and fluorine may be added to water during treatment processes, and must be removed from water for cell culture media preparation.

In water purification, analysis of the feed water source is crucial to determine the proper filtration steps required, and water-processing protocols should be adapted to meet regional requirements. Processing systems include particulate filtration, activated carbon cartridge filtration, reverse osmosis (RO) and electrodeionization (EDI), an ultraviolet

oxidation system, followed by a Milli-Q PF Plus purification before final filtration through a 0.22-mm filter to scavenge any trace particles and prevent reverse bacterial contamination from the environment.

IVF laboratory personnel should be familiar with any subtle variations in their water source, as well as the capabilities of their water purification system, and develop protocols to ensure consistently high-quality ultrapure water supplies, following manufacturers' instructions for monitoring, cleaning, filter replacement and maintenance schedules.

## Supplies

A basic list of supplies is outlined in the Appendix at the end of this chapter; the exact combination required will depend upon the tissue culture system and techniques of manipulation used. Disposable supplies are used whenever possible and must be guaranteed nontoxic tissue culture grade, in particular the culture vessels, needles, collecting system and catheters for oocyte aspiration and embryo transfer. Disposable glass pipettes for gamete and embryo manipulations can be purchased presterilized and packaged. If nonsterile disposable pipettes are purchased, they must be soaked and rinsed with tissue culture grade sterile water and dry heat sterilized before use. In preparing to handle gametes or embryos, examine each pipette and rinse with sterile medium to ensure that it is clean and residue-free.

Important considerations in the selection of supplies include:

- Suitability for intended purpose
- Suitable storage facilities (i.e., storerooms away from excessive heat/direct sunlight)
- Compliance of suppliers to a contract with specified terms and conditions
- Disposable plastics CE marked or mouse embryo tested where possible
- Media with quality certification, mouse embryo tested and proven track record, with validation evidence
- Delivery of perishable items such as media under controlled conditions
- Batch numbers to be recorded for quality assurance purposes
- Health and safety of operators handling potentially infectious bodily fluids

Routine schedules of cleaning, maintenance and servicing must be established for each item of equipment, and checklist records maintained for daily, weekly, monthly and annual schedules of cleaning and maintenance of all items used, together with checks for restocking and expiry dates of supplies.

## Tissue Culture Media

Original IVF culture systems were based on simple media developed for organ explant and somatic cell culture, designed to mimic physiological conditions. Analysis of tubal and uterine fluids, together with research into embryo metabolism, then led to the development of complex media. Many controlled studies have shown fertilization and cleavage to be satisfactory in a variety of simple and complex media (see Poole *et al.*, 2012; Mantikou *et al.*, 2013; Swain *et al.*, 2016 for reviews). However, the culture medium is only one component of a culture system; its efficacy is dependent on numerous other parameters, making it difficult/impossible to assess and compare the contribution of different media formulations to embryo viability. Poole *et al.* (2012) identified a total of over 200 factors that may affect the outcome of an IVF procedure, of which culture media represents only one of >100 variables associated with the laboratory/culture system itself; many of these parameters can also have a direct impact on the efficacy of the culture media itself. Specific culture parameters and their effects on embryonic development have been further reviewed and discussed by Wale & Gardner (2016).

Metabolic and nutritional requirements of mammalian embryos are complex, stage specific and, in many cases, species specific; several decades of research in laboratory and livestock animal systems have shown that, although there are some basic similarities, culture requirements of different species must be considered independently. Understanding metabolic pathways of embryos and their substrate and nutrient preferences has led to major advances in the ability to support embryo development in vitro; the physiological role of the oviduct in vivo, and the composition/role of oviductal fluid should not be neglected (Ménézo *et al.*, 2013, 2014).

---

**Culture Media: Physical Parameters**

- Osmolarity = osmoles of solute particles per liter of solution

  Temperature-dependent (volume changes with temperature)

  Osmolarity of tubal/uterine secretions = 275–305 mOsm/L

- Osmolality = the osmotic concentration of a solution, mOsm/kg of solvent

  Temperature-independent

  One osmole = Avogadro's number of osmotically active particles = $6.02 \times 10^{23}$

- Physiological pH range of body fluids = 7.2–7.5. pH is related to an equilibrium between gas phase $CO_2$ and $CO_2/HCO_3$ dissolved in the medium, with carbonic acid as an intermediate.

  Henderson–Hasselbach equation:

$$CO_2(gas) \leftrightarrow CO_2(dissolved) \leftrightarrow H_2CO_3 + H^+ + HCO_3$$
$$pH = pK_a + \log_{10}[H^+]$$

  = log of the reciprocal of the molar concentration of hydrogen ions

$pK_a$ = ionization constant for the acid

- pH is affected by:
  - Temperature (less $CO_2$ dissolved at higher temperature)
  - Atmospheric pressure (more $CO_2$ in solution at higher pressure)
  - Presence of other solutes such as amino acids and complex salt mixtures, since pKa is a function of salt concentration.

- HEPES buffered medium has been equilibrated to a pH of 7.4 in the presence of bicarbonate; exposure to a $CO_2$ atmosphere will lower the pH, and therefore culture dishes containing HEPES buffered medium should be equilibrated at 37°C only, and not in a $CO_2$ incubator.

- Temperature fluctuations during storage and handling can affect pH, and should therefore be avoided:
  - acid pH destroys glutamine and pyruvate
  - some salts or amino acids may precipitate out of solution and further affect pH.

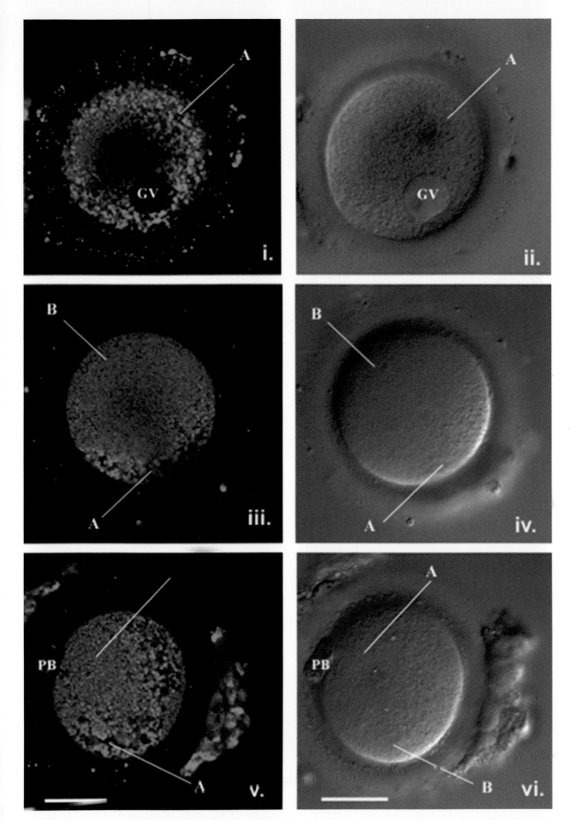

**Figure 1.4** Mitochondrial aggregation patterns in a germinal vesicle (GV) oocyte (top), an MI oocyte (center) and an MII oocyte (bottom). Frames to the left are in fluorescence using the potential sensitive dye JC-1 to show the mitochondria; frames on the right are transmitted light images. The two mitochondrial patterns, A (granular-clumped) and B (smooth), are shown. From Wilding *et al.*, 2001.

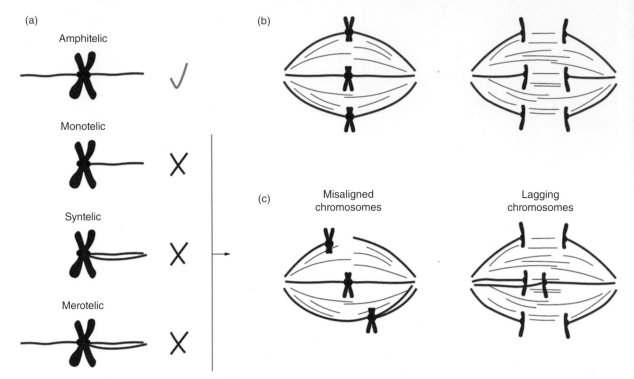

**Figure 1.12** Kinetochore–microtubule attachments. (a) Correct attachment (tick, amphitelic). Incorrect attachments (**X**): monotelic, one kinetochore is unattached; syntelic, both sister kinetochores attached to K-fibers from the same pole; merotelic, one of the kinetochores attached to K-fibers from opposite poles. (b) Balanced, amphitelic attachment: chromosomes are aligned, and sister chromatid separation is synchronized. (c) Incorrect attachments can lead to unbalanced tension and chromosome alignment defects (misaligned chromosomes) or lagging chromosomes during anaphase. Reproduced with kind permission of Bianka Seres, from 'Characterisation of a novel spindle domain in mammalian meiosis,' PhD thesis, University of Cambridge.

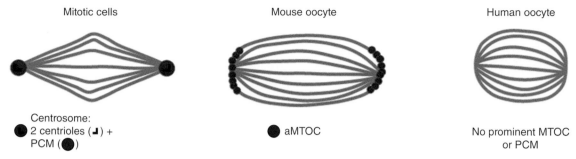

**Figure 1.16** Examples of different types of spindle morphology and location of spindle poles. Bipolar mitotic cell spindles are organized by centrosomes (two centrioles in orthogonal arrangement surrounded by the pericentriolar material [PCM]) with sharp, pointed spindle poles. The barrel-shaped meiotic spindle in mouse oocytes is organized by the coalescence of multiple acentrosomal microtubule-organizing centers made up of PCM components (aMTOCs). The small, barrel-shaped spindle in human oocytes does not contain prominent MTOCs or foci of PCM. Modified from Bennabi *et al.*, 2016 [CC license BY-NC-SA 3.0], with thanks to Bianka Seres.

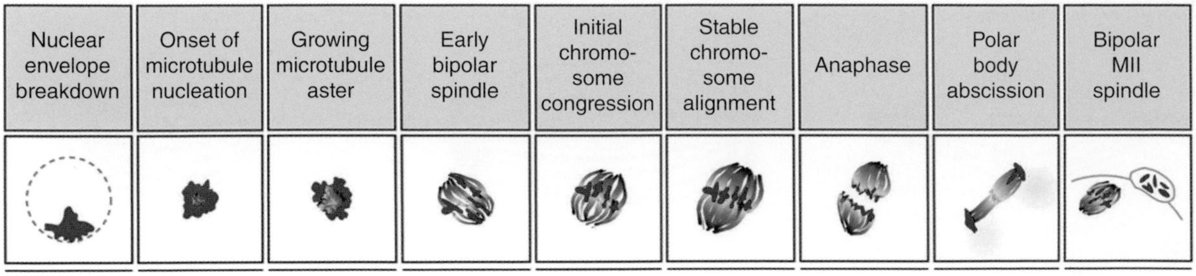

| Nuclear envelope breakdown | Onset of microtubule nucleation | Growing microtubule aster | Early bipolar spindle | Initial chromo-some congression | Stable chromo-some alignment | Anaphase | Polar body abscission | Bipolar MII spindle |
|---|---|---|---|---|---|---|---|---|
| | | | | | | | | |

**Figure 1.17** Schematic representation of the stages of meiosis in human oocytes. Adapted from Holubcova *et al.*, 2015, with permission.

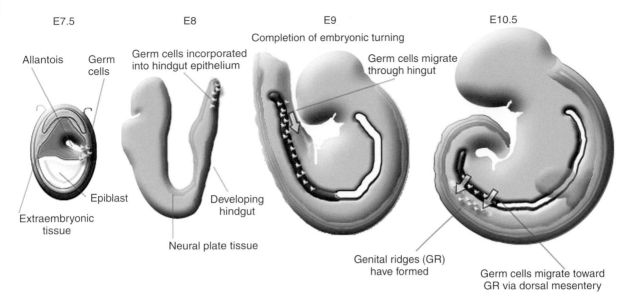

**Figure 3.1** Migration of primordial germ cells in the mouse. PGCs arise at the start of gastrulation, around embryonic Days 7–7.25 (E7–7.5) at the border of the extraembryonic tissue and the epiblast, at the root of the allantois. The PGCs can be identified and distinguished from the surrounding somatic cells by their positive staining for alkaline phosphatase. Expression of the OCT4 transcription factor becomes restricted to PGCs around day E8 and is used as a PGC marker. Adapted diagram courtesy of J. Huntriss, University of Leeds. Modified from Starz-Gaiano & Lehmann, 2001, with permission from Elsevier Ltd.

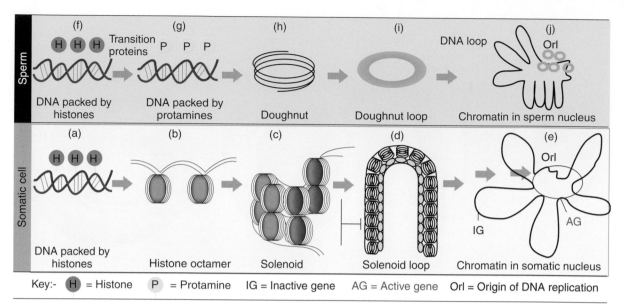

**Figure 3.6** DNA packaging in somatic cells and spermatozoa. Image adapted with permission from Ward, 1993.

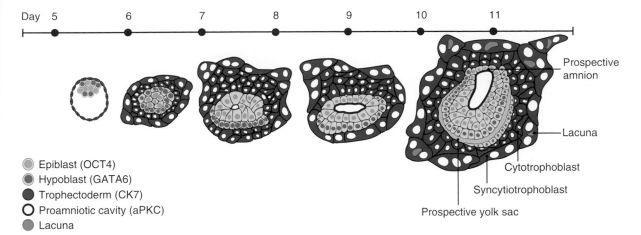

Day 5    6    7    8    9    10    11

Prospective
amnion

Lacuna

Cytotrophoblast

Syncytiotrophoblast

Prospective yolk sac

⬤ Epiblast (OCT4)
⬤ Hypoblast (GATA6)
⬤ Trophectoderm (CK7)
◯ Proamniotic cavity (aPKC)
⬤ Lacuna

**Figure 6.4** Schematic model of human embryo morphogenesis during peri-implantation and early implantation. Day 7: segregation of epiblast and hypoblast progenitors; Day 8–10: polarization and formation of the proamniotic cavity in the epiblast; Day 8–10: differentiation of the trophectoderm (TE) into cytotrophoblast and syncytiotrophoblast cells; Day 10–11: formation of the prospective amniotic epithelium, the prospective yolk sac and the bilaminar disc. Adapted with permission from Shabazi *et al.* (2016), with thanks to Alejandra Ontiveros.

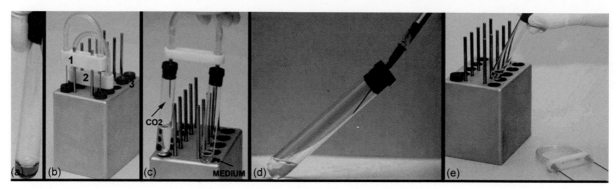

**Figure 8.2** Set up of the simplified culture system and kinetics of atmosphere and pH formation. (a) Phenol red in Global medium is consistent with pH 7.35. (d) Insertion of spermatozoa and cumulus–oocyte complexes. (e) Aluminum block containing closed vacutainer tubes in which IVF and embryo culture took place. (f) Graphic demonstration of the kinetics by which stable $O_2$, $CO_2$ and pH conditions optimal for fertilization and embryogenesis in the simplified culture system were reproducibly generated. The aluminum tube holder shown in (b) allows simultaneous equilibration of medium, fertilization and embryo culture and storage. The equilibrated tubes are fully contained within the block and are ready for IVF, performed in a dark environment that maintains 37°C throughout the length of the tube, such as a covered water bath. Reproduced with permission from van Blerkom *et al.* (2014).

(a)

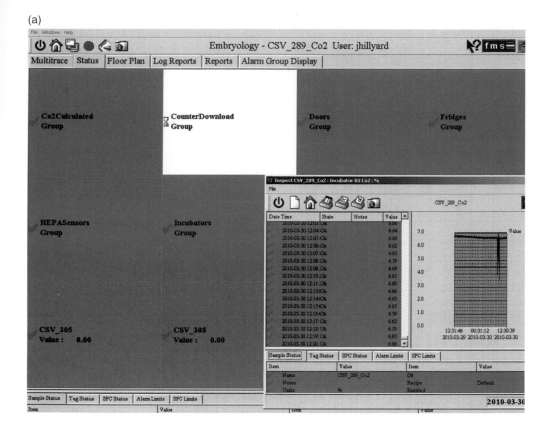

(b)

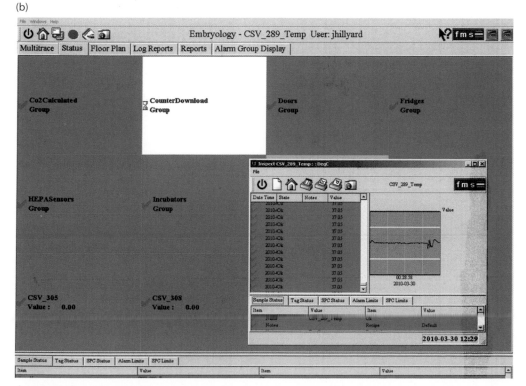

**Figure 9.2** Data from a facilities monitoring system in the IVF laboratory at Bourn Hall Clinic. The background shows the different monitoring modules that can be viewed: $CO_2$ sensors, HEPA sensors, incubator temperature, refrigerators, freezers. Insets: 24-hour records from a single incubator showing (a) $CO_2$ concentration and (b) temperature. Note dips during peak laboratory activity times, 8–10.30 am.

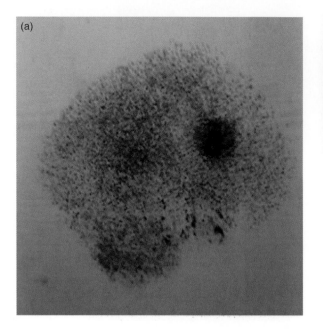

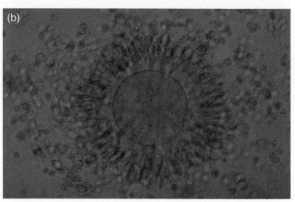

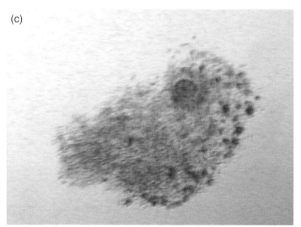

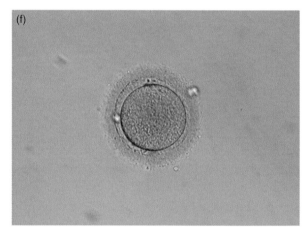

**Figure 11.2** Images after oocyte retrieval, before and after hyaluronidase denudation. Cumulus–oocyte complexes, without denudation: (a) cumulus–oocyte complex visualized under dissecting microscope, ×25 magnification; (b) phase-contrast image of mature metaphase II cumulus–oocyte complex, first polar body visible; (c) cumulus–oocyte complex with clumped refractile areas indicating signs of luteinization; (d) empty zona pellucida. Phase-contrast images after denudation: (e) germinal vesicle; (f) metaphase I oocyte, polar body not extruded; (g) preovulatory metaphase II oocyte, polar body extruded; (h) postmature oocyte, showing granularity in the perivitelline space; (i) dysmorphic metaphase II oocyte showing a large necrotic first polar body. Images (e), (f), (g) courtesy of Julia Uraji; Images (h) and (i) courtesy of Thomas Ebner, Austria.

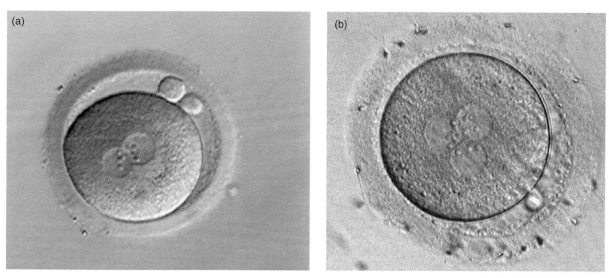

**Figure 11.4** Phase-contrast micrographs of fertilized human oocytes. (a) Normal fertilization: two pronuclei, two polar bodies. (b) Abnormal fertilization: three pronuclei. With thanks to Marc van den Bergh.

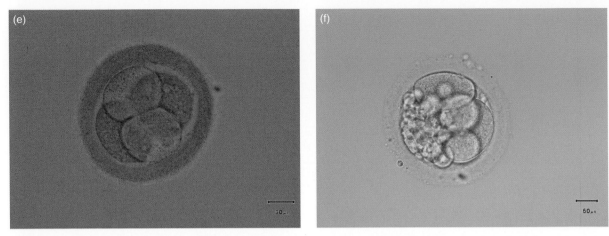

**Figure 11.8** Morphological variations in cleavage stage human embryos. (e) Four-cell embryo on Day 2, Grade 1. (f) Grade 3 embryo on Day 2. Images supplied by Oleksii Barash, Ukraine.

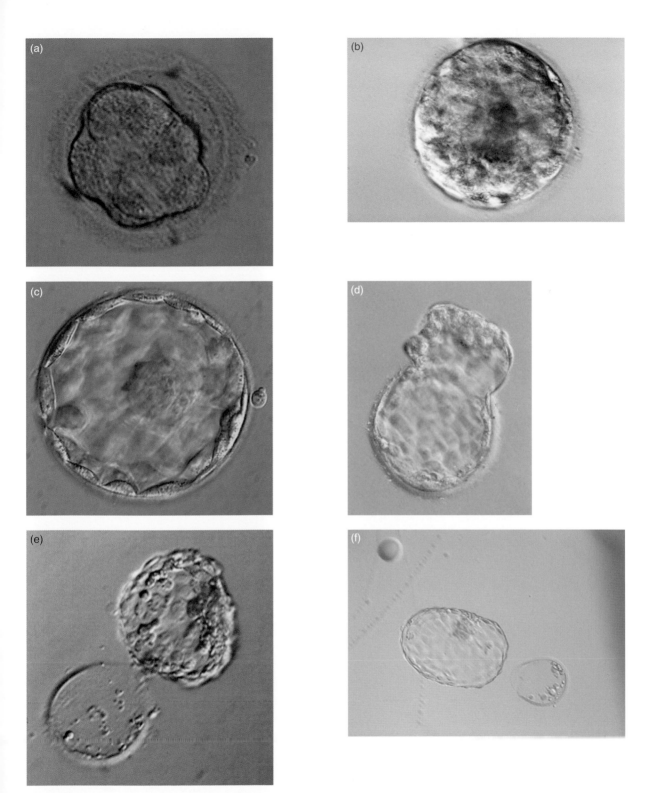

**Figure 11.9** Stages in blastocyst development. (a) Compacting morula. (b) Early stages of cavitation. (c) Fully expanded top-grade blastocyst with well-developed ICM and trophectoderm, thinned zona, hatching process initiated. (d) Top-grade blastocyst in the process of hatching. (e) Hatching blastocyst about to leave the zona. (f) Fully hatched blastocyst and empty zona.

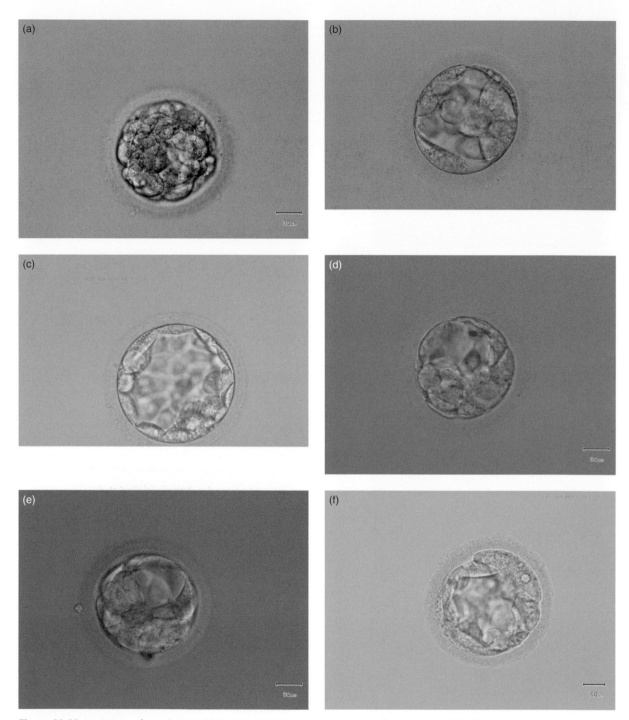

**Figure 11.10** Limitations of morphological blastocyst assessment. Although each of the embryos pictured here would be graded as lesser quality compared with the 'classic' optimal grade blastocysts seen in Figure 11.8, each of these embryos resulted in a healthy live birth after single embryo transfer on Day 5. Image (a) is a thawed embryo. (Two blastocysts were thawed on Day 5 [slow-freeze protocol]; the one pictured here survived and was transferred on the same day). With thanks to Oleksii Barash, Clinic of Reproductive Medicine 'Nadiya,' Ukraine.

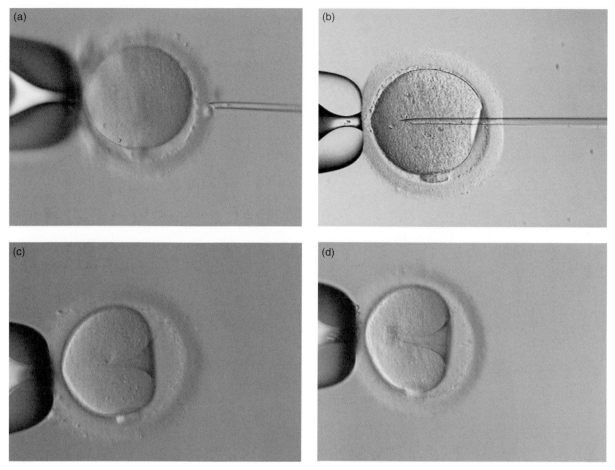

**Figure 13.4** ICSI. (a) Metaphase II oocyte with injection needle in position prior to injection. (b) Injection needle within the cytoplasm, prior to release of sperm. (c) Post-injection illustrating the typical track left following withdrawal of the needle. (d) Post-injection, oocyte with a very elastic membrane. With thanks to Agnese Fiorentino.

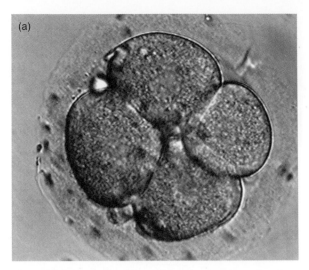

**Figure 13.6** Assisted hatching. (a) Laser-hatched four-cell embryo.

Fertilization can be achieved in very simple media such as Earle's, or a TALP-based formulation, but the situation becomes more complex thereafter. (See Chapter 5 for details of embryo metabolism.) Prior to 1997, single media formulations were used for all stages of IVF. However, research in animal systems during the 1990s led to elucidation of the metabolic biochemistry and molecular mechanisms involved in gamete maturation, activation, fertilization, genomic activation, cleavage, compaction and blastocyst formation. This drew attention to the fact that nutrient and ionic requirements differ during all these different stages. Inappropriate culture conditions expose embryos to cellular stress which could result in retarded cleavage, cleavage arrest, cytoplasmic blebbing, impaired energy production, inadequate genome activation and transcription. Blastocyst formation is followed by an exponential increase in protein synthesis, with neosynthesis of glycoproteins, histones and new surface antigens.

Although the specific needs of embryos during their preimplantation development have by no means been completely defined, both single-step and sequential, stage-specific and chemically defined media are used in IVF systems. Media formulations endeavor to mimic the natural in-vivo situation and take into account the expected theoretical changes in embryo physiology and metabolism that occur during the preimplantation period, although this has largely been based upon mouse embryo culture (see Fleming et al., 1987; Elder et al., 2015; Ménézo et al., 2018). Protocols that have been used include:

1. One-step culture using a single medium formulation (nonrenewal monoculture)
2. Single medium formulation, renewed on Day 2/Day 3 (renewal monoculture)
3. Two-step culture using two different media formulations (sequential media culture).

Although two-step sequential media appeared to have advantages, doubts have been raised as to whether these more complex protocols have any advantage over one-step protocols. (See Biggers and Summers, 2008 for review.) The introduction of time-lapse technology led to the development of new single-step formulations, but it is impossible to assess whether any improvements in outcome might be due to the media itself, or to other factors inherent in the system, such as new incubator design or lowered cellular stress due to less handling for routine observation.

Commercial media is 'ready to use,' with protein supplements added, and may also contain other components or factors. Different formulations are available for sperm preparation, oocyte washing during retrieval, insemination/fertilization, early cleavage, blastocyst development and freezing/thawing. Media containing HEPES, which maintains a relatively stable pH even in ambient air, can be used for sperm preparation, oocyte harvesting and washing, and during ICSI procedures; however, HEPES-buffered medium will become acidic when placed in a $CO_2$ atmosphere, and therefore the gametes should be washed in HEPES-free medium before being placed in the culture incubator.

**Table 8.2** International regulations regarding the use of IVF culture media

| | |
|---|---|
| Australia | Regulated by the Australian Therapeutic Goods Administration (TGA) as a Class III medical device |
| USA | Regulated by the FDA as a Class II medical device with special conditions under the 510k Pre-market notification scheme |
| Japan | Classed as a laboratory reagent in Japan, and as such, has no formal regulatory review or approval |
| China | No official designation of the IVF media as a medical device, but regulatory approval by the Chinese Regulator (SFDA) is required to apply for hospital tenders |
| France | IVF media products are seen as a 'hybrid' product in France (i.e., somewhere between drug and device) and are regulated as a PTA (Product Therapeutique Annexe) by the French Regulatory Authority (AFSSaPS) |
| European Union (excl. France) | IVF cell culture media has not been officially declared a medical device in the EU |

### Media Used Historically in Embryo Culture and Manipulation

See Table 8.2.

### Simple Media: Balanced Salt Solutions (BSS)

- Contain combinations of Na, K, Cl, Ca, Pi, Mg, $HCO_3$, glucose, ± phenol red
- Salt concentrations/balance differ slightly in different formulations:

    Ringer's: contains Na, K, Cl, Ca only

    Earle's, Hank's, Tyrode's, etc.: also contain Pi, Mg, $HCO_3$, glucose.

### Complex Media

Contain the inorganic salts of BSS, as well as amino acids, fatty acids, vitamins, other substrates (nucleotide bases, cholesterol, glutathione, other macromolecules), antibiotics, and other labile substances to be added before use (pyruvate, lactate, glutamine, methionine, bicarbonate):

- Minimal essential medium (MEM)
- Dulbecco's modified MEM
- Ham's F-10, F-12
- BWW, TC199, KSOM, etc.

### Media Optimized for Preimplantation Embryos

- Menezo B2, 'complex,' designed for bovine embryo culture (1976)
- Human tubal fluid (HTF), 'simple,' contains pyruvate and lactate (Quinn, 1995)
- P1, Basal IX HTF: no pyruvate or lactate, contains EDTA and glutamine
- HTF-12: no phosphate, low level of glucose + EDTA, taurine, glutathione
- G1/S1, 'simple,' contains EDTA, lactate/pyruvate, amino acids
- G2/S2, 'complex,' high level of glucose
- Cook IVF: Sydney IVF Cleavage/Sydney IVF Blastocyst medium
- Cooper Surgical

Phosphate buffered saline (PBS) and HEPES buffers: commonly used to stabilize pH solutions used for washing in room atmosphere, e.g., follicle flushing, cryopreservation protocols, sperm preparation.

### Low Oxygen Culture

Oxygen is known to be a powerful regulator of cell function, and decades of extensive research in human and other mammalian embryos confirms that oxygen concentrations during culture exert effects on preimplantation development. As outlined in Chapter 1, any perturbation in the delicate balance of factors that control oxidative stress may affect global methylation patterns, with an impact on gene expression. Variations in embryonic transcriptome and proteome related to oxygen concentrations during culture have been demonstrated, as well as effects on metabolic pathways that alter the ulitization/turnover of culture media components. It is clear that metabolic pathways shift between pre- and postcompaction periods, and effects of different oxygen concentrations appear to be stage-specific. Oxygen concentrations have also been found to affect the physiology of human embryonic stem cells (hESCs), demonstrated by changes in metabolism and gene expression (Harvey et al., 2016).

Physiological concentrations of oxygen in human bodily fluids range between 2 and 8%. Oxygen concentrations within the female reproductive tract are estimated to be around 5%, whereas atmospheric oxygen concentration is much higher at around 21%, depending on altitude. Pioneering studies in human preimplantation culture during the 1970s were carried out in a low oxygen atmosphere of 5% $O_2$, 5% $CO_2$ and 90% $N_2$, achieved by using premixed gas cylinders and sealable chambers such as desiccators for incubation. (See Wale & Gardner, 2016 for review.) With the widespread growth of ART during the 1980s, this cumbersome system was replaced by using tissue culture incubators that could accommodate larger numbers of culture dishes, which were designed to function with an atmosphere of 5% $CO_2$ in air, i.e., atmospheric oxygen at a concentration of 20%. This system was adopted by the majority of clinical IVF laboratories all over the world.

During the 1990s, data began to accumulate describing the benefits of culture under conditions of reduced oxygen, including effects on postimplantation development and live birth rates; more significant effects were noted after extended culture to blastocyst stage. A range of different types of incubators have now been developed (including time-lapse systems) that can maintain both $CO_2$ and $O_2$ concentrations at predetermined levels, with $O_2$ routinely set at around 5%. Using time-lapse evaluation to compare culture in 5% vs 20% $O_2$, Kirkegaard et al. (2013) demonstrated stage-specific differences: the timing of the third cleavage cycle was delayed for embryos cultured in 20% $O_2$, although cumulative development and overall embryo score did not differ between the two groups.

A Cochrane evaluation of data published up to November 2011 concluded: '...culturing embryos under low oxygen concentrations improves the success rates of IVF/ICSI, resulting in an increase in the live birth rate' (Bontekoe *et al.*, 2012). A 2014 meeting of the Association of Clinical Embryologists in the UK (ACE) reviewing commercial culture media also concluded that there is strong evidence that low oxygen concentrations are beneficial during human embryo culture (Bolton *et al.*, 2014).

### Culture Media Preparations

Commercially prepared, pretested, high-quality culture media is available for purchase from a number of suppliers worldwide, so that media preparation for routine use in the laboratory is not necessary, and may not be a cost-effective exercise when time and quality control are taken into account. Quality control is essential in media preparation, including knowledge of the source of all ingredients, especially the water, which must be tested to make sure that it is endotoxin-free, low in ion content, and guaranteed free of organic molecules and microorganisms. Pharmaceutical grade reagents are required in order to follow Good Manufacturing Practice (GMP). Each batch of culture media prepared must be checked for osmolality (285 ± 2 mOsm/kg) and pH (7.35–7.45), and subjected to quality control procedures with a LAL (limulus amebocyte lysate) test for endotoxins and sperm survival or mouse embryo toxicity before use. Culture media can rapidly deteriorate during storage, with a decrease in their ability to support embryo development, and careful attention must be paid to storage conditions and manufacturers' recommended expiry dates.

A 2014 consensus meeting of ACE in the UK concluded that there is no firm scientific evidence that any medium is superior to another in routine IVF. The report also suggests that possible epigenetic and long-term effects of in-vitro culture require further investigation, emphasizing the importance of explicit information regarding the precise composition of all components of the culture media.

Choice of culture media should depend upon considerations such as quality control and testing procedures applied in its manufacture, cost and, in particular, guaranteed efficient supply delivery in relation to shelf life. After delivery, the medium may be aliquoted in suitable small volumes, such that one aliquot can be used for a single patient's gamete preparation and culture (including sperm preparation). Shelf life is dependent on specific composition and

conditions of storage; generally, the more 'complex' the media, the shorter its useful lifespan, with an average of approximately 4–6 weeks. All media must be equilibrated for temperature and pH for 4–6 hours before use, ideally by overnight incubation.

**Important Factors When Choosing Commercial Media**
- Information available about composition (not always easy to obtain)
- Information about quality control during production
- Information about endotoxin testing
- Assurance of regular, reliable delivery under controlled conditions
- Acceptable shelf life
- Delivery of batches well before expiry date
- Validation evidence of use in human IVF – i.e., proven track record
- Tested using appropriate bioassay
- Certificates of analysis available
- Serum or serum derivatives from virally screened sources

### Protein Supplement

Protein, or an equivalent macromolecule (e.g., polyvinyl alcohol, hyaluronate), is required in human IVF for:

- Sperm capacitation – involves the removal of sterols from the plasma membrane, and this requires a sterol acceptor molecule (such as albumin) in the medium.
- Handling – a molecule with surfactant properties is needed to facilitate sperm and embryo handling in order to prevent sticking to pipettes and dishes.
- Proteins also act as lipid and peptide carriers, chelators, cell surface protectors and regulators of redox potential, and are a source of fixed nitrogen/amino acids after hydrolysis.

Bovine serum albumin used for embryo culture is now recognized to carry the risk of disease transmission, including prion disease (Creutzfeldt–Jakob disease, CJD). In domestic animals, media supplemented with whole serum was found to affect embryo development at several different levels (Leese, 1998), and its presence is associated with the development of abnormally large fetuses when used to grow embryos to the blastocyst stage (Thompson *et al.*, 1995). The mechanisms involved are thought to be related to abnormal epigenetic/imprinting mechanisms; the findings led to further concerns about the use of whole serum in human IVF, particularly in extended culture systems, and serum substitutes are used instead.

Serum albumin contains 650 amino acids, with a molecular weight of 65 000 kDa. Albumin and transferrin are major protein constituents of the oviductal embryo environment. Albumin regulates oncotic pressure and acts as a detergent through its capacity to bind lipids: this facilitates gamete and embryo manipulations, by preventing them from sticking to glass or plastic surfaces. It can enter the embryo directly, acting as a carrier for numerous small molecules such as catecholamines, peptides and amino acids, and it may help to bind and stabilize growth factors. Theoretically albumin may not be indispensable, but it does effectively replace serum, and probably acts as a source of embryo nutrition. Commercially prepared media are supplied complete; most contain a serum substitute such as human serum albumin (HSA). Human serum contains approximately 4.5% albumin, i.e., 45 mg/mL. A supplement of 10% HSA provides an albumin concentration of 4.5%. Synthetic serum Substitute (SSS) is a 6% protein solution made up of 84% HSA, 16% alpha- and beta-globulins, plus a trace of gamma globulins. Although disease transmission from commercial preparations of HSA was a concern in the past, recombinant preparations are now available and are used routinely in commercial culture media.

### Growth Factors

Growth factors play a key role in growth and differentiation from the time of morula/blastocyst transition. However, defining their precise role and potential for improving in-vitro preimplantation development is complicated by factors such as gene expression of both the factors and their receptors. There is also the potential of ascribing positive effects to specific factors when the result may in fact be due to a combination of a myriad of other causes. The mammalian blastocyst expresses ligands and receptors for several growth factors, many of which can cross-react, making it difficult to interpret the effects of single factors added to a medium. Insulin, LIF, EGF/TGF-α, TGF-β, PDGG and HB-EGF have all been studied in IVF culture, and, although it is clear that these and other growth factors may influence in-vitro blastocyst development and hatching, further assessment remains an area of research; a comprehensive review was published by Richter in 2008 (Richter, 2008). It has been suggested that the mechanism whereby serum induces abnormalities in domestic animal systems may involve the overexpression of certain growth factors – there is no doubt that complex and delicate regulatory systems are involved.

Culture of embryos in 'groups' rather than singly has been found to improve viability and implantation in some systems: it is possible that autocrine/paracrine effects or 'trophic' factors exist between embryos. However, observed effects of 'group' culture will inevitably be related to the composition of the culture medium and the precise physical conditions used for embryo culture, and in particular the number of embryos in relation to the volume of media used per culture drop.

### Follicular Fushing Media

Ideally, if a patient has responded well to follicular phase stimulation with appropriate monitoring and timing of ovulation induction, the oocyte retrieval will proceed smoothly with efficient recovery of oocytes without the need to flush follicles. If the number of follicles is low or the procedure is difficult for technical reasons, follicles may be flushed with a physiological solution to assist recovery of all the oocytes. Follicles can be flushed with balanced salt solutions such as Earle's (EBSS) or lactated Ringer's solution, and heparin may be added at a concentration of 2 units/mL. HEPES- or MOPS-buffered media can also be used for flushing. Temperature and pH of flushing media must be carefully controlled, and the oocytes recovered from flushing media subsequently washed in culture media before transfer to their final culture droplet or well.

## Tissue Culture Systems

Vessels successfully used for IVF include test-tubes, four-well culture dishes, organ culture dishes and Petri dishes containing microdroplets of culture medium under a layer of clinical grade mineral or silicone oil. Whatever the system employed, it must be capable of rigidly maintaining fixed stable parameters of temperature, pH and osmolarity. Human oocytes are extremely sensitive to transient cooling in vitro, and modest reductions in temperature can cause irreversible disruption of the meiotic spindle, with possible chromosome dispersal. Temperature-induced chromosome disruption may contribute to aneuploidy, and the high rates of preclinical and spontaneous abortion that follow IVF and ICSI. Therefore, it is essential to control temperature fluctuation from the moment of follicle aspiration, and during all oocyte and embryo manipulations, by using heated microscope stages and heating blocks or platforms. Most importantly, the temperature within the media itself must be maintained at the optimal temperature, rather than the temperature of the dish (see Elder *et al.*, 2015, Chapter 6).

An overlay of equilibrated oil as part of the tissue culture system confers specific advantages:

1. The oil acts as a physical barrier, separating droplets of medium from the atmosphere and airborne particles or pathogens.
2. Oil prevents evaporation and delays gas diffusion, thereby keeping pH, temperature and osmolality of the medium stable during gamete manipulations, protecting the embryos from significant fluctuations in their microenvironment. (Aliquots of medium without an oil overlay begin to show an immediate rise in pH as soon as they are removed from the incubator.)
3. Because humidified and pre-equilibrated oil prevents evaporation, nonhumidified incubators can be used, which are easier to clean and maintain.

It has been suggested that oil could enhance embryo development by removing lipid-soluble toxins from the medium; on the other hand, an oil overlay prevents free diffusion of metabolic by-products such as ammonia, and accumulation of ammonia in culture media is toxic to the embryo. The use of an oil overlay also influences oxygen concentration in the medium, with resulting effects on the delicate balance of embryo metabolism; as mentioned previously, it can absorb and concentrate harmful VOCs in the incubator atmosphere. Oil is difficult to sterilize and inappropriate handling can lead it to be a source of fungal contamination.

Two types of oil have been used in culture overlays, from a mineral or a silicone source. Silicone oil, commonly used as a stationary phase in gas chromatography or as an anti-foaming agent, should not be confused with mineral oil, which is obtained from fractionated distillation in the petrol industry.

---

**Types of Oil Used in Culture Overlays**

1. Paraffin oil – also known as white mineral oil or liquid paraffin

   - Merck Index: 'Liquid Petrolatum' (Petrolatum = Vaseline)

   - Is derived from petroleum, and exists in many different forms with differing melting points and viscosities
   - Available in 'light' or 'heavy' forms
   - Light – density = 0.83–0.89
   - Batch-to-batch variations are common, since they are a mixture of hydrocarbons with fluctuating composition

2. Silicone oil (dimethyl-polysiloxane) (Erbach *et al.*, 1995)

   - Polymer, available in many viscosities, from 10 to 600 000 centistokes
   - Composition should be more stable than that of paraffin
   - Problems have been encountered with $Zn^{2+}$ contamination, and toxicity after degradation as a result of exposure to sunlight (Provo and Herr, 1998)

---

## Oil Preparation

Commercial companies now supply washed, sterilized oil that is ready for use in overlays. If obtained from other sources, mineral or silicone oil should be sterile as supplied, and does not require sterilization or filtration. High temperature for sterilization may be detrimental to the oil itself, and the procedure may also 'leach' potential toxins from the container. Provo and Herr (1998) reported that exposure of mineral oil to direct sunlight for a period of 4 hours resulted in a highly embryotoxic overlay, and they recommend that washed oil should be shielded from light and treated as a photoreactive compound. Contaminants have been reported in certain types of oil. Washing procedures remove water-soluble toxins, but non-water-soluble toxins may also be present which will not be removed by washing. Therefore, it is prudent not only to wash, but also to test every batch of oil before use with, at the very least, a sperm survival test as a quality control procedure. Erbach *et al.* (1995) suggested that zinc might be a contaminant in silicone oil, and found that washing the oil with EDTA removed a toxicity factor that may have been due to the presence of zinc. Some mineral oil products may also contain preservatives such as alpha-tocopherol. Oil can be carefully washed in sterile disposable tissue culture flasks (without vigorous shaking) with either Milli-Q water, sterile saline solution or a simple culture medium without protein or lipid-soluble components, in a ratio of 5:1 (oil:aq). The oil can be further 'equilibrated' by bubbling 5% $CO_2$ through the mixture before allowing the phases to separate and settle. Washed oil can be stored either at room temperature or at 4°C in equilibrium with the aqueous layer, or separated before storage, but should be prepared at least 2 days prior to its use.

Oil overlays must be further equilibrated in the $CO_2$ incubator for several hours (or overnight) before introducing media/gametes/embryos. Conaghan (2008) established experimentally that even relatively small volumes of medium (50 µL) with an oil overlay require a minimum of 8 hours equilibration in order to establish a stable pH under normal culture conditions. However, once equilibrated, the oil acts as an effective buffer, maintaining pH for up to 10 minutes after removing dishes from the incubator, whereas media without an oil overlay show a dramatic rise in pH as soon as the dishes are removed from the $CO_2$ atmosphere.

## Simplified IVF

Although a great deal of costly technology has been introduced into the IVF laboratory since the 1980s, the basic science of procedures and protocols used for routine IVF have changed very little. The prevalence of infertility that requires assisted reproductive intervention continues to increase, but this remains out of reach to couples in many 'developing' countries where resources and cost prohibit its availability. Laboratory costs have been estimated to represent over half of the financial outlay associated with routine IVF; the 'Walking Egg Project' (www.thewalkingegg.com) was initiated as a means of making assisted reproductive technologies, including IVF, available and accessible to a wider population in both developed and developing countries (Ombelet, 2014). A highly simplified IVF culture system that does not require a costly 'high-tech' infrastructure was developed that would allow small centers to treat couples with uncomplicated fertility problems such as bilateral tubal occlusion, one of the commonest indications for IVF.

A completely closed system that allows insemination and embryo development in a single container (glass vacutainer) was devised, controlled for pH and temperature. $CO_2$ is created *de novo* via a simple chemical reaction, producing a defined atmosphere; culture medium is equilibrated prior to the IVF cycle, with temperature maintained at 37° C using an aluminum tube holder in a water bath, heating block or basic

incubator. Culture remains undisturbed in the same tube, maintaining sterility and minimizing or eliminating potential changes in temperature, atmosphere or pH that might adversely affect embryo development. Fertilization and embryo development can be observed through the glass vacutainer until day 3, when embryos are selected for transfer without opening the vacutainer. The system is designed for incubation of a single cumulus–oocyte complex/embryo per tube, so that the embryos remain undisturbed until selected for transfer. A sterile field for manipulations is recommended if possible; potential contamination is avoided by using medium containing antibiotics and treating the rubber vacutainer stopper with ethanol prior to each operation (van Blerkom *et al.*, 2014).

An overview of the procedure is outlined below; see van Blerkom *et al.* (2014) for details.

**Materials:**

- Disposable 10-mL glass vacutainers, washed and sterilized
- Aluminum tube holder
- Water bath, heating block, basic warming oven/incubator or high-quality Thermos flask
- Commercial culture medium supplement with 5% human serum albumin
- Citric acid and sodium bicarbonate for $CO_2$ generation
- Tuberculin syringes (0.5–1.0 mL) or 500-µL gas-tight Luer-lock syringe
- 18-g 1.5-inch needles
- Standard Vortex instrument
- Dissecting microscope or inverted microscope with long working distance, 10× objective lens
- Basic centrifuge for sperm preparation
- Embryo transfer catheters

**Method:**

1. Using a 3-mL syringe, rinse a sterile glass vacutainer several times with sterile deionized water, and then remove the water completely with the same syringe. (This also relieves the partial vacuum in the vacutainer.) Add 1 mL of culture medium.

2. $CO_2$ generation: remove the stopper from a sterile but unwashed vacutainer, add 11.5 mg citric acid + 50 mg sodium bicarbonate + 3 mL water, and replace the stopper

   Or: add 50 mg sodium bicarbonate (one-eighth teaspoon) to 3 mL of 10× stock solution of citric acid: $CO_2$ is liberated, with immediate effervescence.

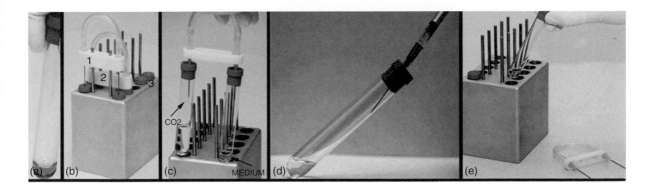

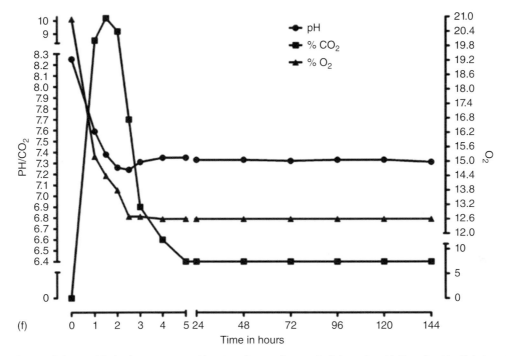

**Figure 8.2** Set up of the simplified culture system and kinetics of atmosphere and pH formation. (a) Phenol red in Global medium is consistent with pH 7.35. (d) Insertion of spermatozoa and cumulus–oocyte complexes. (e) Aluminum block containing closed vacutainer tubes in which IVF and embryo culture took place. (f) Graphic demonstration of the kinetics by which stable $O_2$, $CO_2$ and pH conditions optimal for fertilization and embryogenesis in the simplified culture system were reproducibly generated. The aluminum tube holder shown in (b) allows simultaneous equilibration of medium, fertilization and embryo culture and storage. The equilibrated tubes are fully contained within the block and are ready for IVF, performed in a dark environment that maintains 37°C throughout the length of the tube, such as a covered water bath. Reproduced with permission from van Blerkom *et al.* (2014). See color plate section.

3. Seal both ends of an 8-cm length of plastic tubing with 18-g 1.5-inch needles, and use this to connect the two tubes together after effervescence has ceased in the $CO_2$ generator (Figure 8.2).

4. Incubate the two tubes at 37°C for at least 5 hours; the culture medium is then ready for use or can be stored for up to 2 weeks at 4–15°C.

5. Collect each cumulus–oocyte complex (COC) into the syringe in 25 μL medium followed by 20 μL air buffer; each COC is incubated individually, in separate tubes.

6. Insert the entire length of the needle through the vacutainer stopper, with the opening of the needle on the inner surface of the tube; alternatively, the COC can be deposited directly into the center of the tube, and needle examined after withdrawal and rinsing under a dissecting microscope.

7. Insemination: prepare sperm by routine methods, to a concentration of 1000–5000 sperm/mL. Two

to 3 hours after OCR, clean the surface of the stopper with ethanol and add a 10- to 15-μL aliquot of prepared sperm to the culture tube, swirl gently and incubate so that the tubes are completely surrounded by a darkened 37°C environment, with only the top of the stopper visible.

8. Pronuclear check: vortex tubes for up to 30 seconds, with instrument set between 5 and 6 on a typical scale of 1–10.

9. Observe embryos through the glass vacutainer by holding the tube horizontally in a dissecting microscope or inverted microscope with a long working distance, 10× objective lens.

10. Embryo transfer (ET): wipe the stopper with ethanol and insert ET catheter directly into the vacutainer through a beveled needle with the appropriate gauge, position the catheter above the embryo and withdraw it in 10 μL of medium.

11. After ET, incubate each culture tube for at least 10 days, checking periodically for signs of contamination.

The simplified system eliminates the need for expensive and complex logistical support, such as medical grade gases, reliable electricity supplies, rapid availability of replacement parts, microprocessor-controlled incubators and costly disposable supplies for culture. Each part of the procedure was tested and validated both in mouse and human embryo culture, and pilot studies comparing the system with routine practice carried out in a modern high-resource facility in Belgium demonstrated that acceptable pregnancy and live birth rates can be achieved.

## Co-culture Systems

Historically, co-culture systems played an important role in the evolution of modern culture systems, using a substrate layer of feeder cells in order to support the growth of human embryos and regulate their metabolic turnover processes. A variety of different types of homologous and autologous cells were used as feeder layers in the past, including tubal epithelial cells, explants of endometrial tissue, granulosa cells, as well as the animal cells used in commercial vaccine production, African green monkey kidney (Vero). For the same developmental stage, embryos co-cultured to the blastocyst stage were found to have higher numbers of cells and a fully cohesive inner cell mass when compared with embryos cultured in simple media. It was postulated that improved development occurs as a result of four different possible mechanisms:

1. 'Metabolic locks': co-culture cell layers can provide a supply of small molecular weight metabolites which simpler culture media lack. This supply may assist continued cell metabolism required for genome activation, and divert the potential for abnormal metabolic processes which may lead to cleavage arrest.

2. The feeder cell layer may supply growth factors essential for development.

3. Toxic compounds resulting from cell metabolism can be removed: heavy metal ions may be chelated by glycine produced by feeder cells, and ammonium and urea may be recycled through feeder cell metabolic cycles.

4. Feeder cells can synthesize reducing agents which prevent the formation of free radicals.

The use of feeder cells during the late 1980s played an important role in research into embryo metabolism and preimplantation development, and the observations and data obtained were instrumental in helping to develop more appropriate culture media formulations and systems. However, maintaining a safe and effective co-culture system is difficult and labor intensive, and their use carries the risk of potential disease transmission, or even retrovirus-induced cell transformation in the feeder layer. Accumulated experimental data suggest that the ability of human embryos to develop in vitro during the early cleavage stages is more a measure of their adaptability and survival capabilities than of the suitability of the medium, and media formulations that are now based upon research into early embryo metabolism (see Chapter 5) have made the use of co-culture systems redundant; they also introduce an unacceptable risk in clinical practice.

## Emerging Technologies

Research continues into technologies that will improve the outcome of in-vitro embryo culture, with the goal of minimizing environmental stress imposed upon the embryo during laboratory manipulations. The active integrated workstation was an early approach, aiming to eliminate fluctuations in the physical parameters of the environment. However, carrying out the manipulations in these systems is more difficult for the operator, and involves additional training, experience and a learning curve. An alternative approach is to mimic dynamic in-vivo conditions by exposing them to continuous movement: 'embryo rocking' using a dynamic microfunnel culture system (Heo *et al.*, 2010), tilting platforms (Matsuura *et al.*, 2010) or with microfluidic technology, using chambers or devices that enable continuous fluid movement in a micro- or nano-environment. The gametes/embryos can be perfused with media that gradually changes in composition, providing different chemical substrates for different stages during development. This could have the effect of removing metabolic by-products such as ammonia, or simply disrupting any microgradients that may form in small culture droplets. Although microfluidic platforms for ART procedures have theoretical advantages, and a number of different devices have been tried, there are practical considerations yet to be addressed before they can be successfully implemented (see Monteiro da Rocha & Smith, 2014; Smith *et al.*, 2012; Elder *et al.*, 2015, Chapter 3).

# Appendix
## Equipment and Supplies for Embryology

$CO_2$ incubator

Dissecting microscope

Inverted microscope

Heated surfaces for microscope and manipulation areas

Heating block for test-tubes

Laminar flow cabinet

Oven for heat-sterilizing

Small autoclave

Water bath

Pipette 10–1000 mL Eppendorf Refrigerator

Supply of medical grade $CO_2$

Supply of 5% $CO_2$ in air (or special gas mixtures)

Wash bottle + Millex filter for gas

Rubber tubing

Pipette canisters

Clinical grade mineral or paraffin oil

Culture media

Glassware for media preparation

Tissue culture plastics:

    Flasks for media and oil: 50 mL, 175 mL

    Culture dishes: 60, 35 mm

OCR (oocyte retrieval) needles

Test-tubes for OCR: 17 mL disposable

Transfer catheters and stylets: embryo, GIFT, intrauterine insemination (IUI) syringes

Needles

Disposable pipettes: 1, 5, 10, 25 mL

'Pipetus' pipetting device

Eppendorf tips, small and large

Millipore filters: 0.22, 0.8 mm

Glass Pasteur pipettes

Pipette bulbs

Test-tube racks

Rubbish bags

Tissues

Tape for labeling

7X or Oosafe® disinfectants

70% ethanol

Sterile gloves, latex and non-latex

Oil for culture overlay

Supply of purified water: Milli-Q system or Analar

Glassware for making culture media and solutions: beakers, flasks, measuring cylinder

# Further Reading

### Books and Reviews

ASRM Guidelines: Practice Committee of the American Society for Reproductive Medicine and the Practice Committee of the Society for Assisted Reproductive Technology (2014) Recommended practices for the management of human embryology, andrology and endocrinology laboratories: a committee opinion. *Fertility and Sterility* 102(4): 960–963.

Bolton VN, Cutting R, Clarke H, Brison DR (2014) ACE consensus meeting report: Culture systems. *Human Fertility* 17(4): 239–251.

Bontekoe S, Mantikou E, van Wely M, *et al.* (2012) Low oxygen concentrations for embryo culture in assisted reproductive technologies. *Cochrane Database of Systematic Reviews* 7: CD008950.

Brison DR, Roberts SA, Kimber SJ (2013) How should we assess the safety of IVF technologies? *Reproductive BioMedicine Online* 27: 710–721.

Elder K, Baker DJ, Ribes JA (2004) *Infections, Infertility and Assisted Reproduction*. Cambridge University Press, Cambridge, UK.

Elder K, Van den Bergh M, Woodward B (2015) *Troubleshooting and Problem-Solving in the IVF Laboratory*. Cambridge University Press, Cambridge, UK.

de los Santos, MJ, Apter S, Coticchio G, *et al.* (2016) Revised guidelines for good practice in IVF laboratories (2015). *Human Reproduction* 31(4): 685–686.

Magli MC, Van den Abbeel E, Lundin K, *et al.* (2015) Revised guidelines for good practice in IVF laboratories. *Human Reproduction* 23(6): 1253–1262.

Mantikou E, Youssef MAFM, van Wely M, *et al.* (2013) Embryo culture media and IVF/ICSI success rates: a systematic review. *Human Reproduction* 19(3): 210–220.

Poole TB, Schoolfield J, Han D (2012) Human embryo culture media comparisons. *Methods in Molecular Biology* 912: 367–386.

Summers MC, Biggers JD (2003) Chemically defined media and the culture of mammalian preimplantation embryos: historical perspective and current issues. *Human Reproduction Update* 9(6): 557–582.

Swain, JE (2014) Decisions for the IVF laboratory: comparative analysis of embryo culture incubators. *Reproductive BioMedicine Online* 28: 535–547.

Wale PL, Gardner DK (2016) The effects of chemical and physical factors on mammalian embryo culture and their importance for the practice of assisted human reproduction. *Human Reproduction Update* 22(1): 2–22.

## Website Information

Association of Clinical Embryologists – www.embryologists.org.uk

COSHH – www.hse.gov.uk/coshh

Department of Health – www.dh.gov.uk

The Human Fertilisation and Embryology Authority – www.hfea.gov.uk

## Publications

Almeida PA, Bolton VN (1996) The effect of temperature fluctuations on the cytoskeletal organisation and chromosomal constitution of the human oocyte. *Zygote* 3: 357–365.

Angell RR, Templeton AA, Aitken RJ (1986) Chromosome studies in human in vitro fertilisation *Human Genetics* 72: 333–339.

Ashwood-Smith MJ, Hollands P, Edwards RG (1989) The use of Albuminar (TM) as a medium supplement in clinical IVF. *Human Reproduction* 4: 702–705.

Bavister BD (1995) Culture of preimplantation embryos: facts and artifacts. *Human Reproduction Update* 1(2): 91–148.

Bavister BD, Andrews JC (1988) A rapid sperm motility bioassay procedure for quality control testing of water and culture media. *Journal of In Vitro Fertilization and Embryo Transfer* 5: 67–68.

Biggers JD, Summers MC (2008) Choosing a culture medium: making informed choices. *Fertility and Sterility* 90(3): 473–483.

Blechová R, Pivodová D (2001) LAL test – an alternative method of detection of bacterial endotoxins. *Acta Veterinaria* 70: 291–296.

Bongso A, Ng SC, Ratnam S (1990) Cocultures: their relevance to assisted reproduction. *Human Reproduction* 5: 893–900.

Boone WR, Johnson JE, Locke AJ, Crane MM, Price TM (1999) Control of air quality in an assisted reproductive technology laboratory. *Fertility and Sterility* 71: 150–154.

Campbell S, Swann HR, Aplin JD, *et al.* (1995) CD44 is expressed throughout pre-implantation human embryo development. *Human Reproduction* 10: 425–430.

Cohen J, Gilligan A, Esposito W, Schimmel T, Dale B (1997) Ambient air and its potential effects on conception in vitro. *Human Reproduction* 12(8): 1742–1749.

Conaghan J (2008) Real-time pH profiling of IVF culture medium using an incubator device with continuous monitoring. *Journal of Clinical Embryology* 11(2): 25–26.

Cutting R, Pritchard J, Clarke H, Martin K (2004) Establishing quality control in the new IVF laboratory. *Human Fertility* 7(2): 119–125.

Danforth RA, Piana SD, Smith M (1987) High purity water: an important component for success in in vitro fertilization. *American Biotechnology Laboratory* 5: 58–60.

Davidson A, Vermesh M, Lobo RA, Paulsen RJ (1988) Mouse embryo culture as quality control for human in vitro fertilisation: the one-cell versus two-cell model. *Fertility and Sterility* 49: 516–521.

de los Santos MJ, Ruiz A (2013) Protocols for tracking and witnessing samples and patients in assisted reproductive technology. *Fertility and Sterility* 100(6): 1499–1502.

Dumoulin JC, Land JA, Van Montfoort AP, *et al.* (2010) Effect of in vitro culture of human embryos on birthweight of newborns. *Human Reproduction* 25(3): 605–612.

Dumoulin JS, Menheere PP, Evers JL, *et al.* (1991) The effects of endotoxins on gametes and preimplantation embryos cultured in vitro. *Human Reproduction* 6: 730–734.

Edwards RG, Brody SA (1995) Human fertilization in the laboratory. In: *Principles and Practice of Assisted Human Reproduction*. Saunders, Philadelphia, PA, pp. 351–413.

Elder K, Elliott T (1998) *Troubleshooting and Problem Solving in IVF*. Worldwide Conferences on Reproductive Biology. Ladybrook Publishing, Australia.

Elder K, Van den Bergh M, Woodward B (2015) The IVF culture system. In: Elder K, Van den Bergh M, Woodward B (2015) *Troubleshooting and Problem-Solving in the IVF Laboratory*. Cambridge University Press, Cambridge, UK., pp. 28–43.

Erbach GT, Bhatnagar P, Baltz JM, Biggers JD (1995) Zinc is a possible toxic contaminant of silicone oil in microdrop cultures of preimplantation mouse embryos. *Human Reproduction* 10: 3248–3254.

Fleetham J, Mahadevan MM (1988) Purification of water for in vitro fertilization and embryo transfer. *Journal of In Vitro Fertilization and Embryo Transfer* 5: 171–174.

Fleming TP, Pratt HPM, Braude PR (1987) The use of mouse preimplantation embryos for quality control of culture reagents in human in vitro fertilisation programs: a cautionary note. *Fertility and Sterility* 47: 858–860.

Gardner D (1999) Development of new serum-free media for the culture and transfer of human blastocysts. *Human Reproduction* 13(Suppl. 4): 218–225.

George MA, Braude PR, Johnson MH, Sweetnam DG (1989) Quality control in the IVF laboratory: in vitro and in vivo development of mouse embryos is unaffected by the quality of water used in culture media. *Human Reproduction* 4: 826–831.

Guo KJ (2015) "By the work, one knows the workman": the practice and profession of the embryologist and its translation to quality in the embryology laboratory. *Reproductive BioMedicine Online* 31: 449–458.

Harvey AJ, Rathjen J, Yu LJ, Gardner DK (2016) Oxygen modulates human embryonic stem cell metabolism in the absence of changes in self-renewal. *Reproduction Fertility and Development* 28(4): 446–458.

Heitman RJ, Hill MJ, James AN, Schimmel T, *et al.* (2015) Live births achieved via IVF are increased by improvements in air quality and laboratory environment. *Reproductive BioMedicine Online* 31: 364–371.

Heo YS, Cabrera LM, Bormann CL, *et al.* (2010) Dynamic microfunnel culture enhances mouse embryo development and pregnancy rates. *Human Reproduction* 25(3): 613–622.

Johnson C, Hofmann G, Scott R (1994) The use of oil overlay for in vitro fertilisation and culture. *Assisted Reproduction Review* 4: 198–201.

Kane MT, Morgan PM, Coonan C (1997) Peptide growth factors and preimplantation development. *Human Reproduction Update* 3(2): 137–157.

Kattal N, Cohen J, Barmat L, *et al.* (2007) Role of co-culture in human IVF: a meta-analysis. *Fertility and Sterility* 86(3): S225–S226.

Kimber SJ, Sneddon SF, Bloor DJ, *et al.* (2008) Expression of genes involved in early cell fate decisions in human embryos and their regulation by growth factors. *Reproduction* 135: 635–647.

Kirkegaard K, Hindkjaer JJ, Ingerslev HJ (2013) Effect of oxygen concentration on human embryo development evaluated by time-lapse monitoring. *Fertility and Sterility* 99(3): 738–744.

Korhonen K, Sjövall S, Viitanen J, *et al.* (2009) Viability of bovine embryos following exposure to the green filtered or wider bandwidth light during in vitro embryo production. *Human Reproduction* 24: 308–314.

Leese HJ, Donnay I, Thompson JG (1998) Human assisted conception: a cautionary tale. Lessons from domestic animals. *Human Reproduction* 13: 184–202.

Ma S, Kalousek DK, Zouves C, Yuen BH, Gomel V, Moon YS (1990) The chromosomal complements of cleaved human embryos resulting from in vitro fertilisation. *Journal of In Vitro Fertilization and Embryo Transfer* 7: 16–21.

Marrs RP, Saito H, Yee B, Sato F, Brown J (1984) Effect of variation of in vitro culture techniques upon oocyte fertilization and embryo development in human in vitro fertilization procedures. *Fertility and Sterility* 41: 519–523.

Matson PL (1998) Internal and external quality assurance in the IVF laboratory. *Human Reproduction Supplement* 13(Suppl. 4): 156–165.

Matsuura K, Hayasahi N, Kuroda Y, *et al.* (2010) Improved development of mouse and human embryos using a tilting embryo culture system. *Reproductive BioMedicine Online* 20(3): 358–364.

Meintjes M, Chantilis SJ, Douglas JD, *et al.* (2009) A controlled, randomized trial evaluating the effect of lowered incubator oxygen tension on live births in a predominantly blastocyst transfer program. *Human Reproduction* 24(2): 300–307.

Ménézo Y (1976) Milieu synthétique pour la survie et la maturation des gamètes et pour la culture de l'oeuf fécondé. *Comptes Rendus de l'Académie des Sciences Paris, Serie D* 282: 1967–1970.

Ménézo Y, Dale B, Elder K (2018) Time to evaluate ART protocols in the light of advances in knowledge about methylation and epigenetics. *Human Fertility* 21(3): 156–162.

Ménézo Y, Guerin P, Elder K (2014) The oviduct: a neglected organ due for re-assessment in IVF. *Reproductive BioMedicine Online* 30(3): 233–240.

Ménézo Y, Lichtblau I, Elder K (2013) New insights into human embryo metabolism in vitro and in vivo. *Journal of Assisted Reproduction and Genetics* 30(3): 293–303.

Monteiro da Rocha A, Smith GD (2014) Culture of embryos in dynamic fluid environments. In: Quinn P (ed.) *Culture Media, Solutions, and Systems in Human ART.* Cambridge University Press, Cambridge, UK, pp. 197–210.

Morbeck DE (2015) Air quality in the assisted reproduction laboratory. *Journal of Assisted Reproduction and Genetics* 32: 1019–1024.

Munné S, Howles CM, Wells D (2009) The role of preimplantation genetic diagnosis in diagnosing embryo aneuploidy. *Current Opinion in Obstetrics and Gynecology* 21(5): 442–449.

Naaktgeboren N (1987) Quality control of culture media for in vitro fertilisation. In Vitro Fertilisation Program, Academic Hospital, Vrije Universiteit, Brussels, Belgium. *Annales de Biologie Clinique (Paris)* 45: 368–372.

Ombelet W (2014) Is global access to infertility care realistic? The Walking Egg Project. *Reproductive BioMedicine Online* 28: 267–272.

Ottosen LD, Hindkjaer J, Ingerslev J (2007) Light exposure of the ovum and preimplantation embryo during ART procedures. *Journal of Assisted Reproduction and Genetics* 24(2–3): 99–103.

Pearson FC (1985) *Pyrogens: Endotoxins, LAL Testing, and Depyrogenation.* Marcel Dekker, New York, pp. 98–100, 206–211.

Pellestor F, Girardet A, Andreo B, Anal F, Humeau C (1994) Relationship between morphology and chromosomal constitution in human preimplantation embryos. *Molecular Reproduction and Development* 39: 141–146.

Pickering SJ, Braude PR, Johnson MH, Cant A, Currie J (1990) Transient cooling to room temperature can cause irreversible disruption of the meiotic spindle in the human oocyte. *Fertility and Sterility* 54: 102–108.

Plachot M, De Grouchy J, Montagut J, et al. (1987) Multicentric study of chromosome analysis in human oocytes and embryos in an IVF programme. *Human Reproduction* 2: 29.

Pomeroy K, Reed M (2015) The effect of light on embryos and embryo culture. In: Elder K, Van den Bergh M, Woodward B, *Troubleshooting & Problem Solving in the IVF Laboratory.* Cambridge University Press, Cambridge, UK, pp. 104–106.

Pool TM, Schoolfield J, Han D (2012) Human embryo culture media comparisons. *Methods in Molecular Biology* 912: 367–386.

Provo MC, Herr C (1998) Washed paraffin oil becomes toxic to mouse embryos upon exposure to sunlight. *Theriogenology* 49(1): 214.

Purdy J (1982) Methods for fertilization and embryo culture in vitro. In: Edwards RG, Purdy, JM (eds.) *Human Conception In Vitro.* Academic Press, London, p. 135.

Quinn P (1995) Enhanced results in mouse and human embryo culture using a modified human tubal fluid medium lacking glucose and phosphate. *Journal of Assisted Reproduction and Genetics* 12: 97–105.

Quinn P (2000) Review of media used in ART laboratories. *Journal of Andrology* 21(5): 610–615.

Quinn P, Warner GM, Klein JF, Kirby C (1985) Culture factors affecting the success rate of in vitro fertilization and embryo transfer. *Annals of the New York Academy of Sciences* 412: 195.

Richter KS (2008) The importance of growth factors for preimplantation embryo development and in-vitro culture. *Current Opinion in Obstetrics and Gynecology* 20(3): 292–304.

Rienzi L, Bariani F, Zorza M, et al. (2017) Comprehensive protocol of traceability during IVF: the result of a multicentre failure mode and effect analysis. *Human Reproduction* 32(8):1612–1620.

Rinehart JS, Bavister BD, Gerrity M (1988) Quality control in the in vitro fertilization laboratory: comparison of bioassay systems for water quality. *Journal of In Vitro Fertilization and Embryo Transfer* 5: 335–342.

Rinehart J, Chapman C, McKiernan S, Bavister B (1998) A protein-free chemically defined embryo culture medium produces pregnancy rates similar to human tubal fluid (HTF) supplemented with 10% synthetic serum substitute (SSS). Abstracts of the 14th Annual meeting of the ESHRE, Göteborg 1998. *Human Reproduction* 13: 59.

Smith GD, Takayama, S, Swain J (2012) Rethinking in vitro embryo culture: new developments in culture platforms and potential to improve assisted reproductive technologies. *Biology of Reproduction* 86(3): 62, 1–10.

Staessen C, Van den Abbeel E, Carle M, et al. (1990) Comparison between human serum and Albuminar-20(TM) supplement for in vitro fertilization. *Human Reproduction* 5: 336–341.

Swain J, Pool TB, Takayama S, Smith GD (2008) Microfluidic technology in ART: is it time to go with the flow? *Journal of Clinical Embryology* 11(2): 5–18.

Swain J, Pool TB, Takayama S, Smith GD (2012) Microfluidics in ART. In: Gardner DK, Weissman A, Howles CM, Shoham Z (eds.) *Textbook of Assisted Reproductive Technologies*, 4th edn. Informa Healthcare, London, pp. 396–414.

Swain, JE (2012) Is there an optimal pH for culture media used in clinical IVF? *Human Reproduction Update* 18: 333–339.

Swain JE, Carrell D, Cobo A, *et al.* (2016) Optimizing the culture environment and embryo manipulation to help maintain embryo developmental potential. *Fertility and Sterility* 105(3): 571–587.

Takenaka M, Horiuchi T, Yanagimachi R (2007) Effects of light on development of mammalian zygotes. *Proceedings of the National Academy of Sciences of the USA* 104(36): 14289–14293.

Thompson JG, Gardner DK, Pugh A, MacMillan W, Teruit JJR (1995) Lamb birth weight is affected by culture system utilized during in vitro pre-elongation development of ovine embryos. *Biology of Reproduction* 53: 1385–1391.

Van Blerkom J, Ombelet W, Klerkx E, *et al.* (2014) First births with a simplified culture system for clinical IVF and embryo transfer. *Reproductive BioMedicine Online* 28: 310–320.

Wales RG (1970) Effect of ions on the development of preimplantation mouse embryos in vitro. *Australian Journal of Biological Sciences* 23: 421–429.

Weimer KE, Anderson A, Stewart B (1998a) The importance of water quality for media preparation. *Human Reproduction Supplement* 13(Suppl. 4): 166–172.

Weimer KE, Cohen J, Tucker MJ, Godke A (1998b) The application of co-culture in assisted reproduction: 10 years of experience with human embryos. *Human Reproduction Supplement* 13(Suppl. 4): 226–238.

Yovich JL, Edirisinghe W, Yovich JM, Stanger J, Matson P (1988) Methods of water purification for the preparation of culture media in an IVF-ET programme. *Human Reproduction* 3: 245–248.

Zorn TMT, Pinhal MAS, Nader HB, *et al.* (1995) Biosynthesis of glucosaminoglycans in the endometrium during the initial stages of pregnancy of the mouse. *Cellular and Molecular Biology* 41: 97–106.

# Chapter 9

# Quality Management in the IVF Laboratory

There is no doubt that success in ART is crucially dependent on carefully controlled conditions in every aspect of the IVF laboratory routine (Figure 9.1).

From the beginning of the twenty-first century onwards, laboratories that offer human ART treatment or are involved in the handling of human gametes and/or tissue became subject to increasing demands and precepts set down by regulatory and legislative authorities. The regulations differ from country to country,

and some directives (e.g., the EuropeanTissue Directive 2004/23/EC-2006/86/EC) are subject to interpretation according to legislation or guidelines set down by national authorities in individual countries. In many countries, it has become necessary to obtain accreditation and/or certification by a national or international body that will carry out in-depth assessments and inspections to ensure that all aspects of facilities and treatment meet a required standard.

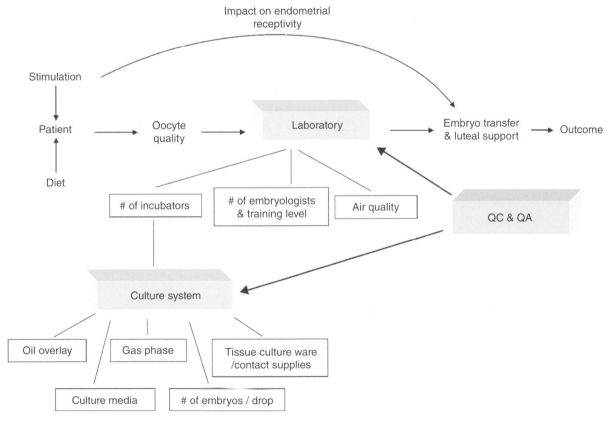

**Figure 9.1** Critical elements of an ART treatment cycle (with thanks to David Gardner, Melbourne, Australia).

## Certification and Accreditation

**Certification**: a neutral independent third party confirms (certifies) that a system complies with an internationally accepted standard, such as an 'ISO Norm.' In practice, this means that laboratories can search for a company that will assess whether or not their quality system has the structure required by the ISO Norm. A wide and varied choice of companies offers this service, and their fees may differ considerably. Certification provides testimony that a correctly structured QMS is in place, according to an internationally accepted standard. Certification is often presented to patients as reassurance and guarantee of the clinic's high quality, but this is not the case. These certificates merely confirm that there is a quality management whose structure corresponds to an internationally recognized ISO standard: the appropriate structure is in place, but there is no guarantee of the content. For example, an IVF laboratory with very poor results can be certified, but will never be accredited because poor treatment outcomes usually indicate a lack of competence.

**Accreditation** requires evidence that your laboratory has the appropriate competencies for the service provided, including adequate facilities/space, equipment/instruments, personnel who are adequately and continuously trained and able to demonstrate the competence to fulfill their tasks. *Accreditation can only be granted by a 'National Accreditation Office,'* and there is no elective choice in selecting the third party who will audit the clinic/laboratory. If the laboratory seeks accreditation in a very specific field, e.g., 'comparative genome hybridization,' a local/national expert might not be available, and the national accreditation office might appeal for an expert from a neighboring country. The national/federal accreditation office is likely to be a member of the International Association for Laboratory Accreditation ILAC (International Laboratory Accreditation Cooperation, https://ilac.org) or EA (European Co-operation for Accreditation, www.european-accreditation.org).

It is important to note that certification and accreditation are valid only for limited time periods of between 2 and 5 years, and re-certification and surveillance are required in order to maintain validity of the acquired certification/accreditation. Nicely framed certificates on display at the clinic entrance are completely meaningless if the date is beyond its period of validity.

## Benefits of Certification/Accreditation

From Elder *et al.* (2015), Chapter 2.

1. Improvement in quality of care provided
2. Recognition of individual training and competencies by providing education
3. Improved management structure
4. Cost reduction via quality improvement policies such as 'Gemba Kaizen,' a Japanese concept of continuous improvement designed to enhance processes and reduce waste (Imai, 1997)
5. Patient satisfaction
6. Third-party recognition for reimbursement of treatments
7. Better market position
8. 'Firewall' in cases of litigation

# ISO9001:2015

The International Organisation for Standardization (ISO) (www.iso.org) is a network of the national standards institutes of 162 countries, consisting of one member per country; a Central Secretariat in Geneva, Switzerland, coordinates the system. The ISO is an independent body, not associated with the government of any particular country. Some of the 162 member institutes (www.iso.org/members.html) may be a part of their country's government structure, but others have been set up by national partnerships of industry associations, and therefore are in the private business domain. The ISO therefore tries to reach a consensus on issues that concern both business requirements and the broader needs of society. Their standard for quality management is published as ISO9001:2015.

In order to obtain ISO certification, a unit with an established quality management system (QMS) is inspected and assessed by an external auditor. If all the requirements of the ISO standard are met, a certificate is issued stating that the QMS conforms to the standards laid down in ISO9001:2015. Many countries now require that IVF clinics and laboratories show evidence such as this, that an effective QMS is in place. ART laboratories in the USA should conform to the American Society for Reproductive Medicine guidelines (ASRM, 2014) and must undergo certification and accreditation by an appropriate agency, such as the College of American Pathologists (CAP) or Joint Commission International (JCI).

In the UK, all IVF clinics must apply for a license from the Human Fertilisation and Embryology Authority (HFEA) and ensure that all of their procedures are compliant with the HFEA Code of Practice. The HFEA monitors all UK data and carries out annual audits and inspections.

The final impact of legislative, regulatory, accreditation and certification requirements is that every ART laboratory should have an effective total quality management (TQM) system. TQM is a system that can monitor all procedures and components of the laboratory; this must include not only pregnancy and implantation rates, but also a systematic check and survey of all laboratory materials, supplies, equipment and instruments, procedures, protocols, risk management and staff training/education (continued professional development, CPD).

---

**Definitions Used in Quality Management**

- Quality: fitness for purpose.
- Quality management system: a system that encompasses quality control, quality assurance and quality improvement by providing defined sets of procedures for the management of each component.
- Quality policy: a statement defining the purpose of the organization and its commitment to a defined quality objective.
- Quality control: inspection of a system to ensure that a product or service is delivered under optimal conditions.
- Quality assurance: monitoring the effectiveness of quality control and indicating preventive and corrective action taken when errors are detected.
- Quality audit: review and checking of the quality management system to ensure its correct operation.
- External quality assurance: testing a product or service against an external standard.

---

Irrespective of the numerous fine details involved in TQM, the first, and ultimate, test of quality control must rest with pregnancy and live birth rates per treatment cycle. An ongoing record of the results of fertilization, cleavage and embryo development provide the best short-term evidence of good quality control (QC). Daily records in the form of a laboratory logbook or electronic database are essential, summarizing details of patients and outcome of laboratory procedures: age, cause of

infertility, stimulation protocol, number of oocytes retrieved, semen analysis, sperm preparation details, insemination time, fertilization, cleavage, embryo transfer and cryopreservation. Details of media and oil batches and all consumables that come into contact with gametes and embryos must also be recorded for reference, and the introduction of any new methods or materials must be documented. It is essential that all records are reviewed on a regular basis.

A QMS in the IVF laboratory aims to achieve specific goals:

1. Identify all of the processes to be included in the QMS:

   - provision and management of resources
   - ART processes
   - evaluation and continual improvement
   - monitoring of key performance indicators (KPIs).

2. Make available the resources and information necessary to operate and support these processes.

3. Implement any actions necessary to ensure that the processes are effective and subject to continual improvement.

4. Document control management (80% of nonconformities concern missing documents).

A QMS ensures continuous assessment and improvement of all component parts of the patient treatment cycle. KPIs to be monitored include rates of fertilization, cleavage, survival of injected oocytes, pregnancy, implantation and live births; satisfaction of patients and referring clinicians with the quality of the service should also be monitored, and suppliers of media, disposables, etc. also monitored and evaluated. Graphic analysis of these parameters can reveal problems early so that corrective action can be taken promptly to minimize the extent of any problem that might arise (Kastrop, 2003).

## Basic Elements of a Quality Management System

A formal QMS should include:

- Scope: a list of all treatments provided and links to the forms and documents used
- Normative reference values, with levels of uncertainty: definition of a successful outcome
- Terms and definitions: those used in IVF

- Management responsibility: organization chart showing lines of responsibility and accountability of all staff
- Resource management: provision of sufficient resources, including staff, to deliver the service
- Provision of sufficient and appropriate facilities, with regular survey of all environmental parameters
- Product realization: treatment plans, procedures, purchasing, traceability, witnessing
- Measurement, analysis, improvement: monitoring of KPIs, risk management with frequency and grade of impact, reporting of adverse incidents, corrective and preventive action to improve service.

# Implementing QMS in the IVF Laboratory

The first key requirement for implementing a formal QMS is appropriately educated and trained personnel, with training records that are regularly updated. Other key requirements include:

1. Complete list/index of standard operating procedures (SOPs)
2. Housekeeping procedures: cleaning and decontamination, with a calendar clearly indicating schedules
3. Correct operation, calibration and maintenance of all instruments with manual and logbook records
4. Proper procedure, policy and safety manuals
5. Consistent and correct execution of appropriate techniques and methods
6. Comprehensive documentation, record keeping, validation and reporting of results
7. System for specimen collection and handling
8. Safety procedures including personnel vaccination and appropriate handling and storage of materials
9. Infection control measures
10. Documentation of suppliers and dates of receipt and expiry of consumables
11. System of performance appraisal, correction of deficiencies and implementation of advances and improvements
12. Quality materials, tested with bioassays when appropriate
13. Quality assurance program

# Laboratory Equipment

Equipment failure or suboptimal operation in an IVF laboratory can seriously jeopardize the prognosis for patients undergoing treatment, and therefore service contracts should be set up with reliable companies. As part of the service, the companies should train all staff regarding routine maintenance and emergency procedures, and provide calibration certificates for the tools that they use in servicing and calibrating the equipment. Alarms should be fitted to all vital equipment, and provision made for emergency call-out. Any defect requiring correction must be documented, with description, date and details of repair. Back-up equipment should be held in reserve.

*Documentation must be available to confirm*:

1. The equipment is installed in an appropriate location and is correctly connected.
2. The equipment has been checked for correct function and has been calibrated.
3. All personnel who will work with the equipment have been trained by the company.

Electrical appliances must be tested for safety before first use (e.g., by portable appliance testing) and then regularly tested by a trained operator. They should be designated as a potential source of fire, and must not be used if faulty; any faults must be reported and repaired immediately. Contracts for service and calibration should be held for:

- Incubators
- Incubator alarms
- Flow cabinets
- Microscopes
- Micromanipulator stations
- Heated surfaces/microscope stages
- Centrifuges
- Refrigerators and freezers
- Embryo/oocyte freezing machines
- Liquid nitrogen storage dewars
- Low-level nitrogen alarms in the dewars
- Air filtration equipment
- Electronic witnessing system.

Key items of equipment in daily use must have systems of continuous monitoring to ensure optimal performance. Numerous systems for computer-controlled data acquisition, including verification of patient identity and chain of custody and monitoring, are available, with continuous monitoring and logging

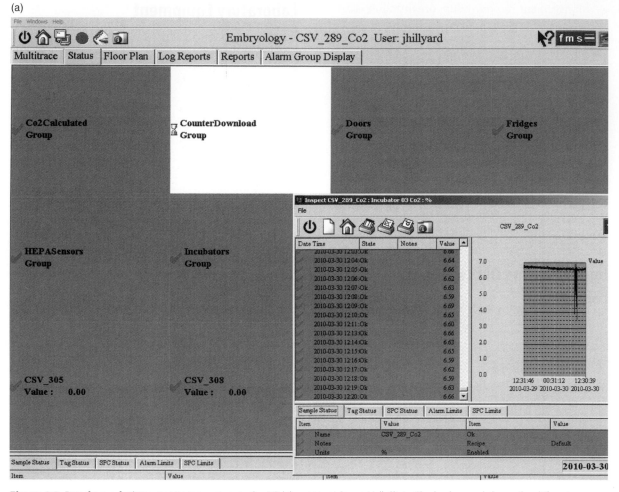

(a)

**Figure 9.2** Data from a facilities monitoring system in the IVF laboratory at Bourn Hall Clinic. The background shows the different monitoring modules that can be viewed: $CO_2$ sensors, HEPA sensors, incubator temperature, refrigerators, freezers. Insets: 24-hour records from a single incubator showing (a) $CO_2$ concentration and (b) temperature. Note dips during peak laboratory activity times, 8–10.30 am. See color plate section.

software systems that support multiple instrument inputs (Figure 9.2). A system such as this can continuously check and record airborne particle counts, as well as data from key equipment such as incubators, freezers, refrigerators and liquid nitrogen storage vessels. The data are monitored in real-time, and the computerized system can display historical data acquisition and analysis, trend-lines, correlation studies and various levels of alarm notification. Variation outside set parameters is covered by an alarm system that is monitored 24 hours a day.

Temperature and pH are known to be critical parameters that must be carefully controlled, and their measurement in an IVF culture system requires special attention:

## Temperature

The temperature of incubators, water baths, heating blocks, heated surfaces and microscope stages should not rely on a digital display from the equipment, but must be independently recorded and controlled, with individual fine tuning for each. Always note that the temperature of the incubator, bath or surface will differ from that in the culture media within a drop, tube or dish; 37°C should be the temperature to aim for within the media, not for the incubator or heating device. As with monitoring of all parameters that can have an impact on results, (pH, temperature, VOC levels, etc.), setpoints and tolerance intervals must be defined for each dish on each separate device, using a

(b)

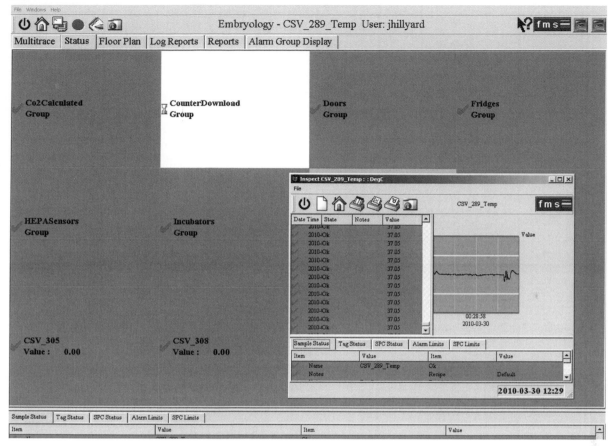

**Figure 9.2** (*cont.*)

calibrated thermometer with type K thermocouple (PT100 or PT1000). Laboratory equipment is affected by environmental temperatures, and therefore regular adjustment according to seasonal variations is to be expected (Butler *et al.*, 2013).

## pH

An 'optimal' pH for in-vitro culture has not been precisely defined or characterized, and according to the manufacturers' information, the range of acceptable pH differs with media type, since the hydrogen ion concentration is determined by the overall composition, including concentrations of amino acids and protein supplement (Swain, 2012). Different media companies advise that incubators are run at different $CO_2$ concentrations in order to optimize the pH for their media.

pH is a number that reflects dynamic culture conditions; it changes rapidly if acid/base concentrations change. Although it is a critical parameter, in practice it is not easy to monitor effectively, especially in microdrop culture under oil. A standard glass probe pH meter is fragile, requires a volume of at least 1 mL that needs to be equilibrated (cannot be used for microdrops) and is not standardized, and therefore readings taken do not represent actual culture conditions. A number of alternative devices are available for use in IVF culture systems, but none provide an ideal solution to the problem of pH monitoring, and the different devices can yield different results when used to test a variety of different media and solutions. Therefore, whatever device is used, careful validation and calibration is essential; it may be unwise to rely on only one method. Although pH measurement is important, and is useful in monitoring manipulation and handling procedures, a change in pH reflecting $CO_2$ concentration takes time, and depends upon the volume and the culture system being used. Please refer to Elder *et al.* (2015) and Pool (2004) for a comprehensive review of the science behind culture media pH and its importance in human IVF.

---

**Devices Used to Monitor pH in Culture Media**

1. ISFET (ion-sensitive field effect transistor) probes:
   - Can be used in small volumes outside the incubator, are simple and fast.
   - Require frequent calibration and cleaning (sensitive to protein deposits), expensive.

2. RI pH meter:
   - Can be used for measurements inside the incubator, but not for microdrop culture.
   - Slow, drifts over time, and calibration is difficult/time consuming.

3. pH Online™, 'fluorescent decay time' pH meter:
   - Allows continuous pH measurement inside the incubator; can be used to monitor pH in up to 10 incubators simultaneously.
   - Requires disposable four-well Nunc dish, with one well fitted with a pH reactive fluorochrome spot.
   - Simple to use, but expensive and slow.

4. Blood gas analyzer:
   - Accurate, but not suitable for microdrops.
   - Method of choice for initial media pH testing.
   - Sampling errors can be a problem.

5. Beckmann pH meter:
   - Can be used to measure pH in 5-mL aliquots of media after overnight incubation in test-tubes with loose-fitting caps (see Pool, 2004).
   - Electrode selection, cleaning and regular replacement are important.
   - Must be correctly calibrated before each use.

6. SAFE Sens (Sterile Automated Fluoroscopic Evaluation):
   - Noninvasive continuous pH monitoring, based on emission of characteristic wavelength spectra at different pH by fluorescent dyes.
   - Uses small disposable cuvettes with a fluorescent membrane that are placed inside the incubator.

---

- Provides accurate real-time pH reading every 30 minutes.
- No user calibration is required.

## Incubator $CO_2$

In contrast to pH measurements, a properly calibrated device can measure $CO_2$ and provide fast and reproducible results, as well as detect rapid changes in gas concentration: very important in case of incubator malfunction. Older Fyrite kits for measuring $CO_2$ are inaccurate, and Fyrite is toxic; these kits should not be used in the IVF laboratory. Infrared gas analyzers are available that can provide accurate measurements of gas concentrations. The devices must be calibrated with a reference gas and should be used at least once per week to measure actual incubator $CO_2$ with reference to the digital display. Incubator gases can also be monitored with calibrated independent probes as part of a facilities monitoring system.

## Equipment Monitoring for QMS

1. Incubators:
   - Independent readings of temperature and gases; calibrated thermometer inside the incubator as standard.
   - Monitor $CO_2$ supply cylinders regularly; ensure that autochangers are functional.
   - For humidified incubators, check water levels daily.
   - Each incubator should have a 24-hour surveillance system, with alarms accessible to staff when at home or at work.
   - A back-up secondary power source should be installed (bearing in mind that most battery-powered systems have limited use, and should be tested before they are used as back-up), and a contingency plan made available to all laboratory staff with back-up arrangements clearly outlined in writing.

2. Heated surfaces and water baths:
   - Record the temperature of water baths daily, using a calibrated thermometer in a tube of water.
   - Use a thermocouple to record the temperature of heated surfaces of flow cabinets and the temperature of media drops in culture dishes

(the temperature of the surface usually differs from the temperature of media in the culture dish).

- Define acceptable limits of maxima and minima, and record action taken when these are exceeded.

3. Refrigerators and freezers approved for storage of medical supplies:

  - Record temperatures daily, using calibrated thermometers.
  - Define acceptable limits of maximum and minimum temperatures, and record any action taken when these are exceeded.

4. Liquid nitrogen dewars:

  - Should always have an alarm to indicate low nitrogen levels (or increasing temperature, or both).
  - Top up nitrogen levels at least once per week (be careful not to overfill, as liquid nitrogen pouring over the top can damage the seal at the neck).
  - Monitor weekly nitrogen usage by recording the liquid $N_2$ level before top up, and plot the readings on a graph in order to detect any gradual increase in usage, indicating a slow vacuum leak.

Records of all readings should be kept and can be plotted on a graph, with acceptable limits and any corrective action noted on the records. A graph provides a useful means of quickly monitoring and analyzing results visually:

1. Dispersion: increased frequency of both high and low numbers
2. Trend: progressive drift (in one direction) from a mean
3. Shift: abrupt change from the mean.

# Bioassays

Guidelines issued by ESHRE (de los Santos *et al.*, 2016) and ASRM (The Practice Committee of the American Society for Reproductive Medicine and the Practice Committee of the Society for Assisted Reproductive Technology, 2014) state that all tissue culture media prepared in the laboratory should undergo quality control testing with an appropriate bioassay system. A range of bioassays to detect toxicity

and suboptimal culture conditions have been tried, including:

1. Human or hamster sperm survival (Critchlow *et al.*, 1989; Nijs *et al.*, 2009)
2. Continued culture of multipronucleate embryos
3. Somatic cell lines: LAL test for endotoxins (Blechová and Pivodová, 2001), HeLa – test for cytotoxins (Painter, 1978)
4. Culture of mouse embryos from either the one-cell or two-cell stage.

The validity of a mouse embryo bioassay has been questioned as a reliable assay for extrapolation to clinical IVF: it assumes that the requirements of human and mouse embryos are the same, and we know that this is a false assumption. The mouse embryo cannot regulate its endogenous metabolic pool before the late two-cell stage; this is not the case for human or bovine embryos. Mouse embryos will develop from the two-cell stage onwards in a wide variety of cell culture media.

Although none of the systems currently available can guarantee the detection of subtle levels of toxicity, they can be helpful in providing baseline data for comparative purposes, and for identifying specific problems. Any bioassay done routinely and frequently with baseline data for comparing deviations from the norm will be helpful in minimizing the random introduction of contaminants into the system, and is a useful investment of time and resources in an IVF laboratory.

New batches of media, oil, material or supplies used in the culture system, if not pretested, should be tested before use. The physico-chemical limits of culture media testing are crucial: osmolarity must be within the limits of 275–305 mOsm, with a total variation of no more than 30 mOsm. pH must be within the limits of 7.2–7.5, with a maximal variation of 0.4 units of pH. Larger variations in either parameter indicate poor technique/technology and inadequate controls during manufacture, leading to poor reproducibility (see Swain *et al.*, 2012; Elder *et al.*, 2015).

Tissue culture plastics have on occasion been found to be subject to variation in quality: well–well variations have been observed even within a single four-well plate, and rinsing plates with media before use may be a useful precaution. Studies have shown that oil can interact with different plastic supports, and this can affect embryo development.

187

Manufacturers of plasticware used for tissue culture may change the chemical formulation of their products without notification, and such changes in manufacture of syringes, filters and culture dishes may sometimes be embryotoxic. It is also important to store plasticware at an ambient room temperature, away from direct sunlight, as this can affect the properties of the plastic.

Embryos are very sensitive quality control indicators: in routine IVF culture a normal fertilization rate in the order of >70% and cleavage rate of >95% is expected. The cleavage rate is important, as a block at the two-pronucleate stage indicates a serious problem. At least 65–75% of inseminated oocytes should result in cleaved embryos on Day 2. The appearance of the blastomeres and the presence of fragmentation are also good indicators: blastomeres in the early human embryo should be bright and clear, without granules in the cytoplasm. During cell division, the nucleo-cytoplasmic ratio is important, and this can be affected by culture medium osmolarity; in the presence of low osmolarity, the size of the embryo increases relative to the volume of the cytoplasm, and cytoplasmic blebs are formed to compensate, in order to achieve an adequate nuclear/cytoplasmic ratio for entry into mitosis. However, in forming blebs, the embryo loses not only cytoplasm but also mRNA and proteins, which are necessary for further development.

Any trend or shift in data should be investigated, with consideration of patient age and activity level: batches of materials (plasticware and media), air quality, temperature/$CO_2$ levels in incubators and flow cabinets, water quality, oil and gloves should all be investigated.

## Useful Routine Quality Control Procedures

### Sperm Survival Test

The test should be performed in protein-free media, since protein may act as a buffer for potential toxicity. Select a normal sample of washed prepared spermatozoa and assess for count, motility and progression. Divide the selected sample into four aliquots: add test material to two aliquots, and equivalent control material (in current use) to the remaining two aliquots. Incubate one control and one test sample at 37°C, and one of each at room temperature. Assess each sample for count, motility and progression after 24 and 48 hours (a computer-aided system can be used if available). Test and control samples should show equivalent survival. If there is any doubt, repeat the test.

## Culture of Surplus Oocytes

Surplus oocytes from patients who have large numbers of oocytes retrieved may be used to test new culture material. Culture at least six embryos in the control media and a maximum of four in test media.

## Multipronucleate Embryo Culture

Oocytes that show abnormal fertilization on Day 1 after insemination can be used for testing new batches of material. Observe, score and assess each embryo daily until Day 6 after insemination.

## Culture of Surplus Embryos

Surplus embryos after embryo transfer that are not suitable for freezing have also been used for testing new culture material, but this practice is not allowed under an HFEA treatment license in the United Kingdom. The HFEA Act as amended in 2009 does now allow surplus embryos to be used for training purposes, provided that written patient consent is obtained (HFEA, 2019).

---

**Key Points in the Use of Bioassays**

- Choice of bioassay
- Selection of materials to test
- Frequency of testing
- Establish a set of standards, routine and schedule
- Establish acceptable performance range
- Document all results
- Review results regularly
- Do not use anything that fails the bioassay
- Write a standard operating procedure for any corrective action required

---

## Risk Assessments and Standard Operating Procedure

The standard IVF unit has many areas of risk which should be assessed (see also Elder *et al.*, 2015, ch 12):

- Transport and storage of liquid nitrogen and compressed gases (e.g., transport of liquid nitrogen in elevators requires the dewar to be transported on its own, with 'hazard' signs on all floors in between, to prevent the elevator from being used by anyone else)

- Fire
- Infection (bacterial, viral) in theater, scan rooms, laboratories, treatment rooms, consultation rooms, waiting area
- Staff health and safety in all clinical areas and during all clinical activities
- Patient health and safety during all procedures including diagnostic
- Patient confidentiality
- Equipment: use, maintenance, assessment, emergency cover
- Regulatory restrictions for:
  - . confidentiality of patients
  - . security and confidentiality of current and archived patient records
  - . storage and confidentiality of data
  - . audit
- IT support
- Security of laboratory stores
- Witnessing (a risk assessment is needed when introducing electronic witnessing in order to ensure that they are effective).
- Sample collection, identification, storage and transport.

**Standard operating procedures** must be listed on a regularly updated document and be available to all laboratory personnel. Each SOP should be accessible to all staff in only one version, with version number, date and author, and must be updated at predefined appropriate intervals, or when any changes are made. They should refer to all associated documentation including patient consent, be part of a document control system, and be archived and no longer available when a new version is created. The Quality Manager should have access to archived versions for reference.

The SOPs should describe in detail:

- The procedures used
- The expected end product
- All equipment and reagents required for each procedure.

They should also include:

- Information on health and safety and infection control

- SOPs for:
  - . housekeeping, cleaning and decontamination
  - . patient identification, chain of custody and witnessing of all procedures
  - . storage and audit of cryopreserved material
- Validation evidence of the procedure described.

---

**Key Points of a QMS**
- Review and update all processes regularly.
- Ensure traceability by recording batch numbers and expiry dates of all consumables, including plastics and culture media.
- Monitor and service equipment frequently, keeping detailed records.
- Monitor KPIs to check laboratory performance.

---

# Basic Housekeeping Procedures in the IVF Laboratory

## Daily Cleaning Routine

During the course of procedures, any spillage should be immediately cleaned with damp tissue and the use of an appropriate VOC-free disinfectant that has been designed and tested for use in the IVF laboratory. No detergent or alcohol should be used whilst oocytes/embryos are being handled. Should it be necessary to use either of the above, allow residual traces to evaporate for at least 20 minutes before removing oocytes/embryos from incubators.

At the end of each day:

1. Heat seal, double bag and dispose of all waste from procedures.
2. Remove all pipette holders for washing and sterilizing before reuse.
3. Reseal and resterilize pipette canisters.
4. Clean flow hoods, work benches and all equipment by washing with a solution of distilled water and 7X laboratory detergent followed by wiping with 70% denatured alcohol or specific detergent sprays developed for IVF laboratories such as Oosafe (www.parallabs.com) or Fertisafe.
5. Prepare each workstation for the following day's work, with clean rubbish bags, pipette holder and Pasteur pipettes.

189

## Washing Procedures

If the laboratory has a system for preparation of ultrapure water, particular attention must be paid to instructions for maintenance and chemical cleaning. Water purity is essential for washing procedures, and the system should be periodically checked for organic contamination and endotoxins.

## Pipettes

Prewashed and sterilized pipettes are available, but the following procedure can be used if necessary:

1. Soak new pipettes overnight in fresh Analar or Milli-Q water, ensuring that they are completely covered
2. Drain the pipettes and rinse with fresh water
3. Drain again and dry at 100°C for 1–2 hours
4. Place in a clean pipette canister (tips forward), and dry heat sterilize for 3 hours at 180°C
5. After cooling, record date and use within 1 month of sterilization.

## Nondisposable Items (Glassware, etc)

Handle with nonpowdered gloves, rinsed in purified water.

1. Soak in distilled water containing 3–5% 7X
2. Sonicate small items for 5–10 minutes in an ultrasonic cleaning bath
3. Rinse eight times with distilled water, then twice with Analar or Milli-Q water
4. Dry, seal in aluminum foil or double wrap in autoclave bags as appropriate
5. Autoclave or dry heat sterilize at 180°C for 3 hours
6. Record date of sterilization, and store in a clean, dust-free area.

## Incubator Maintenance

- Schedule for cleaning should be based on:
  - External environment (climate: humid or dry?)
  - How often the incubator is used
  - Type of incubator
  - Where it is housed (clean room, hospital room?)
- Follow manufacturer's instructions for the particular incubator regarding cleaning agents (hydrogen peroxide can normally be used, followed by rinsing with distilled water)
- Fungal contamination in a humidified incubator can be avoided by placing a piece of autoclaved copper in the water pan.

## Microbiological Testing and Contamination in the Laboratory

The risk of introducing infection into the laboratory can be minimized by screening patients for infectious agents where indicated by medical history and physical examination. The risk of infectious agent transmission in ART procedures varies in different populations and geographical regions; a risk assessment should be carried out according to the prevalence of disease in the specific patient population, bearing in mind the possibility of 'silent' infection prior to detectable seroconversion. National and international guidelines in many countries now recommend that patients attending for ART procedures should undergo routine testing for human immunodeficiency virus (HIV) 1 and 2, and hepatitis B and C at least annually; screening for Zika virus may also be required if patients have been exposed to a high-risk area. In some cases, viral screening for both partners prior to each cycle is mandatory. Human T-cell lymphotropic virus (HTLV-I and -II) has a low prevalence in Western countries, but HTLV-I is principally endemic in Japan, Central Africa, the Caribbean and Malaysia, and HTLV II is prevalent in Central America and the southern USA. Screening for these viruses prior to blood or organ donation is now mandatory in some countries; guidelines for HTLV-I and -II patient screening prior to ART procedures should be adapted to local regulations and epidemiology. Routine screening for genital infections – i.e., syphilis, gonorrhea, chlamydia, cytomegalovirus, herpes simplex, human papilloma virus and vaginal infections – should be assessed within the context of patient population, prevalence of disease and full medical history/physical examination of both partners (e.g., malaria, sickle cell disease, *Trypanosoma cruzi*). For syphilis testing, a validated testing algorithm must be applied to exclude the presence of active infection with *Treponema pallidum*.

Effective handling, cleaning and maintenance schedules, together with strict adherence to aseptic technique should make routine microbiological testing unnecessary, but it may be required in order to identify a source of contamination in a culture system. It is required as part of some of the ISO 9000 series quality management protocols and is recommended by the UK Department of Health for laboratories that offer tissue banking facilities, including ovarian and testicular tissue.

Culture systems should be under constant vigilance to detect early signs of possible microbial contamination, in order to avert serious subsequent problems. Any turbidity or drastic color change in media is a clear reflection of contamination, and an inseminated culture dish that shows all sperm dead or immotile should prompt further investigation for possible microbial contamination. A practical and simple method that can be used for checking bacterial and fungal contamination in the incubator or culture medium is to leave an aliquot of culture medium without an oil overlay in the incubator for 5 days. Organisms contaminating the medium or the incubator that are a hazard under IVF culture conditions will multiply in this optimal growth environment of nutrients, temperature, pH and humidity. The aliquot can then be checked for contamination by looking for turbidity and change in color (if medium with a pH indicator is used), and stained for microscopic observation of bacteria or fungi. This test can be used as an ongoing procedure for sterility testing of the incubator as well as the culture medium. Methods used for microbiological testing of the environment include air sampling, settle plates, contact plates and glove print tests. Although air sampling by either settle plates or Anderson air filtration systems is rarely indicated in an ART laboratory except in evaluating an episode of contamination or outbreak, specific air quality testing is now a requirement under the European Tissue Directive. Table 9.1 shows average values used for guidance in defining acceptable limits for viable particle detection (microbiological contamination) in monitoring areas of different air quality.

Routine culture of bacteria or fungal spores is expected in most environments and does not reflect the environment in the sterile hood where procedures are performed. Settle plates are noninhibitory culture media plates that are left out on a work surface so that bacteria and mold spores can settle out of the air onto the plate. This method represents an unconcentrated air volume assessment, and the procedure used should specify the length of time of exposure for the plate (1 hour vs. 12 or 24 hours). Air filters such as the Anderson air filter apparatus actively collect (suck in) air through a filter. The filter is then placed on a culture medium to allow bacterial and fungal growth. Using this technique, the number of cubic feet of air to be processed must be specified; it is used mainly in clinical transplant areas (e.g., bone marrow transplant). Isolation of spores is expected and usually does not correlate with patient disease.

## Fungal Contamination in the Laboratory

The ability of fungi to form spores that can survive in a wide range of physical extremes makes them a continuous source of potential contamination, and a laboratory that is not kept strictly and rigorously clean at all times provides an ideal environment for them to thrive. Fungal spores may be introduced from the environment, or from central heating/air conditioning systems, and can grow in incubators, water baths, sinks, refrigerators and on walls and surfaces that escape regular thorough cleaning. They thrive in a moist environment where there is a substrate, such as air filters, heat exchangers, humidifiers, water pumps, cooling units, wet carpet, ceiling tiles, condensation on windows – even indoor plants. In most cases, a thorough routine of regular cleaning together with comprehensive visual inspection should eliminate fungal contamination in the laboratory.

**Table 9.1** Average values for limits of microbial detection in areas of defined air quality

| Grade | Air sample (CFU/m³) | Settle plates (90-mm diameter) (CFU/4 hours) | Contact plates (55-mm diameter) (CFU/plate) | Glove print (5 fingers) (CFU/ glove) |
|---|---|---|---|---|
| A | <3 | <3 | <3 | <3 |
| B | 10 | 5 | 5 | 5 |
| C | 100 | 50 | 25 | – |
| D | 200 | 100 | 50 | – |

Contamination in an incubator is usually detected when the same fungus grows in multiple culture dishes. In this case, the incubator must be decontaminated according to the manufacturer's instructions: each manufacturer has specifications about safe and appropriate decontamination procedures. The use of quaternary ammonium compounds, chlorine and alcohol solutions must be dictated by the reactivity of these compounds with the components of the incubator. Following decontamination, the incubators must be wiped down with sterile water to remove any residual cleaning solution that might volatize and contaminate the cultures. Full decontamination procedures should be carried out during laboratory 'down' periods, when no embryos are being cultured. Decontamination should include all surfaces, the water pan and the fan blades (which are very efficient at dispersing spores). Occasionally decontamination may fail; some institutions have been forced to replace the incubators. Many incubators now incorporate an in-built sterilizing cycle to assist in regular decontamination.

## Further Reading

### Books

Bento F, Esteves S, Agarwal A, eds. (2013) *Quality Management in ART Clinics: A Practical Guide*. Springer, New York.

Carson B, Alper M, Keck C (2005) *Quality Management Systems for Assisted Reproductive Technology*. Taylor & Francis, London.

Elder KT, Baker D, Ribes J (2005) *Infections, Infertility and Assisted Reproduction*. Cambridge University Press, Cambridge, UK.

Elder K, Van den Bergh M, Woodward B (2015). *Troubleshooting and Problem-Solving in the IVF Laboratory*. Cambridge University Press, Cambridge, UK.

Keel BA, May JV, De Jonge CJ (eds.) (2000) *Handbook of the Assisted Reproduction Laboratory*. CRC Press, Boca Raton, FL.

Mortimer ST, Mortimer D (2015) *Quality and Risk Management in the IVF Laboratory*, 2nd edn. Cambridge University Press, Cambridge, UK.

### Useful Websites

Association of Clinical Embryologists: www.embryologists.org.uk

College of American Pathologists, Accreditation and Laboratory Improvement: www.cap.org/laboratory-improvement/accreditation

COSHH: www.hse.gov.uk/coshh

Health and Safety: www.hse.gov.uk

Human Fertilisation and Embryology Authority: www.hfea.gov.uk

Human Fertilisation and Embryology Code of Practice 9th edition, 2019: www.hfea.gov.uk/media/2793/2019-01-03-code-of-practice-9th-edition-v2.pdf

International Organization for Standardization (ISO): www.iso.org

Joint Commission International (JCI): www.jointcommissioninternational.org/

Department of Health: www.dh.gov.uk

### ASRM Guidelines

The Practice Committee of the American Society for Reproductive Medicine and the Practice Committee of the Society for Assisted Reproductive Technology (2014) Recommended practices for the management of human embryology, andrology and endocrinology laboratories: a committee opinion. *Fertility and Sterility* 102(4): 0015–0284.

### ESHRE Guidelines

de los Santos MJ, Apter S, Coticchio G, *et al.* (2016) Revised guidelines for good practice in IVF laboratories. *Human Reproduction* 31(4): 685–686.

Magli MC, Van den Abbeel E, Lundin K, *et al.* (2008) Revised guidelines for good practice in IVF laboratories. *Human Reproduction* 23(6): 1253–1262.

### Publications

Alper MA (2013) Experience with ISO quality control in assisted reproductive technology. *Fertility and Sterility* 100(6): 1503–1508.

Blechová R, Pivodová D (2001) LAL test – an alternative method of detection of bacterial endotoxins. *Acta Veterinaria* 70: 291–296.

Butler JM, Johnson J, Boone WR (2013) The heat is on: room temperature affects laboratory equipment; an observational study. *Journal of Assisted Reproduction and Genetics* 30(10): 1389–1393.

Cohen J, Gilligan A, Esposito W, Schimmel T, Dale B (1997) Ambient air and its potential effects on conception in vitro. *Human Reproduction* 12: 1742–1749.

Critchlow JD, Matson PL, Newman MC, *et al.* (1989) Quality control in an in vitro fertilisation laboratory: use of human sperm survival studies. *Human Reproduction* 4: 545–549.

Cutting R, Pritchard J, Clarke H, Martin K (2004) Establishing quality control in the new IVF laboratory. *Human Fertility* 7(2): 119–125.

Gilling-Smith C, Emiliani S, Almeida P, Liesnard C, Englert Y (2005) Laboratory safety during assisted reproduction in patients with blood-borne viruses. *Human Reproduction* 20: 1433–1438.

Imai M (1997) *Gemba Kaizen: A Commonsense, Low-Cost Approach to Management.* McGraw Hill, New York.

Kastrop PM (2003) Quality management in the ART laboratory. *Reproductive BioMedicine Online* 7(6): 691–694.

Meintjes M, Chantilis SJ, Douglas JD, *et al.* (2009) A controlled, randomized trial evaluating the effect of lowered incubator oxygen tension on live births in a predominantly blastocyst transfer program. *Human Reproduction* 24(2): 300–307.

Nijs M, Franssen K, Cox A, *et al.* (2009) Reprotoxicity of intrauterine insemination and in vitro fertilization – embryo transfer disposables and products: a 4-year survey. *Fertility and Sterility* 92(2): 527–535.

Painter RB (1978) DNA synthesis inhibition in HeLa cells as a simple test for agents that damage human DNA.

*Journal of Environmental Pathology and Toxicology* 2(1): 65–78.

Phillips KP, Leveille MC, Klaman P, Baltz JM (2000) Intracellular pH regulation in preimplantation embryos. *Human Reproduction* 15: 896–904.

Pool T (2004) Optimising pH in clinical embryology. *Clinical Embryologist* 7(3): 1–17.

Rinehart JS, Bavister BD, Gerrity M (1988) Quality control in the in vitro fertilization laboratory: comparison of bioassay systems for water quality. *Journal of In Vitro Fertilization and Embryo Transfer* 5: 335–425.

Swain JE (2012) Is there an optimal pH for culture media used in clinical IVF? *Human Reproduction Update* 18: 333–339.

Swain JE, Cabrera L, Smith GD (2012) Microdrop preparation factors influence culture media osmolality which can impair mouse preimplantation embryo development. *Reproductive BioMedicine Online* 2012; 24(2): 142–147.

Tedder RS, Zuckerman MA, Goldstone AH, *et al.* (1995) Hepatitis B transmission from contaminated cryopreservation tank. *Lancet* 346: 137–140.

Tomlinson M (2005) Managing risks associated with cryopreservation. *Human Reproduction* 20: 1433–1438.

# Chapter 10

# Sperm and ART

## Introduction

At least 50% of couples referred for infertility investigation and treatment are found to have a contributing male factor. Male factor infertility can represent a variety of defects, which result in abnormal sperm number, morphology or function. Detailed analysis of sperm assessment and function are important for accurate diagnosis, and are described in detail in numerous textbooks of practical andrology and semen analysis. A comprehensive review of semen analysis is beyond the scope of this book, and only details relevant to assisted conception treatment will be described here.

The *World Health Organization (WHO) Laboratory Manual* (5th edition, 2010) describes standard conditions for the collection of semen samples, their delivery and the standardization of laboratory assessment procedures. This manual represents a major revision over the previous (WHO, 1999) edition and includes new 'Reference Values' to allow decisions to be made about patient management; the latest edition proposes that 'normal' should potentially be defined as the 5th centile of a population of men whose partners conceived within 12 months of stopping contraceptive use. Therefore, the lower reference limits (5th centile and 95% confidence intervals) are $15 \times 10^6$/mL (12–16) for concentration, 32% (31–34) for good forward progressive movement within 60 minutes of ejaculation and 4% (3–4) for normal morphology (see *WHO Manual*, 2010: appendix A1.1). The introduction of external quality control and quality assurance schemes in semen assessment has highlighted the fact that accurate analysis of seminal fluid is notoriously difficult to standardize, with many technical variables, and the quality of semen analysis in different laboratories can be highly variable (Matson, 1995; Pacey 2006). This implies that diagnosis and treatment modality chosen for a patient could differ according to the laboratory carrying out

the assessment. Without accurate semen analysis data, patients may be offered inappropriate treatments or no treatment at all; it is essential that an assisted reproductive service should ensure that laboratory personnel are adequately and correctly trained in basic semen assessment techniques according to WHO guidelines. Even the most confident of laboratories should have a discipline of monitored standards. The routine application of intracytoplasmic sperm injection (ICSI) provides effective treatment for even the most severe cases of male infertility which were previously felt to be beyond hope, and the fact that fertilization can be achieved from semen with 'hopeless' sperm parameters has forced a review of standard semen analysis and sperm function testing. This chapter will address only the basic principles required in the practical features of sperm preparation procedures for assisted conception techniques.

## Semen Assessment

### Sample Collection and Handling

(a) Record information: Before sample production the patients should be asked to confirm their personal details and, if necessary, provide suitable identification. They should be asked when they last ejaculated, and for a history of recent illness, medication taken, smoking and alcohol consumption; this information should be noted on the final report form. Once the sample has been produced, the patient should sign a consent form agreeing to the use of that sample for analysis or treatment.

(b) Provide adequate instructions: patients should be given written instructions about the process involved, including precise details about the location and time that their sample will be required. They should be informed of the need to abstain from sexual intercourse or masturbation for between 3 and 5 days before their sample is to be produced. Care should be taken over language difficulties and for patients with special needs.

(c) Methods of sample production: The sample should ideally be produced by masturbation after the required period of abstinence. However, it is acknowledged that this is not possible for all patients. A small number of men can only produce a sample at intercourse and in these cases they should be provided with a silastic (nonspermicidal) condom. No other condoms are permissible. Samples produced by coitus interruptus without a condom should not be accepted for analysis.

(d) Location of production: Whenever possible, all samples for analysis or treatment should be produced on site. It is unacceptable to ask a patient to produce a sample in a lavatory, and there should be a special room set aside for this purpose. Where it is not possible to produce a sample on site, a sample produced at home should be brought to the laboratory within 1 hour of production.

(e) Specimen container: Samples should be collected into a preweighed wide-necked plastic or glass container. All specimen containers should be cytotoxically tested as some plastics are detrimental to sperm motility (see WHO, 2010, box 2.1, for details). Samples previously assessed as having high viscosity benefit from collection into pots containing 1 mL of medium. Prior to production, the patient should be asked to pass urine and then rinse his hands and penis.

(f) Treatment of samples post-production: Once the sperm sample has been produced, the patient and a member of staff should check that the sample container is identified with the patient's name or identification number, and the time of sample production. The samples should be placed in an incubator at 37°C for up to 1 hour to allow liquefaction.

## Macroscopic Evaluation

Once the process of liquefaction has occurred (usually within 30–60 minutes of ejaculation), the sample should be examined macroscopically, with evaluation of:

- *Appearance and consistency*: Semen should be a grayish opalescent liquid with a neutral odor. Any

unpleasant smell or discoloration (e.g., contains blood), or the presence of mucus or jelly should be reported.

- *Liquefaction and viscosity*: Although semen is ejaculated as a coagulum, it should liquefy within 30 minutes. If a sample fails to liquefy or is highly viscous after liquefaction, this should be noted.
- *Volume*: Volume is measured by weighing the container in which the specimen was ejaculated and subtracting the full weight from the empty weight. The volume can be inferred from the weight assuming the density of semen to be 1 g/mL. The use of volumetric methods to measure semen volume is no longer recommended.
- *pH*: The most convenient way to measure the pH of a sample is to use pH paper.

Macroscopic anomalies can provide important information about the patient and should not be ignored. For example, a low pH can indicate infection of the genital tract, and a low volume could suggest a retrograde ejaculation, a leakage from the sample container or that the patient failed to collect the entire sample he produced.

## Sperm Motility

Since sperm motility decreases with increasing exposure to seminal plasma, this should be the first assessment carried out. There are three important aspects to correctly estimating sperm motility:

- *Observation chamber*: A variety of types are available, but this should have a minimum depth of 20 µm to allow the sperm to move freely. A number of companies produce disposable chambers designed for motility observation (e.g., Microcell), but an alternative strategy is to place a 10-µL drop of semen on a glass microscope slide and cover it with a 22-mm diameter coverslip. NB: the depth of a Makler chamber (10 µm) makes it unsuitable for accurate motility measurements. However, when the purpose of assessment is the selection of an appropriate method of preparing the sample for assisted conception procedures, the Makler chamber does allow simultaneous judgment of approximate motile and immotile concentrations, and a quick assessment of type of sperm motility.
- *Temperature*: The microscope slide should be maintained at 37°C on a heated stage during

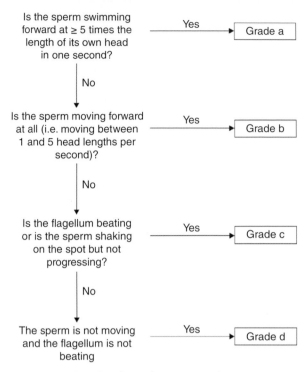

**Figure 10.1** Flow chart for grading sperm motility.

motility assessment for correct identification of motility grade.

- *Microscope*: Observe the sample at ×200 or ×400 magnification using a phase-contrast objective.
- *Grading system*: Approximately 200 sperm should be examined and each sperm classified as belonging to one of four motility grades. Figure 10.1 outlines the difference between the motility grades, with a flow chart explaining how to classify them. A percentage for the number of sperm belonging to each category should be calculated.

### Aggregated or Agglutinated Spermatozoa

- A high number of aggregated or agglutinated spermatozoa can make accurate motility assessment impossible. A motility count should then be performed only on the free-swimming portion, with this noted in the report.

### Less than 50% of the Spermatozoa Are Motile

- If less than 50% of the spermatozoa are motile, a vitality test, such as a hypo-osmotic swelling (HOS) test, is recommended in order to determine whether the nonmotile sperm are dead or alive.

## Sperm Concentration

Methods used to determine sperm concentration have long been a subject of debate. Andrologists tend to agree that using a hemocytometer is the most appropriate, as it provides the most reproducible result with the lowest coefficient of variation when used properly. Since it normally relies upon the use of fixatives to kill spermatozoa before they are placed on the counting chamber, its use is often thought to be in conflict with the principles of trying to reduce chemical contaminants in the IVF laboratory. Many embryologists, however, use water instead of fixative in which to dilute the spermatozoa, and the osmotic shock is sufficient to immobilize sperm sufficiently for a count to be undertaken. Others prefer to use a Makler chamber or disposable chambers such as the Microcell. If an alternative chamber is chosen, then it is important that its accuracy is regularly checked using a thorough internal quality control system. This should preferably be checked against a hemocytometer as the gold standard. Whatever chamber is chosen, it is important to pay special consideration to samples in which no spermatozoa are observed. These samples should be centrifuged at >3000 g for 15 minutes; a sample can be classified as truly azoospermic only if no sperm are observed in the pellet after centrifugation.

Before performing the count, note the presence of agglutination and type if present (H-H, T-T, H-T), and any debris and cells other than spermatozoa, such as red or white blood cells.

Examine the counting grid and count the number of *motile* sperm in 20 squares. If the count appears on initial observation to be less than 10 million/mL, all 100 squares should be counted. Count the total number of sperm in the same group of squares and calculate motility:

> Sperm density in millions/mL = the number of sperm in 10 squares of the grid

The sperm concentration should be reported in millions per milliliter.

## Sperm Antibody Detection

Antibodies directed against sperm can be detected by two methods, the mixed antiglobulin reaction (MAR) test and the immunobead test. They differ slightly in their approach and methodology, but their interpretation is similar in that they rely upon the identification of motile spermatozoa with adherent latex spheres or beads. Kits are available for anti-sperm antibody screening in semen samples; the MAR test will nonspecifically detect IgG, IgA or IgM antibodies, and specific latex particle immuno-beads can be used to distinguish between the different categories of antibody. Although the results of the two tests do not always agree, it is generally considered that a test is clinically significant only if >50% of sperm have antibodies directed against them. In cases where the test cannot be performed due to an insufficient number of motile sperm, the sample can be tested indirectly by using the sperm of a donor (known to have no sperm antibodies in his semen) as part of the test: the donor sperm acts as a reagent in the assay. The percentage of spermatozoa with adherent particles should be recorded on the report form after evaluating 200 sperm.

## Sperm Morphology Estimation

Sperm morphology assessment is one of the most controversial measures in semen analysis. This is due partly to several changes in reporting the dimensions of normal spermatozoa in successive editions of the WHO manual, but is also due to the technical difficulty of making accurate morphology measurements without the aid of a computerized system. All morphology measurements should be made using fixed smears stained by the Papanicolaou method or the Diff-Quick or Shorr stains (prestained slides are also available). Stained slides should be examined by bright-field optics using an oil-immersion objective at ×1000 magnification. At least 200 spermatozoa should be examined; an eyepiece graticule can be used to measure individual spermatozoa if necessary. The normal head has an oval shape with a length:width ratio of 1.50:1.75. A well-defined acrosomal region should cover 40–70% of the head area. No neck, midpiece or tail defects should be evident, and cytoplasmic droplets should constitute no more than one-third the size of a normal sperm head. Figure 10.2 illustrates some examples of typical sperm abnormalities. Count the number of sperm that display:

1. Abnormal heads
2. Tail abnormality
3. Midpiece abnormalities
4. Immature forms.

All borderline forms are classified as abnormal. Calculate the percentage of each abnormal form,

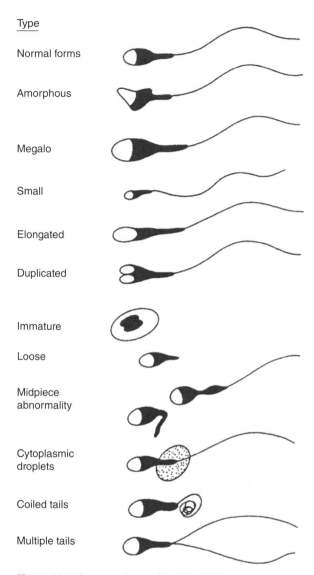

**Figure 10.2** Common abnormalities found in human sperm morphology.

and add together the percentages to yield the total percentage of abnormal forms in the sample.

A normal, fertile semen sample contains a very high proportion of morphologically abnormal forms, and the significance of abnormal sperm morphology is not entirely understood. Although sperm of abnormal morphology evidently have reduced fertilizing potential, the true anomalies present in abnormal sperm cells have been only partially characterized; a correlation has been found with specific deficiencies such as poor zona pellucida binding and penetration, poor response to agonists that modulate intracellular

197

calcium concentrations, and with biochemical markers such as reactive oxygen species production and enhanced creatine phosphokinase activity. The significance of sperm morphology is discussed further in Chapter 13.

## Other Cells in Semen

Other (non-sperm) cells can sometimes be observed during the semen analysis, either in the wet (motility) preparation or in the stained morphology slide. These include epithelial cells from the urethra, erythrocytes, germ cells and leukocytes. Whilst epithelial cells and erythrocytes are easily identifiable from their morphology, germ cells and leukocytes can easily be confused. Therefore, specific stains are needed to discriminate between the two cell types and to correctly enumerate their concentration on the semen analysis report. Leukocytes can be identified using a peroxidase-based stain, or with the use of specific monoclonal antibodies. The concentration of any non-sperm cell can be calculated relative to the sperm concentration using the equation $c = n \times s/100$, where $n$ is the number of a given cell type in the same field as 100 sperm, and $s$ is the sperm concentration in millions per milliliter.

## Internal and External Quality Control Procedures

A final but important part of the semen analysis is the application of internal and external quality control procedures to the semenology laboratory. Several studies have shown that samples analyzed in different laboratories can give rise to radically different results, in some cases leading to an inappropriate diagnosis for the patient. Many techniques have been outlined that can be used to monitor the performance of a laboratory, and these are described in more detail in the 5th edition of the WHO manual. Any laboratory involved in making diagnoses should have such protocols in place and should be members of an external quality assessment scheme for andrology.

## Sperm Kinematics

In the early 1980s several studies used time-lapse photography to analyze detailed movement characteristics of sperm in time and space (sperm kinematics). The motion of spermatozoa can be described in a number of different ways (see Mortimer, 1994):

VSL = straight line velocity

VCL = curvilinear velocity

VAP = average path velocity

ALH = amplitude of lateral head displacement.

These early data led to the suggestion that specific patterns of sperm motility behavior were advantageous. For example, only spermatozoa with a high degree of lateral head displacement are able to penetrate cervical mucus. The development of computerized systems allowed such measurements to be made more rapidly as well as allowing the analysis of more sophisticated behavior patterns, such as sperm hyperactivation. Although the measurement of sperm hyperactivation has been controversial, it has been linked with IVF success. However, this technology is not used routinely as the prognostic value is poor, and the high cost of the machines precludes their use in all but the most specialized laboratories. (See Tomlinson *et al.*, 2010 for review.)

## DNA Fragmentation

As detailed in Chapter 3, spermatogenesis is a complex and dynamic process of proliferation and differentiation, involving mitosis, meiosis, changes in cytoplasmic architecture, replacement of histones with transition proteins and the final addition of protamines, leading to a highly packaged chromatin. It is not surprising therefore that ejaculated spermatozoa have a variety of abnormalities at the nuclear, cytoskeletal and organelle levels. There is now evidence to suggest that sperm DNA integrity may be useful in predicting male fertility potential. The first manuscript describing in-situ detection of sperm DNA fragmentation was published more than 30 years ago, and a surge in published reports about sperm DNA fragmentation then appeared between 2005 and 2010. These studies provide strong evidence that semen samples in which more than a third of the DNA is fragmented have a reduced chance of resulting in clinical pregnancy (Sakkas and Alvarez, 2010). Sperm DNA fragmentation may result from aberrant chromatin packaging during spermatogenesis, apoptosis before ejaculation, excessive production of reactive oxygen species in the ejaculate, exposure to environmental or industrial toxins, genetics, oxidative stress, smoking, etc. Current standard sperm preparation techniques depend on a sedimentation or migration approach to separate spermatozoa based on their motility or density with molecular events being overlooked. Thus, the use of sperm with DNA damage during IVF may be one of the reasons for suboptimal pregnancy and low live birth rates.

## Sperm Chromatin Assays

Sperm condensation quality and sperm morphology studies suggest that the quality of chromatin packaging in human sperm, as assessed by its binding capacity for specific dyes and fluorochromes, can be used as an adjunct to the assessment of morphology. Sperm of poor morphology may possess loosely packaged chromatin, and this may contribute to a failure in sperm decondensation during fertilization.

Damaged chromatin will take up the following dyes:

1. **Chromomycin (CMA3) staining**

   - Fix prepared semen samples or semen smears in 3:1 v/v of methanol/glacial acetic acid, at 4°C for 5 minutes.
   - Treat each slide for 20 minutes with 100 mL CMA3 solution: 0.25 mg/mL in McIlvane's buffer, pH 7.0, containing 10 mM $MgCl_2$.
   - Evaluate the slides using fluorescent microscopy.

2. **Aniline blue staining (AAB)**

   - Fix the samples in 3% buffered glutaraldehyde for 30 minutes.
   - Stain the slides with 5% aqueous aniline blue and mix with 4% acetic acid (pH 3.5) for 7 minutes.
   - Three classes of head staining can be noted: unstained (gray/white), partially stained, entire sperm head dark blue intensity.

## Detection of DNA Fragmentation by the TUNEL Assay

Kits for DNA fragmentation analyses are commercially available from a number of different companies, each with its own protocol to be followed.

- Wash a semen aliquot containing $1-2 \times 10^6$ spermatozoa with phosphate-buffered saline (PBS) by centrifugation at 500 g at room temperature for 5 minutes.
- Remove the seminal plasma and wash the pellet twice in PBS with 1% bovine serum albumin (BSA).
- Suspend the pellet in 100 μL of PBS/BSA 1%, and fix it in 100 μL of 4% paraformaldehyde in PBS

(pH 7.4) for 1 hour at room temperature, with agitation.

- Wash the cells again in PBS/1% BSA, spot a 10-μL aliquot onto a demarcated area on a clean microscope slide and allow this to air dry.
- Rinse the slides twice in PBS, and then permeabilize using 0.1% Triton X100 in 0.1% sodium citrate for 2 minutes on ice.
- Wash again twice with PBS, add terminal deoxyribonucleotidyl transferase (TdT)-mediated dUTP nick-end label in order to allow DNA elongation, and incubate the slides in a humidified chamber at 37°C for 60 minutes.
- Rinse slides twice in PBS and counterstain with 1 mg/mL 4,6 diamidino-2-phenylindole (DAPI) to visualize the nucleus.
- Include negative (omitting TdT from the reaction mixture) and positive (using only DNAse I, 1 mg/mL for 30 minutes at room temperature) controls in each sample tested.
- Evaluate a total of 500 sperm per sample using fluorescence microscopy for fluorescein isothiocyanate (FITC). Count the number of sperm per field stained with DAPI (blue); the number of cells with green FITC fluorescence (TUNEL positive) is expressed as a percentage of the total sample.

# Preparation of Sperm for In-Vitro Fertilization

At the time of oocyte retrieval or intrauterine insemination (IUI), the laboratory should already be familiar with the male partner's semen profile and can refer to features that might influence the choice of sperm preparation method used. Semen is a nonsterile body fluid that can transmit infection, and viral screening tests should be confirmed as negative before the sample is handled for preparation in the laboratory. Aseptic technique should be maintained throughout.

The choice of sperm preparation method or combination of methods depends upon the assessment of:

- motile count
- ratio between motile:immotile counts
- volume
- presence of antibodies, agglutination, pus cells or debris.

199

Ejaculated semen is a viscous liquid composed of a mixture of testicular and epididymal secretions containing spermatozoa, mixed with prostatic secretions produced at the time of ejaculation. This seminal plasma contains substances that inhibit capacitation and prevent fertilization. The purpose of sperm preparation is to concentrate the motile spermatozoa in a fraction that is free of seminal plasma and debris. Early IVF practice involved preparing sperm by simple washing and centrifugaring, but this method also concentrates cells, debris and immotile sperm, which can jeopardize fertilization. Aitken and Clarkson (1987) demonstrated that leukocytes and dead sperm in semen can generate reactive oxygen species (ROS), and these can initiate lipid peroxidation in human sperm membranes. Peroxidation of sperm membrane unsaturated fatty acids leads to a loss of membrane fluidity, which inhibits sperm fusion events during the process of fertilization. When preparing sperm for assisted conception, it is advantageous to separate motile sperm from leukocytes and dead sperm as effectively and efficiently as possible. However, if ICSI is the treatment of choice, sperm fusion events are of course bypassed, and direct high-speed centrifugation of these suboptimal sperm samples does not appear to jeopardize fertilization by ICSI.

Sperm samples that show moderate to high counts ($>35 \times 10^6$ motile sperm/mL) with good forward progression and motility can be prepared using a basic overlay and swim-up technique. Discontinuous buoyant density gradient centrifugation is the method of choice for samples that show:

1. Low motility
2. Poor forward progression
3. Large amounts of debris and/or high numbers of cells
4. Antisperm antibodies.

At the end of each preparation procedure, adjust the pH of the resulting samples by gassing gently with 5% $CO_2$, and store the samples at room temperature until final preparation for insemination.

## Standard Swim-Up or Layering

1. Pipette 2 mL of HEPES-buffered culture medium into a round-bottomed disposable test-tube.
2. Gently pipette approximately 1.5 mL of neat semen underneath the medium (being very careful

not to disturb the interface formed between the semen and the medium).
3. Tightly cap the tube and allow it to stand at room temperature for up to 2 hours. (The ejaculate can also be divided into several tubes for layering if necessary.)
4. Harvest the resulting top and middle clouded layers into a conical test-tube and spin at 200 g for 5 minutes.
5. Remove the supernatant and resuspend the pellet in 2 mL of medium. Centrifuge again, discard the supernatant and resuspend the pellet in 1 mL of medium.
6. Assess this sample for count and motility, gas the surface gently with 5% $CO_2$ in air, and store at room temperature prior to dilution for the insemination procedure.

Alternatively, 2 mL of medium can be gently layered over the semen sample in its pot, which provides a larger interface surface area. After 10–45 minutes, suspend an aliquot of this layer in 1 mL of medium and process as above. The time allowed for swim-up should be adjusted according to the quality of the initial sample: the percentage of abnormal sperm that will appear in the medium increases with time and continues to do so after normal motile density has reached its optimum level.

## Pellet and Swim-Up

This method is used when the semen has been collected into medium or medium + albumin. It is also useful for viscous samples (once the viscosity has been decreased, by vigorous pipetting or syringing) and when the total volume of semen is very low. This method is not recommended when motility is very poor or when there is a large degree of cellular contamination and debris (the sperm will be concentrated with this prior to the swim-up).

1. Mix semen and medium and centrifuge once. Note: In some cases (i.e. oligo/asthenospermia) much more semen will need to be prepared, and the volume of medium used should be increased accordingly. As a general rule, be careful not to take far more of the semen than is required.
2. Carefully remove all the supernatant and then very gently pipette about 0.75 mL of medium over the pellet, taking care not to disturb it.

3. Allow the sperm to swim up into the medium. If the sample has poor motility, it sometimes helps to lay the centrifuge tube on its side.

   - 10 minutes is sufficient for very motile sperm (activity 3–4).
   - 1 hour plus may be required for poorly motile sperm.
   - In general, do not leave for too long, as some cells and debris will become resuspended.

4. Carefully remove the supernatant from the pellet and place in a clean centrifuge tube.
5. Centrifuge again, resuspend in medium, assess count and motility, and gas with $CO_2$ before storing at room temperature.

This method has the disadvantage of exposing motile sperm to peroxidative damage during centrifugation with defective sperm and white cells. Aitken (1990) has shown that unselected sperm exhibit higher levels of ROS production in response to centrifugation than the functionally competent sperm selected prior to centrifugation by the layering method. Sperm that are selected prior to centrifugation produce much lower levels of ROS, and their functional capacity is not impaired.

## Discontinuous Buoyant Density Gradient Centrifugation

Buoyant density gradient 'kits' for sperm preparation are commercially available. These are based upon either coated silica particles, a mixture of Ficoll and iodixanol, or highly purified arabinogalactan. Individual experiences comparing the use of these products have reported no significant differences between them. Buoyant density gradients apparently protect the sperm from the trauma of centrifugation, and a high proportion of functional sperm can be recovered from the gradients. Discontinuous two- or three-step gradients are simple to prepare and highly effective in preparing motile sperm fractions from suboptimal semen samples. A single layer of 90–100% density can also be used for simple filtration by layering the sample on top of the column and allowing the sperm to migrate through the density medium, where they can be harvested from the bottom of the test-tube.

### Methods

Manufacturers' instructions should be followed for the different commercial preparations, but 'recipes'

can be adapted according to each individual semen sample, in particular with respect to volumes, speed of centrifugation and length of centrifugation. In general, a longer centrifugation time increases the recovery of both motile and immotile sperm; normal immotile sperm are only decelerated by the particles, and after long spinning they will reach the bottom of the gradient. Higher centrifugation speeds increase the recovery of motile sperm, and also of lower density particles; therefore, if the gradients are spun at a higher speed, a shorter time should be used. Debris, round cells, and abnormal forms with amorphous heads and cytoplasmic droplets never reach the bottom of the tube because of their low density. Gradients with larger volumes result in improved filtration, but decreased yield. The three layers of a mini-gradient improve filtration, and the smaller volumes improve recovery of sperm from severely oligospermic samples. Large amounts of debris can disrupt gradients and prevent adequate filtration. There is a limit to the number of cells that can be loaded onto any gradient, and samples with high density or a large amount of debris should be distributed in smaller volumes over several gradients. Severely asthenozoospermic samples with a normal sperm density but poor motility can also be distributed over a series of mini-gradients.

The temperature of the prepared gradients also affects the 'merging of gradients,' which is improved at 37°C compared to room temperature.

### Isotonic Gradient Solution

| | |
|---|---|
| 10 × concentrated EBS (or other media concentrate): | 10 mL |
| 5% human serum albumin: | 19 mL |
| Sodium pyruvate: | 113 mg |
| Sodium lactate 60%: | 0·37 mL |
| 1 M HEPES: | 12 mL |
| Gentamicin sulfate, 5 mg/mL: | 12 mL |

Mix, and filter this solution through a 0.22-mm Millipore filter.

Add 90 mL of density gradient preparation media.

Store at +4°C for up to 1 week.

### Two-Step Gradient, 80/40

- Can be used for all samples which contain $> 4 \times 10^6$ motile sperm/mL.

- Should be used for all specimens with known or suspected antisperm antibodies:

  80%: 8 mL isotonic + 2 mL culture medium

  40%: 4 mL isotonic + 6 mL culture medium.

1. Gradients: pipette 2.0–2.5 mL of 80% into the bottom of a conical centrifuge tube, and gently overlay with an equal volume of 40%.
2. Layer up to 2 mL of sample on top of the 40% layer.
3. Centrifuge at 600 g for 20 minutes.
   Cells, debris and immotile/abnormal sperm accumulate at the interfaces, and the pellet should contain functionally normal sperm. Recovery of a good pellet is influenced by the amount of debris and immotile sperm, which impede the travel of the normal motile sperm.
4. Carefully recover the pellet at the bottom of the 80% layer, resuspend in 1 mL of medium and assess (even if there is no visible pellet, a sufficient number of sperm can usually be recovered by aspirating the bottom portion of the 80% layer).
5. If the sample looks sufficiently clean, centrifuge for 5 minutes at 200 g, resuspend the pellet in fresh medium and assess the final preparation.
6. If there is a high percentage of immotile sperm, centrifuge at 200 g for 5 minutes, remove the supernatant, carefully layer 1 mL fresh medium over the pellet and allow the motile sperm to swim up for 15–30 minutes. Collect the supernatant and assess the final preparation.

If at least $10^6$ motile sperm/mL have been recovered, spin at 200 g for 5 minutes and resuspend in fresh medium. This will be the final preparation to be diluted before insemination, therefore the volume of medium added will depend upon the calculated assessment.

### Mini-gradient (95/70/50)

| | |
|---|---|
| 95% | 9.5 mL gradient solution + 0.5 mL culture medium |
| 70% | 7.0 mL + 3.0 mL |
| 50% | 5.0 mL + 5.0 mL |

1. Gradients: make layers with 0.3 mL of each solution: 95, then 70, then 50.
2. Dilute the semen 1:1 with culture medium, and centrifuge at 200 g for 10 minutes.

3. Resuspend the pellet in 0.3 mL of culture medium, and layer over mini-gradient (resuspend in a larger volume if it is to be distributed over several gradients).
4. Centrifuge at 600 g for 20–30 minutes.
5. Recover the pellet(s), resuspend in 0.5 mL of culture medium, and assess count and motility. Proceed exactly as for two-step gradient preparation: either centrifuge at 200 g for 5 minutes and resuspend the pellet, or layer over the pellet for a further preparation by swim-up. The concentration of the final preparation should be adjusted to a sperm density of approximately $10^6$ motile sperm per mL if possible.

If a sample is being prepared for ICSI, note that residual polyvinylpyrrolidone (PVP)-coated particles in the preparation will interact with PVP used for sperm immobilization, resulting in a gelatinous mass from which the sperm cannot be aspirated. Careful washing of the preparation to remove all traces of gradient preparation is essential when handling samples for ICSI (one wash is usually sufficient).

## Sedimentation Method or Layering Under Paraffin Oil

This method is useful for samples with very low counts and poor motility. It is very effective in removing debris, but requires several hours of preparation time.

1. Mix the semen with a large volume of medium, pipetting thoroughly to break down viscosity etc., and wash the sample by dilution and centrifugation twice.
2. Alternatively: process the entire sample (undiluted) on an appropriate discontinuous buoyant density gradient.
3. Resuspend the pellet in a reduced volume of medium so that the final motile sperm concentration is not too dilute.
4. Layer this final suspension under paraffin oil (making one large droplet) in a small Petri dish. Place in a desiccator and gas with 5% $CO_2$.
5. Leave at room temperature for 3–24 hours. The duration of sedimentation depends upon the amount of cells, debris and motile spermatozoa; a longer period is usually more effective in reducing cells and debris, but may also reduce the

number of freely motile sperm in the upper part of the droplet.

6. Carefully aspirate motile sperm by pipetting the upper part of the droplet. Aspiration can be made more efficient by using a fine-drawn pipette and also by positioning the droplet under the stereomicroscope, to ensure that as little debris as possible is collected.

## High-Speed Centrifugation and Washing

Cryptozoospermic (or nearly cryptozoospermic) samples which must be prepared for ICSI can be either centrifuged directly (without dilution) at 1800 g for 5 minutes, or diluted with medium and then centrifuged at 1800 g for 5 minutes.

1. Wash the pellet with a small volume of medium (0.5 mL approximately) and centrifuge at 200 g for 5 minutes.
2. Recover this pellet in a minimal volume of medium (20–50 mL) and overlay with mineral oil. Single sperm for microinjection can then be retrieved from this droplet using the micromanipulator.

It is important to bear in mind that every semen specimen has different characteristics and parameters, and it is illogical to apply an identical preparation technique to each specimen. All preparation methods are adaptable in some way: layering can be carried out in test-tubes, but a wider vessel increases the area exposed to culture medium and decreases the depth of the specimen, increasing the potential return of motile sperm from oligoasthenospermic samples. Centrifugation times for buoyant density gradients may be adjusted according to the quality of the specimen to give optimum results. It is important to tailor preparation techniques to fit the parameters of the semen specimen, rather than to have fixed recipes. A trial preparation prior to oocyte retrieval may be advisable in choosing the suitable technique for particular patients.

## Chemical Enhancement of Sperm Motility Prior to Insemination

Pentoxifylline is a methylxanthine-derived phosphodiesterase inhibitor which is known to elevate spermatozoal intracellular levels of cAMP in vitro. It has been postulated that the resulting increase in intracellular adenosine triphosphate (ATP) enhances sperm motility in samples that are assessed as having poor progressive motility, with an increase in fertilization and pregnancy rates for suboptimal semen samples. 2-De-oxyadenosine has also been used to achieve a similar effect. The protocol involves a 30-minute preincubation of prepared sperm with the stimulant; the resulting sperm suspension is then washed to remove the stimulant, and the preparation is used immediately for insemination.

## Stock Solutions

1 mM PF: dissolve 22 mg of pentoxifylline in 10 mL of medium.

3 mM 2-DA: dissolve 8 mg of 2-deoxyadenosine in 10 mL of medium.

Gas with 5% $CO_2$ to adjust pH.

Store at 4°C for a maximum period of 1 month.

### Procedure

1. Gas and warm PF or 2-DA solutions, and also an additional 10 mL of medium.
2. 35–40 minutes prior to insemination time, add an equal volume of PF or 2-DA solutions to the sperm preparation suspension.
3. Incubate at 37°C for 30 minutes.
4. Centrifuge, 5 minutes at 200 g, and resuspend pellet in warm medium.
5. Analyze the sperm suspension for count and motility, dilute to appropriate concentration for insemination, and inseminate oocytes immediately.

## Determination of Reactive Oxygen Species in Seminal Fluid

Free radicals are atoms or molecules with one or more unpaired electrons, which makes them extremely reactive. Having an incomplete outer valence shell, they attempt to interact with other molecules in order to gain electrons. Once a molecule loses an electron to a free radical, it then itself becomes a free radical, initiating a chain reaction that can potentially be disastrous for cells. ROS are radical and non-radical derivatives of oxygen; the most common ROS in spermatozoa is the superoxide anion radical which eventually forms hydrogen peroxide. Seminal plasma contains two types of antioxidants to combat free radical-induced damage: enzymatic antioxidants, such as superoxide dismutase, catalase and peroxidase, and non-enzymatic antioxidants, such as vitamins, glutathione and pyruvate.

Although excessive generation of ROS is involved in the pathogenesis of a wide range of diseases, such as neurodegenerative disease, cancer and infertility, they are also essential in a variety of physiological functions such as cellular signaling (see Chapter 1). Homeostasis is the key, as in all cell functions, and an excessive use of antioxidants to treat male infertility may be detrimental, triggering, amongst other problems, a decrease in spermatogenesis and fertility (Henkel *et al.*, 2019).

ROS can be detected in seminal fluid via both direct and indirect methods:

*Direct methods:* cytochrome c reduction, electron spin resonance, nitroblue tetrazolium techniques and flow cytometry.

*Indirect methods:* redox potential, measuring the level of lipid peroxidation products or oxidative DNA damage and measuring reactive nitrogen species by fluorescence spectroscopy.

The chemiluminescence assay is the most commonly used technique in andrology laboratories. This relies on the measurement of light after reagents are added to human sperm to cause a reaction:

**Luminol** measures both intracellular and extracellular ROS, such as hydrogen peroxide, superoxide anions and hydroxyl radicals.

**Lucigenin** measures only extracellular ROS, in particular the superoxide anion.

ROS can be measured in ejaculated semen, or in processed sperm following swim-up or density gradient techniques. A variety of luminometers are commercially available, varying in design, features and price.

## Can Sperm Metabolism Be Improved in Vitro?

Spermatozoa have a very small volume of cytoplasm and a high level of mitochondrial activity; these two features make sperm cells extremely vulnerable to oxidative damage that may affect DNA, proteins and the plasma membrane. Mitochondria generate energy for motility, using oxidative phosphorylation to produce large amounts of NADH and $FADH_2$ and moving electrons from NADH to $O_2$. Approximately 1–4% of the oxygen generated escapes, forming ROS. ATP production and leakage of ROS by the electron transport chain depend on the mitochondrial membrane potential.

Damage to sperm membranes may jeopardize many events essential for fertilization, including the acrosome reaction, sperm motility, adhesion and fusion of the gametes. Glutathione is a ubiquitous ROS scavenger, and hypotaurine is a dominant ROS scavenger in the female reproductive tract; both require cysteine for their synthesis, and supplements targeted toward reinforcing the one-carbon cycle in vitro should improve sperm metabolism (see Chapter 1). Adding B vitamins and zinc to human sperm in vitro has been shown to improve sperm kinetics and the mitochondrial membrane potential (Gallo *et al.*, 2018), promising a new direction for generating new culture medium formulations for human IVF.

## Sperm Preparation for ICSI

A combination of sperm preparation methods can be used; extremely oligospermic/asthenozoospermic samples cannot be prepared by buoyant density centrifugation or swim-up techniques.

1. Centrifuge the whole sample, 1800 g, 5 minutes, wash with medium, and resuspend the pellet in a small volume of medium.
2. Apply this sample directly to the injection dish (without PVP/ hyaluronic acid [HA]), or add an aliquot of the suspension to a drop of HEPES-buffered medium.
3. If possible, use the injection pipette to select a moving sperm with apparently normal morphology from this drop, and transfer it into the drop to be used for sperm immobilization.
4. If there is debris attached to the sperm, clean it by pipetting the sperm back and forth with the injection pipette.
5. If the sperm still has some movement in the immobilization drop, immobilize it by crushing the tail and proceed with the injection as described in Chapter 11.
6. It may sometimes be helpful to connect the sperm droplet to another small medium droplet by means of a bridge of medium and allow motile sperm to swim out into the clean droplet. Overloading a PVP/HA droplet with very poor sperm can seriously hamper the selection procedure, due to the presence of excessive amounts of debris. Using a bridge of medium allows motile sperm to swim into the second, clean droplet.

Even if the results of semen analysis show no motile sperm, it may be possible to see occasional slight tail movement in a medium drop without PVP. If absolutely no motile sperm are found, immotile sperm may be used. The fertilization rate with immotile sperm is generally lower than that with motile sperm, and oocytes with a single pronucleus are seen more often in these cases, possibly indicating incomplete oocyte activation. Previous assessment with a vital stain may be helpful before deciding upon ICSI treatment. However, embryologists may be left with the dilemma of making a decision regarding injection in situations where there are only immotile sperm, the vitality stain/HOS test indicates the sperm tested are not alive and there is no donor back-up.

## Hypo-osmotic Swelling Test (HOS)

The HOS test assesses the osmoregulatory ability of the sperm, and therefore the functional integrity of its membranes. It can be used to discriminate viable from nonviable sperm cells in a sample which has zero or little apparent motility. The test is based upon the ability of live spermatozoa to withstand the moderate stress of a hypo-osmotic environment; they react to this stress by swelling of the tail. Dead spermatozoa whose plasma membranes are no longer intact do not show tail swelling. HOS test diluent is a solution of 150 mOsm/kg osmolarity and can be made by dissolving 7.35 g sodium citrate and 13.51 g fructose in 1000 mL of reagent-grade water (alternatively, sperm preparation medium can be diluted 1:1 with reagent-grade water). Mix an aliquot of the sample with approximately 10 times the volume of diluent, incubate at 37°C for 30 minutes, remix and transfer one drop of the mixture to a clean microscope slide. Cover with a coverslip and examine using phase-contrast microscopy at a magnification of ×400–500 for the presence of swollen (coiled) tails. Osmotically incompetent and dead spermatozoa swell so much that the plasma membrane bursts, allowing the tail to straighten out again.

## 100% Abnormal Heads

If the semen analysis shows 100% head anomalies, it may still be possible to find the occasional normal form in the sample. In cases where no normal forms are found, the fertilization and implantation rates may be lower; however, debate continues about this

subject, and individual judgment should be applied to each case, with careful assessment of several different semen samples.

Fertilization and pregnancy have now been demonstrated using samples from men with globozoospermia, a 100% head anomaly where all sperm lack an acrosomal cap; in these cases the oocytes need to be artificially activated post-ICSI for fertilization to occur. However, there is evidence to suggest that such defects which are genetically determined have a high probability of being transmitted to the offspring, and debate continues as to whether it is ethically advisable to offer treatment to these men.

## Sticky Sperm

Sperm that have a tendency to stick to the injection pipette make the injection procedure more difficult. If the sperm is caught in the pipette, try to release it by repeatedly aspirating and blowing with the injection system.

## Excessive Amounts of Debris

Large amounts of debris in the sperm preparation may block the injection pipette or become attached to the outside of the pipette. A blocked pipette may be cleared by blowing a small amount of the air already in the pipette through it. Another useful technique is to insert the injection pipette into the lumen of the holding pipette, and then apply negative suction to the holding pipette and simultaneous positive pressure to the injection pipette. Debris attached to the outside of the injection pipette can be cleaned by rubbing the pipette against the holding pipette, against the oocyte or against the oil at the edge of the medium drop. It may be necessary (and preferable) to change the pipette if it cannot be quickly cleared.

## Sperm Preparation after Retrograde Ejaculation and Electroejaculation

When treating patients with ejaculatory dysfunction, with or without the aid of electroejaculation, both antegrade and retrograde ejaculation (into the bladder) are commonly found. When retrograde ejaculation is anticipated, the patient should first empty his bladder, and then drink an alkaline drink (e.g., bicarbonate of soda), and empty his bladder again 30 minutes later before producing a sample that

205

can then be collected from a urine sample by centrifugation. In cases of spinal cord injury, the bladder is emptied via a catheter and approximately 20 mL of culture medium then instilled. After electroejaculation, the bladder is again emptied and the entire sample centrifuged. The resulting pellet(s) are resuspended in medium and processed on appropriate density gradients. As with all abnormal semen samples, a flexible approach is required in order to obtain a suitable sample for insemination; ICSI is recommended as the treatment of choice.

## Surgical Sperm Retrieval

Until the mid-1990s, virtually all patients with obstructive or nonobstructive azoospermia (see Appendix for list of pathologies) had untreatable male sterility; this situation was completely reversed by the ability to combine ICSI with surgical techniques to recover samples from the epididymis and directly from the testis.

1. Epididymal sperm can be obtained by open microscopic surgery (MESA) or by percutaneous puncture (PESA), using a 21-gauge 'butterfly' or equivalent needle to aspirate fluid. If large numbers of sperm are found, they can be processed by buoyant density gradient centrifugation. Samples with fewer sperm can be washed and centrifuged with IVF medium a number of times, and the concentrated sample is then added to microdroplets in the injection dish. Motile spermatozoa 'swim out' to the periphery of the droplets, where they can be collected and transferred to clean drops of medium for injection later.

2. Testicular sperm is obtained by open biopsy (testicular sperm extraction, TESE) or by percutaneous needle biopsy (testicular fine needle aspiration, TEFNA), and samples can be processed in a variety of ways:

    - Crush the biopsy sample between two microscope slides, and expose sperm by shredding the tissue either with glass slides, by needle dissection, by dissection using microscissors, or by maceration using a microgrinder. Concentrate the debris by centrifugation and examine under high-power microscopy to look for spermatozoa. Large quantities of debris are invariably present, and it may be difficult to find sperm (especially

with cases of focal spermatogenesis). Further processing steps will depend upon the quality of the sample: it may be loaded onto a small single-step buoyant density gradient, or sperm simply harvested 'by hand' under the microscope. Use a large needle, assisted hatching pipette or biopsy pipette to collect and pool live sperm in a clean drop of medium.

    - Tubules in the biopsy sample can be carefully unraveled under the dissecting microscope, using fine watchmakers' forceps. Cut the tubules into small lengths of 1–2 cm and 'milk' the contents by squeezing from the middle to an open end (analogous to squeezing a tube of toothpaste). The cells can be picked out of the dish and examined under the ICSI microscope, or placed into a centrifuge tube of clean medium for further preparation. An alternative approach is to slit the segments of tubule rather than 'milking' to release the cells. Fresh testicular sperm are often immotile and combined with Sertoli cells, but free-swimming sperm are usually seen after further incubation. In cases of obstructive azoospermia, pregnancies have been achieved from testicular sperm incubated for up to 3 days after the biopsy procedure, but the proportion of motile sperm in a testicular biopsy sample is usually highest after 24 hours' incubation. Incubation at 32°C instead of 37°C may also be of benefit (Van den Berg, 1998). If fresh sperm is to be used, the biopsy procedure should be carried out the day before the planned oocyte retrieval. In cryopreserved samples, a higher proportion of frozen testicular sperm have been found to retain their motility on thawing if they have been incubated for 24–48 hours before freezing; however, in cases of nonobstructive azoospermia, incubation for longer than 24 hours is not recommended. When biopsied sperm are processed in advance, any motile sperm found using an injection needle can be stored in empty zonae before freezing (see Chapter 12); this has the advantage that the sperm are then readily available at the time of ICSI, which can save considerable time.

# Spermatid Identification

In some cases of severe testicular dysfunction, no spermatozoa can be found either in the ejaculate or in testicular tissue, but precursor cells (round, elongating or elongated spermatids) may be identified. Although there was initial enthusiasm in the late 1990s with the technique of round spermatid nucleus injection (ROSNI), this was short-lived with the prospect of unresolved genetic concerns and poor activating capacity of the immature sperm cells. Spermatid injection is forbidden by the HFEA in the United Kingdom, and also by regulatory authorities in some other countries. Males with meiotic arrest of spermatogenesis are counseled toward the use of donor sperm.

Using Hoffman Modulation Contrast systems, four categories of spermatids can be observed and identified according to their shape, amount of cytoplasm, and size of tail: round, elongating, elongated and mature spermatids just prior to their release from Sertoli cells. However, in practice it can be difficult to confidently identify immature sperm cells in a wet preparation. Round spermatids must be distinguished from other round cells such as spermatogonia, spermatocytes, polymorphonuclear leukocytes, lymphocytes and erythrocytes. Their diameter (6.5–8 μm) is similar to that of erythrocytes (7.2 μm) and small lymphocytes. Round spermatids may be observed at three different phases: Golgi, cap and acrosome phase (where the nucleus moves toward a peripheral position). When the cell is rotated, a centrally located smooth (uncondensed) nucleus can be seen, and a developing acrosomal structure may be observed as a bright spot or small protrusion on one side of the cell, adjacent to the spermatid nucleus. Sertoli cell nuclei are very flat and transparent, with a prominent central or adjacent nucleus, whereas the round spermatid is a three-dimensional round cell (Figure 10.3a). Phase 3 is a transition between round and elongated forms; elongated spermatids have an elongated nucleus at one side of the cell and a larger cytoplasmic region on the other side, surrounding the developing tail (Figure 10.3b).

# Pathology of Azoospermia

The Johnsen score is an assessment of the degree of spermatogenesis found in a biopsy: a number of tubules are assessed, and each one is given a score for the most advanced stage of spermatogenesis seen:

(a)

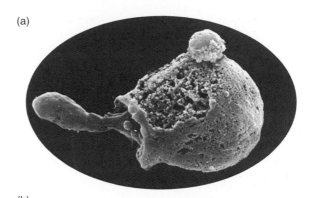

(b)

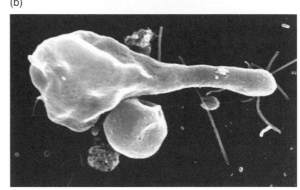

**Figure 10.3** (a and b) Scanning electron micrographs of early spermatid detected in azoospermic ejaculate. Courtesy of Professor B. Bartoov, Israel.

1 = no cells present in the tubule

2 = Sertoli cells

3 = spermatogonia

4–5 = spermatocytes

6–7 = spermatids

8–10 = spermatozoa.

Mean Johnsen Score (MJS) = average of all the tubules assessed, i.e.:

MJS = 2 is the Sertoli cell only syndrome

MJS = 8–10 is normal spermatogenesis

MJS between 2 and 8 represents varying degrees of subnormal spermatogenesis, but a qualitative description is required.

There is a correlation between testicular size and MJS.

## Pathologies

A. Pretesticular: deficient gonadotropin drive – low FSH

B. Androgen resistance: familial pseudohermaphroditism

207

C. Testicular failure: no spermatogenesis – raised FSH

D. Post-testicular duct obstruction: functional sperm usually present, size of testes is normal, FSH is not raised

## Pretesticular

These are pathologies that result in secondary testicular failure (hypogonadotropic hypogonadism) due to decreased gonadotropin release (low serum FSH). Testicular biopsy may show a prepubertal appearance, with precursors of Sertoli cells, prespermatogenic cells and absence of Leydig cells.

1. Congenital

    - partial or complete Kallman's syndrome, GnRH deficiency associated with agenesis of the first cranial nerve and thus anosmia
    - low FSH and LH, small but potentially normal testes.

2. Acquired: space-occupying lesions

    - pituitary tumors
    - craniopharyngioma
    - trauma, meningitis, sarcoidosis
    - Cushing's syndrome (adrenal hypoplasia)
    - congenital adrenal hyperplasia
    - hemochromatosis.

## Androgen Resistance

Familial incomplete male pseudohermaphroditism, type 1: partial or complete defects in amount or function of the androgen receptor. Patients fall into a wide spectrum of disorders, probably due to variable manifestations of a single-gene defect. Cryptorchidism is common, and the testes remain small in size. The testes demonstrate normal Leydig cells and tubules containing both germ cells and Sertoli cells, but there is usually no maturation beyond the primary spermatocyte. Plasma testosterone and LH are high, suggesting that there is a defect in the feedback control of testosterone on the hypothalamus. There are four (phenotypically) separate clinical disorders:

1. Rosewater's syndrome (mildest form)
2. Reinfenstein's syndrome
3. Gilbert–Dreyfus syndrome
4. Lub's syndrome (most severe) – phenotypic females with partial Wolffian duct development and masculine skeletal development.

## Testicular Failure

This can be congenital or acquired, and testicular biopsy can show a wide variation in appearance, e.g., sclerosing tubular degeneration is seen in Klinefelter's syndrome. Disorganization with extensive hyalinization and tubular atrophy is seen after orchitis.

1. Congenital

    - Klinefelter's syndrome (XXY)
    - autosomal abnormalities
    - torsion (maturation arrest)
    - cryptorchidism, anorchia
    - sickle cell disease
    - myotonic muscular dystrophy
    - Noonan's syndrome (male Turner's).

2. Acquired

    - mumps orchitis
    - epididymo-orchitis
    - testicular trauma
    - inguinal/scrotal surgery
    - radiotherapy.

## Post-testicular: Obstructive Causes of Azoospermia

Testicular biopsy shows well-preserved normal spermatogenesis, and there may be sloughing of superficial layers of the seminiferous epithelium. The upper epididymis is the most common site of genital tract obstruction (two-thirds of lesions), and multifocal sites of obstruction may be present. Obstructive lesions can be caused by specific or nonspecific infection, and edema and/or hematoma as a result of trauma can lead to epididymal or vasal obstruction.

1. Congenital:

    - Congenital absence of the vas deferens (CAVD – female partner should be screened for cystic fibrosis mutations)
    - Cystic fibrosis
    - Young's syndrome
    - Zinner's syndrome: congenital absence of the vas deferens, corpus and cauda epididymis, seminal vesicle, ampulla and ejaculatory duct – may be bilateral or unilateral and can be associated with ipsilateral renal agenesis – due to failure of the Wolffian (mesonephric) duct.

2. Acquired

    - TB
    - Gonococcal or chlamydial infection

- surgical trauma
- smallpox
- bilharziasis
- filariasis
- vasectomy.

## Other Causes of Spermatogenic Failure or Disorder

These may be associated with defective testosterone synthesis, decreased metabolic clearance rates, increased binding of testosterone to plasma proteins, increased plasma estradiol and low, normal or moderately elevated serum FSH levels.

1. Systemic illness:
   Fevers, burns, head trauma, chronic renal failure, thyrotoxicosis, diabetes, male anorexia nervosa, surgery, general anesthesia.
2. Drugs/industrial toxins:
   a. Therapeutic: sulfasalazine, nitrofurantoin, cimetidine, niridazole, colchicine, spironolactone, testosterone injections, cytotoxic agents
   b. Occupational: carbon disulfide (rayon), lead, dibromochloropropane, radiation
   c. Recreational abuse: alcohol, opiates, anabolic steroids.
3. Absent spermatogenesis: germinal aplasia or hypoplasia, Sertoli cell only (del Castillo) syndrome. Only Sertoli cells are present in the tubular epithelium; none of the spermatogenic elements remain. In germinal cell hypoplasia, there is a generalized reduction in the numbers of germ cells of all stages. The numbers of more mature cells are greatly reduced, and the germinal epithelium has a loose, poorly populated appearance. There are two forms:
   a. serum FSH is grossly elevated, Sertoli cells show severe abnormalities on electron microscopy – no inhibin production
   b. serum FSH is normal – normal inhibin production.

   Testis size is often not markedly reduced, and this may lead to diagnostic difficulties. These patients are frequently misdiagnosed as having an obstructive lesion, and biopsy is the only means of making a correct diagnosis.

4. Leydig cell failure leads to low testosterone levels, and raised serum FSH and LH. In this situation the testis is atrophied, with gross reduction in size.
5. Immotile sperm: Kartagener's immotile cilia syndrome. Normal numbers of sperm are present in the semen, but they are all immotile. Transmission electron microscopy shows that the central filaments of the tails are absent, and this anomaly may be present in cilia throughout the body, resulting in chronic sinusitis and bronchiectasis.
6. Retrograde ejaculation: diabetes, multiple sclerosis, sympathectomy, prostatectomy, funnel bladder neck.
7. Ejaculatory failure: spinal cord injury, multiple sclerosis, diabetes, abdominal aortic surgery, abdominoperineal resection, psychomimetic/antihypertensive drugs, hypogonadism.

# Chromosomal Anomalies

## Klinefelter's Syndrome

- Bilateral testicular atrophy, signs of hypogonadism with a greater span than height, often with gynecomastia.
- FSH and LH are extremely high, often with low testosterone.
- Diagnosis can be made on clinical and biochemical grounds, and confirmed by buccal smear or karyotype (XXY).
- Affects 1 in 400 live-born males, and is found in around 7% of infertile men.
- Testicular histology: obvious and gross spermatogenic failure with disappearance of all the spermatogenic elements in all the tubules. Marked hyperplasia of the Leydig cells.

## 46XX Klinefelter's

Patients are phenotypically male, with the same clinical and endocrinological features as the XXY patient. H-Y antigen has been demonstrated: despite apparent absence of Y chromosome, there is expression of some Y genes.

## 46XX (Noonan's Syndrome)

Male equivalent of Turner's (XO): normal male phenotype, but are usually cryptorchid and show varying degrees of hypoandrogenization. There is testicular atrophy, raised FSH and LH, and reduced testosterone.

209

## Robertsonian Translocation

A form of chromosomal aberration which involves the fusion of long arms of acrocentric chromosomes at the centromere. Breaks occur at the extreme ends of the short arms of two nonhomologous acrocentric chromosomes; these small segments are lost, and the larger segments fuse at their centromeric region, producing a new, large submetacentric or metacentric chromosome.

'Balanced translocations' (see Chapter 14) may produce only minor deficiencies, but translocation heterozygotes have reduced frequencies of crossing-over and are usually subfertile through the production of abnormal gametes.

# Appendix
## Sperm Preparation: Equipment and Materials

Semen sterile collection pot 60 mL

Microscope (phase is useful)

Counting chamber (Makler, MicroCell or standard haemocytometer)

Centrifuge with swing-out rotor

Centrifuge tubes (15 mL)

Microscope slides

Coverslips

Disposable test-tubes: 4 mL, 10 mL

Culture media

Buoyant density media

Glass Pasteur pipettes

Disposable pipettes: 1, 5, 10 mL

Spirit burner + methanol or gas Bunsen burner

Plastic ampules or straws for sperm freezing

Sperm cryopreservation media (Chapter 12)

Supply of liquid nitrogen and storage dewars

## Further Reading

### Books

Aitken RJ, Comhaire FH, Eliasson R, *et al.* (1999) *WHO Manual for the Examination of Human Semen and Semen-Cervical Mucus Interaction*, 2nd edn. Cambridge University Press, Cambridge, UK.

Björndahl L, Mortimer D, Barratt CL (eds.) (2010) *A Practical Guide to Basic Laboratory Andrology.* Cambridge University Press, Cambridge, UK.

Elder K, Elliott T (1998) *The Use of Testicular and Epididymal Sperm in IVF.* Worldwide Conferences on Reproductive Biology. Ladybrook Publishing, Australia.

Glover TD, Barratt CLR, Tyler JPA, Hennessey JF (1990) *Human Male Fertility and Semen Analysis.* Academic Press, London.

Menkveld R, Oettler EE, Kruger TF, *et al.* (1991) *Atlas of Human Sperm Morphology.* Williams & Wilkins, Baltimore.

Mortimer D (1994) *Practical Laboratory Andrology.* Oxford University Press, New York.

World Health Organization (2010) *WHO Manual for the Examination and Processing of Human Semen,* 5th edn. WHO, Geneva.

### Publications

Agarwal A, Deepinder F (2009) Determination of seminal oxidants (reactive oxygen species). In: Lipshult L, Howards S, Neiderberger C (eds.) *Infertility in the Male*, 4th edn. Cambridge University Press, Cambridge, UK.

Aitken RJ (1988) Assessment of sperm function for IVF. *Human Reproduction* 3: 89–95.

Aitken RJ (1989) The role of free oxygen radicals and sperm function. *International Journal of Andrology* 12: 95–97.

Aitken RJ (1990) Evaluation of human sperm function. *British Medical Bulletin* 46: 654–674.

Aitken RJ (2006) Sperm function tests and fertility. *International Journal of Andrology* 29(1): 69–75.

Aitken RJ, Clarkson JS (1987) Cellular basis of defective sperm function and its association with the genesis of reactive oxygen species by human spermatozoa. *Journal of Reproductive Fertility* 81: 459–469.

Aitken RJ, Gordon E, Harkiss D, *et al.* (1998) Relative impact of oxidative stress on the functional competence and genomic integrity of human spermatozoa. *Biology of Reproduction* 59: 1037–1046.

Barratt CLR, Bolton AE, Cooke ID (1990) Functional significance of white blood cells in the male and female reproductive tract. *Human Reproduction* 5(6): 639–648.

Braude PR, Bolton VN (1984) The preparation of spermatozoa for in vitro fertilization by buoyant density centrifugation. In: Feichtinger W, Kemeter P (eds.) *Recent Progress in Human In Vitro Fertilisation.* Cofese, Palermo, pp. 125–134.

Cohen J, Edwards RG, Fehilly C, *et al.* (1985) In vitro fertilization: a treatment for male infertility. *Fertility and Sterility* 43: 422–432.

Comhaire F, Depoorter B, Vermeulen L, Schoonjans F (1995) Assessment of sperm concentration. In: Hedon B, Bringer J, Mares P (eds.) *Fertility and Sterility: A Current Overview* (IFFS 1995). Parthenon Publishing Group, New York, pp. 297–302.

Donnelly ET, McClure N, Lewis SEM (1999) The effect of ascorbate and alpha-tocopherol supplementation in vitro on DNA integrity and hydrogen peroxide-induced DNA damage in human spermatozoa. *Mutagenesis* 14(5): 505–512.

Dravland JE, Mortimer D (1985) A simple discontinuous Percoll gradient for washing human spermatozoa. *IRCS Medical Science* 13: 16–18.

Edwards RG, Fishel SG, Cohen J, *et al.* (1984) Factors influencing the success of in vitro fertilization for alleviating human infertility. *Journal of In Vitro Fertilization and Embryo Transfer* 1: 3–23.

Elder KT, Wick KL, Edwards RG (1990) Seminal plasma anti-sperm antibodies and IVF: the effect of semen sample collection into 50% serum. *Human Reproduction* 5: 179–184.

Evenson DP, Jost LJ, Marshal D, *et al.* (1999) Utility of the sperm chromatin structure assay as a diagnostic and prognostic tool in the human fertility clinic. *Human Reproduction* 14: 1039–1049.

Fleming SD, Meniru GI, Hall JA, Fishel SB (1997) Semen analysis and sperm preparation. In: *A Handbook of Intrauterine Insemination.* Cambridge University Press, Cambridge, UK.

Franken D (1998) Sperm morphology: a closer look – is sperm morphology related to chromatin packaging? *Alpha Newsletter* 14: 1–3.

Gallo A, Menezo Y, Dale B, *et al.* (2018) Metabolic enhancers supporting 1-carbon cycle affect sperm functionality: an in vitro comparative study. *Scientific Reports* 8: 11769 DOI:10.1038/s41598-018-30066-9.

Grobler GM, De Villiers TJ, Kruger TF, Van Der Merwe JP, Menkveld R (1990) Part Two – The Tygerberg Experience. In: Acosta AA, Swanson RJ, Ackerman SB, *et al.* (eds.) *Human Spermatozoa in Assisted Reproduction.* Williams & Wilkins, Baltimore, pp. 280–285.

Hall J, Fishel S, Green S, *et al.* (1995) Intracytoplasmic sperm injection versus high insemination concentration in-vitro fertilization in cases of very severe teratozoospermia. *Human Reproduction* 10: 493–496.

Hamamah S, Gatti J-L (1998) Role of the ionic environment and internal pH on sperm activity. *Human Reproduction* 13(Suppl. 4): 20–30.

Henkel R, Sandhu IS, Agarwal A (2018). The excessive use of antioxidant therapy: a possible cause of male infertility? *Andrologia* 2019; 51(1): e13162.

Hinsch E, Ponce AA, Hägele W, *et al.* (1997) A new combined in-vitro test model for the identification of substances affecting essential sperm functions. *Human Reproduction* 12(8): 1673–1681.

Hughes CM, McKelvey-Martin VJ, Lewis SE (1999) Human sperm DNA integrity assessed by the Comet and ELISA assays. *Mutagenesis* 14(1): 71–75.

Jager S, Kremer J, Van-Schlochteren-Draaisma T (1978) A simple method of screening for antisperm antibodies in the human male: detection of spermatozoa surface IgG with the direct mixed antiglobulin reaction carried out on untreated fresh human semen. *International Journal of Fertility* 23: 12.

Lessey BA, Garner DL (1983) Isolation of motile spermatozoa by density gradient centrifugation in Percoll. *Gamete Research* 7: 49–52.

Makler A (1978) A new chamber for rapid sperm count and motility evaluation. *Fertility and Sterility* 30: 414.

Matson PL (1995) External quality assessment for semen analysis and sperm antibody detection: results of a pilot scheme. *Human Reproduction* 10: 620–625.

Ménézo Y, Dale B (1995) Paternal contribution to successful embryogenesis. *Human Reproduction* 10: 1326–1327.

Ménézo Y, Entezami F, Lichtblau L, Belloc S, Cohen M, Dale B (2013) Oxidative stress and fertility: incorrect assumptions and ineffective solutions? *Zygote* 20: 1–11.

Ménézo Y, Evenson D, Cohen M, Dale B (2013) Effect of anti-oxidants on sperm genetic damage. In: Baldi E, Muratori M (eds.) *Genetic Damage in Human Spermatozoa.* Advances in Experimental Medicine and Biology. Springer, New York, pp. 173–189.

Mortimer D (1991) Sperm preparation techniques and iatrogenic failures of in-vitro fertilization. *Human Reproduction* 6(2): 173–176.

Pacey AA (2006) Is quality assurance in semen analysis still really necessary? A view from the andrology laboratory. *Human Reproduction* 21(5): 1105–1109.

Pacey AA (2010) Quality assurance and quality control in laboratory andrology. *Asian Journal of Andrology* 12(1): 21–25.

Rainsbury PA (1992) The treatment of male factor infertility due to sexual dysfunction. In: Brinsden PR, Rainsbury PA (eds.) *In Vitro Fertilization and Assisted Reproduction.* Parthenon Publishing Group, Carnforth, UK, pp. 345–360.

Sakkas D, Alvarez JG (2010) Sperm DNA fragmentation: mechanisms of origin, impact on reproductive outcome, and analysis. *Fertility and Sterility* 93(4): 1027–1036.

Sakkas D, Mariethosz E, St John J (1999) Abnormal sperm parameters in humans are indicative of an abortive apoptotic mechanism linked to the FAS-mediated pathway. *Experimental Cell Research* 251: 350–355.

**211**

Sakkas D, Urmer F, Bizzaro D, *et al.* (1998) Sperm nuclear DNA damage and altered chromatin structure: effect on fertilization and embryo development. *Human Reproduction* 13(Suppl. 4): 11–19.

Sato K, Tanaka F, Hasegawa H (2004) Appearance of the oocyte activation of mouse round spermatids cultured in vitro. *Human Cell* 17(4): 177–180.

Sousa M, Barros A, Tesarik J (1998) Current problems with spermatid conception. *Human Reproduction* 13: 255–258.

Stewart B (1998) New horizons in male infertility: the use of testicular and epididymal sperm in IVF. *Alpha Newsletter* 13: 1–3.

Tomlinson MJ, Pooley K, Simpson T, *et al.* (2010) Validation of a novel computer-assisted sperm analysis (CASA) system using multitarget-tracking algorithms. *Fertility and Sterility* 93(6): 1911–1920.

Twigg JP, Fulton N, Gomez E, *et al.* (1998a) Analysis of the impact of intracellular reactive oxygen species generation on the structural and functional integrity of human spermatozoa and functional integrity of human spermatozoa: lipid peroxidation, DNA fragmentation and effectiveness of antioxidants. *Human Reproduction* 13(6): 1429–1436.

Twigg JP, Irvine DS, Aitken RJ (1998b) Oxidative damage to DNA in human spermatozoa does not preclude pronucleus formation at intracytoplasmic sperm injection. *Human Reproduction* 13(7): 1864–1871.

Van den Berg M (1998) Sample preparation. In: Elder K, Elliott T (eds.) *The Use of Epidemiological and Testicular Sperm in IVF*. World Wide Conferences on Reproductive Biology. Ladybrook Publishing, Australia, pp. 51–54.

Van der Ven H, Bhattacharya AK, Binor Z, Leto S, Zaneveld LJD (1982) Inhibition of human sperm capacitation by a high molecular weight factor from human seminal plasma. *Fertility and Sterility* 38: 753–755.

Vanderzwalmen P, Zech H, Birkenfeld A, *et al.* (1997) Intracytoplasmic injection of spermatids retrieved from testicular tissue: influence of testicular pathology, type of selected spermatids and oocyte activation. *Human Reproduction* 12: 1203–1213.

Yovich JL (1992) Assisted reproduction for male factor infertility. In: Brinsden PR, Rainsbury PA (eds.) *In Vitro Fertilization and Assisted Reproduction*. Parthenon Publishing Group, Carnforth, UK, pp. 311–324.

Yovich JM, Edirisinghe WR, Cummins JM, Yovich JL (1990) Influence of pentoxifylline in severe male factor infertility. *Fertility and Sterility* 53: 715–722.

# Oocyte Retrieval and Embryo Culture

## Preparation for Each Case

Every individual treatment cycle involves a number of different stages and manipulations in the laboratory, and each case must be assessed and prepared for in advance; the afternoon prior to the procedure (the day after hCG administration) is a convenient time to make the preparations. The laboratory staff should ensure that all appropriate consent forms have been signed by both partners, including consent for special procedures and storage of cryopreserved embryos. Details of any previous assisted conception treatment should be studied, including response to stimulation, number and quality of oocytes, timing of insemination, fertilization rate, embryo quality and embryo transfer procedure, and judgments regarding whether any parameters at any stage could be altered or improved in the present cycle can be assessed. The risk of introducing any infection into the laboratory via gametes and samples must be absolutely minimized: screening tests such as human immunodeficiency virus (HIV 1 and 2: Anti-HIV 1, 2) and hepatitis B (HbsAg/Anti-HBc) and C (Anti-HCV-Ab) should be confirmed, as well as any other tests indicated by the patients' history (e.g., HTLV-I antibody, RhD, malaria, *Trypanosoma cruzi*, Zika virus). If donor gametes are to be used, additional tests for the donor are required: chlamydia, cytomegalovirus and a validated testing algorithm to exclude the presence of active infection with *Treponema pallidum* for syphilis testing.

---

**Laboratory Preparation: Checklist for Each Case**

- Results of viral screening tests for both partners
- Consent forms signed by both partners
- Specific details or instructions regarding insemination, cryopreservation, number of embryos for transfer, etc.

---

- Results of semen assessments; note any special features or precautions for semen collection or preparation
- Previous history, current response to stimulation; note any special features of ultrasound scans, endocrine assays or IVF laboratory results
- Current cycle history: number of follicles, endocrine parameters, potential ovarian hyperstimulation syndrome (OHSS)

---

Laboratory case notes, media, culture vessels and tubes for sperm preparation, with clear and adequate labeling throughout, are prepared in advance of each case. All labeling should have a minimum of the patient's full name and a unique identifier, for example, patient number. When donor sperm is used, the donor code must uniquely identify that specific donor. Tissue culture dishes or plates can be equilibrated in the culture incubator overnight. The choice of culture system used is a matter of individual preference and previous experience; microdroplets under oil, four-well dishes and organ culture dishes are amongst those most commonly used.

## Culture Dish Preparation: General Considerations

### Osmolality

*In vitro*, gametes and embryos are very sensitive to even small external increases in the osmolality of their environment, with potentially dramatic effects on viability. Inappropriate handling of the culture system can lead to changes in osmolality that are sufficient to jeopardize embryonic development, and osmolality of a culture system is influenced by the methods used in dish preparation. Minimizing the risk of evaporation is crucial when preparing culture dishes: time, temperature, air flow, volume of media and oil overlay, as well as the method of preparation, must all be considered in order to avoid osmolality increases that may jeopardize embryo development (see Swain *et al.*, 2012; Elder *et al.*, 2015, Chapter 4). Evaporation can be minimized by taking culture media directly from the refrigerator immediately prior to dish preparation, so that the droplets are prepared with cold medium. In open cultures (without oil), a humidified atmosphere in the incubator is essential to prevent evaporation and increase in osmolality.

A number of systems are now available that differ from the traditional methods of placing droplets onto flat dish surfaces, such as microwell dishes with indents manufactured into the surface, GPS Corral dishes and dishes designed for use with time-lapse systems and incubators. Osmolality is an important factor that will influence the successful application of these systems. The depth of medium, surface area exposed to the oil overlay and depth of the overlay may all influence the osmolality of the culture medium. Preparation of dishes for time-lapse imaging requires special care in order to make sure that no bubbles are present. Devices used for microfluidic culture are particularly vulnerable to detrimental osmolality shifts due to evaporation; thin hybrid polydimethylsiloxane (PDMS)-Parylene membranes are recommended to circumvent this problem (Heo *et al.*, 2007).

### Practical Tips for Keeping Osmolality Constant during Preparation of Dishes

1. Take note of the osmolality and osmolyte content of the medium to be used; osmolytes act to maintain fluid balance within oocytes/blastomeres, and some media may have a lower concentration of osmolytes than others (HTF has no osmolytes). If there is a risk of increase in osmolality during preparation, consider using a medium that has a lower osmolality.

2. Work at room temperature, using medium that has been taken out of the refrigerator immediately prior to dish preparation.

3. Consider droplet size. Using larger volumes of media in the culture system will minimize the chance of large shifts in osmolality; droplet sizes less than 20 µl are not recommended.

4. Carefully note the date of first opening the bottle of medium in relation to the date of dish

preparation: osmolality can change if the bottle has been opened repeatedly.

5. Note the time/date of dish preparation: the likelihood of evaporation with resulting rise in osmolality is higher in dishes that have been in the incubator for long periods.

6. Prepare droplets as quickly as possible, reducing the number of droplets per dish if necessary.

7. If droplets are made before adding the oil overlay, replace original droplets with droplets of fresh medium in exactly the same spot after overlaying with oil.

8. If sufficient staff are available, the dishes can be prepared by two technicians: one to pipette the droplets into the dish and the second to immediately cover the droplets with oil. Ensure that good laboratory practice and sterility is rigorously maintained throughout.

9. Be aware that osmolality will change more rapidly with 'open' culture and without humidified incubators.

10. Reduce airflow during dish preparation by turning the laminar air flow off. However, this is recommended only if background air has a suitable grade of purity. Since it is essential that sterility is maintained during dish preparation, an alternative to consider is reducing the air flow velocity by setting it to the lowest level during dish preparation.

11. Use washed/humidified oil: in general, there is always an equilibrium between the components of two liquid phases. Unless the oil is first washed with the same medium, an oil interface with albumin-carrying lipids in the medium may extract all lipophilic elements present in the medium. Washing can be carried out by gently shaking oil with medium in a ratio of 1(oil):2(medium) and leaving the mixture to settle overnight, until the two phases are clearly separate.

## Microdroplets under Oil

- Pour previously equilibrated mineral oil into 60-mm Petri dishes that are clearly marked with each patient's full name.

- Using either a Pasteur pipette or adjustable pipettor and sterile tips, carefully place eight or nine droplets of medium around the edge of the dish. One or two droplets may be placed centrally, to be used as wash drops (alternatively, droplets can be placed first, and then overlaid with oil – see above).

- Examine the follicular growth records to assess approximately how many drops/dishes should be prepared; each drop may contain one or two oocytes. Droplet size can range from 50 to 250 μL per droplet.

## Four-Well Plates

This system may also be used in combination with an overlay of equilibrated mineral oil.

- Prepare labeled and numbered plates containing 0.5–1 mL of tissue culture medium; each well is normally used to incubate up to three oocytes.
- Equilibrate overnight: If used without an oil overlay, the incubator must be humidified.
- Small Petri dishes with approximately 2 mL of HEPES-containing medium may also be prepared, to be used for washing oocytes immediately after identification in the follicular aspirates (media containing HEPES should not be equilibrated in a $CO_2$ atmosphere).

Organ culture (center well) dishes can also be used for group culture: place three 250-μL drops in the center well, and three to four oocytes in each drop.

## New Directions for Culture Systems

The quest for defining better media and culture systems has traveled from simple salt solutions in gas-filled desiccators to computer-controlled microchambers with continuous renewal of media (Figure 11.1). Microfluidic systems extend the strategy behind sequential media by aiming to mimic dynamic changes in the tubal environment of the embryo during its transit toward the uterus (Swain et al., 2012, 2013; da Rocha & Smith, 2012, 2014). At present, the use of such chambers is limited by high costs, and by problems associated with maintaining sterile conditions in pumps and tubing. Dynamic culture platforms that involve tilting and vibrating ('rock and roll') have also been proposed as being of potential benefit, by disrupting media gradients that form around cells or stimulating mechano-sensitive signaling pathways that might stimulate embryo growth (Swain, 2013).

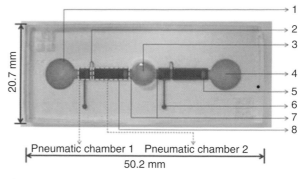

**Figure 11.1** Example of a microfluidic device used for embryo culture. 1: Reservoir for fresh medium; 2: pneumatic microchannel; 3: cell culture chamber; 4: waste medium reservoir; 5: normally closed valve; 6: airtube insertion hole; 7: microchannel for medium; 8: pneumatically driven membrane-based micropump. Adapted from da Rocha & Smith (2012), with kind permission from Springer Science+Business Media.

**Laboratory Supplies for Labeling and Preparation**

- Pots for semen collection
- Test-tubes for sperm preparation: conical tubes, small and large round-bottomed tubes
- Aliquots of media for each patient
- Culture vessels for overnight equilibration
- Paperwork for recording case details and results

## Oocyte Retrieval (OCR) and Identification

A Class II biological safety cabinet is recommended for handling of follicular aspirates to avoid risk of infection, but be aware that the laminar flow of air can have a dramatic cooling effect on the samples.

Prior to the follicle aspiration procedure:

1. Ensure: heating blocks, stages and trays are warmed to a temperature that will maintain the medium in the dishes at 37°C; media to be used for flushing/rinsing must also be warmed and equilibrated to correct pH.
2. Prewarm collection test-tubes and 60-mm Petri dishes for scanning aspirates.
3. Prepare a sterile Pasteur pipette plus holder, a fine-drawn blunt Pasteur pipette as a probe for manipulations, and 1-mL syringes with attached needles for dissection.
4. Check patient ID, confirm names and unique identifiers on dishes and laboratory case notes with medical notes.

**215**

If follicular aspirates cannot be examined immediately, they should be collected into test-tubes that are completely filled with fluid, tightly sealed and rigorously maintained at 37°C until they reach the laboratory. Aliquot the contents of each test-tube into two or three Petri dishes, forming a thin layer of fluid that can be quickly, carefully and easily scanned for the presence of an oocyte, using a stereo dissecting microscope with transmitted illumination base and heated stage. Low-power magnification ($\times6$–12) can be used for scanning the fluid, and oocyte identification verified using higher magnification ($\times25$–50). Always work quickly and carefully, with rigid attention to sterile technique, maintaining correct temperature and pH at all times.

## Oocyte Identification

The oocyte usually appears within varying quantities of cumulus cells and, if very mature, may be pale and difficult to see. (Immature oocytes are dark and also difficult to see.) Granulosa cells are clearer and more 'fluffy,' present in amorphous, often iridescent clumps. Blood clots, especially from the collection needle, should be carefully dissected with 23-gauge needles to check for the presence of cumulus cells.

The presence of blood clots within the cumulus–oocyte complex (COC) may be a reflection of poor follicular development, with an effect on the competence of the corresponding oocyte (Ebner, 2008). When a COC is identified, assess its stage of maturity by noting the volume, density and condition of the surrounding cumulus cells and the expansion of coronal cells. It is unlikely that the oocyte itself can be seen, since it will most commonly be surrounded by cumulus cells. However, when an oocyte can be observed with minimal cumulus cells, the presence of a single polar body indicates that it has reached the stage of metaphase II. The appearance of the COC can be used to classify the oocyte according to the following scheme (Figure 11.2):

1. *Germinal vesicle*: the oocyte is very immature. There is no expansion of the surrounding cells, which are tightly packed around the oocyte. A large nucleus (the germinal vesicle) is still present and may occasionally be seen with the help of an inverted microscope. Maturation may occasionally take place in vitro from this stage, and the COC can be assessed later in the day prior to insemination (Figure 11.2e).

2. *Metaphase I*: the oocyte is surrounded by a tightly apposed layer of corona cells; tightly packed cumulus with little extracellular matrix may surround this with a maximum size of approximately five oocyte diameters. If the oocyte can be seen, it no longer shows a germinal vesicle. The absence of a polar body indicates that the oocyte is in metaphase I, and these immature oocytes may be preincubated for 6–24 hours before insemination (Figure 11.2f).

3. *Metaphase II*:

   a. *Preovulatory* (harvested from Graafian follicles): this is the optimal level of maturity, appropriate for successful fertilization. Coronal cells are still apposed to the oocyte but are fully radiating; one polar body has been extruded. The cumulus has expanded into a fluffy viscous mass that can be easily stretched, with abundant extracellular matrix (Figure 11.2a and b).

   b. *Mature*: the oocyte can often be seen clearly as a pale orb; little coronal material is present and is dissociated from the oocyte. The cumulus is very profuse but is still cellular. The latest events of this stage involve a condensation of cumulus into small black (refractile) drops, as if a tight corona is reforming around the oocyte. The perivitelline space often shows granularity (Figure 11.2h).

   c. *Luteinized*: the oocyte is very pale and often is difficult to find. The cumulus has broken down and becomes a gelatinous mass around the oocyte. These oocytes have a low probability of fertilization, and are usually inseminated with little delay (Figure 11.2).

   d. *Atretic*: the oocyte is very dark and can be difficult to identify. Granulosa cells are fragmented and have a lace-like appearance.

Gross morphological assessment of oocyte maturity is highly subjective and open to inaccuracies. In preparation for intracytoplasmic sperm injection (ICSI), the oocytes are completely denuded of surrounding cells using hyaluronidase, allowing accurate assessment of nuclear maturity and cytoplasm; this process has made it apparent that gross COC morphology does not necessarily correlate with nuclear maturity, and there is considerable conflict in the data

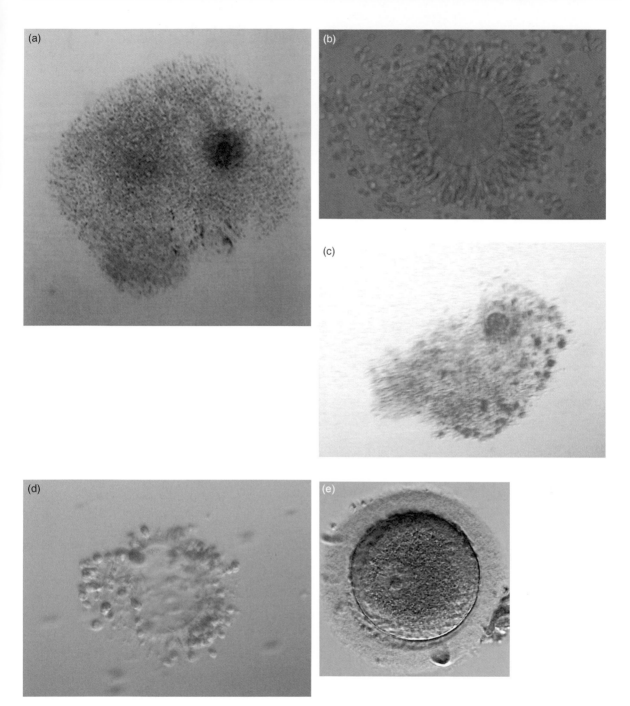

**Figure 11.2** Images after oocyte retrieval, before and after hyaluronidase denudation. Cumulus–oocyte complexes, without denudation: (a) cumulus–oocyte complex visualized under dissecting microscope, ×25 magnification (see color plate section); (b) phase-contrast image of mature metaphase II cumulus–oocyte complex, first polar body visible (see color plate section); (c) cumulus–oocyte complex with clumped refractile areas indicating signs of luteinization (see color plate section); (d) empty zona pellucida. Phase-contrast images after denudation: (e) germinal vesicle; (f) metaphase I oocyte, polar body not extruded; (g) preovulatory metaphase II oocyte, polar body extruded; (h) postmature oocyte, showing granularity in the perivitelline space, (i) dysmorphic metaphase II oocyte showing a large necrotic first polar body. Images (e), (f), (g) courtesy of Julia Uraji; Images (h) and (i) courtesy of Thomas Ebner, Austria.

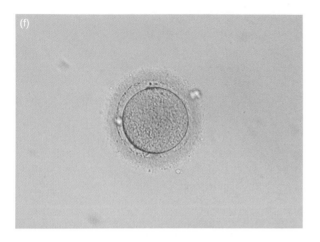

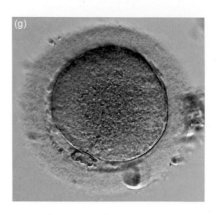

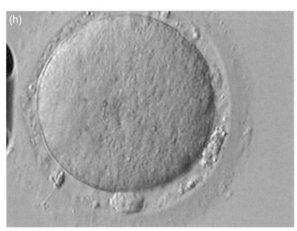

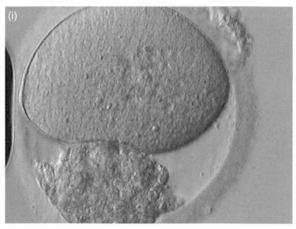

**Figure 11.2** *(cont.)*

available regarding the association between oocyte morphology and treatment outcome (see Ebner, 2006, for review). A number of dysmorphic features can be identified in denuded oocytes, including areas of necrosis, organelle clustering, vacuolation or accumulating aggregates of smooth endoplasmic reticulum (sER). Anomalies of the zona pellucida and nonspherical oocytes can also be seen. In practice, a wide variety of unusual and surprising dysmorphisms are often observed. A collection of interesting photographs, together with patient clinical details and histories, can be seen in the *Atlas of Oocytes, Zygotes and Embryos in Reproductive Medicine* by Van den Bergh *et al.* (2012).

Some features of dysmorphism may be associated with the endocrine environment during ovarian stimulation, in particular the structure of the zona pellucida and/or oolemma (Ebner, 2002, 2006). Although aberrations in the morphology of oocytes are not necessarily of any consequence to fertilization or early cleavage after ICSI, it is possible that embryos generated from dysmorphic oocytes have a reduced potential for implantation and further development. Repeated appearance of some dysmorphic features such as sER aggregation, central granulation or vacuoles in an individual patient's oocyte cohort may indicate an underlying intrinsic problem in the process of oocyte development within the ovary.

**Dysmorphic Oocyte Features**

See Figure 11.3.

- Irregular shape
- Areas of necrosis in the cytoplasm
- Cytoplasmic granularity
- Organelle clustering
- Aggregates of sER
- Vacuoles/vesicles
- Anomalies of the zona pellucida

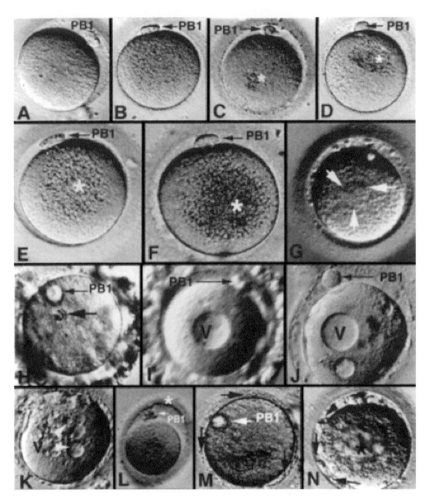

**Figure 11.3** Normal and dysmorphic oocytes (A, B). Normal appearing oocytes with no visually outstanding features (C–F). Varying degrees of organelle clusters (*) (central granularity) observed from mild to very severe. (G, N) Aggregation (arrows) of smooth endoplasmic reticulum as a flat, clear disc in the middle of the cytoplasm of the oocyte. (H) A dark 'horse-shoe-shaped' (large arrow) cytoplasmic inclusion. (I, J, K) Varying degrees (mild to severe) of fluid-filled vacuoles within the cytoplasm. (L) Organelle cluster with fragmented polar body (arrow) and increased perivitelline debris (*) and space. (K–M) Combination of cytoplasmic dysmorphisms and extracytoplasmic phenotypes. PB1 = first polar body. From Meriano *et al.* (2001), with permission from Oxford University Press.

Van Blerkom and Henry (1992) reported aneuploidy in 50% of oocytes with cytoplasmic dysmorphism; it is not clear whether oocyte aneuploidy is a fundamental developmental phenomenon or a patient-specific response to induced ovarian stimulation. In 1996, the same group related the oxygen content of human follicular fluid to oocyte quality and subsequent implantation potential. They propose that low oxygen tension associated with poor blood flow to follicles lowers the pH and produces anomalies in chromosomal organization and microtubule assembly, which might cause segregation disorders. Measurement of blood flow to individual follicles by power color Doppler ultrasound (Gregory and Leese, 1996) confirmed the observations of Van Blerkom *et al.* (1997) in correlating follicular blood flow with implantation; the incidence of triploid zygotes was also found to be significantly higher when oocytes were derived from follicles with poor vascularity. Follicular vascularity may also influence free cortisol levels in follicular fluid by promoting its diffusion across the follicle boundary. However, a robust model that can be applied for clinical assessment is not yet available (Mercé *et al.*, 2006).

## Insemination

Oocytes are routinely inseminated with a concentration of 100 000 progressively motile sperm per milliliter. If the prepared sperm show suboptimal parameters of motility or morphology, the insemination concentration may be accordingly increased. Some reports have suggested that the use of a high insemination concentration of up to 300 000 progressively motile sperm per milliliter may be a useful prelude before deciding upon ICSI treatment for male factor patients. Traditionally, inseminated oocytes were incubated overnight in the presence of the prepared sperm sample; however, sperm binding to the zona pellucida normally takes place within 1–3 hours of insemination, and fertilization occurs very rapidly thereafter. A few hours of sperm–oocyte contact yields the same time course of events that is observed after overnight incubation, and oocytes can be washed free of excess sperm after 3 hours' incubation (Gianaroli *et al.*, 1996; Ménézo and Barak, 2000).

For a culture system of microdroplets under oil, each oocyte is transferred into a drop containing motile sperm at a concentration of approximately 100 000 sperm/mL. In a four-well system, a measured volume of prepared sperm is added to each well, to a final concentration of approximately 100 000 progressively motile sperm per well.

---

**Insemination**

For microdroplets under oil, the oil overlays for insemination dishes must be prepared earlier, so that there is at least 4–6 hours of equilibration time.

1. Prepare a dilution of prepared sperm, containing 100 000 motile sperm/mL

   - Assess a drop of the dilution on a glass slide, under ×10 magnification; at least 20 motile sperm should be visible in the field.
   - Equilibrate the suspension at 37°C for 30 minutes, 5% $CO_2$.
   - Place droplets of the sperm suspension under the previously prepared and equilibrated oil overlays.
   - Examine each oocyte before transfer to the insemination drop, and dissect the cumulus to remove bubbles, large clumps of granulosa cells or blood clots if necessary.

2. If oocytes are in premeasured culture droplets, e.g., 240 μL, add 10 μL of a prepared sperm suspension that has been adjusted to $2.5 \times 10^6$/mL.

   - Final concentration = approximately 100 000 sperm/mL, or 25 000 sperm per oocyte.

3. Prepare labeled 35-mm Petri dishes containing equilibrated oil, to be used for culture of the zygotes after scoring for fertilization the following day.

---

**Four-well dishes and organ culture dishes**

- Add 0.5–1.0 mL of prepared sperm suspension to each well or drop.
- Total: approximately 100 000 motile sperm per well/drop.

---

# Scoring of Fertilization on Day 1

## Dissecting Fertilized Oocytes

Inseminated oocytes are dissected 17–20 hours following insemination in order to assess fertilization. Oocytes at this time are normally covered with a layer of dispersed coronal and cumulus cells, which must be carefully removed so that the cell cytoplasm can be examined for the presence of two pronuclei and two polar bodies, indicating normal fertilization. The choice of dissection procedure is a matter of individual preference, and sometimes a combination of methods may be necessary for particular cases. Whatever the method used, it must be carried out carefully, delicately and speedily, taking care not to expose the fertilized oocytes to changes in temperature and pH. Scoring for pronuclei should be carried out within the appropriate time span, before pronuclei merge during syngamy: cleaved embryos with abnormal fertilization are indistinguishable from those with two pronuclei.

## Dissection Techniques

1. Narrow-gauge pipetting: narrow-gauge pipettes can be made (see below), but commercial hand-held pipetting devices are simpler and more convenient. 'Flexipet' and 'Stripper' are hand-held pipetting devices for cumulus/corona removal, with sterile disposable polycarbonate capillaries of specified inner diameters ranging from 135 up to 175 or 600 μm. Variations that incorporate a capillary that attaches to a tiny pressure 'bulb' inserted into a hollow metal tube are also available.

   - Use the microscope at ×25 magnification, and choose a tip with a diameter slightly larger than the oocyte. (A tip that is too small will damage the oocyte; therefore, take care in selecting the appropriate diameter.)

- Aspirate approximately 2 cm of clean culture medium into the tip, providing a protective buffer. This allows easy flushing of the oocyte and prevents it from sticking to the inside surface of the tip.
- Place the tip over the oocyte and gently aspirate it into the shaft.
- If the oocyte does not easily enter, change to a larger diameter pipette. (However, if the diameter is too large, it will be ineffective for cumulus removal.)
- Gently aspirate and expel the oocyte through the pipette, retaining the initial buffer volume, until sufficient cumulus and corona is removed to allow clear visualization of the cell cytoplasm and pronuclei.

2. Needle dissection: use two 26-gauge needles attached to 1-mL syringes, microscope at ×25 magnification. Use one needle as a guide, anchoring a piece of cellular debris if possible; slide the other needle down the first one, 'shaving' cells from around the zona pellucida, with a scissors-like action.

Before commercial hand-held denudation devices were available, a technique known as 'Rolling' was sometimes used, and a description of this method is included here for historical interest only.

- Use one 23-gauge needle attached to a syringe, and a fine glass probe.
- With the microscope at ×12 magnification, use the needle to score lines in each droplet on the base of the plastic dish.
- Adjust the magnification to ×25, and push the oocyte gently over the scratches with a fire-polished glass probe until the adhering cells are teased away. This technique was useful in removing adherent sticky blood clots.

Great care must be taken with any technique to avoid damaging the zona pellucida or the oocyte either by puncture or overdistortion. Breaks or cracks in the zona can sometimes be seen, and a small portion of the oocyte may extrude through the crack. (This may have occurred during dissection or during the aspiration process.) Occasionally the zona is very fragile, fracturing or distorting at the slightest touch; it is probably best not to continue the dissection in these cases.

### Making Narrow-Gauge Pipettes

The preparation of finely drawn pipettes with an inner diameter slightly larger than the circumference of an oocyte is an acquired skill which requires practice and patience.

- Hold both ends of the pipette, and roll an area approximately 2.5 cm below the tapered section of the pipette over a gentle flame (Bunsen or spirit burner).
- As the glass begins to melt, quickly pull the pipette in both directions to separate.
- Before the glass has a chance to cool, carefully and quickly break the pipette at an appropriate position.
- The tip must have a clean break, without rough or uneven edges; these will damage the oocyte during dissection.
- Examine the tip of each pipette to ensure that it is of accurate diameter, with smooth clean edges.

## Pronuclear Scoring

An inverted microscope is recommended for accurate scoring of fertilization; although the pronuclei can be seen with dissecting microscopes, it can often be difficult to distinguish normal pronuclei from vacuoles or other irregularities in the cytoplasm. Normally fertilized oocytes should have two pronuclei, two polar bodies, regular shape with intact zona pellucida and a clear healthy cytoplasm. A variety of different features may be observed: the cytoplasm of normally fertilized oocytes is usually slightly granular, whereas the cytoplasm of unfertilized oocytes tends to be completely clear and featureless. The cytoplasm can vary from slightly granular and healthy-looking, to brown or dark and degenerate. The shape of the oocyte may also vary, from perfectly spherical to irregular (see Figure 11.3). A clear halo of peripheral cytoplasm 5–10 mm thick is an indication of good activation and reinitiation of meiosis. The pattern and alignment of nucleoli has also been thought to be significant (Scott and Smith, 1998; Tesarik and Greco, 1999).

Approximately 5% of fertilized oocytes in human IVF routinely show abnormal fertilization, with three or more pronuclei visible; this is attributed to polyspermy, or nonextrusion of the second polar body. Fluorescent in-situ hybridization (FISH) analysis indicates that 80–90% of these zygotes are mosaic after cleavage. Single pronucleate zygotes obtained after conventional IVF analyzed by FISH to determine their ploidy reveal that a proportion of these zygotes are diploid (Levron *et al.*, 1995). It seems that during the course of their interaction, it is possible for human gamete nuclei to associate together and form diploid, single pronucleate zygotes. These findings may indicate a variation of human pronuclear interaction during syngamy, and the authors suggest that single pronucleate zygotes which develop with normal cleavage may be selected for transfer in cases where no other suitable embryos are available.

Details of morphology and fertilization should be recorded for each zygote, for reference when choosing embryos for transfer. Remove zygotes with normal fertilization at the time of scoring from the insemination drops or wells, transfer into new dishes or plates containing pre-equilibrated culture medium, and return them to the incubator for a further 24 hours of culture. Those with abnormal fertilization such as multipronucleate zygotes should be discarded, so that there is no possibility of their being selected for embryo transfer; after cleavage, these are indistinguishable from normally fertilized oocytes.

Although the presence of two pronuclei confirms fertilization, their absence does not necessarily indicate fertilization failure, and may instead represent either parthenogenetic activation or a delay in timing of one or more of the events involved in fertilization (Figure 11.4). Numerous studies have accumulated evidence to demonstrate that up to 40% of oocytes with no sign of fertilization 17–27 hours after insemination may have the appearance of morphologically normal embryos on the following day, with morphology and cleavage rate similar to that of zygotes with obvious pronuclei on Day 1. However, around a third of these zygotes may subsequently arrest on Day 2 (Plachot *et al.*, 1993). Cytogenetic analysis of these embryos reveals a higher incidence of chromosomal anomalies and a high rate of haploidy, confirming parthenogenetic activation (Plachot *et al.*, 1988, 1993).

Delayed fertilization with the appearance of pronuclei on Day 2 may also be observed, and these embryos also tend to have an impaired developmental potential. Delayed fertilization can be attributed to morphological or endocrine oocyte defects in some cases, and to sperm defects in others. No obvious association with either oocyte or sperm defects can be found in a number of cases (Oehninger *et al.*, 1989).

## Reinsemination

Reinsemination of oocytes that fail to demonstrate clear pronuclei at the time of scoring for fertilization is a practice that has been widely questioned scientifically. Fertilization or cleavage may subsequently be observed on Day 2, but this may be as a consequence of the initial insemination, and the delay in fertilization may be attributed either to functional disorders of the sperm, or maturation delay of the oocyte. These embryos generally have a poor prognosis for implantation.

## 'Rescue' ICSI

In cases of total failure of fertilization after IVF or ICSI, 'rescue' is sometimes attempted as a last resort by injecting the oocytes on Day 1. This practice is banned in some countries such as the United Kingdom, since it cannot be certain if a sperm has already entered the oocyte and fertilization is delayed. Others reserve rescue ICSI only for cases where there is complete failure to fertilize following conventional IVF. However, it is now clear that successful embryo development is crucially dependent upon events surrounding the timing of fertilization, as well as on cytoplasmic maturity: extended culture risks numerous negative effects on the oocyte. Although fertilization can sometimes be achieved via 'rescue ICSI,' developmental potential of the embryos is very poor, with minimal chance of pregnancy (see Beck-Fruchter *et al.*, 2014, for review).

## Selection of Pronucleate Embryos for Cryopreservation

Legislation in some countries forbids embryo freezing but allows cryopreservation at the zygote stage, before syngamy. Zygotes to be frozen should have a regular outline, distinct zona and clearly visible pronuclei. The cryopreservation procedure must be initiated while the pronuclei are still visible, before the onset of syngamy (see Chapter 12).

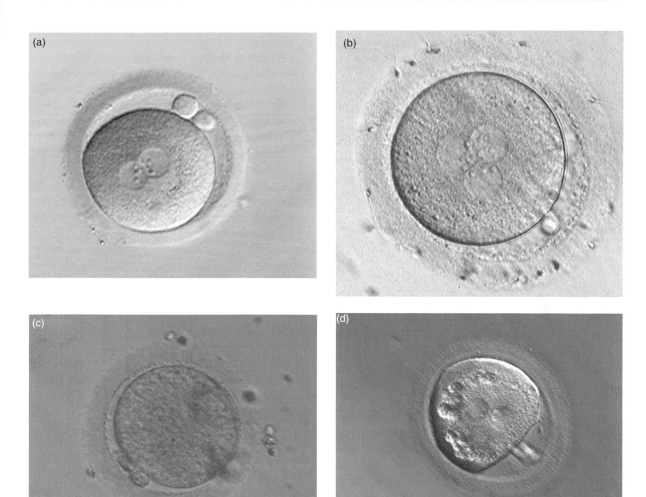

**Figure 11.4** Phase-contrast micrographs of fertilized human oocytes. (a) Normal fertilization: two pronuclei, two polar bodies. See color plate section. (b) Abnormal fertilization: three pronuclei. See color plate section. (c) Abnormal fertilization, no pronuclei, two polar bodies. (d) Zygote showing two pronuclei, numerous vacuoles and irregular perivitelline space, illustrating that severely dysmorphic oocytes are capable of fertilization. With thanks to Marc van den Bergh.

## Selection of Embryos for Transfer

Historically, embryo transfer was carried out 2 days (approximately 48–54 hours) after oocyte retrieval, but transfer has been carried out from as early as 1 hour post-ICSI (AOT, activated oocyte transfer, Dale *et al.*, 1999) to 5 days later, at the blastocyst stage. Trials of zygote transfer on Day 1 also achieved acceptable pregnancy rates (Scott and Smith, 1998; Tesarik and Greco, 1999; Tesarik *et al.*, 2000); it seems that the specific timing of transfer may not be crucial for the human implantation process. On Day 2, cleaved embryos may contain from two to six blasto-

meres. Embryo transfer 1 day later, on Day 3, or on Day 5 at the blastocyst stage is advocated as a means of selecting embryos with higher implantation potential, by the elimination of those that arrest at earlier cleavage stages in vitro.

Two major problems continue to hinder the effectiveness of ART treatment: low implantation rates and a high incidence of multiple pregnancies. Poor endometrial receptivity and adverse uterine contractions can both contribute to early embryo loss, but the low efficiency of assisted conception is widely attributed to genetic defects in the embryo.

More than 40% of ART-derived embryos are known to harbor chromosomal abnormalities. Errors in meiotic and mitotic segregation of chromosomes in the oocyte and during the cleavage of early embryos can lead to different patterns of aneuploidy, including polyploidy and chaotic mosaics, which account for around one-third of aneuploidies involving more than one chromosome per cell. However, despite the fact that grossly abnormal chromosome complements are lethal, in most cases the morphology of embryos that are genetically normal does not differ markedly from those with aneuploid, polyploid or mosaic chromosomal complements. Consequently, genetically abnormal embryos after IVF or ICSI may be graded as suitable for transfer using subjective selection criteria. Developing a reliable diagnostic test that can be used to identify embryos with the greatest developmental competence continues to be a major priority in human ART, in the hope of eventually selecting a single embryo that is likely to result in a healthy live birth following transfer.

In selecting embryos for transfer, the limitations of evaluating embryos based on morphological criteria alone are well recognized: correlations between gross morphology and implantation are weak and inaccurate, unless the embryos are clearly degenerating/fragmented. Objective criteria for evaluating embryos are available in laboratories with research facilities, but may be out of reach for a routine clinical IVF laboratory without access to specialized equipment and facilities. Objective measurements of human embryo viability that have been applied historically include:

- High-resolution videocinematography
- Computer-assisted morphometric analysis
- Blastomere or polar body biopsy for cytogenetic analysis
- Culture of cumulus cells
- Oxygen levels in follicular fluid/perifollicular vascularization
- Distribution of mitochondria and ATP levels in blastomeres
- Molecular approaches:
  - Metabolic assessment of culture media (amino acid profiling, metabolomics)
  - Gene expression/expression of messenger RNA (mRNA) in cumulus cells and/or embryos.

### Sequence of Events Observed by Time-Lapse Cinematography

From Mio and Maeda (2008).

Day 0 = day of OCR, insemination approximately 4–5 hours post OCR.

| Hours post-insemination: | Observation: |
| --- | --- |
| 1.5 ± 0.2 | Sperm penetrated |
| 2.0 ± 0.2 | Sperm incorporated |
| 2.5 ± 1.2 | Second polar body extruded |
| 2.5 ± 0.5 | Cone appearance (interaction between sperm midpiece and oocyte plasma membrane) |
| 3.7 ± 0.7 | Appearance of cytoplasmic flare (may represent sperm aster) |
| 4.5 ± 0.8 | Cone disappears |
| 5.5 ± 0.5 | Cytoplasmic flare disappears |
| 6.6 ± 0.3 | Male pronucleus formed |
| 6.8 ± 0.3 | Female pronucleus formed |
| 8.8 ± 0.7 | Both pronuclei abutted |
| 9.0 ± 0.5 | Halo appears |
| 19.2 ± 1.1 | Halo disappears |
| 24.8 ± 1.0 | Syngamy |
| 27.3 ± 1.0 | First cleavage commenced |
| 37.2 ± 1.2 | Second cleavage commenced |

Activation of the zygote genome begins at this stage, with massive increase in transcription and translation; this cell cycle requires a full 24 hours.

By 96 hours post-insemination, on Day 4: compacting morula stage (around 32 cells).

Day 5: differentiation to blastocyst stage. Cell number may vary considerably, from 50 to 100–120 cells for early expanding blastocysts.

Hatching may start as early as the morning of Day 5 but is usually observed on Day 6/7.

## High-Resolution Videocinematography

As early as 1989, Cohen *et al.* carried out a classic experiment that aimed to clearly define morphological criteria that might be used for embryo assessment, using a detailed analysis of videotaped images. Immediately before embryo transfer, embryos were recorded on VHS for 30–90 seconds, at several focal points, using Nomarski optics and an overall magnification of ×1400. The recordings were subsequently analyzed by observers who were unaware of the outcome of the IVF procedure, and they objectively assessed a total of 11 different parameters:

| Objective Parameters Assessed on Videocinematography | |
|---|---|
| Cell organelles visible | Cellular extrusions |
| Blastomeres all intact | Cytoplasmic vacuoles |
| Identical blastomere size | Blastomeres contracted |
| Smooth membranes | % variation in zona thickness |
| Dark blastomeres | % extracellular fragments |
| Cell–cell adherence | |

Nine parameters were judged (+) or (–), and variation in zona thickness and percentage of extracellular fragments were given a numerical value. Analysis of these criteria showed no clear correlation with any intracellular features of morphology, but that the most important predictor of fresh embryo implantation was the percentage of variation in thickness of the zona pellucida. Embryos with a thick, even zona had a poor prognosis for implantation; those whose zona had thin patches also had 'swollen,' more refractile blastomeres, and had few or no fragments. This observation was one of the parameters that led the group to introduce the use of assisted hatching (see Chapter 13). In analyzing frozen-thawed embryos, the best predictor of implantation was cell–cell adherence. The proportion of thawed embryos with more than one abnormality (77%) was higher than that of fresh embryos (38%) despite similar implantation rates (18% versus 15%).

Nearly 30 years have elapsed since these observations were published, and the quest to identify specific morphological markers of embryo implantation potential still continues – now with the help of more sophisticated technology to measure both properties of the zona and detailed embryo morphology.

## Zona Pellucida Birefringence

Polarized microscopy allows three layers to be distinguished in the zona, with the innermost layer showing the greatest birefringence (i.e., a higher level of light retardance). Several studies have investigated a possible correlation between this zona property and implantation potential (Montag et al., 2008; Madaschi et al., 2009); there is no doubt that properties of the zona may be important in assessing oocyte/embryo potential, particularly in response to exogenous FSH stimulation, but further studies are required in order to establish a clear correlation.

## Computer-Assisted Morphometric Analysis

High-resolution digital images of embryos can be assessed in detail with the help of computer-assisted multilevel analysis, which provides a three-dimensional picture of embryo morphology. A system with a computer-controlled motorized stepper mounted on the microscope will automatically focus through different focal planes in the embryo to produce a sequence of digital images. Automatic calculations of morphometric information from the image sequences describe features and measurements of each embryo, including size of nucleus and blastomeres and their spatial positions within the embryo, as well as features of the zona pellucida; all of the information is stored in a database. Preliminary results indicated that implantation was affected by the number and size of blastomeres on Day 3, and prediction of embryo implantation was superior to that of traditional manual scoring systems (Paternot et al., 2009). Additional information about morphology and embryo development has also accumulated from the use of modern systems that allow time-lapse photography in combination with culture systems.

## Aneuploidy Screening

Cytogenetic analysis of a biopsied polar body or blastomere has been used to screen embryos in order to detect those with an abnormal chromosome composition, a strategy known as aneuploidy screening or preimplantation genetic screening (PGS). The techniques employed for biopsy and diagnosis are described in Chapters 13 and 14, as well as the associated pros and cons. PGS continues to be a subject of considerable debate (Kuliev and Verlinsky, 2008; Mastenbroek et al., 2008; Sermondade and Mandelbaum, 2009; Dale et al., 2016; Gleicher and Orvieto, 2017): time-lapse studies have demonstrated that removing a single blastomere has a negative effect on embryo development (Kirkegaard et al., 2012b). Guidelines issued by the European Society for Human Reproduction and Embryology (ESHRE) and the American Society for Reproductive Medicine (ASRM) currently discourage the use of PGS.

## Follicular Indicators of Embryo Health

Each assisted conception cycle generates a number of waste products: luteinized granulosa cells, follicular fluids harvested from follicles at the time of oocyte retrieval and cumulus cells that can be removed and separated from the oocytes. These products have all been assayed to provide indices of embryo developmental competence. Biomarkers quantified in serum and follicular fluid include cytokines, C-reactive protein and leptin (Wunder *et al.*, 2005), inhibin B (Chang *et al.*, 2002) and reactive oxygen species (Das *et al.*, 2006). Cumulus cell gene expression profiles have also been linked to the implantation potential of oocytes and embryos (McKenzie *et al.*, 2004). While many of these parameters are indicative of follicular differentiated status at the time of oocyte harvest, follicular fluid is a highly concentrated cellular exudate, which is accumulated over an extended period. Consequently, to date neither follicular fluid nor granulosa cell assays at the time of oocyte collection have provided a consistent measure for assessing the implantation potential of individual embryos. The degree of follicular vascularization and its relationship to mitochondrial segregation in embryonic blastomeres has also been promoted as a determinant of embryo developmental competence (Van Blerkom *et al.*, 2000).

## Secreted Factors

Assessment of products secreted by the embryo, the embryonic 'secretome,' may be a better indicator of embryo development in vitro and in vivo than measurements of the follicular environment. For example, secretion of factors that regulate gamete transport and/or prepare the female tract for implantation has been used to predict embryo health. In this context, measurement of the amount of soluble human leukocyte antigen-G (HLA-G) into embryo culture media has been directly related to embryo quality and viability (Sher *et al.*, 2004). mRNAs for HLA-G can be detected in human blastocysts, but the cellular origins and biology of soluble HLA-G are not clear (Sargent, 2005). The suitability of HLA-G as a predictor of embryo developmental potential has also been questioned, as the amount of HLA-G measured in embryo culture media appears to exceed the total protein content of the embryo itself (Ménézo *et al.*, 2006).

## Molecular Approaches to Embryo Assessment

Analysis of medium that has been used for embryo culture offers further approaches to determine embryo 'health'/viability. Three different types of substance have been studied as potential biomarkers:

1. Proteins translated from specific gene expression products (proteomics)
2. Products of embryo metabolism, the metabolome: amino acids, oxidation products, carbohydrates, carboxylic acids (metabolomics)
3. RNA-based regulators of gene expression (small noncoding interference RNA, micro messenger RNA [miRNA]).

Since such molecules may be found in only minute quantities, assay methods must be highly sensitive, with cost efficiency and methodology that can be applied in clinical IVF. Apart from small sample volumes and low analyte concentrations, the presence of albumin in the media also makes it difficult to detect other proteins in a 60- to 70-kDa range.

Advances in technology facilitated noninvasive measurement of amino acid uptake/output into the spent culture medium of individual embryos, and products of embryo metabolism have been quantified and used in attempts to identify healthy embryos. During early development in vivo and in vitro, each preimplantation embryo will utilize numerous substrates from its immediate environment: oxygen for respiration, sugars, energy sources such as glucose and proteins/amino acids. The embryo also secretes many waste products of metabolism into its immediate environment. The turnover of these substrates and products has been measured in embryos themselves and in their culture environment (Gardner, 2007). Development of technologies to measure embryo metabolism led to the science of 'embryo metabolomics,' defined as 'the systematic analysis of the inventory of metabolites – as small molecule biomarkers – that represent the functional phenotype at the cellular level' (Posillico *et al.*, 2007). Amino acid turnover in spent embryo culture media has been measured noninvasively using high performance liquid chromatography (HPLC), gas chromatography and mass spectrometry, nuclear magnetic resonance spectroscopy and Raman near infrared spectroscopy. Embryo oxygen consumption by respirometry has also been used to quantify embryo metabolism. Details of the advantages and disadvantages associated with each of these different methods are reviewed by Rødgaard *et al.* (2015). Potential biomarkers were identified in different trials, but none have proved to be consistently helpful for clinical use.

The use of amino acid turnover to predict the developmental competence of individual embryos is based on the premise that metabolism is intrinsic to early embryo health and that the embryonic metabolome is immediately perturbed when embryos are stressed (Houghton and Leese, 2004; Lane and Gardner, 2005, Leese, 2012). Amino acid profiling has been extensively tested as a valid clinical diagnostic test for embryo selection in animal species, including mice, cows and pigs, as well as humans (Houghton *et al.*, 2002). Collectively the data on amino acid metabolism across these species indicate that:

1. The net rates of depletion or appearance of amino acids by individual embryos vary between amino acids and the stage of preimplantation development.
2. There is no difference between the turnover of essential and nonessential amino acids as defined by Eagle in 1959.
3. The turnover of amino acids is moderated by the concentrations of the amino acids in the embryo culture media.

The association of metabolic profiles of certain amino acids (particularly asparagine, glycine and leucine) with embryo viability is based on a variety of complex interactions that involve energy production, mitochondrial function, regulation of pH and osmolarity. Nevertheless, on the basis of the turnover of three to five key amino acids, morphologically similar cleavage stage human embryos which are metabolically 'quiet' were identified (Leese, 2002). These were identified to have the capacity to undergo zygotic genome activation and blastocyst development, and were compared with embryos which are metabolically active but are destined to undergo cleavage arrest (Houghton *et al.*, 2002). Interestingly, amino acid turnover by early cleavage embryos appears to be linked to embryo genetic health (Picton *et al.*, 2010). In this context inadequate energy production has been postulated as a cause of aneuploidy induction, due to errors during the energy-dependent processes of chromosome alignment, segregation and polar body formation (Bielanska *et al.*, 2002a; Ziebe *et al.*, 2003).

Preliminary trials of in-vitro amino acid profiling suggested that this strategy might be used to identify cleavage stage embryos with high implantation potential (Brison *et al.*, 2004). Metabolic profiles of developmentally competent, frozen-thawed human embryos were also consistent with those of fresh embryos (Brison *et al.*, 2004), and metabolic profiles could be used to identify frozen-thawed embryos with the potential to develop to the blastocyst stage in vitro.

Although underlying principles and concepts may be valid and initial results were encouraging, the technical demands of the assays and complexity of diagnosis have so far restricted their clinical application.

## Micro Messenger RNA (miRNA)

miRNAs are small, stable noncoding RNA molecules of 18–22 nucleotides that are thought to be negative regulators of gene expression, driving numerous cellular processes by repressing translation of mRNA. They are secreted from cells into the extracellular environment, where they may act as signaling molecules, and have been detected in urine, milk, saliva, semen and blood plasma. Their role in embryogenesis and development both in humans and in other species has been reviewed by Galliano & Pellicer (2014). The types and amounts of miRNA secreted into culture medium has been analyzed by quantitative real-time polymerase chain reaction (qPCR), with initial results suggesting that differences between viable and nonviable embryos can be detected (Kropp *et al.*, 2014; Rosenbluth *et al.*, 2014). The qPCR method is fast, relatively inexpensive and can be used with small sample volumes, but several logistic challenges still remain before it can be applied in routine clinical IVF.

## Mitochondrial DNA (mtDNA)

Studies examining the levels of mtDNA in blastocyst trophectoderm have suggested that embryos with high levels of mtDNA do not implant, and quantification of mtDNA in blastocyst trophectoderm has been proposed as another biomarker of embryo viability (Fragouli *et al.*, 2017; see Cecchino & Garcia-Velasco, 2019 for review). However, conflicting results continue to challenge the potential significance of mtDNA in human embryo implantation, and a number of studies have not been able to confirm this observation (Humaidan *et al.*, 2018). Methods used to quantify mtDNA have technical limitations, in particular due to the challenge of quantification in a small number of cells, as well as the fact that the number of cells in a trophectoderm biopsy varies from sample to sample. To compensate for this factor, the amount of mtDNA detected must be normalized against reference DNA sequences in the nuclear genome, and this crucial parameter can differ between protocols/studies. Our current understanding is inadequate in many areas, and further validation of protocols is essential. The technical challenges of mtDNA quantification must be fully appreciated in order to understand the significance of study results (Wells, 2017).

High levels of mtDNA are thought to be a reflection of cellular stress, and the levels could be influenced by factors specific to their in-vitro culture, such as culture medium, handling procedures or ovarian stimulation protocols, as well as by patient-specific parameters. It is possible that the phenomenon of elevated mtDNA as an indicator of embryo stress might be usefully applied in attempts to optimize aspects of IVF treatment.

## Gene Expression Studies

The activity of individual genes in an embryo change continuously in response to fluctuating intrinsic requirements or environmental conditions. Embryonic gene expression has been assessed at different stages of preimplantation development, using real-time PCR analysis of cDNA fragments as a measure of mRNA transcripts as well as by single-cell RNA-sequence profiling (Adjaye et al., 1998, Yan et al., 2013). More recently, in-vitro transcription techniques have been developed that allow oocyte and embryo mRNA to be amplified to a level that can be analyzed by microarrays (Wells, 2007). Factors related to patient or treatment have been shown to have an effect on gene expression in oocytes, morulae and blastocysts (Mantikou et al., 2016), and different patterns of gene expression have been associated with the use of different types of culture media (Kleijkers et al., 2015). Although the technology is far from routine clinical application, as a research tool it is hoped that data accumulated from gene expression studies over time may eventually lead to the identification of markers for embryo viability and implantation potential.

Overall, the search for biomarkers as predictors of developmental potential has highlighted important fundamental principles, in particular the fact that there may be differences between different patient populations, or even between individual embryos in a single cohort. It is now clear that early stage embryos have a high degree of plasticity, reflected by the effect of culture conditions on patterns of gene expression. Sophisticated analytical methods are capable of producing hundreds or thousands of variables that can mask a drift in accuracy; there are no simple 'standards,' and different analytical methods can produce varying results, making them difficult to standardize. Although the technologies continue to contribute to our basic knowledge about early embryo development, such concerns make the techniques difficult/impossible to introduce into clinical routine, and morphological assessment continues to be the most appropriate tool in selecting embryos for transfer in a routine IVF laboratory.

## Embryo Grading

Divergent national strategies define the maximum number of embryos that can be transferred in any one cycle, and elective single embryo transfer (eSET) is recommended for selected patient populations, in order to decrease the incidence of multiple births associated with ART. In the United Kingdom, the HFEA introduced a 'Multiple Births, Single Embryo Transfer Policy' in 2009, setting a target multiple birth rate for each UK clinic of 10%.

In routine practice, embryo selection for transfer continues to be based primarily on morphological assessment, often with multiple observations over the course of the embryo's development. Disturbance to the embryo culture system should be minimized, with assessment no more than once per day; some laboratories skip assessment on Day 2 or Day 4. Embryo development should also be checked within a time period that is appropriate to the laboratory workload.

Routine morphological assessment is highly subjective, with both inter- and intraobserver variation repeatedly documented. In addition, embryo development is affected by differences in culture media and environment, as well as by handling procedures. These two factors make it difficult to compare embryo scores/success rates between different units, and embryo assessment procedures should be validated both within laboratories and for each individual carrying out the assessment. Online external quality control schemes provide an extremely useful tool for training and validation procedures.

For cleavage stage embryos, assessment criteria include:

- rate of division judged by the number of blastomeres
- size, shape, symmetry and cytoplasmic appearance of the blastomeres

- presence of anucleate cytoplasmic fragments
- appearance of the zona pellucida.

Criteria are frequently combined to produce composite scoring systems which may incorporate pronuclear scoring of zygotes. Online quality control schemes are available, where participants can compare their scoring criteria for embryo assessments with those of others (www.fertaid.com, www.embryologists.org.uk/).

Although morphological assessment is recognized to be highly subjective, arbitrary and unsatisfactory, it is quick, noninvasive, easy to carry out in routine practice, and does help to eliminate those embryos with the poorest prognosis. Evaluation of blastomere shape, size and number will reflect synchronous cleavage of the blastomeres, and embryos with asynchrony in either the timing of cleavage or the process of blastomere division will be given lower scores. Unfortunately embryo cleavage in vitro rarely follows the postulated theoretical timing of early development, and computer-assisted morphometric analyses confirm that large variations in blastomere size and fragmentation are frequently observed; large variations in blastomere size have been linked to increased chromosomal errors (Hnida and Ziebe, 2007).

## Zygote Scoring

Schemes for identifying healthy viable embryos at the zygote stage were proposed by Scott et al. (2000) and Tesarik and Greco (1999). Criteria suggested as predictive of optimal implantation potential include:

- close alignment of nucleoli in a row
- adequate separation of pronuclei
- heterogeneous cytoplasm with a clear 'halo'
- cleavage within 24–26 hours.

The scoring systems were reviewed by James (2007) and are compared in Table 11.1. The timing of assessment is critical, as pronuclear development is a dynamic process, and zygote scoring should therefore be used with caution and only in conjunction with other methods of evaluation.

## Early Cleavage

Timing of the first cell division of the embryo has been investigated as a predictor of developmental competence, with the suggestion that 'early cleavage' is associated with higher pregnancy rates. However, there is only a certain window where true early cleavage can be seen, and this extra assessment may be difficult to fit into the normal routine of an IVF laboratory. Once the embryos have undergone the second division to the four-cell stage, those that might have cleaved a few hours earlier will have similar morphology to those that did not, and it is not possible to differentiate between them.

## Multinucleation

Multinucleated blastomeres can sometimes be observed at early cleavage stages, most easily on Day 2 (Figure 11.5). Studies have revealed that blastocysts developing from embryos showing multinucleation at early cleavage stages have similar aneuploidy rates to blastocysts that resulted from embryos that did not have multinucleation. Transfer of binucleated and multinucleated frozen-thawed embryos does not apparently increase the incidence of congenital anomalies and chromosomal defects in newborns (Seikkula et al., 2018). Aneuploidy activates a spindle-apparatus checkpoint in different types of cells (Wenzel & Singh, 2018), and it is possible that blastomere multinucleation may represent the activation of a cell cycle checkpoint that can convert a mosaic embryo to one that is euploid (Tesarik, 2018).

## Cumulative Scoring Systems

Multi-day scoring systems can enhance embryo selection by combining both developmental rate and morphological assessment (Skiadas and Racowsky, 2007). These should provide a more accurate picture of developmental progression than can be obtained from a single observation. However, the ultimate combination of morphological features required for optimal evaluation of developmental competence has yet to be resolved. The optimal timing of embryo transfer will be more accurately determined when agreement on this is reached. In addition, multi-day assessment requires repeated embryo handling and exposure to potentially hazardous conditions outside of the incubator (see section 'Time-Lapse Systems (TLS)').

## Fragments

Fragmentation in the human embryo is very common, affecting up to 75% of all embryos developed in vitro (Alikani, 2007); it is not clear whether this is an effect of culture conditions and follicular stimulation, or a characteristic of human development (Figure 11.6).

**Table 11.1** Comparison of pronuclear morphology scoring systems, with a representative illustration of pronuclei in each scoring group

| Scott et al., 2000 Series 1 | Scott et al., 2000 Series 2 | Scott, 2003 | Tesarik and Greco, 1999 | Tesarik et al., 2000 | Pronuclear morphology |
|---|---|---|---|---|---|
| Grade 1 | Z1 | Z2 | Pattern O | Pattern O | |
| Grade 3 | Z2 | Z2 | Pattern O | Pattern O | |
| Grade 2 | Z3 | Z3–2 | Pattern 2 | Non-pattern 0 | |
| Grade 4 | Z3 | Z3–1 | Pattern 5 | Non-pattern 0 | |
| Grade 4 | Z3 | Z3–4 | Pattern 1 | Non-pattern 0 | |
| Grade 4 | Z3 | Z3–4 | Pattern 3 | Non-pattern 0 | |
| Grade 5 | Z3 | Z3–1 | Pattern 4 | Non-pattern 0 | |
| Grade 5 | Z4 | Z4–2 | Pattern 4 | Non-pattern 0 | |
| Grade 5 | Z4 | Z4–1 | NA | Non-pattern 0 | |

Extensive fragmentation is known to be associated with implantation failure, but the relationship between the degree of fragmentation and the developmental potential of the embryo is far from clear. Alikani et al. (1999) found that when embryos with more than 15% fragmentation were cultured to blastocyst stage, they formed fewer morulae, fewer cavities and fewer blastocysts compared to those embryos with less than 15% fragmentation. When fragmentation was greater than 35%, all processes were compromised. Retrospective analysis of embryo transfer data revealed that nearly 90% of embryos

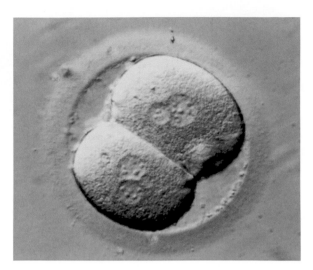

**Figure 11.5** A two-cell embryo showing two nuclei in each blastomere. Reprinted with permission from Meriano *et al.* (2004).

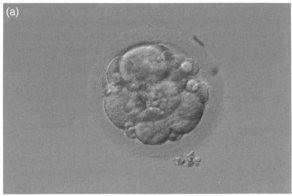

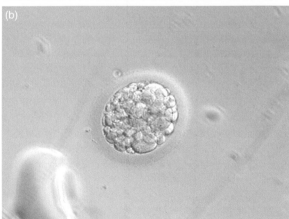

**Figure 11.6** (a) Day 3 human embryo with type 3 fragments. (b) Day 3 embryo with type 4 fragmentation.

selected for transfer were developed from embryos with less than 15% fragmentation observed on Day 3.

Alikani and Cohen (1995) used an analysis of patterns of cell fragmentation in the human embryo as a means of determining the relationship between cell fragmentation and implantation potential, with the conclusion that not only the degree, but also the pattern of embryo fragmentation determine its implantation potential. Five distinct patterns of fragmentation which can be seen by Day 3 were identified:

Type I: <5% of the volume of the perivitelline space (PVS) occupied by fragments.

Type II: small, localized fragments associated with one or two cells.

Type III: small, scattered fragments associated with multiple cells.

Type IV: large, scattered fragments associated with several unevenly sized cells and scattered throughout the PVS.

Type V: fragments throughout the PVS, appearing degenerate such that cell boundaries are invisible, associated with contracted and granular cytoplasm.

Some embryos have no distinct pattern of fragmentation.

No definite cause of fragmentation has been identified, although speculations include high spermatozoal numbers and consequently high levels of free radicals, temperature or pH shock, and stimulation protocols. Apoptosis has been suggested as a possible cause, and a progressive shortening of telomere length, which induces apoptosis, has been linked with fragmentation (Keefe *et al.*, 2005); however, this study was not definitive. Mitotically inactive cells do not exhibit fragmentation (Liu *et al.*, 2002), and it has been suggested that aberrant cytokinesis in the presence of spindle and cytoskeletal abnormalities may be associated with fragmentation.

Observed via the scanning electron microscope, the surface of fragments is made up of irregularly shaped blebs and protrusions, very different to the regular surface of blastomeres, which is organized into short, regular microvilli (Figure 11.7).

Interestingly, programmed cell death in somatic cells also starts with surface blebbing, and is caused, in part, by a calcium-induced disorganization of the cytoskeleton. We can speculate that similar mechanisms operate within human embryos, but there is so far no scientific evidence that this is the case.

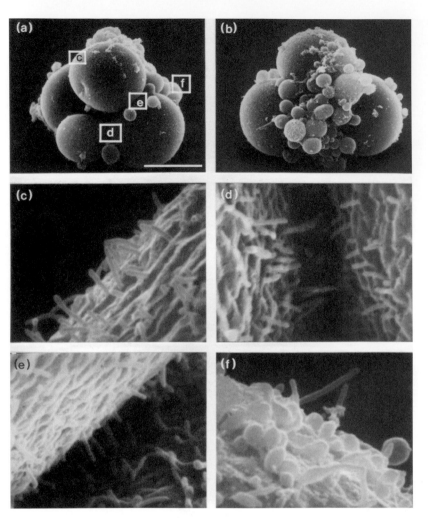

**Figure 11.7** Scanning electron micrographs. (a, b) Two views of a human four-cell embryo showing 20% fragmentation. (c–e) Magnification of corresponding areas showing regular short microvilli of vital blastomeres and intercellular areas. (f) Magnification of the surface of a cytoplasmic fragment showing irregular blebs and protrusions. Reproduced with permission from Dale *et al.* (1995).

There does appear to be an element of programming in this partial embryonic autodestruction, as embryos from certain patients, irrespective of the types of procedure applied in successive IVF attempts, are always prone to fragmentation. Surprisingly, fragmented embryos, repaired or not, do implant and often come to term. Time-lapse photography technology has clearly demonstrated that an individual embryo can radically change its morphological appearance in a short period of time: fragments that are apparent at a particular moment in time can be subsequently absorbed with no evidence of their prior existence (Hamberger *et al.*, 1998; Hashimoto *et al.*, 2009; Mio and Maeda, 2008). This demonstrates the highly regulative nature of the human embryo, as it can apparently lose over half

of its cellular mass and still recover, and also confirms the general consensus that the mature oocyte contains much more material than it needs for development. The reasons why part, and only part, of an early embryo should become disorganized and degenerate are a mystery. Different degrees of fragmentation argue against the idea that the embryo is purposely casting off excess cytoplasm, somewhat analogous to the situation in annelids and marsupials that shed cytoplasmic lobes rich in yolk, and favor the idea of partial degeneration. Perhaps it involves cell polarization, where organelles gather to one side of the cell. It is certain that pH, calcium and transcellular currents trigger cell polarization, which may in certain cases lead to an abnormal polarization, and therefore to fragmentation. Describing fragmentation as a degenerative process may not be justified, but more research is needed to elucidate whether the implantation of embryos with extensive fragmentation at the cleavage stages has any long-term effects.

## Embryo Grading: Cleavage Stages

Despite the introduction of extended culture and sophisticated monitoring and genetic screening technologies, a significant number of apparently high-quality and chromosomally normal embryos still do not implant, and selecting embryos for transfer remains an ongoing challenge in routine clinical IVF. After more than 40 years, and the birth of close to 10 million babies, the basic selection criteria in a routine IVF laboratory without research facilities continue to be based on assessment of morphology, despite numerous attempts to find new biomarkers and variables (Figure 11.8). Preimplantation genetic screening has shown a surprising discrepancy between gross morphology and genetic normality of embryos. Even the most 'beautiful' Grade 1 embryos may have numerical chromosomal anomalies, whilst those judged to be of 'poorer' quality, with uneven blastomeres and fragments, may have a normal chromosome complement. The variables that continue to prove consistently useful as predictors of viability remain: numbers of cells and fragmentation, cell symmetry and nucleation. (See Van den Bergh *et al.* [2012] for an atlas of >1000 embryo images together with their clinical/IVF histories and cycle outcomes.)

### Grade 1/A

- Even, regular spherical blastomeres
- Moderate refractility (i.e., not very dark)
- Intact zona
- No, or very few, fragments (less than 10%)

Allowance should be made for the appearance of blastomeres that are in division or that have divided asynchronously with their sisters, e.g., three-, five-, six- or seven-cell embryos, which may be uneven. As always, individual judgment is important, and this is a highly subjective assessment.

### Grade 2/B

- Uneven or irregularly shaped blastomeres
- Mild variation in refractility
- No more than 10% fragmentation of blastomeres

### Grade 3/C

- Fragmentation of no more than 50% of blastomeres
- Remaining blastomeres must be at least in reasonable (Grade 2) condition
- Refractility associated with cell viability
- Intact zona pellucida

### Grade 4/D

- More than 50% of the blastomeres are fragmented
- Gross variation in refractility
- Remaining blastomeres appear viable

### Grade 5

- Zygotes with two pronuclei on Day 2 (delayed fertilization or reinsemination on Day 1)

### Grade 6

- Nonviable: fragmented, lysed, contracted or dark blastomeres
- No viable cells

It is important to bear in mind that the time during which the assessment and judgment is made represents only a tiny instant of a rapidly evolving process of development. Embryos can be judged quite differently at two different periods in time, as may be seen if a comparison is made between assessments made in the morning, and later in the day immediately before transfer. Individual judgment should be exercised in determining which embryos are selected. In general, those embryos at later stages and of higher grades are preferred, but the choice is often not clear cut. The Grade 2 category covers a wide range of morphological states but, provided the blastomeres are not grossly abnormal, a later stage Grade 2 embryo may be selected in preference to an earlier stage Grade 1 embryo. Attention should also be paid to the appearance of the zona pellucida and to the pattern of fragmentation. Embryos of Grade 3 or 4 are transferred only where no better embryos are available. If only pronucleate embryos are available on Day 2, they should be cultured further and transferred only if cleavage occurs.

## Blastocyst Transfer

The transfer of blastocysts on Day 5 or 6 has the advantage of allowing better synchrony between the embryo and endometrium, as well as eliminating embryos that cannot develop after activation of the

233

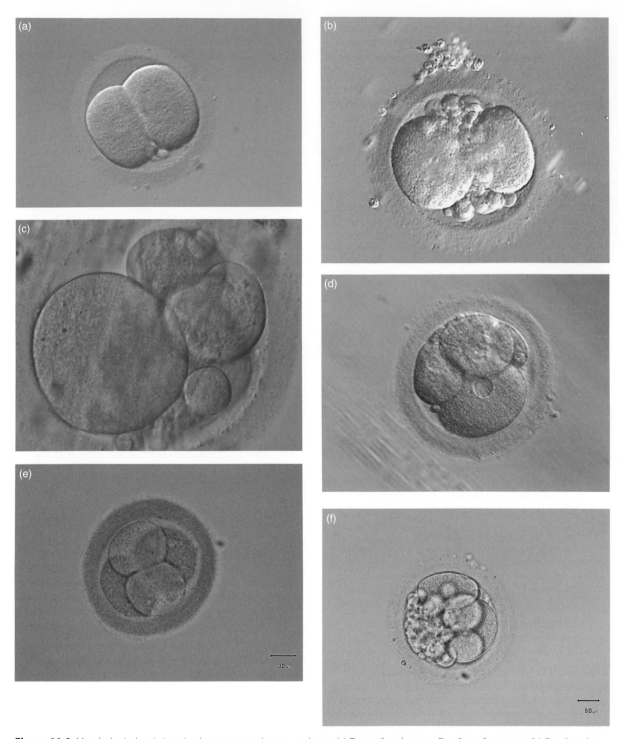

**Figure 11.8** Morphological variations in cleavage stage human embryos. (a) Two-cell embryo on Day 2, no fragments. (b) Day 2 embryo, Grade 3. (c) Day 2 embryo, uneven blastomeres with one large dominant blastomere. (d) Day 2 embryo, one blastomere shows large vacuole, Grade 2/3. (e) Four-cell embryo on Day 2, Grade 1. See color plate section. (f) Grade 3 embryo on Day 2. See color plate section. (g) Grade 4 embryo on Day 2. (h) Day 3 six-cell embryo, Grade 1. (i) Day 3 eight-cell embryo, Grade 1. Images (c) and (g) kindly supplied by Thomas Ebner, Austria; (g) by Marc van den Bergh, Switzerland; (e) and (f) by Oleksii Barash, Ukraine; (h) by Gemma Fabozzi, Naples. Despite the extreme difference in their morphology, the single transfer of embryos (e) and (f) both led to healthy live births (photos and history courtesy of Oleksii Barash, Ukraine).

234

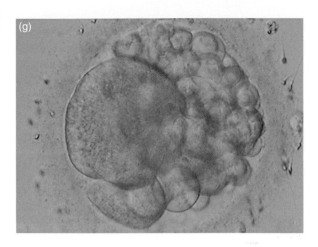

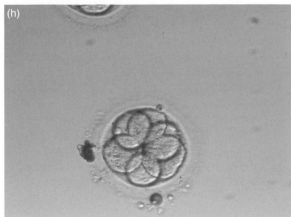

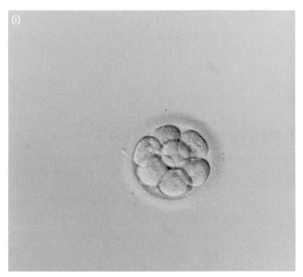

**Figure 11.8** (*cont.*)

zygote genome due to genetic or metabolic defects. Following the development of new generation sequential embryo culture media, single blastocyst transfer has been promoted as a means of improving the success of IVF, while at the same time reducing multiple birth rates. An important prerequisite for blastocyst culture is an optimal IVF laboratory culture environment; there is no advantage in extended culture unless satisfactory implantation rates are already obtained after culture to Day 2 or 3. Published literature indicates that a policy of careful embryo evaluation at cleavage stages can lead to success rates after Day 3 transfer that broadly match the success rates achieved with blastocyst transfer. Concern has also been expressed about the safety of prolonged culture to the blastocyst stage and the risk of potential

aberrant epigenetic programming during extended in-vitro development (Huntriss and Picton, 2008; see Chapter 15). In the past, the poor survival rate for supernumerary blastocysts after slow freezing was a disadvantage of blastocyst culture, but blastocyst vitrification and its associated high survival rate (see Chapter 12) has made single blastocyst transfer a more viable option; this also facilitates a policy for elective single embryo transfer (eSET).

The ability to identify healthy viable blastocysts is an important factor in the success of blastocyst transfer, and a grading system for their assessment takes into consideration the degree of expansion, hatching status, the development of the inner cell mass (ICM) and the development of the trophectoderm (Gardner and Schoolcraft, 1999; Richardson *et al.*, 2015).

Careful assessment of all morphological parameters available will optimize the chance of achieving satisfactory implantation rates after blastocyst transfer.

---

**Potential Benefits of Blastocyst Transfer**

From Gardner *et al.* (2007).

- True embryo viability can be assessed, post embryonic genome activation.
- Embryos with limited developmental potential are eliminated.
- Embryonic stage is synchronized with the uterus, reducing cellular stress on the embryo.
- Exposure of the embryo to a hyperstimulated uterine environment is minimized.
- Possibility of uterine contractions is reduced, minimizing the chance of embryo expulsion.
- High implantation rate; reduces the need to transfer multiple embryos.
- Single embryo transfer reduces the rate of multiple gestation.

---

Blastocysts are initially graded on the basis of volume/expansion (this can be performed under a dissecting microscope):

1. Early blastocyst: the blastocoele occupies less than half the volume of the embryo.
2. Blastocyst: the blastocoele occupies half the volume of the embryo or more.
3. Full blastocyst: the blastocoele completely fills the embryo, but the zona has not thinned.
4. Expanded blastocyst: the volume of the blastocoele is larger than that of the ICM, and the zona is thinning.
5. Hatching blastocyst: the trophectoderm has started to herniate through the zona.
6. Hatched blastocyst: the blastocyst has completely escaped from the zona.

The morphology of the ICM and trophectoderm are then assessed under an inverted microscope:

| ICM | Trophectoderm |
| --- | --- |
| A. Tightly packed, many cells | A. Many cells forming a cohesive epithelium |
| B. Loosely grouped, several cells | B. Few cells forming a loose epithelium |
| C. Very few cells | C. Very few large cells |

Examples of stages of human blastocyst development are illustrated in Figure 11.9; Figure 11.10 illustrates the limitations of morphological assessment.

Blastocyst transfer has also been used as a strategy for the treatment of patients who carry chromosomal translocations; chromosome translocations cause a delay in the cell cycle, and abnormal or slowly developing embryos are eliminated during in-vitro culture. Several normal pregnancies have been successfully established after transfer of healthy blastocysts in a group of patients carrying translocations (Ménézo *et al.*, 2001).

## Remaining Embryos

After cleavage stage embryo transfer, remaining embryos of Grades 1 or 2 which show less than 20% fragmentation at the time of assessment may be cryopreserved on Day 2 or Day 3. Embryos of suboptimal morphology at this time can be further cultured until Day 6, with daily assessment. Those that develop to blastocysts on Days 5 or 6 can also be cryopreserved.

## Time-Lapse Systems (TLS)

A time-lapse system takes digital images at set time intervals, e.g., every 5 to 15 minutes. In the IVF laboratory, TLS can be installed into an existing embryo incubator or can be used as a separate stand-alone system that combines incubation with time-lapse. Specialist software compiles the images to create a timed sequence of embryo development that can be digitally displayed on a monitor. Specific events such as timing of cleavage divisions, irregular cleavage, fragmentation, fragment resorption, blastocoele formation, and blastocyst expansion can be visualized without disturbing the culture system. Objective and accurate information is recorded, which can be analyzed in detail.

Early studies using TLS assessed the sequence and timing of morphological events up to formation of pronuclei in ICSI-generated human zygotes (Payne *et al.*, 1997). After further refinements in technology, optics, software, etc., their use in IVF laboratories on a larger scale was introduced from around 2010 onwards. Embryo development is a highly dynamic process, driven by fundamental molecular and cellular mechanisms that regulate the kinetics of the cell cycle. Static periodic observations necessary in routine IVF culture cannot truly reflect the details of such a dynamic process, and important events that are

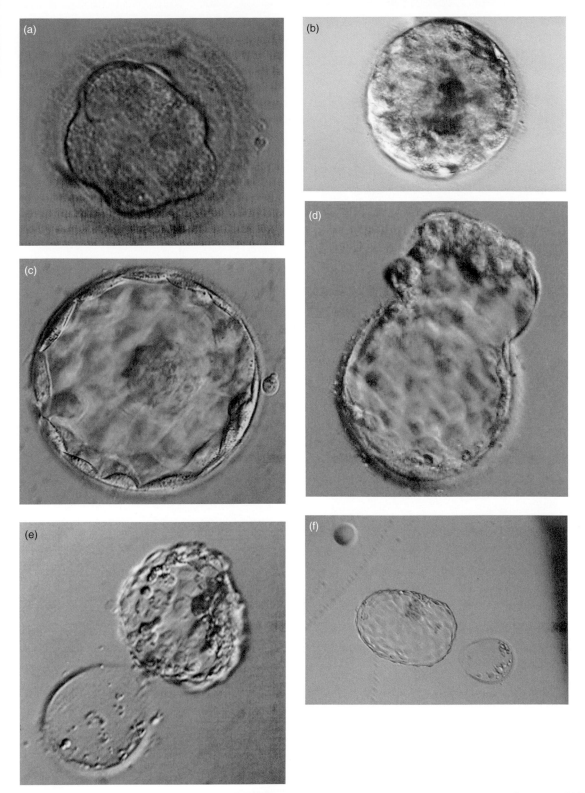

**Figure 11.9** Stages in blastocyst development. (See color plate section.) (a) Compacting morula. (b) Early stages of cavitation. (c) Fully expanded top-grade blastocyst with well-developed ICM and trophectoderm, thinned zona, hatching process initiated. (d) Top-grade blastocyst in the process of hatching. (e) Hatching blastocyst about to leave the zona. (f) Fully hatched blastocyst and empty zona. See color plate section.

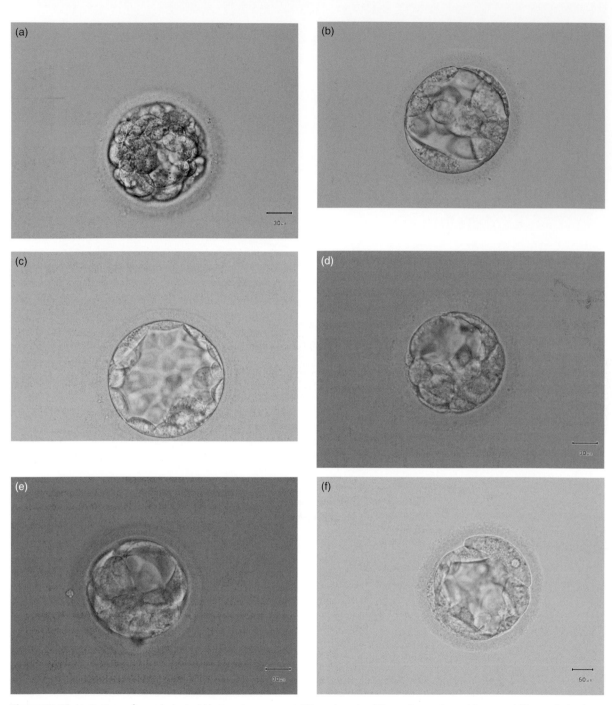

**Figure 11.10** Limitations of morphological blastocyst assessment. Although each of the embryos pictured here would be graded as lesser quality compared with the 'classic' optimal grade blastocysts seen in Figure 11.8, each of these embryos resulted in a healthy live birth after single embryo transfer on Day 5. Image (a) is a thawed embryo. (Two blastocysts were thawed on Day 5 [slow-freeze protocol]; the one pictured here survived and was transferred on the same day.) See color plate section. With thanks to Oleksii Barash, Clinic of Reproductive Medicine 'Nadiya,' Ukraine.

crucial to normal development may be missed or over-looked. Continuous monitoring by TLS provides a more complete picture, including pronuclear patterns, timing of cell divisions, intervals between cell cycles, presence of multinucleation and blastomere symmetry, allowing potential dynamic markers of embryo development to be identified. Embryos that have shown aberrant cleavage patterns or have a high potential of developmental arrest can be excluded from transfer.

The systems can provide a stable tightly controlled closed culture environment, avoiding fluctuations in light, pH and temperature that are inevitably associated with removing culture dishes from the incubator for routine intermittent microscopic assessment. Sample handling is minimized, and this may also reduce the risk of human error. However, embryos may sometimes move out of the microscope's field of view, or air bubbles may form that prevent adequate image capture. Embryos are exposed to light during each image acquisition, and a potential for harm due to UV radiation cannot so far be excluded (Pomeroy & Reed, 2015). Modern systems incorporate a reduced oxygen atmosphere, and this had been shown to have an effect on rates of embryo development (Gomes Sobrinho *et al.*, 2011).

Some systems offer computer-assisted assessment of morphokinetic parameters and developmental milestones, incorporating algorithms to improve selection of embryos with the highest implantation potential. Numerous studies and trials have so far documented a great deal of information about embryo development, identifying several phenomena whose detailed analysis could ultimately improve the outcome of treatment cycles. Parameters that have been investigated in detail include:

- Duration of time for: visible pronuclei, syngamy, timing of each cell division, initiation of compaction, initiation of blastulation, completion of blastulation.
- Analysis of abnormal cleavage patterns: abnormal syngamy, direct cleavage, reverse cleavage, absent cleavage in the presence of karyokinesis, chaotic cleavage, and cell lysis.
- Early prediction of blastocyst development.
- Negative parameters: multinucleation, micronuclei, fragmentation, blastomere asymmetry, direct cleavage from 1 to 3 cells.
- Association between morphokinetic parameters and aneuploidy.

However, the parameters observed and correlations identified have varied widely between different investigators, with contradictory results published. Embryo development is highly subject to biological and technical variations, and the algorithms for embryo selection differ: timings that are prognostic for one laboratory may not be directly applicable in another laboratory setting. It is clear that prediction models based on morphokinetics are more complicated than first anticipated, and it may not be feasible to establish a universal algorithm for embryo selection. Each IVF unit should instead work toward building a specific model based on its own patients and practice (Meseguer *et al.*, 2011).

Although TLS technology has undoubtedly contributed a great deal to the field of IVF as a research tool, a 2018 Cochrane review (Armstrong *et al.*, 2018) concluded: 'There is as yet insufficient evidence of differences in live birth, miscarriage, stillbirth or clinical pregnancy to choose between TLS, with or without embryo selection software, and conventional incubation. The studies were at high risk of bias for randomisation and allocation concealment, the results should be interpreted with extreme caution.'

## Embryo Transfer Procedure

### Materials

1. Pre-equilibrated, warmed culture medium
2. 1-mL disposable syringe
3. Embryo transfer catheter
4. Sterile disposable gloves (nonpowdered)
5. Clean Petri dish
6. Sterile Pasteur pipette and glass probe
7. Dissecting microscope with warm stage

Although it may seem obvious that correct identification of patient and embryos is vital, errors in communication do happen and can lead to a disastrous mistake, especially should there be patients with similar names undergoing treatment at the same time. Electronic identity/witnessing systems are now available to confirm identities of doctor, nurse, embryologist and patient, but if such a system is not available, a routine discipline of identification should be followed to ensure that there is no possibility of mistaken identity.

1. Ensure that medical notes always accompany a patient who is being prepared for embryo transfer.

2. Name and medical numbers on medical notes and patient identity bracelet should be checked by two people, i.e., the clinician in charge of the procedure and the assisting nurse.

3. The doctor should also check name and number verbally with the patient, and doctor, nurse and patient may sign an appropriate form confirming that the details are correct.

4. The duty embryologist should check the same details with the embryology records, and also sign the same form in the presence of the doctor.

## Preparation of Embryos for Transfer

The rate of multiple gestation resulting from IVF/ET is unacceptably high, and legislation in the UK and other European countries now prohibits the transfer of more than two embryos in a treatment cycle for certain patient groups. Elective single embryo transfer (eSET) is recommended for selected patients with a good prognosis, i.e., young age, tubal infertility only, first attempt or previous history of pregnancy and/or delivery.

1. Prepare a droplet (or well) of fresh medium for the selected embryos.

2. When the embryos for transfer have been identified and scored, and their details recorded (number, developmental stage and grade), place them together in the pre-equilibrated droplet or well. No more than two embryos should be selected. If medium with a higher density is used (i.e., with 50–75% serum), this transfer should be carried out carefully, as the embryos will 'float' in the higher density medium and must be allowed to settle before aspiration into the embryo transfer catheter.

3. After gently pushing the embryos together, leave them under low power on the heated stage of the microscope, in focus.

4. Turn off the microscope light.

5. Wash your hands with a surgical scrub preparation, and don sterile gloves.

6. Fill a 1-mL sterile syringe with warm medium, and eject any air bubbles.

7. Check that the catheter to be used moves freely through its outer sheath, attach it to the syringe and eject the medium from the syringe through the catheter, discarding the medium. Syringes designed specifically for embryo transfer are available, and these allow better control than a standard 1-mL syringe.

8. Draw up warm medium through the catheter into the syringe, and then push the piston down to the 0.1-mL mark, ejecting excess medium and again discarding it.

9. Pour some clean warm medium into the warm Petri dish on the microscope stage (for rinsing the catheter tip).

10. Place the end of the catheter into the drop or well, away from the embryos, and inject a small amount of medium to break the boundary of surface tension that may appear at the end of the catheter. Aspirate the embryos into the catheter, so that the volume to be transferred is 15–20 µL.

11. If the embryos have been loaded from a droplet under oil, rinse the tip of the catheter in the Petri dish containing clean warm medium.

Hand the catheter and syringe to the clinician for transfer to the patient. When the catheter is returned after the procedure, carefully inspect it, rotating under the microscope. It is especially important to ensure that no embryo is buried in any mucus present; note and record the presence of mucus and/or blood. Loosen the Lueur fitting, and allow the fluid in the catheter to drain into the clean Petri dish while continuing to observe through the microscope. Inform the doctor and patient as soon as you have confirmed that no embryos have been returned. If any embryos have been returned, they should be reloaded into a clean catheter, and the transfer procedure repeated. If difficulties arise during the transfer procedure causing delay, return the embryos to the culture drop in the interim, until the physician is confident that they can be safely transferred to the uterus of the patient.

Implantation is a complex and multistep process that requires successful interplay between several factors: not only a competent embryo and receptive endometrium, but also a competent embryologist as well as the personnel carrying out the transfer procedure. Although the technique of embryo transfer may appear to be a simple and straightforward procedure, its correct management is absolutely critical in safe delivery of the embryos to the site of their potential implantation. Studies repeatedly show that pregnancy rates can vary in the hands of different operators and with the use of different embryo transfer catheters. In a study of embryo transfer procedures under ultrasound-guided control, Woolcott and Stanger (1998) observed guiding cannula and transfer catheter placement in relation to the endometrial surface and uterine fundus during embryo transfer. Their results indicated that tactile assessment of the embryo transfer catheter was unreliable, in that the cannula and the catheter could be seen to abut the fundal endometrium, and indent or embed in the endometrium in a significant number of cases. Endometrial movement due to subendometrial myometrial contraction was obvious in 36% of cases, and this movement was associated with a reduced pregnancy rate. Their studies highlight the fact that 'blind' embryo transfer procedures may often lead to an unsatisfactory outcome, and they recommend the use of ultrasound guidance as a routine during embryo transfer.

## Transport IVF and Transport ICSI

The facilities of a central expert IVF laboratory can be used to offer treatment in hospitals that do not have the necessary laboratory space and personnel. Carefully selected patients undergo ovarian stimulation, monitoring and oocyte retrieval under the care and management of a gynecologist who has a close liaison with an IVF laboratory team in a location that can be reached ideally within 2 hours of the hospital or clinic where the oocyte retrieval procedure takes place. It is an advantage to select patients with simple, uncomplicated infertility and good ovarian response, and close communication and coordination between the patient, physician and IVF laboratory team are essential.

A GnRH agonist/FSH long protocol for superovulation has the advantage that a simplified monitoring regimen can be used (ultrasound assessment and optional serum estradiol levels). This protocol also allows scheduled admission of patients into the stimulation phase, as well as latitude in the administration of hCG so that the timing of oocyte retrieval can be scheduled in a routine operating list. Ovulation is induced by hCG administration 36 hours prior to the planned follicular aspiration.

The couple under treatment must visit the central unit before hCG is given, both to receive detailed information and consent forms, and to familiarize themselves with the journey and the facilities. The husband will return to the central unit on the morning of oocyte retrieval to produce a semen sample and to collect a prewarmed portable incubator. The portable incubator, plugged into a car cigarette lighter, is then used to transport the

follicular aspirates which have been collected in the peripheral hospital or clinic. Follicular aspirates are collected under ultrasound-guided control into sterile test-tubes (without flushing). It is essential that each test-tube is filled completely and tightly capped in order to prevent pH fluctuations. A heated test-tube rack during aspiration must be used to prevent temperature fluctuations in the aspirates. At the end of the oocyte retrieval procedure, the partner transports the follicular aspirates, together with the treatment records, to the central laboratory for oocyte identification and subsequent insemination and culture.

The embryo transfer procedure is carried out at the central unit, either on Day 2/3 or when embryos reach the blastocyst stage. Patient follow-up is carried out by the physician at the peripheral unit. Provided that the instructions and inclusion criteria are strictly adhered to, a highly motivated, well-coordinated team working in close liaison can achieve success rates comparable to those obtained in the specialist center, and IVF treatment can thus be offered to couples to whom it might otherwise be unavailable. Transport ICSI can also be successfully offered on a similar basis (see Chapter 13).

---

**Selection Criteria for Transport IVF/ICSI**
1. Women 35 years of age or less
2. Tubal damage as the sole cause of subfertility

**Exclusion Criteria**
1. Women over 35 years of age
2. Patients with LH:FSH ratio higher than 3:1
3. Patients with laparoscopically proven moderate or severe endometriosis
4. Patients requesting oocyte donation or donor insemination
5. Three previously unsuccessful IVF treatment cycles

---

## In-Vitro Maturation (IVM)

In-vitro maturation technology has been successfully used in farm animals for decades, and collection of immature animal oocytes continues to be routine. Pincus and Enzmann (1935) were the first to show that immature rabbit oocytes removed from their natural ovarian environment were capable of undergoing spontaneous maturation and fertilization in vitro. Robert Edwards made similar observations in human oocytes in 1965 (see Thompson & Gilchrist, 2013). Veeck and colleagues (1983) matured human oocytes in the laboratory that had been retrieved from COH cycles in 1983, and these subsequently fertilized and resulted in live births. However, such 'rescued' oocytes were often suboptimal, showing a high incidence of aneuploidy as well as other defects. Robert Edwards had previously anticipated this challenge as early as 1969:

> Problems of embryonic development are likely to accompany the use of human oocytes matured and fertilized in vitro. When oocytes of the rabbit and other species were matured in vitro and fertilized in vivo, the pronuclear stages appeared normal but many of the resulting embryos had sub-nuclei in their blastomeres, and almost all of them died during the early cleavage stages. When maturation of rabbit oocytes was started in vivo by injecting gonadotrophins into the mother, and completed in the oviduct or in vitro, full-term rabbit fetuses were obtained.

(Edwards *et al.*, 1969: 634–635)

The phrase 'cytoplasmic maturity' was coined by Delage in 1901, to point out that it was not necessarily synchronous with nuclear maturity. This is certainly true for human oocytes, where a metaphase II nucleus does not guarantee developmental competence. Whereas nuclear maturation is relatively visible, cytoplasmic maturity is much more difficult to assess microscopically. The aim of IVM is to retrieve and rescue immature oocytes before they are affected by the endocrine and paracrine influences of the growing dominant follicle. Studies in the bovine have shown that oocytes retrieved in later phases of follicular development have more mRNA transcripts of mtDNA compared with oocytes from less developed follicles, correlated with good embryonic developmental potential. Data from animals suggest that mRNA instability and the absence or abundance of certain transcripts such as LH and FSH receptors, connexin 43 and cyclooxygenase-2 in the cumulus of oocytes from small antral follicles after resumption of meiosis in vitro are predictors of oocyte quality. The presence of other key components that have been described in rodents, such as growth differentiation factor-9 (GDF-9) and bone morphogenetic protein-15 (BMP-15), mediate important biochemical changes in oocytes that are required for normal postmeiotic events.

Current IVM technology aims to retrieve immature oocytes from unstimulated or slightly stimulated small antral follicles; retrieved cumulus-enclosed oocytes are cultured in a specifically designed medium. In-vitro maturation of human oocytes from antral follicles has advantages over traditional controlled ovarian hyperstimulation (COH) for IVF: the risk of OHSS for patients with polycystic ovaries (PCO) is eliminated, and it also reduces side-effects of gonadotropin treatments and lowers the costs of treatment. However, these advantages may come at the expense of clinical success rates compared with standard IVF. PCO patients have numerous antral follicles and respond well to IVM regimes. An IVM treatment cycle aims to recover immature (GV) oocytes that can successfully complete meiosis during in vitro culture, achieving both nuclear and cytoplasmic competence that will enable fertilization, embryo development and ultimately a healthy live birth. Although implantation and pregnancy rates may be lower compared with routine controlled ovarian stimulation protocols, this can be improved via careful and appropriate patient selection. Cha *et al.* (1991) reported the first human live births after retrieval of immature oocytes from antral follicles; in 2015, it was estimated that at least 5000 children had been born following the use of this technique (Sauerbrun-Cutler *et al.*, 2015). A review of the literature published between 1999 and 2013 reported clinical pregnancy rates of up to 35% in young women, with obstetric and perinatal outcomes comparable to standard IVF/ICSI (Ellenbogen *et al.*, 2014). IVM can thus be considered as an alternative treatment strategy for selected patient groups, and for PCO patients in particular; it has now also become another option for fertility preservation (see Chapter 12).

Protocols include initial priming of the ovaries with low doses of recombinant follicle-stimulating hormone (rFSH) (100–150 IU) for 3–6 days with or without administration of hCG or a GnRH agonist (see Chapter 2). Monitoring by vaginal ultrasound scan is carried out on Day 6 of the cycle, recording all follicles of 4 mm, and oocyte collection scheduled within 72 hours once a follicle of 10 mm is observed.

There are several considerations to be taken into account while handling immature oocytes: since the volume of follicular fluid retrieved in IVM procedures is small and often contains blood, it is advisable to use heparin (2–5 IU/mL) in HEPES-buffered medium to minimize blood clotting. As in traditional IVF technology, attention should be given to pH and temperature settings. Oocytes from small antral follicles differ morphologically from mature oocytes and are often found enclosed within a compacted mass of surrounding granulosa cells. The degree of expansion of the cumulus cells may be influenced by the size of the follicle, as well as by the exposure to gonadotropins and/or hCG in vivo.

Immediately after retrieval, cumulus-enclosed immature oocytes are placed in IVM medium for 24–48 hours. Numerous IVM media formulations are commercially available, composed of standard IVF medium with the addition of recombinant FSH and LH or hCG. Patient-inactivated serum or follicular fluid is often added to the maturation media as an exogenous protein source. Growth factors, lipids, glycoproteins, steroid hormones, cytokines and other factors in the serum or follicular fluid may be instrumental in the regulation of oocyte maturation and account for its preference over synthetic serum substitute or human albumin.

ICSI is the preferred method of insemination in IVM, since oocytes are frequently denuded of granulosa cells for evaluation of maturational status and there are fears of zona pellucida hardening during the IVM process. Early studies comparing ICSI versus IVF for the insemination of IVM oocytes suggested that ICSI results in higher rates of fertilization than IVF; however, the developmental potential of the fertilized oocytes was similar irrespective of the insemination method. A more recent study using sibling oocytes that compared rates of fertilization, embryo development and clinical pregnancy found no difference between ICSI and IVF oocytes (Walls et al., 2012). Fewer usable embryos are generated with IVM protocols, and live birth rates per embryo transferred may be lower compared with standard IVF.

The complexities of oocyte maturation, in particular the unknowns in cytoplasmic maturity and the potential effect of in-vitro maturation on the organization of the meiotic spindle and chromosome alignment (see Chapter 4), remain areas for research. The inherent problems of aberrant methylation that may be induced by suboptimal culture conditions (Ménézo et al., 2010; Anckaert et al., 2013) also warrant consideration and caution in the use of IVM.

## In-Vitro Growth (IVG)

Whereas IVM targets immature oocytes arrested at the germinal vesicle stage in preantral follicles, In-Vitro Growth attempts to obtain viable oocytes by growing them from a far earlier immature state: primary oocytes in primordial follicles. These oocytes are arrested in the dictyate stage of prophase 1, with bivalent chromosomes enclosed within the germinal vesicle nucleus (see Chapters 1 and 3). Primary oocytes can remain arrested in meiosis I for up to 50 years, with a few gradually released after puberty to initiate their growth phase under endocrine control. IVG therefore requires a far longer and more complex, sophisticated and carefully orchestrated dynamic process than does IVM: this concept has been the subject of a great deal of research for at least 30 years (McLaughlin et al., 2018).

A dynamic culture system designed to sustain in-vitro growth must support three main steps:

1. Activation of primordial follicles to induce growth
2. Isolation and culture of growing follicles to promote their maturation and continued growth to the preantral stage
3. Removal of oocytes from the follicular environment and culture to mature oocyte–cumulus complexes.

Live births after complete growth from primordial oocytes followed by IVF has so far been achieved only in the mouse. The process of mouse oocyte development has also been demonstrated in vitro starting from primordial germ cells and induced pluripotent stem cells (see Chapter 7).

Contact between the oocyte and its somatic cells must be maintained in order to support oocyte development, and this aspect has proved to be a challenge in IVG systems. Preliminary studies reported primordial follicle activation and growth to the secondary/multilaminar stage within pieces of ovarian cortex in a two-step culture system (Telfer et al., 2008). Growing follicles removed from the cortex developed to the antral stage when cultured individually in the presence of activin. Other groups also isolated multilaminar secondary follicles that successfully grew in vitro to produce oocytes capable of resuming meiosis and reaching metaphase II (Xiao et al., 2015). Telfer's group in Edinburgh then extended their two-step culture to develop a culture system that sustained growth from primordial/unilaminar to antral follicles, producing mature oocytes after 20 days in culture (McLaughlin et al., 2018).

Fresh cortical ovarian biopsies were donated by patients undergoing elective cesarean section deliveries. Histology confirmed that 97.1% of follicles in the biopsies were unilaminar.

1. **Step 1**: Primordial to early antral stage: cortical biopsies were dissected into ~1 × 1 × 0.5 mm$^3$ fragments; unilaminar follicles with a mean diameter >40 μm were excised with fine needles and cultured individually in 24-well culture plates at 37°C in humidified air with 5% $CO_2$ for 8 days. Histological examination on Day 8 showed a progressive increase in growing primary and secondary follicles, with a corresponding decrease in nongrowing follicles compared with Day 0.

2. **Step 2**: Mechanical dissection of growing multilaminar follicles observed on the tissue surface after 8 days of culture. Follicles of 100- to 150-μm diameter were dissected using 25-G needles, and those with an intact basement membrane were selected for further individual culture for a further 8 days in 96-well V-bottomed culture plates, replacing half of the medium every 2 days.

3. **Step 3**: COCs were recovered from individual follicles showing antral cavities, using gentle pressure. After selecting complexes with complete cumulus and adherent mural granulosa cells (in order to maintain contact between the oocyte and its somatic cells), these were cultured in the presence of Activin and rFSH on track-etched nucleopore membranes in four-well culture plates. Oocyte diameter was monitored for 4 days; any that had not reached a diameter of 100 μm were cultured for a further 2 days (total of 20 days in vitro).

4. **Step 4**: Complexes containing oocytes >100 μm in diameter were selected for IVM, cultured in medium containing FSH and LH, examined for polar body extrusion after 24 hours and investigated in detail using confocal microscopy.

At least 30% of the follicles that survived the extended culture formed antral cavities and produced oocytes >100 μm in diameter; 10% of the complexes cultured for IVM extruded polar bodies after 24 hours. This study provided initial proof of concept that complete development of human oocytes from primordial follicles can be achieved in vitro, but further research is needed to optimize each stage and understand the effects of culture on development, and in particular epigenetic effects on potential embryos formed from IVG oocytes. In all cases, the polar bodies were larger, and cumulus expansion was less than is normally observed with in-vivo matured oocytes. Oocytes that lacked a polar body were arrested at GV or metaphase I; those arrested at MI showed chromosomes associated with aberrant spindles.

This IVG culture system can provide a multistep model to increase our understanding of human oogenesis, with potential applications such as screening for gonadotoxic therapies or environmental toxins; its most important clinical application in the future may be in fertility preservation, as an alternative to autologous transplantation (see Chapter 12).

# Conclusion

In view of the complex and elegant biochemistry and physiology involved in the development of a competent oocyte that will fertilize and develop successfully in vitro, as well as the delicate balance that must be required within each contributing component and compartment, it seems miraculous indeed that the application of essentially ill-defined strategies has led to the successful birth of so many children. Although success rates have improved significantly over the past two decades, there continues to be a wastage of embryos that fail to implant. A great deal more research is required to identify and define factors involved in the development of competent oocytes and viable embryos, and new data from the application of current research using the latest advances in molecular biology and culture technology are awaited.

# Further Reading

## Books and Reviews

Armstrong S, Arroll N, Cree LM, *et al.* (2015) Time-lapse systems for embryo incubation and assessment in assisted reproduction. *Cochrane Database of Systematic Reviews* 2: CD011320.

Armstrong S, Bhide P, Jordan V, Pacey A, Farquhar C (2018) Time-lapse systems for embryo incubation and embryo assessment for couples undergoing IVF and ICSI. *Cochrane Database of Systematic Reviews* 5: CDO11230.

Beck-Fruchter R, Lavee M, Weiss A, Geslevich Y, Shalev E (2014) Rescue intracytoplasmic sperm injection: a systematic review. *Fertility and Sterility* 101(3): 690-698.

Campbell A, Fishel S (2015) *Atlas of Time Lapse Embryology*. Taylor & Francis Group, LLC, Boca Raton, FL.

Dale B, Ménézo Y, Elder K (2016) Who benefits from PGS? *Austin Journal of In Vitro Fertilization* 3: 1026.

Edwards RG, Purdy JM (1982) *Human Conception In Vitro*. Academic Press, London.

Elder K, Cohen J (eds.) (2007) *Preimplantation Embryo Evaluation and Selection*. Informa Press, London.

Elder K, Van den Bergh M, Woodward B (2015) *Troubleshooting and Problem-Solving in the IVF Laboratory*. Cambridge University Press, Cambridge, UK.

Gleicher N, Orvieto R (2017) Is the hypothesis of pre-implantation genetic screening (PGS) still supportable? A review. *Journal of Ovarian Research* 10: 1–7.

Gomes Sobrinho DB, Oliveira JBA, Petersen CG, *et al.* (2011) IVF/ICSI outcomes after culture of human embryos at low oxygen tension: a meta-analysis. *Reproductive Biology and Endocrinology* 9: 143.

Leese HJ (2012) Metabolism of the preimplantation embryo: 40 years on. *Reproduction* 143: 417–427.

Pasquale P, Tucker MJ, Guelmann V (eds.) (2003) *A Color Atlas for Human Assisted Reproduction*. Lippincott Williams & Wilkins, Philadelphia.

Van den Bergh M, Ebner T, Elder K (2012) *Atlas of Oocytes, Zygotes and Embryos in Reproductive Medicine*. Cambridge University Press, Cambridge, UK.

Veeck L (1998) *An Atlas of Human Gametes and Conceptuses*. Parthenon Publishing, New York.

## Publications

Adjaye J, Daniels R, Monk M (1998) The construction of cDNA libraries from human single preimplantation embryos and their use in the study of gene expression during development. *Journal of Assisted Reproduction and Genetics* 15(5): 344–348.

Alikani M (2007) The origins and consequences of fragmentation in mammalian eggs and embryos. In: Elder K, Cohen J (eds.) *Preimplantation Embryo Evaluation and Selection*. Informa Press, London, pp. 89–100.

Alikani M, Cohen J (1995) Patterns of cell fragmentation in the human embryo in vitro. *Journal of Assisted Reproduction and Genetics* 12(Suppl.): 28s.

Alikani M, Cohen J, Tomkin G, *et al.* (1999) Human embryo fragmentation in vitro and its implications for pregnancy and implantation. *Fertility and Sterility* 71(5): 836–842.

Alikani M, Palermo G, Adler A, Bertoli M, Blake M, Cohen J (1995) Intracytoplasmic sperm injection in dysmorphic human oocytes. *Zygote* 3: 283–288.

Alikani M, Weimer K (1997) Embryo number for transfer should not be strictly regulated. *Fertility and Sterility* 68: 782–784.

Almeida PA, Bolton VN (1993) Immaturity and chromosomal abnormalities in oocytes that fail to develop pronuclei following insemination in vitro. *Human Reproduction* 8: 229–232.

Almeida PA, Bolton VN (1995) The effect of temperature fluctuations on the cytoskeletal organisation and chromosomal constitution of the human oocyte. *Zygote* 3: 357–365.

Anckaert E, De Rycke M, Smitz J (2013) Culture of oocytes and risk of imprinting defects. *Human Reproduction Update* 19: 52–66.

Angell RR, Templeton AA, Aitken RJ (1986) Chromosome studies in human in vitro fertilization. *Human Genetics* 72: 333.

Barrie A, Homburg R, McDowell G, *et al.* (2017) Preliminary investigation of the prevalence and implantation potential of abnormal embryonic phenotypes assessed using time-lapse imaging. *Reproductive BioMedicine Online* 34(5): 455–462.

Ben-Rafael Z, Kopf G, Blasco L, Tureck RW, Mastoianni L (1986) Fertilization and cleavage after reinsemination of human oocytes in vitro. *Fertility and Sterility* 45(1): 58–62.

Bielanska M, Tan SL, Ao A (2002a) High rate of myxoploidy among human blastocysts cultured in vitro. *Fertility and Sterility* 78(6): 1248–1253.

Bielanska M, Tan SL, Ao A (2002b) Different probe combinations for assessment of postzygotic chromosomal imbalances in human embryos. *Journal of Assisted Reproduction and Genetics* 19(4): 177–182.

Biggers JD, McGinnis LK, Lawitts JA (2005) One-step versus two-step culture of mouse preimplantation embryos: is there a difference? *Human Reproduction* 20(12): 3376–3384.

Bolton VN, Hawes SM, Taylor CT, Parsons JH (1989) Development of spare human preimplantation embryos in vitro: an analysis of the correlations among gross morphology, cleavage rates, and development to the blastocyst. *Journal of In Vitro Fertilization and Embryo Transfer* 7: 186.

Brison DR (2000) Apoptosis in mammalian preimplantation embryos: regulation by survival factors. *Human Fertility* 3: 36–47.

Brison DR, Houghton FD, Falconer D, *et al.* (2004) Identification of viable embryos in IVF by non-invasive measurement of amino acid turnover. *Human Reproduction* 19(10): 2319–2324.

Campbell A, Fishel S, Bowman N, Duffy S, Sedler M, Hickman CFL (2013) Modelling a risk classification of aneuploidy in human embryos using non-invasive morphokinetics. *Reproductive BioMedicine Online* 26: 477–485.

Canipari R, Epifano O, Siracusa G, Salustri A (1995) Mouse oocytes inhibit plasminogen activator production by ovarian cumulus and granulosa cells. *Developmental Biology* 167: 371–378.

Caro C, Trounson A (1986) Successful fertilization and embryo development, and pregnancy in human in vitro fertilization (IVF) using a chemically defined culture medium containing no protein. *Journal of In Vitro Fertilization Embryo Transfer* 3: 215–217.

Cecchino GN, Garcia-Velasco JA (2019) Mitochondrial DNA copy number as a predictor of embryo viability. *Fertility and Sterility* 111(2): 205–211.

Chamayou S, Patrizio P, Storaci G, *et al.* (2013) The use of morphokinetic parameters to select all embryos with full capacity to implant. *Journal of Assisted Reproduction and Genetics* 30: 703–710.

Chang CL, Wang TH, Horng SG, *et al.* (2002) The concentration of inhibin B in follicular fluid: relation to oocyte maturation and embryo development. *Human Reproduction* 17(7): 1724–1728.

Chian RC, Cao YX (2014) In vitro maturation of immature human oocytes for clinical application. *Methods in Molecular Biology* 1154: 271–288.

Clyde JM, Hogg JE, Rutherford AJ, Picton HM (2003) Karyotyping of human metaphase II oocytes by multifluor fluorescence in situ hybridization. *Fertility and Sterility* 80(4): 1003–1011.

Cohen J, Inge KL, Suzman M, Wiker SR, Wright G (1989) Videocinematography of fresh and cryopreserved embryos: a retrospective analysis of embryonic morphology and implantation. *Fertility and Sterility* 51: 820.

Combelles CMH, Fissore RA, Albertini DF, Racowsky C (2006) In vitro maturation of human oocytes and cumulus cells using a co-culture three-dimensional collagen gel system. *Human Reproduction* 20(5): 1349–1358.

Dale B, Fiorentino A, De Stefano RD, *et al.* (1999) Pregnancies after activated oocyte transfer: a new alternative for infertility treatment. *Human Reproduction* 14: 1771–1772.

Dale B, Ménézo Y, Elder K (2016) Who benefits from PGS? *Austin Journal of In Vitro Fertilization* 3: 1026–1027.

Dale B, Tosti E, Iaccarino M (1995) Is the plasma membrane of the human oocyte reorganised following fertilisation and early cleavage? *Zygote* 3(1): 31–36.

D'Amour K, Gage FH (2000) New tools for human developmental biology. *Nature Biotechnology* 18(4): 381–382.

Das S, Chattopadhyay R, Ghosh S, *et al.* (2006) Reactive oxygen species level in follicular fluid – embryo quality marker in IVF? *Human Reproduction* 21(9): 2403–2407.

de los Santos MJ, Juan AD, Mifsud A, *et al.* (2017) Variables associated with mitochondrial copy number in human blastocysts: what can we learn from trophectoderm biopsies? *Fertility and Sterility* 109: 110–117.

De Vos M, Smitz J, Thompson JG (2016) The definition of IVF is clear: variations need defining. *Human Reproduction* 31(11): 2411–2415.

Diamond MP, Rogers BJ, Webster BW, Vaughn WK, Wentz AC (1985) Polyspermy: effect of varying stimulation protocols and inseminating sperm concentrations. *Fertility and Sterility* 43(5): 777–780.

Eagle H (1959) Amino acid metabolism in mammalian cell cultures. *Science* 130: 432–437.

Ebner T (2006) Is oocyte morphology prognostic of embryo developmental potential after ICSI? *Reproductive BioMedicine Online* 12(4): 507–512.

Ebner T (2008) Blood clots in the cumulus-oocyte complex predict poor oocyte quality and post-fertilization development. *Reproductive BioMedicine Online* 16(6): 801–807.

Ebner T, Moser M, Sommergruber M, *et al.* (2002) First polar body morphology and blastocyst formation rate in ICSI patients. *Human Reproduction* 17(9): 2415–2418.

Edwards RG, Bavister BD, Steptoe PC (1969) Early stages of fertilization in vitro of human oocytes matured in vitro. *Nature* 221: 632–635.

Elder K, Elliott T (1999) *Blastocyst Update*. Worldwide Conferences in Reproductive Biology. Ladybrook Publications, Australia.

Ellenbogen A, Shavit T, Shalom-Paz E (2014) IVM results are comparable and may have advantages over standard IVF. *Facts, Views and Vision in ObGyn* 6(2): 77–80.

Englert Y, Puissant F, Camus M, Degueldre M, Leroy F (1986) Factors leading to tripronucleate eggs during human in vitro fertilization. *Human Reproduction* 1(2): 117–119.

Falcone P, Gambera L, Pisoni M, *et al.* (2008) Correlation between oocyte preincubation time and pregnancy rate after intracytoplasmic sperm injection. *Gynecological Endocrinology* 24(6): 25–29.

Fragouli E, McCaffrey C, Ravichandran K, *et al.* (2017) Clinical implications of mitochondrial DNA quantification on pregnancy outcomes: a blinded prospective non-selection study. *Human Reproduction* 32: 2340–2347.

Freour T, Le FLeuter N, Lammers J, *et al.* (2015) External validation of a time-lapse prediction model. *Fertility and Sterility* 103(4): 917–922.

Galliano D, Pellicer A (2014) MicroRNA and implantation. *Fertility and Sterility* 101: 1531–1544.

Gardner DK (1999) Development of serum-free media for the culture and transfer of human blastocysts. *Human Reproduction* 13(Suppl. 4): 218–225.

Gardner DK (2007) Noninvasive metabolic assessment of single cells. *Methods in Molecular Medicine* 132: 1–9.

Gardner DK, Schoolcraft WB (1999) In vitro culture of human blastocysts. In: Jansen R, Mortimer D (eds.) *Towards Reproductive Certainty: Infertility and Genetics beyond 1999*. Parthenon Publishing Group, Carnforth, UK, pp. 378–388.

Gardner DK, Schoolcraft WB, Wagley L, *et al.* (1998) A prospective randomized trial of blastocyst culture and transfer in in-vitro fertilization. *Human Reproduction* 13(12): 3434–3440.

Gardner DK, Stevens J, Sheehan CB, Schoolcraft WB (2007) Analysis of blastocyst morphology. In: Elder K, Cohen J (eds.) *Human Preimplantation Embryo Evaluation and Selection*. Taylor-Francis, London, pp. 79–88.

Gianaroli L, Magli C, Ferraretti A, *et al.* (1996) Reducing the time of sperm-oocyte interaction in human IVF improves the implantation rate. *Human Reproduction* 11: 166–171.

Gott AL, Hardy K, Winston RML, Leese HJ (1990) Noninvasive measurement of pyruvate and glucose uptake and lactate production by single human preimplantation embryos. *Human Reproduction* 5: 104–110.

Gregory L (1998) Ovarian markers of implantation potential in assisted reproduction. *Human Reproduction* 13(Suppl. 4): 117–132.

Gregory L, Leese HJ (1996) Determinants of oocyte and pre-implantation embryo quality metabolic requirements and the potential role of cumulus cells. *Human Reproduction* 11: 96–102.

Grifo JA, Boyle A, Fischer E (1990) Preembryo biopsy and analysis of blastomeres by in situ hybridisation. *American Journal of Obstetrics and Gynecology* 163: 2013–2019.

Hamberger L, Nilsson L, Sjögren A (1998) Microscopic imaging techniques: practical aspects. *Human Reproduction* 13: Abstract book 1: 15.

Harrison K, Wilson L, Breen T, *et al.* (1988) Fertilization of human oocytes in relation to varying delay before insemination. *Fertility and Sterility* 50(2): 294–297.

Hashimoto S, Iwamoto D, Taniguchi S, *et al.* (2009) Successful culture and time-lapse photography of individual human embryos using non-porous poly-(dimethylsiloxane) micro-well plates. *Fertility and Sterility* 92(3): S36–S36.

Heo YS, Cabrera LM, Song JW, *et al.* (2007) Characterization and resolution of evaporation-mediated osmolality shifts that constrain microfluidic cell culture in poly(dimethylsiloxane) devices. *Analytical Chemistry* 79(3): 1126–1134.

Hnida C, Ziebe S (2007) Morphometric analysis of human embryos. In: Elder K, Cohen J (eds.) *Preimplantation Embryo Evaluation and Selection*. Informa Press, London, pp. 89–100.

Hollywood K, Brison DR, Goodacre R (2006) Metabolomics: current technologies and future trends. *Proteomics* 6(17): 4716–4723.

Hook EB (1983) Down syndrome rates and relaxed selection at older maternal ages. *American Journal of Human Genetics* 35(6): 1307–1313.

Hook EB, Cross PK (1987) Rates of mutant and inherited structural cytogenetic abnormalities detected at amniocentesis: results on about 63,000 fetuses. *Annals of Human Genetics* 51 (Pt 1): 27–55.

Houghton FD, Hawkhead JA, Humpherson PG, *et al.* (2002) Non-invasive amino acid turnover predicts human embryo developmental capacity. *Human Reproduction* 17(4): 999–1005.

Houghton FD, Leese HJ (2004) Metabolism and developmental competence of the preimplantation embryo. *European Journal of Obstetrics, Gynecology and Reproductive Biology* 115(Suppl. 1): S92–96.

Huang TTF, Chinn K, Kosasa T, *et al.* (2016) Morphokinetics of human blastocyst expansion in vitro. *Reproductive BioMedicine Online* 33: 659–667.

Humaidan P, Kristensen SG, Coetzee K (2018) Mitochondrial DNA, a new biomarker of embryonic implantation potential: fact or fiction? *Fertility and Sterility* 109(1): 61–62.

Huntriss J, Picton H (2008) Epigenetic consequences of assisted reproduction and infertility on the human preimplantation embryo. *Human Fertility* 11(2): 85–94.

Hurley J, Huntriss J, Adjaye J (2000) Molecular approaches to the study of gene expression during human preimplantation development. *Human Fertility* 3: 48–51.

James A (2007) Human pronuclei as a mode of predicting viability. In: Elder K, Cohen J (eds.) *Human Preimplantation Embryo Evaluation and Selection.* Taylor & Francis, London, pp. 31–40.

Kahraman S, Yakin K, Dönmez E, *et al.* (2000) Relationship between granular cytoplasm of oocytes and pregnancy outcome following intracytoplasmic sperm injection. *Human Reproduction* 15(11): 2390–2393.

Kaser DJ, Racowsky C (2014) Clinical outcomes following selection of human preimplantation embryos with time-lapse monitoring: a systematic review. *Human Reproduction Update* 20(5): 617–631.

Katz-Jaffe MG, McReynolds S (2013) Embryology in the era of proteomics. *Fertility and Sterility* 99: 1073–1077.

Keefe DL, Franco S, Liu L, *et al.* (2005) Telomere length predicts embryo fragmentation after in vitro fertilization in women – toward a telomere theory of reproductive aging in women. *American Journal of Obstetrics and Gynecology* 192(4): 1256–1260; discussion 1260–1261.

Khan I, Staessen C, Van den Abbeel E, *et al.* (1989) Time of insemination and its effect on in vitro fertilization, cleavage and pregnancy rates in GnRH agonist/HMG-stimulated cycles. *Human Reproduction* 4(5): 531–535.

Kimber SJ, Sneddon SF, Bloor DJ, *et al.* (2008) Expression of genes involved in early cell fate decisions in human embryos and their regulation by growth factors. *Reproduction* 135: 635–647.

Kirkegaard K, Agerholm IE, Ingerslev HJ (2012a) Time-lapse monitoring as a tool for clinical embryo assessment. *Human Reproduction* 27: 1277–1285.

Kirkegaard K, Hindkjaer JJ, Ingerslev HJ (2012b) Human embryonic development after blastomere removal: a time-lapse analysis. *Human Reproduction* 27: 97–105.

Kirkegaard K, Hindkjaer JJ, Ingerslev HJ (2013) Effect of oxygen concentration on human embryo development evaluated by time-lapse monitoring. *Fertility and Sterility* 99: 738–744.e4.

Kleijkers SHM, Eijssen LMT, Coonen E, *et al.* (2015) Differences in gene expression profiles between human preimplantation embryos culture in two different IVF culture media. *Human Reproduction* 30(10): 2302–2311.

Kropp J, Salih SM, Khatib H (2014) Expression of microRNAs in bovine and human pre-implantation embryo culture media. *Frontiers in Genetics* 5: 91.

Kruger TF, Stander FSH, Smith K, Van Der Merue JP, Lombard CJ (1987) The effect of serum supplementation on the cleavage of human embryos. *Journal of In Vitro Fertilization and Embryo Transfer* 4: 10.

Kuliev A, Verlinsky Y (2008) Impact of preimplantation genetic diagnosis for chromosomal disorders on reproductive outcome. *Reproductive BioMedicine Online* 16(1): 9–10.

Lane M, Gardner DK (2005) Understanding cellular disruptions during early embryo development that perturb viability and fetal development. *Reproduction and Fertility Development* 17(3): 371–378.

Leese HJ (1987) Analysis of embryos by noninvasive methods. *Human Reproduction* 2: 37–40.

Leese HJ (2002) Quiet please, do not disturb: a hypothesis of embryo metabolism and viability. *Bioessays* 24(9): 845–849.

Leese HJ, Baumann CG, Brison DR, McEvoy TG, Sturmey RG (2008) Metabolism of the viable mammalian embryo: quietness revisited. *Molecular Human Reproduction* 14(12): 667–672.

Leese HJ, Donnay I, Thompson JG (1998) Human assisted conception: a cautionary tale. Lessons from domestic animals. *Human Reproduction* 13(Suppl. 4): 184–202.

Lesny P, Killick SR (2004) The junctional zone of the uterus and its contractions. *British Journal of Obstetrics and Gynaecology* 111(11): 1182–1189.

Levron J, Munné S, Willadsen S, Rosenwaks Z, Cohen J (1995) Male and female genomes associated in a single pronucleus in human zygotes. *Journal of Assisted Reproduction and Genetics* 12(Suppl): 27s.

Lin YC, Chang SY, Lan KC, *et al.* (2003) Human oocyte maturity in vivo determines the outcome of blastocyst development in vitro. *Journal of Assisted Reproduction and Genetics* 20(12): 506–512.

Liu L, Blasco MA, Keefe DL (2002) Requirement of functional telomeres for metaphase chromosome alignments and integrity of meiotic spindles. *EMBO Reports* 3(3): 230–234.

Lundin K, Ahlström A (2015) Quality control and standardization of embryo morphology scoring and viability markers. *Reproductive BioMedicine Online* 31: 459–471.

Lundqvist M, Johansson Ö Milton K, Westin C, Simberg N (2001) Does pronuclear morphology and/or early cleavage rate predict embryo implantation potential? *Reproductive BioMedicine Online* 2: 12–16.

Ma S, Kalousek DK, Zouves C, *et al.* (1990) The chromosomal complements of cleaved human embryos resulting from in vitro fertilization. *Journal of In Vitro Fertilization and Embryo Transfer* 7: 16–21.

Madaschi C, Aoki T, de Almeida Ferreira Braga DP, *et al.* (2009) Zona pellucida birefringence score and meiotic spindle visualization in relation to embryo development and ICSI outcomes. *Reproductive BioMedicine Online* 18(5): 681–686.

Mantikou E, Jonker MJ, Wong KM, *et al.* (2016) Factors affecting the gene expression of in vitro cultured human preimplantation embryos. *Human Reproduction* 31(2): 298–311.

Marrs RP, Saito H, Yee B, Sato F, Brown J (1984) Effect of variation of in vitro culture techniques upon oocyte fertilization and embryo development in human in vitro fertilization procedures. *Fertility and Sterility* 41: 519–523.

Mastenbroek S, Twisk M, van der Veen F, Repping S (2008) Preimplantation genetic screening. *Reproductive BioMedicine Online* 17(2): 293.

McKenzie LJ, Pangas SA, Carson SA, *et al.* (2004) Human cumulus granulosa cell gene expression: a predictor of fertilization and embryo selection in women undergoing IVF. *Human Reproduction* 19(12): 2869–2874.

McLaughlin M, Albertini DD, Wallace WHB, *et al.* (2018) Metaphase II oocytes from human unilaminar follicles grown in a multi-step culture system. *Molecular Human Reproduction* 24(3): 135–142.

Ménézo Y, Barak Y (2000) Comparison between day-2 embryos obtained either from ICSI or resulting from short insemination IVF: influence of maternal age. *Human Reproduction* 15(8): 1776–1780.

Ménézo Y, Chouteau J, Veiga A (2001) In vitro fertilization and blastocyst transfer for carriers of chromosomal translocation. *European Journal of Obstetrics, Gynecology and Reproductive Biology* 96(2): 193–195.

Ménézo Y, Dumont M, Hazout A, *et al.* (1995) Culture and co-culture techniques. In: Hedon B, Bringer J, Mares P. (eds.) *Fertility and Sterility*, IFFS-95. Parthenon Publishing Group, New York, pp. 413–418.

Ménézo Y, Elder K, Viville S (2006) Soluble HLA-G release by the human embryo: an interesting artefact? *Reproductive BioMedicine Online* 13(6): 763–764.

Ménézo Y, Guerin JF, Czyba JC (1990) Improvement of human early embryo development in vitro by co-culture on monolayers of Vero cells. *Biological Reproduction* 42: 301–305.

Ménézo Y, Hazout A, Dumont M, Herbaut N, Nicollet B (1992) Coculture of embryos on Vero cells and transfer of blastocyst in human. *Human Reproduction* 7: 101–106.

Ménézo Y, Janny L (1997) Influence of paternal factors in early embryogenesis. In: Barratt C, De Jonge C, Mortimer D, Parinaud J (eds.) *Genetics of Human Male Infertility*. EDK, Paris, pp. 246–257.

Ménézo Y, Testart J, Perrone D (1984) Serum is not necessary in human in vitro fertilization, early embryo culture, and transfer. *Fertility and Sterility* 42: 750.

Ménézo Y, Veiga A, Benkhalifa M (1998) Improved methods for blastocyst formation and culture. *Human Reproduction* 13 (Suppl. 4): 256–265.

Mercé, LT, Bau, S, Barco, MJ, *et al.* (2006) Assessment of the ovarian volume, number and volume of follicles and ovarian vascularity by three-dimensional ultrasonography and power Doppler angiography on the HCG day to predict the outcome in IVF/ICSI cycles. *Human Reproduction* 21: 1218–1226.

Meriano JS, Alexis J, Visram-Zaver S, Cruz M, Casper RF (2001) Tracking of oocyte dysmorphisms for ICSI patients may prove relevant to the outcome in subsequent patient cycles. *Human Reproduction* 16(10): 2118–2123.

Meriano JS, Clark C, Kadesky K, Laskin CA (2004) Binucleated and multinucleated blastomeres in embryos derived from human assisted reproduction cycles. *Reproductive BioMedicine Online* 9(5): 511–520.

Meseguer M, Herrero J, Tejera A, Hilligsoe KM, Ramsing NB, Remohi J (2011) The use of morphokinetics as a predictor of embryo implantation. *Human Reproduction* 26: 2658–2671.

Michael AE, Gregory L, Piercy EC, *et al.* (1995) Ovarian 11β-hydroxysteroid dehydrogenase activity is inversely related to the outcome of in vitro fertilization-embryo transfer treatment cycles. *Fertility and Sterility* 64(3): 590–598.

Mio Y, Maeda K (2008) Time-lapse cinematography of dynamic changes occurring during in vitro development of human embryos. *American Journal of Obstetrics and Gynecology* 199: 660.e1–660.e5.

Montag M, Schimming T, Koster M, *et al.* (2008) Oocyte zona birefringence intensity is associated with embryonic implantation potential in ICSI cycles. *Reproductive BioMedicine Online* 16(2): 239–244.

Montag M, Toth B, Strowitzky T (2013) New approaches to embryo selection. *Reproductive BioMedicine Online* 27: 539–546.

da Rocha AM, Smith GD (2012) Culture systems: fluid dynamic embryo culture systems (microfluidics). In: Smith G, Swain J, Pool T (eds.) *Embryo Culture. Methods in Molecular Biology (Methods and Protocols)*, vol 912. Humana Press, Totowa, NJ, pp. 355–365.

Monteiro da Rocha A, Smith GD (2014) Culture of embryos in dynamic fluid environments. In: Quinn P (ed.) *Culture Media, Solutions, and Systems in Human ART*. Cambridge University Press, Cambridge, UK, pp. 197–210.

Muggleton-Harris AL, Findlay I, Whittingham DG (1990) Improvement of the culture conditions for the development of human preimplantation embryos. *Human Reproduction* 5: 217–520.

Munné S, Alikani M, Levron J, *et al.* (1995a) Fluorescent in situ hybridisation in human blastomeres. In: Hedon B, Bringer J, Mares P (eds.) *Fertility and Sterility*. IFFS-95. Parthenon Publishing Group, New York, pp. 425–438.

Munné S, Alikani M Tomkin G, Grifo J, Cohen J (1995b) Embryo morphology, developmental rates, and maternal age are correlated with chromosomal abnormalities. *Fertility and Sterility* 64: 382–391.

Munné S, Cohen J (1998) Chromosome abnormalities in human embryos. *Human Reproduction Update* 4(6): 842–855.

Munné S, Lee A, Rosenwaks Z, Grifo J, Cohen J (1993) Diagnosis of major chromosome aneuploidies in human preimplantation embryos. *Human Reproduction* 8: 2185–2191.

Munné S, Wells D (2003) Questions concerning the suitability of comparative genomic hybridization for preimplantation genetic diagnosis. *Fertility and Sterility* 80(4): 871–872; discussion 875.

Oehninger S, Acosta AA, Veeck LL, Simonetti S, Muasher SJ (1989) Delayed fertilisation during in vitro fertilization and embryo transfer cycles: analysis of cause and impact of overall results. *Fertility and Sterility* 52: 991–997.

Pampiglione JS, Mills C, Campbell S, *et al.* (1990) The clinical outcome of reinsemination of human oocytes fertilized in vitro. *Fertility and Sterility* 53: 306–310.

Paternot G, Devroe J, Debrock S, D'Hooghe TM, Spiessens C (2009) Intra- and inter-observer analysis in the morphological assessment of early-stage embryos. *Reproductive Biology and Endocrinology* 7: 105.

Payne D, Flaherty SP, Barry MF, Matthews DC (1997) Preliminary observations on polar body extrusion and pronuclear formation in human oocytes using time-lapse video cinematography. *Human Reproduction* 12(3): 532–541.

Pickering SJ, Braude PR, Johnson MH, Cant A, Currie J (1990) Transient cooling to room temperature can cause irreversible disruption of the meiotic spindle in the human oocyte. *Fertility and Sterility* 54: 102–108.

Picton HM, Elder K, Houghton FD, *et al.* (2010) Association between amino acid turnover and chromosome aneuploidy during human preimplantation embryo development in vitro. *Molecular Human Reproduction* 16: 557–569.

Plachot M, de Grouchy J, Montagut J, *et al.* (1987) Multi-centric study of chromosome analysis in human oocytes and embryos in an IVF programme. *Human Reproduction* 2: 29.

Plachot M, Mandelbaum J, Junca AM, Cohen J, Salat-Baroux J (1993) Coculture of human embryo with granulosa cells. *Contraception, Fertility and Sex* 19: 632–634.

Plachot M, Veiga A, Montagut J, *et al.* (1988) Are clinical and biological IVF parameters correlated with chromosomal disorders in early life: a multicentric study. *Human Reproduction* 3: 627–635.

Platteau P, Staessen C, Michiels A, *et al.* (2006) Which patients with recurrent implantation failure after IVF benefit from PGD for aneuploidy screening? *Reproductive BioMedicine Online* (3): 334–339.

Pomeroy K, Reed M (2015) The effect of light on embryos and embryo culture. In: Elder K, Van den Bergh M, Woodward B (eds.) *Troubleshooting & Problem Solving in the IVF Laboratory.* Cambridge University Press, Cambridge, UK, pp. 104–116.

Posillico JT, and The Metabolomics Study Group for Assisted Reproductive Technologies (2007) Selection of viable embryos and gametes by rapid, noninvasive metabolomic profiling of oxidative stress biomarkers. In: Elder K, Cohen J (eds.) *Human Preimplantation Embryo Evaluation and Selection.* Taylor & Francis, London, pp. 245–262.

Purdy JM (1982) Methods for fertilization and embryo culture in vitro. In: Edwards RG, Purdy JM (eds.) *Human Conception In Vitro.* Academic Press, London, p. 135.

Quinn P, Warner GM, Klein JE, Kirby C (1985) Culture factors affecting the success rate of in vitro fertilization and embryo transfer. *Annals of the New York Academy of Sciences* 412: 195.

Richardson A, Brearley S, Ahitan S (2015) A clinically useful simplified blastocyst grading system. *Reproductive BioMedicine Online* 31: 523–530.

Rienzi L, Capalbo A, Stoppa M, *et al.* (2015) No evidence of association between blastocyst aneuploidy and morphokinetic assessment in a selected population of poor-prognosis patients: a longitudinal cohort study. *Reproductive BioMedicine Online* 30: 57–66.

Rødgaard T, Heegaard PM, Callesen H (2015) Non-invasive assessment of in vitro embryo quality to improve transfer success. *Reproductive BioMedicine Online* 31(5): 585–592.

Roert J, Verhoeff A, van Lent M, Hisman GJ, Zeilmaker GH (1995) Results of decentralised in vitro fertilization treatment with transport and satellite clinics. *Human Reproduction* 10: 563–567.

Rosenbluth EM, Shelton DN, Wells LM, Sparks AET, Van Voorhis BJ (2014) Human embryos secrete microRNAs into culture media: a potential biomarker for implantation. *Fertility and Sterility* 101: 1493–1500.

Salha O, Nugent D, Dada T, *et al.* (1998) The relationship between follicular fluid aspirate volume and oocyte maturity in in vitro fertilization cycles. *Human Reproduction* 13(7): 1901–1906.

Sargent IL (2005) Does 'soluble' HLA-G really exist? Another twist to the tale. *Molecular Human Reproduction* 11(10): 695–698.

Sauerbrun-Cutler MT, Vega M, Keltz M, McGovern PG (2015) In vitro maturation and its role in clinical assisted reproductive technology. *Obstetric and Gynecology Surveys* 70: 45–57.

Scott L (2003) Pronuclear score as a predictor of embryo development. *Reproductive BioMedicine Online* 6: 201–214.

Scott L, Alvero R, Leondires M, *et al.* (2000) The morphology of human pronuclear embryos is positively related to blastocyst development and implantation. *Human Reproduction* 15: 2394–2403.

Scott L, Smith S (1998) The successful use of pronuclear embryo transfers the day following oocyte retrieval. *Human Reproduction* 13: 1003–1013.

Seikkula J, Oksjoki S, Hurme S, Mankonen H, Polo-Kantola P, Jokimaa V (2018) Pregnancy and perinatal outcomes after transfer of binucleated or multinucleated frozen-thawed embryos: a case control study. *Reproductive BioMedicine Online* 36(6): 607–613.

Sermondade N, Hugues JN, Cedrin-Durnerin I, *et al.* (2010) Should all embryos from day 1 rescue intracytoplasmic sperm injection be transferred during frozen-thawed cycle? *Fertility and Sterility* 94(3): 1157–1158.

Sermondade N, Mandelbaum J (2009) Mastenbroek controversy or how much ink is spilled on preimplantation genetic screening subject? *Gynécologie Obstétrique & Fertilité* 37(3): 252–256.

Sher G, Keskintepe L, Nouriani M, Roussev R, Batzofin J (2004) Expression of sHLA-G in supernatants of individually cultured 46-h embryos: a potentially valuable indicator of 'embryo competency' and IVF outcome. *Reproductive BioMedicine Online* 9(1): 74–78.

Skiadas CC, Racowsky C (2007) Development rate, cumulative scoring and embryonic viability. In: Elder K, Cohen J (eds.) *Human Preimplantation Embryo Evaluation and Selection*. Taylor & Francis, London, pp. 101–122.

Smith GD, Takayama, S, Swain J (2012) Rethinking In Vitro embryo culture: new developments in culture platforms and potential to improve assisted reproductive technologies. *Biology of Reproduction* 86(3): 62.

Son WY, Chung JT, Demirtas E, *et al.* (2008) Comparison of in-vitro maturation cycles with and without in-vivo matured oocytes retrieved. *Reproductive BioMedicine Online* 17(1): 59–67.

Sturmey RG, Brison DR, Leese HJ (2008) Symposium: innovative techniques in human embryo viability assessment. Assessing embryo viability by measurement of amino acid turnover. *Reproductive BioMedicine Online* 17(4):486–496.

Swain J (2013) Shake, rattle and roll: bringing a little rock to the IVF laboratory to improve embryo development. *Journal of Assisted Reproduction and Genetics* 89(4): 105.

Swain JE, Cabrera L, Smith GD (2012) Microdrop preparation factors influence culture media osmolality which can impair mouse preimplantation embryo development. *Reproductive BioMedicine Online* 24(2): 142–147.

Swain JE, Lai D, Takayama S, Smith GD (2013) Thinking big by thinking small: application of microfluidic technology to improve ART. *Lab on a Chip* 13(7): 1213–1224.

Tesarik J (2018) Is blastomere multinucleation a safeguard against aneuploidy? Back to the future. *Reproductive BioMedicine Online* 28(4): 506–507.

Tesarik J, Greco E (1999) The probability of abnormal preimplantation development can be predicted by a single static observation on pronuclear stage morphology. *Human Reproduction* 14: 1318–1323.

Tesarik J, Junca AM, Hazout A, *et al.* (2000) Embryos with high implantation potential after intracytoplasmic sperm injection can be recognized by a simple, non-invasive examination of pronuclear morphology. *Human Reproduction* 15: 1396–1399.

Thompson JG, Gilchrist RB (2013) Pioneering contributions by Robert Edwards to oocyte in vitro maturation (IVM). *Molecular Human Reproduction* 19: 794–798.

Van Blerkom J (1996) The influence of intrinsic and extrinsic factors on the developmental potential of chromosomal normality of the human oocyte. *Journal of the Society of Gynecological Investigation* 3: 3–11.

Van Blerkom J, Atczak M, Schrader R (1997) The developmental potential of the human oocyte is related to the dissolved oxygen content of follicular fluid: association with vascular endothelial growth factor concentrations and perifollicular blood flow characteristics. *Human Reproduction* 12: 1047–1055.

Van Blerkom J, Davis P, Alexander S (2000) Differential mitochondrial distribution in human pronuclear embryos leads to disproportionate inheritance between blastomeres: relationship to microtubular organization, ATP content and competence. *Human Reproduction* 15(12): 2621–2633.

Van Blerkom J, Henry G (1992) Oocyte dysmorphism and aneuploidy in meiotically mature human oocytes after ovarian stimulation. *Human Reproduction* 7: 379–390.

Veeck LL (1986) Insemination and fertilization. In: Jones HW Jr., Jones GS, Hodgen GD, Rosenwaks Z (eds.) *In Vitro Fertilization – Norfolk*. Williams & Wilkins, Baltimore, p. 183.

Veeck LL (1988) Oocyte assessment and biological performance. *Annals of the New York Academy of Sciences* 541: 259–262.

Verlinsky Y, Cieslak J, Freidine M, *et al.* (1995) Pregnancies following pre-conception diagnosis of common aneuploidies by fluorescent in situ hybridisation. *Molecular Human Reproduction* 10: 1927–1934.

Verlinsky Y, Strom C, Cieslak J, *et al.* (1996) Birth of healthy children after preimplantation diagnosis of common aneuploidies by polar body fluorescent in situ hybridisation analysis. *Fertility and Sterility* 66: 126–129.

Walls ML, Hunter T, Ryan JP, Keelan JA, Nathan E, Hart RJ (2015) In vitro maturation as an alternative to standard in vitro fertilization for patients diagnosed with polycystic ovaries: a comparative analysis of fresh, frozen and cumulative cycle outcomes. *Human Reproduction* 30: 88–96.

Weimer KE, Cohen J, Tucker MJ, Godke A (1998) The application of co-culture in assisted reproduction: 10 years of experience with human embryos. *Human Reproduction* 13(Suppl. 4): 226–238.

Wells D (2007) Future genetic and other technologies for assessing embryos. In: Elder K, Cohen J (eds.) *Preimplantation Embryo Evaluation and Selection.* Informa Press, London, pp. 287–300.

Wenzel ES, Singh ATK (2018) Cell-cycle checkpoints and aneuploidy on the path to cancer. *In Vivo* 32(1): 1–5.

Woolcott R, Stanger J (1997) Potentially important variables identified by trans-vaginal ultrasound guided embryo transfer. *Human Reproduction* 12: 963–966.

Woolcott R, Stanger J (1998) Ultrasound tracking of the movement of embryo-associated air bubbles on standing after transfer. *Human Reproduction* 13(8): 2107–2109.

Wunder DM, Mueller MD, Birkhäuser MH, Bersinger NA (2005) Steroids and protein markers in the follicular fluid as indicators of oocyte quality in patients with and without endometriosis. *Journal of Assisted Reproduction and Genetics* 22(6): 257–264.

Xiao S, Zhang J, Romero MM, Smith KN, Shea LD, Woodruff TK (2015) In vitro follicle growth supports human oocyte meiotic maturation. *Scientific Reports* 5: 17323.

Yan L, Yang M, Guo H, *et al.* (2013) Single-cell RNA-Seq profiling of human preimplantation embryos and embryonic stem cells. *Nature Structural & Molecular Biology* 20: 1131–1139.

Ziebe S, Loft A, Petersen JH, *et al.* (2001) Embryo quality and developmental potential is compromised by age. *Acta Obstetricia et Gynecologica Scandinavica* 80(2): 169–174.

Ziebe S, Lundin K, Janssens R, Helmgaard L, Arce JC (2007) MERIT (Menotrophin vs Recombinant FSH in vitro Fertilisation Trial) Group. Influence of ovarian stimulation with HP-hMG or recombinant FSH on embryo quality parameters in patients undergoing IVF. *Human Reproduction* 22(9): 2404–2413.

Ziebe S, Lundin K, Loft A, *et al.* (2003) CEMAS II and Study Group; FISH analysis for chromosomes 13, 16, 18, 21, 22, X and Y in all blastomeres of IVF pre-embryos from 144 randomly selected donated human oocytes and impact on pre-embryo morphology. *Human Reproduction* 18(12): 2575–2581.

## In-vitro Maturation

Albertini DF, Sanfins A, Combelles CM (2003) Origins and manifestations of oocyte maturation competencies. *Reproductive BioMedicine Online* 6: 410–415.

Barnes FL, Sirard MA (2000) Oocyte maturation. *Seminars in Reproductive Medicine* 18: 123–131.

Cha KY, Han SY, Chung HM, *et al.* (2000) Pregnancies and deliveries after in vitro maturation culture followed by in vitro fertilization and embryo transfer without stimulation in women with polycystic ovary syndrome. *Fertility and Sterility* 73: 978.

Cha KY, Koo JJ, Ko JJ, *et al.* (1991) Pregnancy after in vitro fertilization of human follicular oocytes collected from nonstimulated cycles, their culture in vitro and their transfer in a donor oocyte program. *Fertility and Sterility* 55: 109–113.

Chian RC, Buckett WM, Tan SL (2004a) In-vitro maturation of human oocytes. *Reproductive BioMedicine Online* 8: 148–166.

Chian RC, Buckett WM, Tulandi T, Tan SL (2000) Prospective randomized study of human chorionic gonadotrophin priming before immature oocyte retrieval from unstimulated women with polycystic ovarian syndrome. *Human Reproduction* 15: 165–170.

Chian RC, Gulekli B, Buckett WM, Tan SL (2001) Pregnancy and delivery after cryopreservation of zygotes produced by in-vitro matured oocytes retrieved from a woman with polycystic ovarian syndrome. *Human Reproduction* 16: 1700–1702.

Chian RC, Lim JH, Tan SL (2004b) State of the art in in-vitro oocyte maturation. *Current Opinion in Obstetrics and Gynecology* 16: 211–219.

Child TJ, Abdul-Jalil AK, Gulekli B, Tan SL (2001) In vitro maturation and fertilization of oocytes from unstimulated normal ovaries, polycystic ovaries, and women with polycystic ovary syndrome. *Fertility and Sterility* 76: 936–942.

Child TJ, Phillips SJ, Abdul-Jalil AK, Gulekli B, Tan SL (2002) A comparison of in vitro maturation and in vitro fertilization for women with polycystic ovaries. *Obstetrics and Gynecology* 100: 665–670.

Combelles CMH, Fissore RA, Albertini DF, Racowsky C (2006) In vitro maturation of human oocytes and cumulus cells using a co-culture three-dimensional collagen gel system. *Human Reproduction* 20(5): 1349–1358.

Edwards RG (1965) Maturation in vitro of human ovarian oocytes. *Lancet* 2: 926–969.

Hreinsson J, Rosenlund B, Frid B, *et al.* (2003) Recombinant LH is equally effective as recombinant hCG in promoting oocyte maturation in a clinical in-vitro maturation programme: a randomized study. *Human Reproduction* 18(10): 2131–2136.

Lagalla C, Tarozzi N, Sciajno R, *et al.* (2017) Embryos with morphokinetic abnormalities may develop into euploid blastocysts. *Reproductive BioMedicine Online* 34(2): 137–146.

Ménézo Y, Elder K, Benkhalifa M, Dale B (2010) DNA methylation and gene expression in IVF. *Reproductive BioMedicine Online* 20(6): 709–710.

Moor RM, Dai Y, Lee C, Fulka J Jr. (1998) Oocyte maturation and embryonic failure. *Human Reproduction Update* 4: 223–236.

Picton H, Briggs D, Gosden R (1998) The molecular basis of oocyte growth and development. *Molecular and Cellular Endocrinology* 145: 27–37.

Pincus G, Enzmann EV (1935) Comparative behavior of mammalian eggs in vivo and in vitro. *Journal of Experimental Medicine* 62: 665–678.

Roberts R, Franks S, Hardy K (2002) Culture environment modulates maturation and metabolism of human oocytes. *Human Reproduction* 17: 2950–2956.

Sutton ML, Gilchrist RB, Thompson JG (2003) Effects of in-vivo and in-vitro environments on the metabolism of the cumulus–oocyte complex and its influence on oocyte developmental capacity. *Human Reproduction Update* 9: 35–48.

Tan SL, Child T (2001) In-vitro maturation of oocytes from unstimulated polycystic ovaries. *Reproductive BioMedicine Online* 4(Suppl. 1): 18–23.

Telfer EE, McLaughlin M, Ding C, Thong KJ (2008) A two-step serum-free culture system supports development of human oocytes from primordial follicles in the presence of activin. *Human Reproduction* 23(5): 1151–1158.

Trounson A, Wood C, Kausche A (1994) In vitro maturation and the fertilization and developmental competence of oocytes recovered from untreated polycystic ovarian patients. *Fertility and Sterility* 62: 353–362.

Veeck LL, Wortham JW Jr, Witmyer J, *et al.* (1983) Maturation and fertilization of morphologically immature human oocytes in a program of in vitro fertilization. *Fertility and Sterility* 39: 594–602.

Walls M, Hunter T, Ryan JP, *et al.* (2015) In vitro maturation as an alternative to standard in vitro fertilization for patients diagnosed with polycystic ovaries: a comparative analysis of fresh, frozen and cumulative cycle outcomes. *Human Reproduction* 30(1): 88–96.

Walls M, Junk S, Ryan J, Hart R (2012) IVF versus ICSI for the fertilization of in vitro matured human oocytes. *Reproductive BioMedicine Online* 25: 603–607.

Wells D (2017) Mitochondrial DNA quantity as a biomarker for blastocyst implantation potential. *Fertility and Sterility* 108(5): 742–747.

253

# Cryopreservation of Gametes and Embryos

## Principles of Cryobiology

The first live births following frozen-thawed embryo transfer were reported in 1984 and 1985 by groups in Australia, the Netherlands and the United Kingdom. Since that time, the original protocols have been modified and simplified such that cryopreservation with successful survival of sperm, oocytes and embryos is now an essential component of every routine IVF program. Pregnancy and live birth rates after frozen embryo transfer contribute significantly to cumulative conception rates after fresh transfer. In recent years, traditional methods of freezing and thawing have been increasingly replaced by protocols for vitrification/warming. For both slow freezing and vitrification, an understanding of the basic principles of cryobiology involved is essential to ensure that the methodology is correctly and successfully applied, in order to minimize cell damage during the processes of freezing/vitrification and thawing/warming. There are two major classes of physical stresses that cells are exposed to during cryopreservation:

1. Direct effects of reduced temperature
2. Physical changes associated with ice formation.

## Direct Effects of Reduced Temperatures

'Chilling injury' is the damage to cell structure and function caused by cooling; the type and extent of damage, associated with modifications in membrane permeability and changes in the cytoskeletal structure, differ between different types of mammalian cells (reviewed by Watson & Morris, 1987 and Fahy & Wowk, 2015). The effect is species-specific and well documented for spermatozoa (cattle, pig), oocytes and embryos (pig). Oocytes are particularly susceptible to damage, and sublethal injuries can also occur during cryopreservation of oocytes and ovarian and testicular tissue, particularly in relation to breakdown of the cellular spindle apparatus.

## Physical Changes Associated With Ice Formation

Temperature changes observed during the freezing of an aqueous solution are illustrated in Figure 12.1. Water and aqueous solutions have a strong tendency to cool below their melting point before nucleation of ice occurs: this phenomenon is referred to as super-cooling, or more correctly undercooling. For example, whilst 0°C is the melting point of ice, the temperature of water may be reduced significantly below 0°C before ice formation occurs, and in carefully controlled conditions water may be cooled to approximately −40°C before ice nucleation becomes inevitable. The homogeneous nucleation temperature ($T_h$) is the lowest temperature to which small samples can be cooled without ice formation; $T_h$ decreases with increasing solute concentration.

Following ice nucleation and initial crystal growth, the temperature rises to its melting point and remains relatively constant at that temperature during the subsequent phase change to ice ('latent

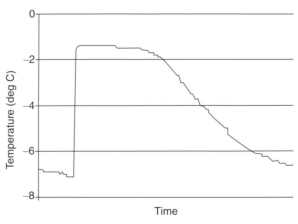

**Figure 12.1** Temperature changes during the freezing of an aqueous solution of glycerol (5% w/v).

heat plateau'), when the temperature then changes more rapidly to the environment temperature.

The tendency of a system to supercool is related to a number of factors including temperature, rate of cooling, volume, exclusion of atmospheric ice nuclei and purity of particulates. In cryopreservation of cells and tissues in IVF systems, there is thus a strong tendency for supercooling to occur. In order to avoid the damaging effects of supercooling on cells and in particular embryos (see below), slow-freezing protocols initiate ice formation in a controlled manner. This is commonly referred to as 'seeding' – although, strictly speaking, this term refers to the introduction of a crystal to an under-cooled solution. 'Nucleation'

is the initiation of ice other than by seeding, and this is the process generally practiced in slow-freezing protocols for IVF.

## Supercooling and Cell Survival

Controlled ice formation during freezing is recognized to be a key factor in determining the viability of embryos following freezing and thawing (see Whittingham, 1977). In a carefully controlled series of experiments, samples which were nucleated below –9°C had a low viability, whilst nucleation at higher subzero temperatures of –5°C to –7.5°C resulted in much higher viability (Figure 12.2).

An analysis of the spontaneous nucleation behavior of straws (Figure 12.3) clearly demonstrates that if nucleation is not controlled, a poor recovery of embryos would be expected.

The physical basis of this injury is clear from examining thermal histories of supercooled straws (Figure 12.4). The differences between laboratories that achieve good results and those that are less successful can often be attributed to the practical step of ice nucleation, or 'seeding.' Straws can be frozen horizontally or vertically – this has no effect on viability or ease of ice nucleation. Embryos sink in the cryoprotective additive and will always be found at the wall of the straw when frozen horizontally, or at the bottom of the column of liquid when frozen vertically. Following thermal equilibration ('holding') at the nucleation temperature (–7°C), ice formation is initiated by touching the outside of the straw or ampule with a liquid nitrogen cooled spatula, forceps,

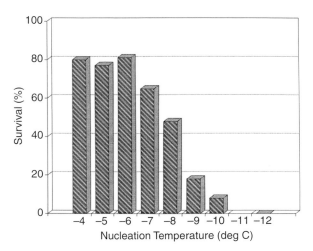

**Figure 12.2** The survival of mouse cell embryos after seeding at various subzero temperatures. Redrawn with permission from Whittingham (1977).

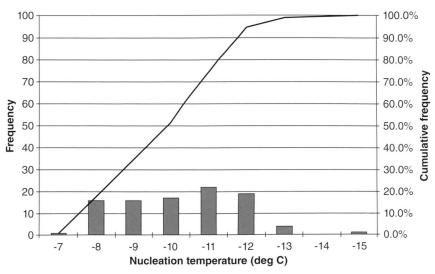

**Figure 12.3** The measured nucleation temperatures within 0.25-mL straws cooling at 0.3°C/min.

**Table 12.1** Factors associated with cooling and cryopreservation that contribute to cellular injury and death in biological systems

| System | Type/cause of damage |
|--------|----------------------|
| All | Intracellular ice formation, extracellular ice formation, apoptosis, toxicity, calcium imbalance, free radicals, ATP levels, general metabolism, fertilization failure, cleavage failure, intracellular pH, parthenogenetic activation, cleavage |
| Membrane | Rupture, leakage, fusion, microvilli, phase transition |
| Chromosomes | Loss/gain, polyspermy, polygny (failure to extrude polar body), tetraploidy |
| DNA | Apoptosis, fusion, rearrangements |
| Cytoskeleton | Microtubules dissolve, actin |
| Proteins/enzymes | Dehydration, loss of function |
| Ultrastructure | Microvilli, mitochondria, vesicles, cortical granules, zona pellucida |
| Zona pellucida | Hardening, fracture |
| Lipids | Free radicals? |

Reproduced with permission from Shaw *et al.* (2000).

cotton bud etc., at the level of the meniscus (seeding at both ends of a horizontal straw has also been advocated). This causes a local cold spot on the vessel wall, which leads to ice nucleation. Immediately following ice nucleation, the temperature will rise rapidly (cf. Figure 12.1), and the ice front will propagate through the sample. Following ice formation, the temperature returns at a rate of 2.5°C/min to –7°C. Cellular dehydration then occurs during subsequent slow cooling.

By contrast, in a straw supercooled to –15°C, spontaneous ice formation again results in a temperature rise followed by a rapid rate of cooling at 10°C/min to –5°C. The combination of a rapid rate of cooling and a large reduction in temperature does not allow the cell to dehydrate, and lethal intracellular ice formation is then inevitable (Table 12.1). This has been observed by direct cryomicroscopy.

Ice crystallization in an aqueous solution effectively removes some water from solution. The remaining aqueous phase becomes more concentrated, and a two-phase system of ice and concentrated solution coexists. As the temperature is reduced, more ice forms and the residual unfrozen phase becomes increasingly concentrated. For example, in glycerol and water a two-phase system occurs at all temperatures to –45°C. At –45°C the nonfrozen phase solidifies, with a glycerol concentration of 64% w/v; this is the eutectic temperature. In dilute aqueous solutions

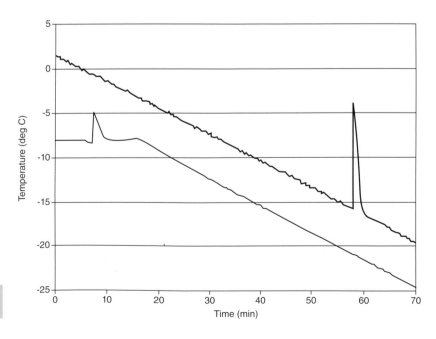

**Figure 12.4** Measured temperatures within straws. During conventional cryopreservation, the straws are held at a temperature of –7°C and nucleated; the resultant rise in temperature following ice nucleation is small. In the absence of induced nucleation the straws may reach very low temperatures before spontaneous nucleation occurs. A large rise in temperature to the melting point of the suspending medium then occurs followed by a rapid reduction in temperature; this will inevitably result in intracellular ice formation within embryos or oocytes.

such as culture media, there is a dramatic increase in ionic composition following ice formation and by −10°C the salt concentration reaches *c.* 3 molal – not surprisingly, this is lethal to cells. Cryoprotective additives reduce cellular damage during freezing and thawing by simply increasing the volume of the residual unfrozen phase. This reduces the ionic composition of the solution at any subzero temperature. It must also be noted that all other physical parameters of the solution change following the formation of ice, including gas content, viscosity and pH.

## Cryoprotectants

The addition of cryoprotectant agents (CPAs) is thought to protect cells by stabilizing intracellular proteins, reducing or eliminating lethal intracellular ice formation, and by moderating the impact of concentrated intra- and extracellular electrolytes. The first successful use of a cryoprotectant was in 1949, when Polge *et al.* used glycerol to freeze semen; glycerol is still commonly used as a cryoprotectant today. All cryoprotectants are low molecular weight compounds, are completely miscible with water, easily permeate cell membranes and depress the freezing point of water to very low subzero temperatures, e.g., $< -60°$ C. Some (but not all) are nontoxic when the cells are exposed to them at room temperature for limited times, even at high concentrations. All are hyperosmotic, and they can be divided into two groups:

1. *Permeating*: glycerol, ethylene glycol, 1,2-propanediol (PROH) and dimethylsulfoxide (DMSO) penetrate the cell membrane, although more slowly than water. Inside the cell, they stabilize intracellular proteins, reduce the temperature at which intracellular ice forms and minimize osmotic damage due to electrolyte concentration effects. Glycerol penetrates tissue less readily than DMSO, PROH and EG. These cryoprotectants have high water solubility, rapid tissue penetration and induce less osmotic damage at high concentrations.

2. *Non-permeating*: a variety of sugars, polymers and amphipathic compounds have been used as non-permeating cryoprotectants. Raffinose and lactose decrease the percentage of unfrozen water and/or decrease salt concentrations. Glycine, proline and trehalose are amphipathic compounds that interact with membrane lipids and proteins to alter phase transitions and hydration status.

Cryoprotectants should always be used in combination with nonpermeating osmolytes such as sucrose or mannitol. These partially dehydrate the cells and act as osmotic buffers to protect against cell swelling during the addition/removal of cryoprotectants. Egg yolk has been added to cryopreservation medium used to preserve animal sperm, since the low-density lipoprotein fraction of egg yolk is thought to protect against cold shock. However, this is not recommended for freezing human cells, as it introduces batch-to-batch variation and the possibility of bacterial contamination.

The pioneering studies on mammalian embryo cryopreservation used either glycerol or DMSO as cryoprotectants, but these were subsequently superseded by the protocol of Lasalle *et al.* (1985), which uses PROH. PROH is considered to have a higher permeability to human embryos than either glycerol or DMSO, and is less toxic than DMSO. The real toxicity of cryoprotectants in cells is largely unknown; Stanic *et al.* (2000) reported that most of the decrease in sperm motility during cryopreservation was due to exposure to cryoprotectants rather than to the freezing process.

## Factors That Affect Cellular Response to Freezing

### Permeability to CPA

Studies investigating the permeability coefficients of oocytes and zygotes demonstrate that the oocyte is much less permeable to CPAs than the zygote, and the activation energy of oocyte permeability is higher than that of the zygote. This means that as temperature is lowered, a CPA will penetrate an oocyte far more slowly than it will penetrate a zygote, with resulting effects on the rates of water loss from the cells. The permeability of oocytes has also been found to vary between individuals, with differences ranging from 3- to 6-fold, i.e., cohorts of oocytes from different women may differ in their permeability to CPAs. This feature has also been demonstrated in mice and in cattle, suggesting that properties of cell membranes may have a genetic basis (see Leibo & Pool, 2011 for review).

### Surface Area

The ratio of surface area to volume in a cell influences permeability characteristics, and this will determine the optimum cooling rate for that cell. In general, the larger the cell, the slower it must be cooled to survive

257

freezing. For example, a human oocyte, the largest cell in the body, is a sphere measuring 120 μm in diameter with a large volume, whereas the flattened paddle-shaped sperm cell has a much higher surface area to volume ratio. Consequently, when exposed to CPAs, spermatozoa reach osmotic equilibrium much faster than oocytes, and optimum cooling rates for spermatozoa are much higher than those for oocytes and embryos. However, although oocytes and zygotes have nearly identical surface area/volume ratios, the oocyte is less permeable to CPAs than the zygote. Germinal vesicle stage oocytes differ from metaphase II oocytes in their activation energy of water permeability, so that decreasing temperature has a greater effect on the osmotic response of a GV oocyte than on a metaphase II oocyte, although both are equally susceptible to chilling injury.

## Cell Volume Changes

At temperatures near 0°C, abrupt changes in volume can immediately damage cells and also make them more susceptible to stress during subsequent cooling or thawing procedures; therefore, extreme fluctuations in cell volume must be avoided during CPA equilibration. The duration of exposure to these potentially toxic chemicals should also be minimized: CPA toxicity can be reduced by lowering the temperature of exposure, but this would require a longer exposure time.

## Cooling to Subzero Temperature

When large cells such as oocytes are frozen in molar concentrations of CPAs, their survival is strongly dependent on cooling rate, and the specific optimum cooling rate depends on both the type and the concentration of CPA. Cell survival is equally dependent on warming rate, and the optimum warming rate depends on both the CPA and its concentration, as well as on the cooling rate that preceded it. Cryobiology studies have shown that different types of cell have different optimal cooling rates, even when frozen in the same solution. This is especially relevant to the cryopreservation of tissues such as ovarian cortex that are made up of many different types of cell, each with its own characteristic size, shape and permeability properties. Cooling and warming conditions that are optimal for one cell type may be harmful to others; warming rate rather than cooling rate is more important in determining ultimate viability of the cell (Jin *et al.*, 2014).

## Osmotic Events

As mentioned above, when aqueous solutions are frozen, water is removed in the form of ice, causing the cells to become increasingly concentrated as the temperature falls. The reverse occurs during thawing. Cells in suspension are not punctured by ice crystals (see Figure 12.5), nor are they mechanically damaged by ice. Cells partition into the unfrozen fraction and are exposed to increasing hypertonic solutions. Varying amounts of water may be removed osmotically from the cell, dependent on the rate of cooling. At 'slow' rates of cooling, cells may remain essentially in equilibrium with the external solution. As the rate of cooling is increased, there is less time for water to move from the cell, which becomes increasingly supercooled until eventually intracellular ice is formed. An optimum rate of cooling results from the balance of these two phenomena. At rates of cooling slower than the optimum, cell death is due to long periods of exposure to hypertonic conditions. At rates of cooling faster than the optimum, cell death is associated with intracellular ice formation, which is inevitably lethal. The actual value of the optimum rate is determined by a number of biophysical factors, including cell volume

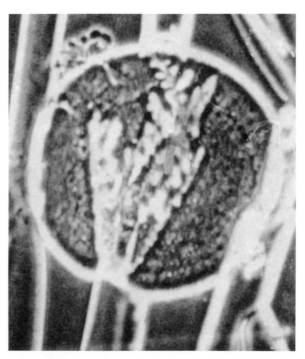

**Figure 12.5** Light microscopy of a human oocyte following ice nucleation in the extracellular medium. The oocyte is not punctured by ice crystals.

and surface area, permeability to water, Arrhenius activation energy, and type and concentration of cryoprotective additives. As the cells are frozen, they must respond osmotically to large changes in extracellular fluid concentrations: the efflux of water during slow freezing (<2°C/min) causes oocytes to undergo osmotic dehydration, with resulting contraction.

### Removal of Cryoprotectant

Although cells in suspension can tolerate exposure to very high concentrations of CPAs, whether or not they survive the freeze–thaw process depends on how the CPA solution is removed. When frozen cells are warmed rapidly, the melting process is equivalent to rapid dilution of the CPA that was concentrated during the freezing process. As the extracellular milieu begins to melt, the rapid influx of water into the cells can cause osmotic shock at subzero temperatures. Sensitivity to osmotic shock is therefore a function of the cell's permeability to water and solutes. This shock can be reduced by using a nonpermeating substance such as sucrose as an osmotic buffer. Tissues are even more sensitive to osmotic effects than are cell suspensions, because cells located in the interior of a piece of tissue can respond osmotically only when the neighboring cells have also responded.

*In summary*, cells that are cooled too slowly can be damaged by changes in solution composition and osmotic effects of shrinkage; cells that are cooled too quickly can be damaged by ice formation. The formation of ice during either cooling or warming depends upon how much time is available for ice nucleation and growth: optimal high cooling and warming rates can 'outrun' the kinetics of ice formation, minimizing the chance of injury. CPAs change the optimal cooling rate in a manner that is dependent on the cell type.

# Cryopreservation Protocols

Two basic types of cryopreservation are used for cells and tissues: slow freezing and vitrification.

## Equilibrium Freezing (Slow Freezing)

The procedures used for slow freezing of oocytes, embryos and ovarian cortex are generally quite similar. The cells or tissues are equilibrated in an aqueous solution containing an optimal concentration (1.0–1.5 M) of cryoprotectant and sucrose (0.1 M) and frozen in straws or ampules. Following CPA exposure, the temperature is slowly lowered, and ice crystal growth is initiated in the

solution ('seeding'). The ampules or straws are seeded at −6.5 to −7°C, cooled slowly at 0.3–0.5°C/min to approximately −40°C, then quickly cooled to −150°C before final transfer into liquid nitrogen for storage. Embryos and spermatozoa do not deteriorate when stored even for decades in liquid nitrogen.

---

**Definitions**

**Freezing:** Water molecules are reorganized into ice crystals.

**Thawing:** Melting of ice.

**Nucleation:** A small number of ions, atoms or molecules arrange into a crystalline pattern, forming a site for crystal growth by addition of further particles.

*Homogeneous:* does not involve foreign particles or atoms, takes place away from surfaces. Homogeneous nucleation temperature ($T_h$) is the lowest temperature to which small samples can be cooled without ice formation.

*Heterogeneous:* a different substance, such as dust particle or wall of the container, acts as the center for crystal formation; takes place at nucleation sites such as interfaces, surface of impurities, etc. Heterogeneous nucleators mimic the structure of ice, with a lower surface energy.

**Cryoprotectant agent (CPA):** An agent that reduces or prevents chilling/freezing injury.

**Critical cooling rate (CCR):** The rate above which ice formation is not observed.

**Critical warming rate (CWR):** Warming rate that suppresses ice formation during warming.

CCR and CWR depend on total solute content and the chemical nature of the solute.

**Vitrification:** Transition of a solution from liquid to glass phase.

**Glass transition temperature ($T_G$):** The temperature at which vitrification takes place on cooling.

**Devitrification:** Formation of ice during warming after previous devitrification.

**Rewarming:** Warming of a previously cryopreserved system, whether frozen or vitrified.

**Recrystallization:** Transfer of water molecules from small ice crystals to larger crystals, which cause greater damage.

## Vitrification/Ultra-rapid Freezing

Vitrification combines the use of concentrated cryoprotectant solutions with ultra-rapid cooling in order to avoid the formation of ice. The high osmotic pressure of concentrated CPAs causes rapid dehydration, and the contracted samples are placed into a vitrification device that can be immediately plunged into liquid nitrogen. Samples reach very low temperatures ($-196^\circ$C) in a state that has the molecular structure of a viscous liquid without crystals, forming an amorphous glassy solid. The transition from liquid to glass phase is a kinetic phenomenon: increased viscosity delays thermodynamic intermolecular rearrangements and 'locks in' a non-equilibrium thermodynamic state. The goal of vitrification is to completely eliminate ice formation in the medium containing the sample throughout all stages of cooling, storage and warming.

Since rapid cooling is effected via direct contact with liquid nitrogen, programmable freezing machines are not needed. There is an inverse correlation between the cryoprotectant concentrations and cooling rates required, and successful vitrification is based on applying extremely high cooling rates in combination with very high concentrations of cryoprotectant or cryoprotectant mixtures. Cooling is too rapid for ice to form or grow appreciably, and the solute concentration remains constant during cooling.

- A balance must be achieved between the lowest level of least hazardous CPA and maximal cooling rate: higher CPA concentrations allow lower cooling rates, and vice versa. Since highly concentrated CPAs may cause toxic and osmotic damage, a preferred strategy is to use the highest possible cooling and warming rates, and then use the lowest concentration of CPA that will prevent ice formation.

- Adequate dehydration and permeation of cells is essential, and therefore exposure time is important.

- In order to avoid the formation of both intracellular and extracellular ice, the initial cooling rate must exceed the critical cooling rate (CCR) of the solution.

- Warming rates are critical to survival: total development of ice is much more rapid during warming, and warming rates required to avoid significant devitrification are far higher than cooling rates required to achieve vitrification.

The cooling rate is affected by several parameters, and different methods have been employed in order to find an effective and practical solution, by varying cryoprotectant solutions, combinations, exposure times and temperature. The addition of sugars (sucrose, trehalose, fructose, sorbitol saccharose, raffinose) reduces the concentration of CPA required; the permeability of mixtures is higher than that of individual components, and different combinations of CPA have also been tried. Vitrification solutions are developed with the lowest possible concentration of CPA compatible with achieving glass formation. Reducing volume to a minimum reduces potential toxicity and osmotic damage, and methods have been devised to reduce the volume of CPA down to between 0.1 μL and 2 μL. Reducing the drop size or increasing the number of embryos per drop risks diluting the CPA with medium carried over from the culture drop, and this could allow the sample to freeze, with lethal results.

---

**Comparison of Slow Cooling vs. Vitrification**

**Slow Freezing**
- Low concentrations of permeating + nonpermeating cryoprotectants (1.5/0.1–0.3), PROH or DMSO/sucrose.
- Requires controlled rate freezing machine, 2°C/min, then 0.3°C/min.
- Nucleation (seeding) and transfer to liquid nitrogen is critical.
- Well-established protocols and techniques.

**Vitrification**
- Avoids formation of ice that can damage membranes.
- Rapid method, simple equipment.
- No specialized controlled rate freezer required.
- Application in clinical practice has been slow, due to concerns about toxicity of high CPA concentrations (up to 6 M).
- Use of very low volumes reduces toxicity risk.
- Requires critical process control: zero tolerance to any changes/fluctuations.
- Samples must be handled and moved very rapidly.
- Avoid accidental warming: stored samples are very fragile and could be susceptible to mini-devitrification cycles during routine dewar use in a busy IVF laboratory.
- 'Open' systems: direct contact with liquid nitrogen.

The thawing rate must also be rapid, in order to prevent devitrification and ice crystal formation during the transition state. The samples are kept in air (room temperature) for 1–3 seconds; for open systems, the sample is then immersed in dilution medium at 37°C, and for closed systems, the carrier is immersed in a 37°C water bath before transferring the sample to the dilution medium. The CPA is diluted in several steps, in order to counterbalance osmotic effects as the CPA leaves the cell.

Although the methodology and protocols that accompany vitrification systems for IVF appear deceptively simple, the principles that ensure viability after warming are a highly complex combination of thermodynamics and cell and molecular biology. Numerous kinetic variables surrounding the physics of aqueous solutions and biological survival can jeopardize success. (See Fahy & Wowk, 2015 for detailed review.) Different types of vitrification systems are available which involve different principles:

1. *Unstable vitrification*: solute concentrations that are too low to prevent homogeneous ice nucleation will nucleate at large numbers of points in the solution, i.e., $>2500/\mu m^3$. Cooling requires thousands of degrees per minute or more, to prevent high ice nucleation and growth rates of homogeneous nucleation. Cells can survive if warming is sufficiently rapid.

2. *Metastable vitrification*: solute concentrations are high enough to avoid homogeneous nucleation, but low enough to thermodynamically favor ice formation. Cells can be supercooled to glass transition without necessarily nucleating ice, but ice can be formed in discrete locations where heterogeneous nucleators are present. Cooling rates on the order of 10°C/minute are possible.

3. *Stable/equilibrium vitrification:* solute concentrations are so high that ice cannot exist in the solution; arbitrarily low cooling rates are possible, but complete stability requires high concentrations of solute.

4. *Kinetic vitrification*: ultrafast cooling ($>10,000$°C/min) usually requires very small sample volumes but lower CPA concentrations.

The basic principles regarding CPA concentrations/cooling rates outlined above were brought into question by Jin & Mazur (2015), who demonstrated >90% survival of mouse oocytes and embryos when cooled at much slower rates, in solutions containing one-third of the 'standard' solute concentrations, provided that they are warmed ultra-rapidly ($10^7$°C/min) using a laser pulse. They suggest that survival of a cell after vitrification is highly dependent on its dehydration, due to the fact that the rate of recrystallization of intracellular ice on warming is highly sensitive to its residual intracellular water content after vitrification: i.e., the osmotic withdrawal of a large fraction of intracellular water prior to cooling is the most important feature during vitrification, provided that warming is ultra-rapid.

Vitrification instead of slow freezing is now routinely used for human oocytes and embryos. However, questions remain about potential external contamination, as well as the long-term stability of the 'glassy state' of the vitrified cells, which are prone to fracture; this may be a hazard under normal working conditions in the IVF laboratory with routine access to storage tanks.

At least 30 different carrier tools have been described in published literature, and at least 15 versions are commercially available (see Vajta *et al.*, 2015 for review).

1. *'Fully open'* systems allow direct contact between the sample and liquid nitrogen, so that both cooling and warming rates can be extremely high. These types of open tools carry potential contamination risks. Examples include Open-pulled straw (OPS), Cryotop, Cryolock, Cryoleaf, Vitri-Anga and Cryoloop.

2. *Open cooling and closed storage*: after cooling, the carrier tool is inserted into a precooled sterile container that is resistant to extreme changes in temperature and then sealed (Cryotop SC).

3. *Semiclosed*: vitrification takes place on the surface of a metal block (Cryohook) or a container straw (Rapid I) that is partially submerged in liquid nitrogen. Samples are exposed to nitrogen vapor, with the risk of vapor-mediated contamination.

4. *Closed thin-walled narrow capillaries*: the device is heat sealed before cooling, and opened only after warming (Cryotip, Cryopette). The devices are warmed in a water bath, then cut to allow contents to be expelled into the medium. The surface of the straw may be contaminated either from the liquid nitrogen or from the water bath. Cooling and warming rates are slower than those obtained with open devices, and CPA dilution after warming is delayed.

5. *Carrier tools* are sealed into a container that separates them from liquid nitrogen during cooling, storage and warming (OPS high security, Vitrisafe); these offer the highest protection, but cooling rates may be seriously compromised.

A novel device (KrioBlast$^{TM}$) has recently been introduced that provides a platform for hyperfast cooling (kinetic vitrification) based on hyperfast spray cooling. The system provides cooling rates of 100,000–600,000°C/min and can be used for sample volumes up to 4000 μl using 15% glycerol as CPA, thus eliminating the need for more toxic agents. Initial trials with human pluripotent stem cells and spermatozoa show promising results (Katkov *et al.*, 2018).

---

### Practical Tips for Vitrification

From Elder *et al.* (2015)

1. Pre-equilibrate all media to the correct temperature prior to dispensing, and invert the vials immediately before use to make sure that the solutions are fully mixed.
2. Label each vitrification device fully prior to use. Remember that timing is crucial to effective vitrification and warming, and make sure that everything is 'ready to go' prior to starting the procedure.
3. Prepare a liquid nitrogen (LN$_2$) bath and place it next to the flowhood, ready for plunging the loaded vitrification devices. The vessel should be a properly functioning container dedicated for the purpose of holding LN$_2$. Portable insulated containers ('eskies') used for media transport/ deliveries are not designed for use as LN$_2$ baths, and using them for this purpose is highly inadvisable. Any leak of LN$_2$ could have disastrous consequences. Place the LN$_2$ bath on a flat secure surface; do not use a chair or stool!
4. Carry out all vitrification/warming procedures in an area that will remain free of distraction throughout.
5. Adhere to the correct timings strictly, using a timer. Using two separate timers can prevent the loss of vital seconds in resetting a single timer. It is also helpful to have a second embryologist to assist with the timings, etc.
6. If a straw sealer is used, make sure that it is switched on and ready to use before starting the vitrification process.
7. Some media companies recommend using 1- to 2-mL solution volumes for each vitrification/ warming event, but 100- to 200-μl droplets are equally effective, provided that the oocyte/ embryo is fully equilibrated in each solution. Larger volumes for warming have the advantage that the vitrification device can be easily submerged into a large volume, making removal of the oocyte/embryo easier. Using larger volumes of the initial equilibration solutions also means that they can be warmed for up to 30 minutes without major pH or osmolality disturbance.
8. Ensure that there are no air bubbles on the surface of the initial warming solutions, as embryos tend to adhere to bubbles; this will hinder full submersion into the solution and also affect the precise timing of the warming process.
9. The speed of warming (at least 20,000°C/min) is more important in avoiding lysis than is the cooling speed. If warming is too slow, the intracellular CPA concentration is too low to prevent ice from re-crystallizing, and the supercooled liquid forms lethal ice crystals.
10. Embryo survival may not be immediately obvious after warming, and survival/morphology is routinely assessed after a minimum period of 2 hours in culture. This is particularly important in the case of blastocysts, which may appear collapsed immediately after warming but will re-expand within 2 hours when cultured under optimal conditions.

---

## Potential Contamination during Cooling and Storage of Cryopreserved Samples

During the early 1990s the transmission of hepatitis B virus between frozen bone marrow samples in a liquid nitrogen storage tank was demonstrated. This incident raised the possibility of pathogen transmission between samples in ART laboratories and led to further consideration of potential sources of contamination and strategies to avoid the transmission of infection. Although no disease transmission caused by liquid nitrogen or other source related to cryopreservation has been reported in mammalian and human assisted reproduction, theoretical sources of contamination include:

1. Within the freezing apparatus. Vapor phase-controlled rate freezers spray nonsterile liquid nitrogen directly onto the samples. This may be

further compounded by liquid condensation that may accumulate within ducting between freezing runs. Ideally, a freezing apparatus should have the capability of being sterilized between freezing runs, but this is not a practical option.

2. During storage. Straws may be contaminated on the outside, or seals and plugs may leak. Particulates may then transfer via the liquid nitrogen within the storage vessel.

3. From liquid nitrogen. Generally, liquid nitrogen has a very low microbial count when it is manufactured. However, contamination may occur during storage and distribution. Any part of the distribution chain that periodically warms up, in particular transfer dewars or dry shippers, may become heavily contaminated. The microbial quality of the liquid nitrogen when delivered from the manufacturer varies widely with geographical region, and more extreme reports of microbial contamination may reflect local industrial practices. Although this raised concern about the safety of 'open' devices used for vitrification, no infection attributable to the procedures has yet been reported (Vajta *et al.*, 2015).

The HFEA in the United Kingdom prepared a consultation document with guidelines for safe storage of human gametes in liquid nitrogen (Human Fertilisation and Embryology Authority, 1998); basic recommendations include patient screening for hepatitis B, hepatitis C and HIV, careful hygiene throughout, double containment of storage straws and the use of sealed ampules. The risks of cross-contamination during the quarantine period need to be assessed and procedures put in place to minimize these risks. However, the literature, as well as experience in both animal models and human IVF, suggests that in practice, the risk of cross-contamination in IVF working conditions is negligible (Pomeroy *et al.*, 2009; Vajta *et al.*, 2015).

## Embryo Cryopreservation Policies

Following fresh embryo transfer in a stimulated IVF cycle, supernumerary embryos are available for cryopreservation in a large number of cycles. In a routine IVF practice, more than half of stimulated IVF cycles may yield surplus embryos suitable for cryopreservation (although this is now subject to legislative control in particular countries of the world). In addition to enhancing the clinical benefits and cumulative conception rate possible for a couple following a single cycle of ovarian stimulation and IVF, a successful cryopreservation program offers other benefits including the possibility of avoiding fresh embryo transfer in stimulated cycles with a potential for ovarian hyperstimulation syndrome, or in which factors that may jeopardize implantation are apparent (e.g., bleeding, unfavorable endometrium, polyps or an extremely difficult embryo transfer).

---

### Consent to Storage after Cryopreservation

A unit that offers embryo cryopreservation must also be aware of logistic, legal, moral and ethical problems that can arise, and ensure that all patients are fully informed and counseled. Both partners must sign comprehensive consent forms indicating how long the embryos are to be stored, and define legal ownership in case of divorce or separation, death of one of the partners, or loss of contact between the Unit and the couple. Cryopreserved samples cannot in practice be maintained in storage indefinitely, and there must be a clear clinic policy to ensure that records are correctly maintained, with regular audits of the storage banks. Clinic administration may mandate that all couples with cryopreserved embryos in storage must be contacted annually and asked to return a signed form indicating whether they wish to continue storage. In the United Kingdom, options for couples include:

1. Continue storage.
2. Return for frozen embryo transfer.
3. Donate their embryos for research projects approved by appropriate ethics committees/Internal Review Boards and the HFEA.
4. Donate their frozen embryos for transfer to another infertile couple.
5. Have the embryos thawed and disposed of.

---

## Selection of Embryos for Slow Freezing

Using PROH as cryoprotectant, embryos can be frozen at either the pronucleate or early cleavage stages. Careful selection of viable embryos will optimize their potential for surviving freeze-thawing.

### Pronucleate

The cell should have an intact zona pellucida and healthy cytoplasm with two distinct pronuclei clearly visible. Accurate timing of zygote freezing is essential to avoid periods of the cell cycle that are highly sensitive to cooling. For example, during the period when pronuclei start to migrate before syngamy, with DNA synthesis and formation of the mitotic spindle, the microtubular system is highly vulnerable to temperature fluctuation, leading to possible scattering of the chromosomes. Zygotes processed for freezing at this stage will no longer survive cryopreservation. The timing of pronucleate freezing is crucial, and the process must be initiated while the pronuclei are still distinctly apparent, no later than 20–22 hours after insemination.

## Cleavage

Two- to eight-cell embryos should be of good quality, Grade 1 or 2, with less than 20% cytoplasmic fragments. Uneven blastomeres and a high degree of fragmentation jeopardize survival potential; embryos with damage after thawing may still be viable and result in pregnancies, but their prognosis for implantation is reduced.

## Embryo Cryopreservation: Method

Details of each patient and the associated embryos must be carefully recorded on appropriate data sheets. Meticulous and complete record keeping is crucial, and must include the patient's date of birth, medical number, date of oocyte retrieval (OCR), date of cryopreservation, number and type of embryos frozen, and number of straws or ampules used, together with clear and accurate identification of storage vessel and location within the storage vessel. The data sheets should also confirm that both partners have signed consent forms. Ampules and straws have been successfully used for embryo storage, and each has advantages and disadvantages. The choice between them is a matter of individual preference, as well as availability of storage space and laboratory time to prepare and sterilize ampules. When straws are used, they must be handled with care to avoid external contamination, and to avoid inadvertent temperature fluctuations during seeding or transfer to the storage dewar. The measured temperature excursions within straws can be very dramatic (see Figure 12.6). It is likely that in straws frozen

horizontally the embryos will be adjacent to the wall, where they will be exposed to the highest thermal gradient; great care must be taken in handling cryopreserved material. Plastic cryovials are not recommended for embryo freezing.

Ready-to-use media for freezing and thawing embryos are available from the majority of companies who supply culture media. Individual methods and protocols vary slightly with the different preparations, and manufacturers' instructions should be followed for each.

- Ensure that no air bubbles are trapped within the freezing medium after the sample has been loaded, into either ampules or straws. Air bubbles can sometimes be seen in both vessels on thawing, and these present a hazard to the fragile dehydrated embryo. Warming solutions to 37°C before starting the procedure may effectively act as a 'degassing' mechanism.

- It is common practice to cool human embryos within the controlled rate freezing apparatus down to below −100°C after the slow cooling to −30°C, before transfer to liquid nitrogen. In veterinary IVF cryopreservation, straws are often transferred to liquid nitrogen directly from −30°C. This procedure would give equally good results for human embryos and is indeed used by some laboratories with no reduction in viability. However, it is essential that the transfer is carried out rapidly (within 5 seconds) because the temperature of the straws may rise very quickly when they are removed from the controlled rate device (see Figure 12.6). Cooling to temperatures below −100°C within the freezing machine carries less risk, but does consume considerably more liquid nitrogen.

## Ice Nucleation: Practical Points

1. Because straws have a large surface area, small diameter and a thin wall, very rapid warming occurs when they are removed from a cold environment. Measured temperature excursions that occur at different points of the cryopreservation procedure are illustrated in Figure 12.6. If straws are removed from the controlled rate freezing apparatus for excessive

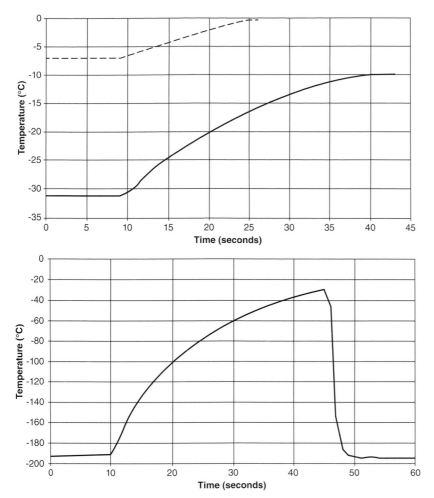

**Figure 12.6** Measured temperatures within straws following removal from a controlled rate freezer or from a liquid nitrogen vessel at various points during the freezing cycle. Prior to nucleation the temperature rise within 5 seconds is sufficient to prevent ice nucleation. At −30°C the sample temperature may rise very quickly and if transfer to liquid nitrogen is carried out at this point of the freezing program, care must be taken to ensure that the increase in temperature is minimized. Following liquid nitrogen immersion, the temperature of straws may rise by 130°C within 20 seconds.

lengths of time during the nucleation procedure, they can warm to a temperature that is too high for ice nucleation to occur. Ice nucleation may occur because of the local cooling induced by the nucleating tool, but it is possible that the bulk temperature of the fluid may not allow ice crystal growth to propagate through the sample. In some laboratories, it is common practice to check that ice propagation has occurred throughout the sample, usually 1 minute after the seeding procedure. If straws are removed from the controlled rate cooling equipment, this in itself may cause melting of the nucleated ice.

2.  Thermal control of the freezing apparatus may not be sufficiently accurate or stable at the nucleation temperature. The temperature achieved may allow nucleation to occur because of the thermal mass of the nucleating tool, but may not be sufficiently low to allow subsequent ice propagation. Any thermal fluctuations within the freezing apparatus may also lead to ice melting.

3.  Within straws, nucleation of ice at temperatures very close to the melting point results in a very slow propagation of ice through the sample. In some cases, ice propagation can actually become blocked, and embryos are then effectively supercooled. In this case the embryos would not be expected to survive further cooling.

## Sample Protocols

### Sample Protocol for Embryo Slow Freezing

1. Equilibrate selected and washed embryos in 1,2-propanediol (1.5 M) at room temperature, to allow uptake of the CP into the cells. This is usually done in two steps, the second step incorporating 0.1 M sucrose.
2. Load equilibrated embryos into straws or ampules.
3. Cool the samples at a rate of 2°C/min to −7°C, and 'hold' at this temperature to allow thermal equilibration before ice nucleation (seeding).
4. Following seeding, with initiation and growth of ice crystals, cool the samples at a slow rate, −0.3°C/min, down to −30°C.
5. Cool the samples rapidly to $LN_2$ temperatures, then plunge and store in $LN_2$.

### Sample Protocol for Embryo Thawing after Slow Freezing

1. Samples are thawed in two stages: hold straws in air for 40 seconds, and then transfer to a 30°C water bath for a further minute.
2. Remove cryoprotectant by dilution through solutions containing 0.2 M sucrose, and then wash three times in culture medium.

The thawing protocol is carried out at room temperature, and the embryos placed in equilibrated culture medium at room temperature before being allowed to warm gradually to 37°C in the incubator. Pronucleate embryos may be cultured overnight to confirm continued development, and cleavage stage embryos are incubated for a minimum of 1 hour before transfer.

# Blastocyst Cryopreservation

The first reports of successful human blastocyst cryopreservation were published in 1985 (Cohen *et al.*, 1985; Fehilly *et al.*, 1985), but blastocyst freezing became routine in IVF only after media for effective extended culture became available during the 1990s. Using Vero cell co-culture to enhance extended culture, Ménézo *et al.* (1992) explored the use of a combination of glycerol and sucrose as cryoprotectants to freeze surplus expanded blastocysts, and the protocols were later modified to obtain satisfactory freeze–thaw rates. Inconsistent success rates were reported initially, but this may have been partly due to lack of experience with selection criteria for freezing, and also a need to understand the subtleties of cryopreservation and the impact that even the

slightest variation might have on consistency. Extended culture to blastocyst stage is now routine in many IVF laboratories, and slow-freezing protocols using glycerol as cryoprotectant have largely been replaced by the more successful technique of blastocyst vitrification.

Using strict criteria to select potentially viable blastocysts is crucial to success:

- Growth rate: expanded blastocyst stage on Day 5/Day 6.
- Overall cell number >60 cells (depending on day of development).
- Relative cell allocation to trophectoderm/inner cell mass.
- Original quality of early stage embryo: pronucleus formation and orientation, blastomere regularity, mono-nucleation, fragmentation, appropriate cleavage stage for time of development.

## Use of Glass Ampules

Tissue culture washed borosilicate glass ampules with a fine-drawn neck can be used for embryo cryostorage.

- Fill the ampule with approximately 0.4 mL of the sucrose/PROH solution using a needle and syringe.
- Carefully transfer the embryos using a fine-drawn Pasteur pipette.
- Using a high-intensity flame, carefully heat seal the neck of the ampule. It is important to ensure (under the microscope) that the seal is complete, without leaks: leakage of $LN_2$ into the ampule during freezing will cause it to explode immediately upon thawing. It is often impossible to detect whether the glass neck is completely sealed, and the possibility of explosion can be avoided by opening the ampule under $LN_2$ before thawing.

# Blastocyst Vitrification

Blastocyst vitrification protocols now yield very favorable survival, implantation and clinical pregnancy rates. Commercial kits for blastocyst vitrification are available – as always, the ultimate success of the protocol will be related to the operator's experience and careful attention to detail. In common with all aspects of human ART, careful research into the consequences of such new therapies continues to be essential. In large expanded blastocysts, collapsing the blastocoelic cavity with an ICSI needle immediately before processing increases survival rates after both slow freezing and vitrification (Kader *et al.*, 2009). Poor morphology and delayed expansion (to Day 7) have a negative impact on survival post-vitrification.

## Assisted Hatching and Cryopreservation

Freeze-thawing is known to cause hardening of the zona pellucida, and the application of assisted hatching, particularly at the blastocyst stage, has been suggested as beneficial to implantation after freeze-thawing (Tucker, 1991). In some cases, zona pellucida fracture can be a routine result of some cryopreservation protocols (Van den Abbeel *et al.*, 2000). Embryos with existing holes in the zona pellucida following PGD procedures can successfully survive and implant (Magli *et al.*, 2006). A recent systematic review confirmed that assisted hatching is consistently of benefit after thawing frozen/vitrified blastocysts (Alteri *et al.*, 2018).

## Thawing/Warming Protocols

Parmegiani *et al.* (2014) postulated that the same warming procedure could be used for both slow-frozen and vitrified oocytes, and carried out a prospective study to investigate this proposal. Using slow-frozen sibling oocytes randomized for either conventional thawing or rapid vitrification warming, their results showed better survival with rapid warming (90%) than with conventional thawing (75%). Chromosomal configuration and the meiotic spindle examined by confocal microscopy showed no differences using either procedure. The authors suggest that a single warming protocol/solution may be used for both slow-frozen and vitrified oocytes; slow-frozen oocytes thawed with this protocol show increased survival rates that are comparable to those obtained after vitrification. This substitution can also potentially be applied for slow-frozen zygotes and embryos (Kojima *et al.*, 2012).

## Clinical Aspects of Frozen Embryo Transfer

Freeze-thawed embryos must be transferred to a uterus that is optimally receptive for implantation, in a postovulatory secretory phase. Patients with regular ovulatory cycles and an adequate luteal phase may have their embryos transferred in a natural cycle, monitored by ultrasound and blood or urine luteinizing hormone (LH) levels in order to pinpoint ovulation. Older patients or those with irregular cycles may have their embryos transferred in an artificial cycle: hormone replacement therapy with exogenous steroids is administered after creating an artificial menopause by downregulation with a gonadotropin-releasing hormone (GnRH) agonist.

---

**Schedule for Frozen Embryo Transfer in a Hormone Replacement Cycle**

1. Patient selection: oligomenorrhea/irregular cycles, or age >38 years.
2. Downregulate with GnRH analog (buserelin or nafarelin) for at least 14 days; continue downregulation until the time of embryo transfer.
3. Administer estradiol valerate:

   | | |
   |---|---|
   | Days 1–5 | 2 mg |
   | Days 6–9 | 4 mg |
   | Days 10–13 | 6 mg |
   | Days 14 onwards | 4 mg |

4. Progesterone from Day 15 to 16, choice between:

   - Gestone 50 mg intramuscular or
   - Cyclogest pessaries 200 mg twice daily or
   - Utrogestan pessaries 100 mg three times daily or
   - 8% Crinone gel per vaginam, once daily.
   - Double the dose from Day 17 onwards (100 mg Gestone, 400 mg twice daily Cyclogest, 200 mg three times daily Utrogestan, 8% Crinone gel PV, twice daily).

5. Embryo transfer:

   (a) Pronucleate: thaw on Day 16 of the artificial cycle, culture overnight before transfer on Day 17 or 18.
   (b) Cleavage stage embryos: thaw and replace on Day 17 or 18.
   (c) Blastocysts: thaw and replace on Day 19 or 20.

6. If pregnancy is established, continue hormone replacement therapy (HRT) with 8 mg estradiol valerate and the higher dose of progesterone supplement daily until Day 77 after embryo transfer. Gradually withdraw the drugs with monitoring of blood P4 (progesterone) levels. This protocol is also successfully used for the treatment of agonadal women who require ovum or embryo donation. In combination with prior GnRH pituitary suppression, the artificial cycle can be timed to a prescheduled program according to the patient's (or clinic's) convenience.

## Transfer in a Natural Menstrual Cycle

1. Patient selection: regular cycles, 28 ± 3 days, previously assay luteal phase progesterone to confirm ovulation. A commercially available ovulation 'kit' can also be used in a previous cycle to confirm that the patient has regular ovulatory cycles.

2. Cycle monitoring from Day 10 until ovulation is confirmed by ultrasound scan and plasma LH. Ultrasound scan should also confirm appropriate endometrial development; the cycle should be canceled if the endometrial thickness is <8 mm at the time of the LH surge.

3. Timing of the embryo transfer:

   a. Pronucleate embryos: thaw on Day 1 after ovulation (3 days after the LH surge: LH + 3), culture overnight

   b. Cleavage stage embryos: thaw and transfer on Day 2 or 3 after ovulation (LH + 4/5)

   c. Blastocysts: thaw and transfer on Day 4 or 5 after ovulation (LH + 6/7).

Patients with irregular cycles may be induced to ovulate using clomifene citrate or gonadotropins, and embryo transfer timed in relation to the endogenous LH surge or following administration of human chorionic gonadotropin (hCG). Although it is possible to estimate embryo transfer time using an ovulation 'kit' to detect the LH surge, this may be less accurate, and does present a risk of inappropriate timing.

## Oocyte Cryopreservation

Prior to 1997, the options for preserving a young woman's fertility after treatment for malignant disease were very limited: a full IVF treatment cycle with cryopreservation of embryos prior to the initiation of chemotherapy, or oocyte or embryo donation following recovery from the malignant disease. The first option is available only to women with partners to provide a semen sample for fertilization of the harvested oocytes. However, the success of frozen embryo cryopreservation in a competent IVF program is such that these patients maintain a very good chance of achieving a pregnancy after transfer of frozen-thawed embryos following recovery from their disease. On the other hand, this strategy also raises the risk of creating embryos with a higher than average chance of being orphaned. Many of the legal and ethical problems created by the cryopreservation and storage of embryos can be overcome by preserving oocytes, especially for young women about to undergo treatment for malignant disease that will result in loss of ovarian function. Oocyte cryopreservation is also indicated in patients with a known family history of premature ovarian failure, and can be advantageous in various clinical scenarios, such as in ovarian hyperstimulation syndrome, unexpected lack of sperm following oocyte retrieval, egg donation programs and in order to extend the duration of natural fertility.

Human oocytes are particularly susceptible to freeze–thaw damage due to their size and complexity. They must not only survive thawing, but also preserve their potential for fertilization and development. The first pregnancies with human oocyte freezing were reported in the 1980s (Chen, 1986; Al-Hasani et al., 1987), but the procedure was abandoned for approximately 10 years due to low survival and fertilization rates, thought to be due primarily to hardening of the zona pellucida and to spindle damage causing aneuploidy. Since 1997, focus intensified on modifying protocols to increase survival rates, in particular to avoid activation/premature release of cortical granules, zona pellucida hardening and the detection/avoidance of spindle damage and aneuploidy. In 2009, Noyes et al. reported the birth of more than 900 babies after oocyte cryopreservation, with no apparent increased incidence of congenital anomalies (Noyes et al., 2009). Attempts to monitor alterations in the permeability of the plasma membrane, assess warming and rehydration protocols, and use ICSI to improve fertilization rates have resulted in significant clinical progress.

Several intrinsic difficulties are associated with human oocyte freezing, due mainly to their high volume:surface area ratio and low membrane permeability. Intracellular ice formation causes critical damage to the cytoskeleton, which is also sensitive to osmotic stress. Disruption of the meiotic spindle can cause chromosome defects and aneuploidy. Lowering the temperature, or the cryoprotectant agents themselves, may cause an increase in intracellular $Ca^{2+}$ leading to changes in the intracellular signaling mechanisms and oocyte activation. Finally, since the zona pellucida hardens after freezing, it is necessary to employ ICSI for fertilization of the thawed oocyte.

Freezing can result in parthenogenetic activation, leading to premature release of cortical granules (CGs). It is also important to consider the cytoplasmic maturity of the oocyte at freezing and the potentially toxic effects of cryoprotectants.

Modifications found to improve the effectiveness of oocyte freezing include:

1. Complete removal of the cumulus and coronal mass, which increases survival rates.

2. Alteration of sucrose concentrations from 0.1 to 0.2, 0.3 or 0.5 mol/L, which increases oocyte dehydration and survival.

3. Choline has been used as a substitute for sodium (Boldt *et al.*, 2006; Stachecki *et al.*, 2006) on the basis that cryodamage to the $Na^+/K^+$ pump might lead to high intracellular concentrations of $Na^+$ with a resulting efflux of protons. Choline does not cross the plasma membrane, is less toxic than high sucrose and does not affect osmotic pressure of the cell.

Not surprisingly, damage caused by oocyte freezing appears to be protocol-dependent (Rienzi *et al.*, 2004). Using a Polscope to observe the meiotic spindle following freeze–thaw procedures, these authors observed that the spindle disintegrates during freeze-thawing, and oocytes must reconstruct their spindles after thawing. Other authors using confocal or electron microscopy have shown that elevated sucrose concentrations may prevent spindle damage (Coticchio *et al.*, 2006; Nottola *et al.*, 2008). The timing of freezing after oocyte retrieval also seems to be important, with lower pregnancy rates reported from oocytes that were frozen more than 2 hours after OCR (Parmegiani *et al.*, 2009). Germinal vesicle stage oocytes show better survival (Sereni *et al.*, 2000), and retrieval of immature oocytes has now become another option for fertility preservation. The protocols require minimal hormonal stimulation, and oocytes can be collected within a short time following the diagnosis of cancer

The thawing process is equally fraught with difficulties. Osmotic stress caused by rehydration must be minimized in order to prevent degeneration, and reassembly of the spindle post-thaw takes at least 3–4 hours.

Vitrification of human oocytes has proved to be superior to slow freezing, and this is now the routine method used for oocyte cryopreservation. The first live birth was reported by Kuleshova *et al.* in 1999,

and numerous studies with favorable results were published between 2005 and 2009. The main concerns with vitrification are the toxicity of high concentrations of cryoprotectant and extreme osmotic changes. Huang *et al.* (2007) showed less damage to the spindle and chromosomes after vitrification compared to slow freezing. Cobo *et al.* (2008) compared sibling fresh oocytes with vitrified donor oocytes using the Cryotop method, reporting very high survival rates after warming (97%), and fertilization, blastocyst development and pregnancy rates for recipients that were equivalent to those obtained with the use of fresh donor oocytes. Differences in participant characteristics and study design, as well as ethical and legal issues related to oocyte cryopreservation in different countries, mean that heterogeneous results can be observed in different studies. Nevertheless, a systematic review and meta-analysis carried out for results published between 1980 and 2013 confirmed that vitrified oocytes have better survival, fertilization and cleavage rates compared with slow-freezing protocols (see Potdar *et al.*, 2014 for review).

## Ovarian Tissue Cryopreservation

Cryopreservation and banking of ovarian tissue has become an interesting and effective strategy for fertility conservation, indicated primarily for young women who will suffer anticipated loss of ovarian function due to premature ovarian failure, cancer or other diseases. Since follicle number diminishes with age, this option is open only to patients who are less than 30 years old and have had no previous chemo- or radiotherapy. The uterus must be functional, and the patient should have a high probability of long-term survival after treatment. The type of malignancy is also important, as any risk of ovarian metastasis must be avoided. Aspiration of immature GV oocytes is also an option for women wishing to preserve their fertility. The oocytes are then matured in vitro and used for IVF or oocyte cryopreservation. Oocytes can be aspirated in the luteal phase of the cycle, and can also be collected from excised ovarian tissue.

Successful fertility preservation is dependent upon a high level of expertise and collaboration between reproductive medicine and oncology specialists, as well as networking between different oncology specialists. It can therefore be offered to young cancer patients only in a multidisciplinary and multicentre network: national and international networks and societies have been initiated in Europe and in the USA in order to facilitate collaboration (reviewed by von Wolff *et al.*, 2015).

## Strategies

Freezing ovarian tissue rather than oocytes offers several advantages:

1. Small pieces of tissue contain very large numbers of primordial follicles and can be stored for children as well as for young adults.
2. Laparoscopic ovarian biopsy/oophorectomy can be carried out rapidly before chemotherapy, any time during the menstrual cycle, thereby avoiding delays in initiating therapy.
3. Germline cells are removed from cytotoxic harm, and the entire tissue can be returned to the patient by grafting.
4. Storing cortical tissue theoretically preserves natural cell–cell interactions and intra-ovarian signals, and grafting can potentially restore both steroidogenic and gametogenic function – both important factors for the quality of life of the patient.

However, this strategy is not suitable for all patients due to concerns about re-transplanting cancer cells after recovery from the disease. Careful patient selection is essential to minimize the risk of contamination by cancer cells.

There are several options for freezing ovarian tissues (Figure 12.7), which depend on permeability properties, optimal cooling rates, susceptibility to cryo-injury and potential options after thawing.

## Fragments or Thin Slices of Ovarian Cortex

The amount of ovarian tissue removed is dependent upon the estimated risk of ovarian failure, related to existing ovarian volume and planned treatment. Very young girls have very small ovaries, and oophorectomy is recommended. In adults, biopsy of one-half to two-thirds of an ovary followed by dissection into small slices for cryopreservation is a technique that is commonly applied. The biopsy should be at least 1.0–1.5 mm thick, as primordial follicles may be difficult or impossible to find in biopsies that are superficial or very thin.

A number of technical problems are associated with the cryopreservation of ovarian tissues compared to isolated oocytes. Tissues respond very differently to ice formation than do cell suspensions. Cells in tissues are usually closely packed, and they also have interacting connections with each other and with basement membranes. Tissues have a three-dimensional structure and are traversed by fine capillaries or other blood vessels. Changes in extracellular ice surrounding the tissue during the freezing process and re-crystallization during warming of the tissue are both hazardous. In the hands of experienced cryobiologists morphological assessments of cryopreserved human ovarian cortex at the light microscope (Gook *et al.*, 1999) and electron microscope (Picton *et al.*, 2000; Kim *et al.*, 2001) have confirmed that cellular damage in the tissue can be minimal. However, the choice of an inappropriate CPA together with poor laboratory practice can lead to extensive cellular damage which will compromise tissue viability on thawing (Picton *et al.*, 2000). The problems of achieving adequate

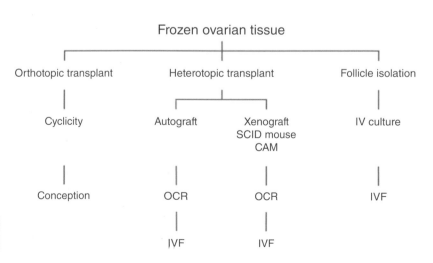

**Figure 12.7** Options for ovarian tissue preservation. OCR = oocyte retrieval; SCID = Severe Combined Immunodeficiency; CAM = chorioallantoic membrane.

permeation of tissue fragments with CPA can be overcome either by preparing thin strips of tissue <1 mm thick, which provides maximal surface area for solute penetration (Newton *et al.*, 1998), or by dissociating the tissue into follicles or isolated cells before freezing (Cox *et al.*, 1996). Most procedures stipulate that ovarian cortex slices are thawed rapidly by being swirled in a water bath at ~20°C or 37°C, and the CPA is progressively diluted from the tissue by repeated rinses with fresh medium.

### Hemi-ovaries or Whole Ovaries

Conserving the whole ovary has the advantage of retaining the entire primordial population, and the cells and oocytes remain in their natural environment. There is also the potential for restoring endocrine function and the menstrual cycle, preventing meno-pausal symptoms and improving quality of life. The main challenge with whole ovary preservation is that permeation is difficult and requires perfusion via the ovarian artery or vascular pedicle. The tissue is denser, with a complex structure of different cell types, a high cell density, a low surface area/volume ratio and decreased efficiency of heat transfer. Vitrification is particularly difficult since large amounts of cryopro-tectant are required and different parts of the ovary will vitrify at different times. The cortex and primor-dial follicles are sustained by very small capillaries which are easily damaged, and this can lead to ischemic follicle loss and death of cortical tissue. The vessels can also fracture during warming, and pedicle lacerations can lead to possible thrombosis. Finally, revasculariza-tion is a time-consuming surgical procedure.

### Dissected Intact Isolated Primordial Follicles and Denuded Primordial Oocytes from Isolated Primordial Follicles

While it may be possible to store ovarian tissue for young cancer patients, where there is any risk of reintroducing malignant cells in the tissue graft (Shaw and Trounson, 1997), a far safer strategy is to culture the follicles to maturity in vitro (Picton *et al.*, 2000). Following fertilization by IVF or ICSI, embryos that are free from contamination could be transferred back to the patient. Freezing isolated primordial follicles has several advantages over freezing metaphase II oocytes, including their availability, size, lack of accessory cells, nuclear status (prophase I with intact nuclear membrane), absence of zona pellucida, CGs and low

metabolic rate. The disadvantage of the technique is that prolonged in-vitro maturation is required, and follicle culture is difficult and unreliable – the growth from primordial to antral follicle takes approximately 70–90 days. Human follicle culture is still an emerging technology, but recent data are encouraging, and it may eventually be possible to grow primordial follicles to antral stages after cryopreservation (Picton *et al.*, 2000; McLaughlin *et al.*, 2018). Nonetheless, a consid-erable amount of research is still needed to confirm that this strategy is safe, and that it does not induce epigenetic alterations in the female gametes, a possi-bility that has already been confirmed in a murine model system (Eppig *et al.*, 2009).

# Techniques for Cryopreservation of Ovarian Tissue

Both slow freezing and vitrification have been suc-cessful in preserving primordial and primary follicles, but vitrification techniques were found to better pre-serve secondary follicles and stroma, based on hist-ology (Amorim *et al.*, 2011, 2012).

Tissue vitrification involves difficult challenges:

- Delivery of high intracellular concentrations of cryoprotectant in order to achieve high levels of dehydration.
- Contact time with solutions must be controlled so that rapid cooling and high heat transfer rates can be achieved whilst avoiding toxicity.

The outcome of the procedure depends on the sample size, the logistics of cooling and storage, direct contact with the liquid nitrogen and specialized containers. Protocols are either 'open' (direct contact with liquid nitrogen) or 'closed' (container in contact with liquid nitrogen). 'Open' protocols are advantageous for rapid cooling:

- Direct cover vitrification (DCV; Chen *et al.*, 2006)
- Solid surface vitrification (SSV; Huang *et al.*, 2008)
- 'Carrier-less' (Li *et al.*, 2007) – drop tissue into shallow container of liquid nitrogen
- Copper grids, 42-mm holes (Isachenko *et al.*, 2007)
- Cryotissue – metal strip full of holes (Kagawa *et al.*, 2008).

Since tissue is involved, the danger of contamination using the open methods is much greater than in the case of oocytes.

271

Several closed devices offer an alternative: Cryotube, Cryobag, Straw, Crovial, Cryotip, Cryopette and the Ohio-Cryo (Kader *et al.*, 2008).

---

**Current Status of Ovarian Transplantation (2018)**

- Restoration of natural fertility is possible, with a mean duration of 4–5 years.
- Graft follicle content is influenced by patient age and previous treatment and possibly by graft location.
- Lipid peroxidation occurs in murine and human ovarian grafts; vitamin E can significantly reduce lipid peroxidation and increase follicle survival.
- Gonadotropin environment probably has no effect on graft survival although low gonadotropins may be detrimental.
- Follicle survival has been demonstrated in orthotopic and heterotopic human autografts.
- More than 100 live births after autotransplantation have been reported (Anderson *et al.*, 2017), with live birth rates ranging from 24–31% per patient.

---

## Success of Ovarian Tissue Preservation

There are varying degrees of success with all the above techniques. Intact or denuded follicles survive the thaw, but do not grow well after isolation, whereas tissue fragments or slices may show signs of injury/necrosis after culture. Tissues may be xenotransplanted in a Severe Combined ImmunoDeficiency (SCID) mouse or in chick embryo chorioallantoic membrane (CAM). In whole ovaries, ultrastructural and apoptotic analyses have been used to assess viability after thaw/recovery. To date there has been success with cryo/transplant in rodents, rabbits, sheep and marmoset monkeys, and successful restoration of fertility in sheep after orthotopic transplantation of cortical strips to the ovarian pedicle. These grafts continue to function for up to 2 years. Cryopreservation experiments that used whole ovaries led to tissue survival in rats, rabbits, dogs, sheep and humans (Martinez-Madrid *et al.*, 2004). Whole ovary vitrification and transplantation has been successfully performed in infantile rats, mice, rabbits, pigs and sheep.

Cryopreserved ovarian cortical tissue may be orthotopically or heterotopically autotransplanted. Heterotopic sites include the rectus abdominis muscle, the abdominal wall, the breast or the forearm; oocytes must be retrieved from the graft for IVF. Orthotopic sites include the pelvic peritoneum, the ovary or the ovarian fossa; if the fallopian tubes are intact, natural conception is possible. Follicular development usually occurs within 4–5 months of transplantation, but variability has been found, with a window of 8 to 26 weeks. Endocrine function after transplantation has also shown individual variation, with a mean duration of 4 to 5 years if sufficient follicle density has been retained in the thawed tissue.

## Human Autotransplantation

Donnez *et al.* (2004) reported the first live birth after orthotopic transplantation of human cryopreserved ovarian tissue; they detected live follicles from 16 to 26 weeks after grafting, and some of the grafts still functioned after 3 years. Silber *et al.* (2015) compared autotransplantation of fresh with cryopreserved ovarian tissue transplantation in a single center, using the same technique: 95% of the women had restoration of endocrine and ovarian function at approximately 4.5 months after surgery. Eight recipients of cryopreserved tissue delivered six babies, and 11 healthy babies were born to 11 recipients of fresh ovary transplants. Half of the babies born were as a result of natural conception.

Overall results to date are very encouraging: more than 100 live births were reported in 2017, and numbers continue to increase steadily, with reported live birth rates ranging from 24 to 31% per patient: around 50% of these are after natural conception. Two different groups have reported delivery of three healthy babies to single patients after cryopreservation and reimplantation (Donnez *et al.*, 2013). Gellert *et al* (2018) reviewed results from 21 different countries, confirming a live birth rate of 25%.

Considering the experimental status of this new technique in ART, it is paramount for each center to test and optimize freeze-thawing results before offering a service to patients. Post-thaw tissue integrity, follicle counts and viability stains should be carried out, as well as investigating the potential of residual malignant cells. The EU Tissue Banking Directive regulations ask for centralized specialized cryobanks with rigid quality control to prevent transmission of disease. Clinical, psychological and ethical concerns must be considered, since transplantation can only be performed as an experimental procedure and there is a potential risk of re-seeding tumor cells. On a more sober note, consent forms must be adequate and discussed with the patient in the event of death. In conclusion, cryopreservation of ovarian tissue is in its infancy but is already successful as a tool for fertility preservation.

## Semen Cryopreservation

Cryopreserved semen has long been used successfully for artificial insemination (AI), intrauterine insemination (IUI) and IVF. Although freeze–thawing does produce damage to the cells with loss of up to 50% of pre-freeze motility, since large numbers of cells are available, successful fertilization can be achieved even with low cryosurvival rates. There is, however, a noticeable difference in sperm cryosurvival rates between normal semen and semen with abnormal parameters such as low count and motility; samples from men who require sperm cryopreservation prior to chemotherapy treatment for malignant disease frequently show very poor cryosurvival rates. The routine introduction of ICSI into IVF practice has surmounted this problem, so that successful fertilization using ICSI is possible even with extremely poor cryosurvival of suboptimal samples.

## Effects of Cryopreservation on Sperm

Sperm membranes have an unusual lipid composition, with relative proportions of phospholipids, glycolipids and sterols that differ from those of other cell membranes. Reduction in temperature alters the membrane lipid organization and modifies the kinetics or intramembrane proteins, leading to lowered permeability and loss of fluidity. This loss of fluidity is associated with lower sperm survival on thawing. Morris et al. (Morris, 2006; Morris et al., 2012) demonstrated that intracellular ice cannot form within sperm cells at any cooling rates, or during the thawing process. Figure 12.8 illustrates the ultrastructure of human sperm following freezing with 10% glycerol as cryoprotectant. Frozen/thawed sperm behave in a similar way to capacitated sperm, which may lead to a shortened lifespan within the female tract; therefore, the timing of insemination is important when using frozen sperm samples.

Semen can be successfully cryopreserved using either glycerol alone at a concentration of 10–15% or a commercially available complex cryoprotective medium. Adding the cryoprotectant gradually, drop-wise, helps to minimize potential damage due to volume changes within the cell. Cooling and freezing can be carried out by using a programmed cell freezer or by simply suspending the prepared specimens in liquid nitrogen vapor for a period of 30 minutes.

Vitrification techniques have been applied for sperm cryopreservation, but results have not demonstrated any significant advantage; it is very time-consuming, and may be useful for low-volume samples, but is not suitable for normal ejaculates with high volume (Agha-Rahimi et al., 2014).

## Method

Samples should be prepared and frozen within 1–2 hours of ejaculation.

1. Allow the sample to liquefy and perform semen analysis according to standard laboratory technique; label two plastic conical tubes and an appropriate number of 0.5-mL freezing straws or ampules for each specimen. Record all details on appropriate record sheets.
2. Add small aliquots of cryoprotectant medium (CPM) to the semen at room temperature over a period of 2 minutes, to a ratio of 1:1. If the ejaculated volume is greater than 5 mL, divide the sample into two aliquots before mixing with CPM.
3. Aliquot the diluted sample into straws or ampules, labeling aliquots for assessment of post-thaw count and motility.
4. Dilute specimens with CPM according to count:

| | |
|---|---|
| 60 million/mL | dilute 1:1 semen/CPM |
| 20–60 million/mL | dilute 2:1 semen/CPM |
| 20 million/mL | dilute 4:1 semen/CPM |

5. Reassess the number of motile sperm/mL, which should ideally be 10 million or above.
6. Aliquot into prelabeled straws.

## Manual Freezing

1. Place the ampules or straws (in goblets) on a metal cane.
2. Refrigerate at 4°C for 15 minutes.
3. Place into liquid nitrogen vapor for 25 minutes.
4. Plunge into liquid nitrogen for storage, and record storage details.

273

(a)

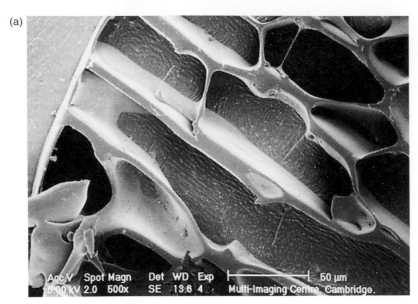

**Figure 12.8** Ultrastructure of human sperm following freezing in a 0.25-mL straw; cells were suspended in glycerol (10%). (a) Freeze fracture followed by etching reveals the structure of ice crystals; cells are entrapped within the freeze concentrated material and few cell structures are evident. (b) Freeze substitution followed by sectioning shows cells entrapped within the freeze concentrated matrix.

(b)

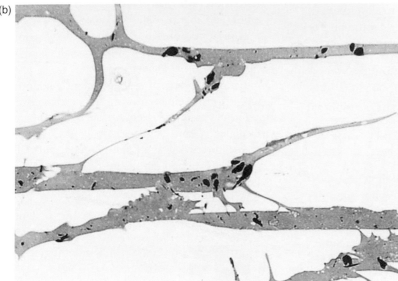

The sample must be carefully washed or prepared by density gradient centrifugation to remove all traces of cryoprotectant medium before it is used for insemination by intrauterine insemination (IUI) or IVF.

## Methods to Improve Sperm Survival

Sperm survival and pregnancy rates are lower when the frozen samples used are from infertile men compared with samples from fertile donors, and there is evidence to suggest that sperm preparation in order to remove immotile and damaged sperm prior to freezing may help to select a population of sperm with a better chance of survival. The use of stimulants such as pentoxifylline may also improve survival after thawing (see Chapter 10).

## Cryopreservation of Testicular and Epididymal Sperm

Whereas the relatively poor survival rates (50%) obtained after freeze–thawing semen samples have not in the past presented a major problem due to the abundance of cells in the original specimens, it is not always possible to obtain an ejaculated semen sample; the current use of suboptimal ejaculate, epididymal and testicular samples in combination with ICSI demands a different approach in order to recover as many sperm cells as possible from each sample. Sample cryopreservation in cases of epididymal and testicular aspiration or biopsy has considerable advantages both to the patient and to the clinical and laboratory staff, in that sperm and oocyte retrieval procedures may be carried out on separate occasions; this strategy is now a successful routine in the majority of ART programs offering this form of treatment. Generally, epididymal and testicular samples are cryopreserved using protocols developed for ejaculated sperm: this may not be optimal. Many changes to the membranes of sperm occur during maturation, and it is likely that the water permeability of testicular sperm, a major factor in determining the cellular response to freezing, is very different from that of ejaculated sperm.

In cases where prolonged washing and searching yield only very few sperm, sperm can be frozen individually or in small groups by injecting them into empty zona pellucida 'shells,' using a crude freezing solution with 8% glycerol in phosphate-buffered saline supplemented with 3% human serum albumin. Samples are recovered after washing the zonae through droplets, and more than 70% of sperm survive using this procedure with resulting successful pregnancy rates (Walmsley *et al.*, 1999).

The criteria for sperm freezing have now changed, in that even the most inadequate samples can be frozen/thawed for successful ICSI. It is no longer necessary to do testicular sperm aspiration/percutaneous epididymal sperm aspiration on the same day as the oocyte retrieval – numerous groups report success with frozen/thawed testicular and epididymal samples. All biopsy samples can be successfully frozen. The use of cryopreservation buffers without egg yolk is recommended for testicular and epididymal samples.

## Testicular Biopsy Samples

Freezing whole biopsy samples without prior processing is not recommended, as cryoprotectant solution will not equilibrate evenly throughout the tissue. Pieces of macerated or minced tissue can, however, be frozen with some success. It has also been reported that a higher proportion of testicular sperm retain their motility on thawing if they have been incubated

24–48 hours before freezing, and Van den Berg (1998) suggests that incubation at 32°C may be beneficial. If there is doubt about sperm viability after thawing, a simple hypo-osmotic swelling test will identify viable sperm before injection.

## Cryopreservation of Semen for Cancer Patients

Patients who are to be treated with combined chemotherapy for various types of cancer, such as Hodgkin's disease and testicular tumors, are frequently young or even adolescent. Recent progress in oncology has given these patients a greatly improved prognosis for successful recovery, and cryopreservation of spermatozoa before initiating treatment can preserve fertility for the majority of patients.

All cancer treatment regimens are toxic to spermatogenesis, and the majority of patients will be azoospermic after 7–8 weeks of treatment. In some cases spermatogenesis is restored after some years, but in others there is minimal recovery even after a decade. Animal studies have indicated that spermatogenesis may be protected from the adverse effects of chemotherapy by inhibiting pituitary control of spermatogenesis with GnRH agonists, androgens or male contraceptive regimens. Similar protective regimens in humans are currently ineffective, and the strategy remains experimental.

Currently, there are no pretreatment parameters that can predict a patient's prognosis for recovery of fertility; the possibility of erectile dysfunction after treatment should also be borne in mind. Patients should be given general advice about the need for contraception when recovery is unpredictable and advised to seek medical help early if fertility is required. Informed consent forms should be signed after discussion and counseling. Ideally, three sperm samples are collected before chemotherapy is initiated; animal studies suggest that chemotherapy may have a mutagenic effect on late-stage germinal cells, but in the absence of a known clinical significance in humans, sample collection after the start of treatment is preferable to no storage at all. Patients should be informed of the potential risks and receive appropriate counseling in such cases. Spermatogenesis is often already impaired due to the effects of the disease: many demonstrate hypothalamic dysfunction, and in severe cases pituitary gonadotropin secretion is altered. Semen quality is commonly compromised pre-treatment in patients with testicular cancer, leukemia, brain tumor and sarcoma. The tremendous stress caused by cancer reduces fertility potential by the action of stress hormones in the brain, leading to altered catecholamine secretion and a rise in prolactin and corticotropin-releasing factor, which in turn suppress the release of GnRH. However, in the light of ICSI treatment success rates, semen samples should be frozen regardless of their quality. Prior to sample collection for storage, patients should be screened for hepatitis B and C and HIV.

Patients are naturally concerned that their cancer treatment might cause an increased risk of congenital malformation in a subsequent pregnancy: the results of studies to date are reassuring, although insufficient data have been accumulated for each cancer or treatment regimen. There are now numerous published reports of successful treatment for couples using sperm stored prior to treatment; type of treatment depends upon the quality of the sample, but pregnancies and live births are reported after AI, IUI, IVF and ICSI (Ukita *et al.*, 2018).

In the future, autotransplantation of cryopreserved testicular tissue may become an alternative option for young men who are not yet producing sperm or who are unable to produce an ejaculate. Research has shown that gonocytes from immature mice injected into the tubules of sterilized hosts restore spermatogenesis and produce fertile spermatozoa; hopefully, this strategy may one day provide another option for cancer patients, especially for children.

# Further Reading

## Principles of Cryobiology

Fahy GM, Wowk B (2015) Principles of cryopreservation by vitrification. In: Wolkers WF, Oldenhof H (eds.) *Cryopreservation and Freeze-Drying Protocols*, Methods in Molecular Biology, vol 1257. Springer Science + Business Media, New York, pp. 21–82.

Fogarty NM, Maxwell WM, Eppleston J, Evans G (2000) The viability of transferred sheep embryos after long-term cryopreservation. *Reproduction, Fertility and Development* 12: 31–37.

Fuller BJ (2003) Gene expression in response to low temperatures in mammalian cells: a review of current ideas. *Cryo Letters* 24(2): 95–102.

Lasalle B, Testart J, Renard JP (1985) Human embryo features that influence the success of cryopreservation

with the use of 1,2 propanediol. *Fertility and Sterility* 44: 645–651.

Leibo SP (1976) Freezing damage of bovine erythrocytes: simulation using glycerol concentration changes at sub-zero temperatures. *Cryobiology* 13: 587–598.

Leibo SP, Oda K (1993) High survival of mouse zygotes and embryos cooled rapidly or slowly in ethylene glycol plus polyvinylpyrrolidone. *Cryo Letters* 14: 133–144.

Leibo SP, Pool TB (2011) The principal vairables of cryopreservation: solutions, temperatures, and rate changes. *Fertility and Sterility* 96(2): 269–275.

Leibo SP, Semple ME, Kroetsch TG (1994) In vitro fertilization of oocytes by 37-year-old bovine spermatozoa. *Theriogenology* 42: 1257–1262.

Liebermann J, Nawroth F, Isachenko V, *et al.* (2002) Potential importance of vitrification in reproductive medicine. *Biology of Reproduction* 67(6): 1671–1680.

Mazur P (1963) Kinetics of water loss from cells at subzero temperatures and the likelihood of intracellular freezing. *Journal of General Physiology* 47: 347–369.

Mazur P (1970) Cryobiology: the freezing of living systems. *Science* 168: 93–94.

Mazur P (1984) Freezing of living cells: mechanisms and implications. *American Journal of Physiology* 247: 125–142.

McWilliams RB, Gibbons WE, Leibo SP (1995) Osmotic and physiological responses of mouse and human ova to mono- and disaccharides. *Human Reproduction* 10: 1163–1171.

Morató R, Izquierdo D, Paramio MT, Mogas T (2008) Cryotops versus open-pulled straws (OPS) as carriers for the cryopreservation of bovine oocytes: effects on spindle and chromosome configuration and embryo development. *Cryobiology* 57(2): 137–141.

Parks JE (1997) Hypothermia and mammalian gametes. In: Karow A, Critser JK (eds.) *Reproductive Tissue Banking: Scientific Principles.* Academic Press, San Diego, pp. 229–261.

Pegg DE (1996) Cryopreservation: a perspective. In: Hervé P, Rifle G, Vuitton D, Dureau G, Bechtel P, Justrabo E (eds.) *Organ Transplantation and Tissue Grafting.* John Libbey, London, pp. 375–378.

Pegg DE (2002) The history and principles of cryopreservation. *Seminars in Reproductive Medicine* 20(1): 5–13.

Pegg DE (2015) Principles of cryopreservation. In: Wolkers W, Oldenhof H (eds.) *Cryopreservation and Freeze-Drying Protocols*, Methods in Molecular Biology (Methods and Protocols), vol 1257. Springer, New York, NY, pp. 3–19.

Pegg DE, Karow AM (1987) *The Biophysics of Organ Cryopreservation.* Plenum, New York.

Smith AU (1952) Behaviour of fertilized rabbit eggs exposed to glycerol and to low temperatures. *Nature* 170: 373.

Tucker MJ, Liebermann J (2007) *Vitrification in Assisted Reproduction: A User's Manual and Troubleshooting Guide.* Informa Healthcare, New York.

Vajta G, Rienzi L, Ubaldi FM (2015) Open versus closed systems for vitrification of human oocytes and embryos. *Reproductive BioMedicine Online* 30: 325–333.

Watson PF, Morris GJ (1987) Cold shock injury in animal cells. In: Bowler P, Fuller J (eds.) *Temperature and Animal Cells.* Symposia of the Society for Experimental Biology no. 41. Company of Biologists, Cambridge, UK, pp. 311–340.

Whittingham DG (1977) Some factors affecting embryo storage in laboratory animals. *Ciba Foundation Symposium* 52: 97–127.

Whittingham DG, Leibo SP, Mazur P (1972) Survival of mouse embryos frozen to –196°C and –269°C. *Science* 178: 411–414.

## Storage of Cryopreserved Samples

Bahadur G, Tedder RS (1997) Safety during sperm banking. *Human Reproduction* 12: 198.

British Andrology Society (1993) British Andrology Society guidelines for the screening of semen donors for donor insemination. *Human Reproduction* 8: 1521–1523.

Department of Health (1997) *Guidance on the processing, storage and issue of bone marrow and blood stem cells.* NHS Executive, Health Service Guidelines 97(19).

Fountain D, Ralston M, Higgins N, *et al.* (1997) Liquid nitrogen freezers: potential source of hematopoietic stem cell components. *Transfusion* 37: 585–591.

Hawkins AE, Zuckerman MA, Briggs M, *et al.* (1996) Hepatitis B nucleotide sequence analysis – linking an outbreak of acute Hepatitis B to contamination of a cryopreservation tank. *Journal of Virological Methods* 60: 81–88.

Human Fertilisation and Embryology Authority (1998) *Consultation on the Safe Cryopreservation of Gametes and Embryos.* HFEA, London.

Hunt CJ, Pegg DE (1996) Improved temperature stability in gas phase nitrogen refrigerators: use of a copper heat shunt. *Cryobiology* 33: 544–551.

McKee TA, Avery S, Majid A, *et al.* (1996) Risks for transmission of hepatitis C virus during artificial insemination. *Fertility and Sterility* 66: 161–163.

Pomeroy KO, Harris S, Conaghan J, *et al.* (2009) Storage of cryopreserved reproductive tissues: evidence that cross-contamination of infectious agents is a negligible risk. *Fertility and Sterility* 94(4): 1181–1188.

Russell PH, Lyaruu VH, Millar JD, Curry MR, Watson PF (1997) The potential transmission of infectious agents by semen packaging during storage for artificial insemination. *Animal Reproduction Science* 47: 337–342.

Tedder RS, Zuckerman AH, Goldstone AH, *et al.* Hepatitis B transmission from contaminated cryopreservation tank. *Lancet* 1995; 346: 137–140.

Tomlinson M, Sakkas D (2000) Safe and effective cryopreservation: should sperm banks and fertility centres move toward storage in nitrogen vapour? *Human Reproduction* 15(12): 2460–2463.

## Embryo Cryopreservation

Alteri A, Vigano P, Maizar AA, Jovine L, Giacomini E, Rubino P (2018) Revisiting embryo assisted hatching approaches: a systematic review of the current protocols. *Journal of Assisted Reproduction and Genetics* 35(3): 367–391.

Ashwood-Smith MJ (1986) The cryopreservation of human embryos. *Human Reproduction* 1: 319–332.

Cimadonmo D, Capalbo A, Levi-Setti PE, Soscia DD, Orland G (2018) Associations of blastocyst features, trophectoderm biopsy and other laboratory practice with post-warming behavior and implantation. *Human Reproduction* 33(11): 1992–2001.

Cohen J, Devane GW, Elsner CW, *et al.* (1988) Cryopreservation of zygotes and early cleaved human embryos. *Fertility and Sterility* 49: 2.

Cohen J, Simons RF, Edwards RG, Fehilly CB, Fishel SB (1985) Pregnancies following the frozen storage of expanding human blastocysts. *Journal of In Vitro Fertilization and Embryo Transfer* 2: 59–64.

Elder K, Van den Bergh M, Woodward B (2015) *Troubleshooting and Problem-Solving in the IVF Laboratory.* Cambridge University Press, Cambridge, UK, Chapter 10.

Fehilly CB, Cohen J, Simons RF, Fishel SB, Edwards RG (1985) Cryopreservation of cleaving embryos and expanded blastocysts in the human: a comparative study. *Fertility and Sterility* 44: 638–644.

Givens C, Markun L, Chenette P, *et al.* (2009) Outcomes of natural cycles versus programmed cycles for 1677 frozen-thawed embryo transfers. *Reproductive BioMedicine Online* 19(3): 380–384.

Guerif F, Cadoret V, Poindron J, Lansac J, Royere D (2003) Overnight incubation improves selection of frozen-thawed blastocysts for transfer: preliminary study using supernumerary embryos. *Theriogenology* 60(8): 1457–1466.

Hartshorne GM, Elder K, Crow J, Dyson H, Edwards RG (1991) The influence of in vitro development upon post-thaw survival and implantation of cryopreserved human blastocysts. *Human Reproduction* 6: 136–141.

Hartshorne GM, Wick K, Elder K, Dyson H (1990) Effect of cell number at freezing upon survival and viability of cleaving embryos generated from stimulated IVF cycles. *Human Reproduction* 5: 857–861.

Jin B, Kleinhaus FW, Mazur P (2014) Survivals of mouse oocytes approach 100% after vitrification in 3-fold diluted media and ultra-raid warming by an IR laser pulse. *Cryobiology* 68(3): 419–430.

Jin B, Mazur P (2015) High survival of mouse oocytes/embryos after vitrification without permeating cryoprotectants followed by ultra-rapid warming with an IR laser pulse. *Scientific Reports* 5: 9271.

Jones HW Jr., Veeck LL, Muasher SJ (1995) Cryopreservation: the problem of evaluation. *Human Reproduction* 10: 2136–2138.

Kader AA, Choi A, Orief Y, Agarwal A (2009) Factors affecting the outcome of human blastocyst vitrification. *Reproductive Biology and Endocrinology* 7: 99.

Katkov II, Bolyukh VF, Sukhikh GT (2018) *KrioBlast*™ as a new technology of ultrafast cryopreservation of cells and tissues. 2. Kinetic vitrification of human pluripotent stem cells and spermatozoa. *Bulletins in Experimental Biological Medicine* 165: 171.

Kojima E, Fukunaga N, Nagai R, Kitasaka H, Ohno H, Asada Y (2012) The vitrification method is significantly better for thawing of slow-freezing embryos. *Fertility and Sterility* 98: S124.

Lassalle B, Testart J, Renard JP (1985) Human embryo features that influence the success of cryopreservation with the use of 1, 2, propanediol. *Fertility and Sterility* 44: 645–651.

Loutradi KE, Kolibianakis EM, Venetis CA, et al. (2008) Cryopreservation of human embryos by vitrification or slow freezing: a systematic review and meta-analysis. *Fertility and Sterility* 90(1): 186–193.

Magli MC, Gianaroli L, Grieco N, et al. (2006) Cryopreservation of biopsied embryos at the blastocyst stage. *Human Reproduction* 21(10): 2656–2660.

Martino A, Songsasen N, Leibo SP (1996) Development into blastocysts of bovine oocytes cryopreserved by ultra-rapid cooling. *Biology of Reproduction* 54: 1059–1069.

Ménézo Y, Nicollet B, Herbaut N, André D (1992) Freezing cocultured human blastocysts. *Fertility and Sterility* 58(5): 977–980.

Noyes N, Reh A, McCaffrey C, Tan O, Krey L (2009) Impact of developmental stage at cryopreservation and transfer on clinical outcome of frozen embryo cycles. *Reproductive BioMedicine Online* 19(Suppl. 3): 9–15.

Parmegiani L, Tatone C, Cognigni GE, et al. (2014) Rapid warming increases survival of slow-frozen sibling oocytes: a step towards a single warming procedure irrespective of the freezing protocol? *Reproductive BioMedicine Online* 28: 614–623.

Pribenszky C, Losonczi E, Molnár M, et al. (2010) Prediction of in-vitro developmental competence of early cleavage-stage mouse embryos with compact time-lapse equipment. *Reproductive BioMedicine Online* 20(3): 371–379.

Rall WF (1987) Factors affecting the survival of mouse embryos cryopreserved by vitrification. *Cryobiology* 24: 387–402.

Rall WF, Fahy GM (1985) Ice-free cryopreservation of mouse embryos at –196°C by vitrification. *Nature* 313: 573–575.

Rama Raju GA, Jaya Prakash G, Murali Krishna K, Madan K (2009) Neonatal outcome after vitrified day 3 embryo transfers: a preliminary study. *Fertility and Sterility* 92(1): 143–148.

Riggs R, Mayer J, Dowling-Lacey D, et al. (2010) Does storage time influence post-thaw survival and pregnancy outcome? An analysis of 11,768 cryopreserved human embryos. *Fertility and Sterility* 93(1): 109–115.

Schmidt CL, Taney FH, de Ziegler D, et al. (1989) Transfer of cryopreserved-thawed embryos: the natural cycle versus controlled preparation of the endometrium with gonadotropin-releasing hormone agonist and exogenous estradiol and progesterone (GEEP). *Fertility and Sterility* 52: 1609–1616.

Schuster TG, Hickner-Cruz K, Ohl DA, Goldman E, Smith GD (2003) Legal considerations for cryopreservation of sperm and embryos. *Fertility and Sterility* 80(1): 61–66.

Sher G, Keskintepe L, Mukaida T, et al. (2008) Selective vitrification of euploid oocytes markedly improves survival, fertilization and pregnancy-generating potential. *Reproductive BioMedicine Online* 17(4): 524–529.

Shu Y, Watt J, Gebhardt J, et al. (2009) The value of fast blastocoele re-expansion in the selection of a viable thawed blastocyst for transfer. *Fertility and Sterility* 91(2): 401–406.

Testart J, Belaisch Allart J, Lassalle B, et al. (1987) Factors influencing the success rate of human embryo freezing in an in vitro fertilization and embryo transfer program. *Fertility and Sterility* 48: 107–112.

Trounson A, Mohr L (1983) Human pregnancy following cryopreservation, thawing, and transfer of an eight-cell embryo. *Nature* 305: 707–709.

Tucker MJ, Cohen J, Massey JB, et al. (1991) Partial dissection of the zona pellucida of frozen-thawed human embryos may enhance blastocyst hatching, implantation, and pregnancy rates. *American Journal of Obstetrics and Gynecology* 165(2): 341–344.

Vajta G, Holm P, Kuwayama M, *et al.* (1998) Open pulled straw (OPS) vitrification: a new way to reduce cryoinjuries of bovine ova and embryos. *Molecular Reproduction and Development* 51: 53–58.

Van den Abbeel E, Camus M, Verheyen G, *et al.* (2005) Slow controlled-rate freezing of sequentially cultured human blastocysts: an evaluation of two freezing strategies. *Human Reproduction* 20(10): 2939–2945.

Van den Abbeel E, Van Steirteghem A (2000) Zona pellucida damage to human embryos after cryopreservation and the consequences for their blastomere survival and in-vitro viability. *Human Reproduction* 15(2): 373–378.

Wennerholm UB, Söderström-Anttila V, Bergh C, *et al.* (2009) Children born after cryopreservation of embryos or oocytes: a systematic review of outcome data. *Human Reproduction* 24(9): 2158–2172.

Youssry M, Ozmen B, Zohni K, Diedrich K, Al-Hasani S (2008) Current aspects of blastocyst cryopreservation. *Reproductive BioMedicine Online* 16(2): 311–320.

## Oocyte Cryopreservation

Al-Hasani S, Diedrich K, van der Ven H, *et al.* (1987) Cryopreservation of human oocytes. *Human Reproduction* 2: 695–700.

Al-Hasani S, Ludwig M, Diedrich K, *et al.* (1996) Preliminary results on the incidence of polyploidy in cryopreserved human oocytes after ICSI. *Human Reproduction* 11: Abstract book 1, 50–51.

Amorim CA, Gonçalves PB, Figueiredo JR (2003) Cryopreservation of oocytes from pre-antral follicles. *Human Reproduction Update* 9(2): 119–129.

Amorim CA, Van Langendonckt A, David A, Dolmans MM, Donnez J (2009) Survival of human pre-antral follicles after cryopreservation of ovarian tissue, follicular isolation and in vitro culture in a calcium alginate matrix. *Human Reproduction* 24(1): 92–99.

Balkenende EME, Dahhan T, van der Veen F, Repping S, Goddijn M (2018). Reproductive outcomes after oocyte banking for fertility preservation. *Reproductive BioMedicine Online* 37(4):425–433.

Boldt J, Tidswell J, Sayer A, Kilani R, Cline D (2006) Human oocyte cryopreservation: Five-year experience with a sodium-depleted slow freezing method. *Reproductive BioMedicine Online* 13: 96–100.

Cao YX, Xing Q, Li L, *et al.* (2009) Comparison of survival and embryonic development in human oocytes cryopreserved by slow-freezing and vitrification. *Fertility and Sterility* 92(4): 1306–1311.

Chen C (1986) Pregnancy after human oocyte cryopreservation. *Lancet* 1: 884–886.

Chen SU, Lien YR, Chao KH, *et al.* (2003) Effects of cryopreservation on meiotic spindles of oocytes and its dynamics after thawing: clinical implications in oocyte freezing – a review article. *Molecular and Cellular Endocrinology* 202(1–2): 101–107.

Chen SU, Lien YR, Chen HF, *et al.* (2005) Observational clinical follow-up of oocyte cryopreservation using a slow-freezing method with 1,2-propanediol plus sucrose followed by ICSI. *Human Reproduction* 20(7): 1975–1980.

Cobo A, Kuwayama M, Perez S, *et al.* (2008) Comparison of concomitant outcome achieved with fresh and cryopreserved donor oocyte vitrified by the cryotop method. *Fertility and Sterility* 89(6): 1657–1664.

Coticchio G, De Santis L, Rossi G, *et al.* (2006) Sucrose concentration influences the rate of human oocytes with normal spindle and chromosome configurations after slow-cooling cryopreservation. *Human Reproduction* 21(7): 1771–1776.

Edgar DH, Gook DA (2007) How should the clinical efficiency of oocyte cryopreservation be measured? *Reproductive BioMedicine Online* 14(4): 430–435.

Eppig JJ, O'Brien MJ, Wigglesworth K, *et al.* (2009) Effect of in vitro maturation of mouse oocytes on the health and lifespan of adult offspring. *Human Reproduction* 24(4): 922–928.

Gook DA, Osborn SM, Bourne H, Johnston WIH (1994) Fertilization of human oocytes following cryopreservation: normal karyotypes and absence of stray chromosomes. *Human Reproduction* 9: 684–691.

Gook DA, Osborn SM, Johnston WIH (1993) Cryopreservation of mouse and human oocytes using 1,2-propanediol and the configuration of the meiotic spindle. *Human Reproduction* 8: 1101–1109.

Gook DA, Osborn SM, Johnston WIH (1995a) Parthenogenetic activation of human oocytes following cryopreservation using 1,2-propanediol. *Human Reproduction* 10: 654–658.

Gook DA, Schiewe MC, Osborn SM, *et al.* (1995b) Intracytoplasmic sperm injection and embryo development of human oocytes cryopreserved using 1,2-propanediol. *Human Reproduction* 10: 2637–2641.

Hong S, Sepilian V, Chung H, Kim T (2009) Cryopreserved human blastocysts after vitrification result in excellent implantation and clinical pregnancy rates *Fertility and Sterility* 92(6): 2062–2064.

Huang J, Chen H, Tan S, Chian R (2007) Effect of choline-supplemented sodium-depleted slow freezing versus vitrification on mouse oocytes meiotic spindles and chromosome abnormalities. *Fertility and Sterility* 88(2): 1093–1110.

279

Kuleshova L, Gianaroli L, Magli C, Ferraretti A, Trounson A (1999) Birth following vitrification of a small number of human oocytes: case report. *Human Reproduction* 14: 3077–3079.

Kuwayama M, Vajta G, Kato O, Leibo SP (2005) Highly efficient vitrification method for cryopreservation of human oocytes. *Reproductive BioMedicine Online* 11(3): 300–308.

Lane M, Bavister BD, Lyons EA, Forest KT (1999) Containerless vitrification of mammalian oocytes and embryos: adapting a proven method for flash-cooling protein crystals to the cryopreservation of live cells. *Nature Biotechnology* 17: 1234–1236.

Nottola S, Coticchio G, De Santis L, *et al.* (2008) Ultrastructure of human mature oocytes after slow cooling cryopreservation with ethylene glycol. *Reproductive BioMedicine Online* 17(3): 368–377.

Noyes N, Porcu E, Borini A (2009) Over 900 oocyte cryopreservation babies born with no apparent increase in congenital anomalies. *Reproductive BioMedicine Online* 18(6): 769–776.

Parmegiani L, Bertocci F, Garello C, Salvarani MC, Tambuscio G, Fabbri R (2009) Efficiency of human oocyte slow freezing: results from five assisted reproduction centres. *Reproductive BioMedicine Online* 18(3): 352–359.

Parmegiani L, Cognigni GE, Bernardi S, *et al.* (2008) Freezing within 2 h from oocyte retrieval increases the efficiency of human oocyte cryopreservation when using a slow freezing/rapid thawing protocol with high sucrose concentration. *Human Reproduction* 23(8): 1771–1777.

Paynter SJ, Borini A, Bianchi V, *et al.* (2005) Volume changes of mature human oocytes on exposure to cryoprotectant solutions used in slow cooling procedures. *Human Reproduction* 20(5): 1194–1199.

Pickering SJ, Braude PR, Johnson MH, Cant A, Currie J (1990) Transient cooling to room temperature can cause irreversible disruption of the meiotic spindle in the human oocyte. *Fertility and Sterility* 54: 102–108.

Porcu E, Fabbri R, Seracchioli R, *et al.* (1997) Birth of a healthy female after intracytoplasmic sperm injection of cryopreserved human oocytes. *Fertility and Sterility* 68: 724–726.

Rienzi L, Martinez F, Ubaldi F, *et al.* (2004) Polscope analysis of meiotic spindle changes in living metaphase II human oocytes during the freezing and thawing procedures. *Human Reproduction* 19(3): 655–659.

Sereni E, Bonu M, Borini A (2000) High survival rates after cryopreservation of human prophase oocytes. *Fertility and Sterility* 74(Suppl. 1): S161.

Stachecki JJ, Cohen J, Willadsen SM (1999) Cryopreservation of mouse oocytes: the effect of replacing sodium with choline in the freezing medium. *Cryobiology* 37: 346–354.

Stachecki J, Cohen J, Garrisi J, Munné S, Willadsen SM (2006) Cryopreservation of unfertilized human oocytes. *Reproductive BioMedicine Online* 13(2): 222–227.

Van den Abbeel E, Schneider U, Liu J, *et al.* (2007) Osmotic responses and tolerance limits to changes in external osmolalities, and oolemma permeability characteristics, of human in vitro matured MII oocytes. *Human Reproduction* 22(7): 1959–1972.

Yoon TK, Kim TJ, Park SE, *et al.* (2003) Live births after vitrification of oocytes in a stimulated in vitro fertilization-embryo transfer program. *Fertility and Sterility* 79(6): 1323–1326.

## Gonadal Tissue Preservation

Amorim CA, Curaba M, Van Langendonckt A, Dolmans MM, Donnez J (2011) Vitrification as an alternative means of cryopreserving ovarian tissue. *Reproductive BioMedicine Online* 23: 160–186.

Amorim CA, Dolmans MM, David A, *et al.* (2012) Vitrification and xenografting of human ovarian tissue. *Fertility and Sterility* 98: 1291–1298.e1–2.

Andersen CY, Rosendahl M, Byskov AG, *et al.* (2008) Two successful pregnancies following autotransplantation of frozen/thawed ovarian tissue. *Human Reproduction* 23(10): 2266–2272.

Anderson RA, Wallace WHB, Telfer EE (2017) Ovarian tissue cryopreservation for fertility preservation: clinical and research perspectives. *Human Reproduction Open* 1: hox001, https://doi.org/10.1093/hropen/hox001.

Chen SU, Chien CL, Wu MY, *et al.* (2006) Novel direct cover vitrification for cryopreservation of ovarian tissues increases follicle viability and pregnancy capability in mice. *Human Reproduction* 21(11): 2794–2800.

Chian RC, Uzelac PS, Nargund G (2013) In vitro maturation of human immature oocytes for fertility preservation. *Fertility and Sterility* 99: 1173–1181.

Cox SL, Shaw J, Jenkin G (1996) Transplantation of cryopreserved fetal ovarian tissue to adult recipients in mice. *Journal of Reproduction and Fertility* 107(2): 315–322.

Demeestere I, Simon P, Buxant F, *et al.* (2006) Ovarian function and spontaneous pregnancy after combined heterotopic and orthotopic cryopreserved ovarian tissue transplantation in a patient previously treated with bone marrow transplantation: case report. *Human Reproduction* 21(8): 2010–2014.

Demeestere I, Simon P, Emiliani S, Delbaere A, Englert Y (2007) Fertility preservation: successful transplantation of cryopreserved ovarian tissue in a young patient previously treated for Hodgkin's disease. *Oncologist* 12(12): 1437–1442.

Demirci B, Lornage J, Salle B, *et al.* (2003) The cryopreservation of ovarian tissue: uses and indications in veterinary medicine. *Theriogenology* 60(6): 999–1010.

Dolmans MM, Donnez J, Camboni A, *et al.* (2009) IVF outcome in patients with orthotopically transplanted ovarian tissue. *Human Reproduction* 24(11): 2778–2787.

Donnez J, Dolmans MM (2015) Ovarian cortex transplantation: 60 reported live births brings the success and worldwide expansion of the technique towards routine clinical practice. *Journal of Assisted Reproduction and Genetics* 32: 1167–1170.

Donnez J, Dolmans MM (2017) Fertility preservation in women. *New England Journal of Medicine* 377: 1657–1665.

Donnez J, Dolmans MM, Demylle D, *et al.* (2004) Livebirth after orthotopic transplantation of cryopreserved ovarian tissue. *Lancet* 364(9443): 1405–1410.

Donnez J, Dolmans MM, Pellicer A, *et al.* (2013) Restoration of ovarian activity and pregnancy after transplantation of cryopreserved ovarian tissue: a review of 60 cases of reimplantation. *Fertility and Sterility* 99(6): 1503–1513.

Donnez J, Jadoul P, Squifflet J, *et al.* (2009) Cryopreservation and autotransplantation of human ovarian tissue prior to cytotoxic therapy – a technique in its infancy but already successful in fertility preservation. *European Journal of Cancer* 45(9): 1547–1553.

Donnez J, Martinez-Madrid B, Jadou Pl, *et al.* (2006) Ovarian tissue cryopreservation and transplantation: a review. *Human Reproduction Update* 12: 519–535.

Gellert SE, Pors SE, Kristensen SG, Bay-Bjørn AM, Ernst E, Yding Andersen C. (2018) Transplantation of frozen-thawed ovarian tissue: an update on worldwide activity published in peer-reviewed papers and on the Danish cohort. *Journal of Assisted Reproduction and Genetics* 35: 561–570.

Gook DA, Edgar DH, Stern C (1999) Effect of cooling rate and dehydration regimen on the histological appearance of human ovarian cortex following cryopreservation in 1,2-propanediol. *Human Reproduction* 14: 2061–2068.

Gosden RG (2002) Gonadal tissue cryopreservation and transplantation. *Reproductive BioMedicine Online* 4(Suppl. 1): 64–67.

Gosden RG, Oktay K, Radford JA, *et al.* (1997) Ovarian tissue banking. *Human Reproduction Update* 3: CD-ROM, item 1, video.

Hovatta O (2004) Cryopreservation and culture of human ovarian cortical tissue containing early follicles. *European Journal of Obstetrics, Gynecology, and Reproductive Biology* 113(Suppl. 1): S50–54.

Huang L, Mo Y, Wang W, Li Y, Zhang Q, Yang D (2008) Cryopreservation of human ovarian tissue by solid-surface vitrification. *European Journal of Obstetrics, Gynecology and Reproductive Biology* 139(2): 193–198.

Isachenko V, Isachenko E, Kreienberg R, Woriedh M, Weiss J (2010) Human ovarian tissue cryopreservation: quality of follicles as a criteria of effectiveness. *Reproductive BioMedicine Online* 20(4): 441–442.

Isachenko V, Isachenko E, Reinsberg J, *et al.* (2007) Cryopreservation of human ovarian tissue: comparison of rapid and conventional freezing. *Cryobiology* 55(3): 261–268.

Isachenko V, Lapidus I, Isachenko E, *et al.* (2009) Human ovarian tissue vitrification versus conventional freezing: morphological, endocrinological, and molecular biological evaluation. *Reproduction* 138(2): 319–327.

Kader A, Biscotti C, Agarwal A, Sharma R, Falcone T (2008) Comparison of post-warming degeneration and apoptosis of porcine ovarian tissue following vitrification using the Ohio-Cryo device and slow cryopreservation. *Fertility and Sterility* 90: S288–S288.

Kagawa N, Kuwayama M, Silber S, *et al.* (2008) Successful vitrification method for bovine and human ovarian tissue: the cryotissue method. *Human Reproduction* 23(Suppl. 1): 145.

Kagawa N, Silber S, Kuwayama M (2009) Successful vitrification of bovine and human ovarian tissue. *Reproductive BioMedicine Online* 18(4): 568–577.

Kim SS, Battaglia DE, Soules MR (2001) The future of human ovarian cryopreservation and transplantation. *Fertility and Sterility* 75: 1049–1056.

Kim SS, Lee WS, Chung MK, *et al.* (2009) Long-term ovarian function and fertility after heterotopic autotransplantation of cryobanked human ovarian tissue: Eight-year experience in cancer patients. *Fertility and Sterility* 91(6): 2349–2354.

Li YB, Zhou CQ, Yang GF, Wang Q, Dong Y (2007) Modified vitrification method for cryopreservation of human ovarian tissues. *Chinese Medical Journal (Engl.)* 120(2): 110–114.

Martinez-Madrid B, Dolmans MM, Van Langendonckt A, Defrère S, Donnez J (2004) Freeze-thawing intact human ovary with its vascular pedicle with a passive cooling device. *Fertility and Sterility* 82(5): 1390–1394.

McLaughlin MM, Albertini DF, Wallace DHB, *et al.* (2018) Metaphase II oocytes from human unilaminar follicles grown in a multi-step culture system *Molecular Human Reproduction* 24(3): 135–142.

Newton H, Aubard Y, Rutherford A, Sharma V, Gosden RG (1996) Low temperature storage and grafting of human ovarian tissue. *Human Reproduction* 11: 487–491.

Newton H, Fisher J, Arnold JR, *et al.* (1998) Permeation of human ovarian tissue with cryoprotective agents in preparation for cryopreservation. *Human Reproduction* 13: 376–380.

Nugent D, Meirow D, Brook PF, Aubard Y, Gosden RG (1997) Transplantation in reproductive medicine: previous experience, present knowledge, and future prospects. *Human Reproduction Update* 3: 267–280.

Nugent D, Newton H, Gosden RG, Rutherford AJ (1998) Investigation of follicle survival after human heterotopic grafting. *Human Reproduction* 13(1): 22–23.

Oktay K, Newton H, Aubard Y, Salha O, Gosden RG (1998) Cryopreservation of immature human oocytes and ovarian tissue: an emerging technology? *Fertility and Sterility* 69: 1–7.

Oktay K, Nugent D, Newton H (1997) Isolation and characterisation of primordial follicles from fresh and cryopreserved human ovarian tissue. *Fertility and Sterility* 67: 481–486.

Onions VJ, Webb R, McNeilly AS, Campbell BK (2009) Ovarian endocrine profile and long-term vascular patency following heterotopic autotransplantation of cryopreserved whole ovine ovaries. *Human Reproduction* 24(11): 2845–2855.

Picton HM, Kim SS, Gosden RG (2000) Cryopreservation of gonadal tissue and cells. *British Medical Bulletin* 56: 603–615.

Potdar N, Gelbaya TA, Nardo LG (2014) Oocyte vitrification in the 21st century and post-warming fertility outcomes: a systematic review and meta-analysis. *Reproductive Biomedicine Online* 29(2): 159–176.

Shaw J, Trounson AO (1997) Ovarian banking for cancer patients: oncological implications in the replacement of ovarian tissue. *Human Reproduction* 12: 403–405.

Shaw JM, Oranratnachai A, Trounson AO (2000) Fundamental cryobiology of mammalian oocytes and ovarian tissue. *Theriogenology* 53: 59–72.

Silber S, Pineda J, Lenahan K, *et al.* (2015) Fresh and cryopreserved ovary transplantation and resting follicle recruitment. *Reproductive Biomedicine Online* 30(6): 643–650.

Smitz J, Dolmans MM, Donnez J, *et al.* (2010) Current achievements and future research directions in ovarian tissue culture, in vitro follicle development and transplantation: implications for fertility preservation. *Human Reproduction Update* 16: 395–414.

Tryde Schmidt KL, Yding Andersen C, Starup J, *et al.* (2004) Orthotopic autotransplantation of cryopreserved ovarian tissue to a woman cured of cancer – follicular growth, steroid production and oocyte retrieval. *Reproductive BioMedicine Online* 8(4): 448–453.

von Wolff M, Dittrich R, Liebenthron J, et al (2015) Fertility-preservation counselling and treatment for medical reasons: data from a multinational network of over 5000 women. *Reproductive BioMedicine Online* 31: 605–612.

## Sperm Freezing

Agha-Rahimi A, Khalili MA, Nabi A, Ashourzadeh S (2014) Vitrification is not superior to rapid freezing of normozoospermic spermatozoa: effects on sperm parameters, DNA fragmentation and hyaluron binding. *Reproductive BioMedicine Online* 28: 352–358.

Gilbert K, Nangia AK, Dupree JM, Smith JF, Mehta A (2018) Fertility preservation for men with testicular cancer: is sperm cryopreservation cost effective in the era of assisted reproductive technology? *Urological Oncology* 36(3): 92e1–92e9.

Gilmore JA, Liu J, Gao DY, Critser JK (1997) Determination of optimal cryoprotectants and procedures for their addition and removal from human spermatozoa. *Human Reproduction* 12: 12–18.

Giraud MN, Motta C, Boucher D, Grizard G (2000) Membrane fluidity predicts the outcome of cryopreservation of human spermatozoa. *Human Reproduction* 15: 2160–2164.

Hammerstedt RH, Graham JK, Nolan JP (1990) Cryopreservation of human sperm. *Journal of Andrology* 11(1): 73–88.

Kawai K, Nishiyama H (2018) Preservation of fertility of adult male cancer patients treated with chemotherapy. *International Journal of Oncology* Oct 23. doi: 10.1007/s10147-018-1333-0 [Epub ahead of print].

Leibo SP, Bradley L (1999) Comparative cryobiology of mammalian spermatozoa. In: Gagnon C (ed.) *The Male Gamete: From Basic Knowledge to Clinical Applications.* Cache River Press, Vienna, IL, pp. 501–516.

Mahadevan M, Trounson A (1983) Effects of CPM and dilution methods on the preservation of human spermatozoa. *Andrologia* 15: 355–366.

McLaughlin EA, Ford WCL, Hill MGR (1990) A comparison of the freezing of human semen in the uncirculated vapour above liquid nitrogen and in a commercial semi-programmable freezer. *Human Reproduction* 5: 734–738.

Meirow D, Schenker JG (1995) Cancer and male infertility. *Human Reproduction* 10: 2017–2022.

Morris GJ (2006) Rapidly cooled human sperm: no evidence of intracellular ice formation. *Human . Reproduction* 21: 2075–2083.

Morris GJ, Acton E, Murray BJ, Fonseca F (2012) Freezing injury: the special case of the sperm cell. *Cryobiology* 64: 71–80.

Polge C, Smith AU, Parkes AS (1949) Revival of spermatozoa after vitrification and dehydration at low temperatures. *Nature* 164: 666–667.

Stanic P, Tandara M, Sonicki Z, *et al.* (2000) Comparison of protective media and freezing techniques for cryopreservation of human semen. *European Journal of Obstetrics, Gynecology and Reproductive Biology* 91: 65–70.

Ukita Y, Wakimoto Y, Sugiyama Y, *et al.* (2018) Fertility preservation and pregnancy outcomes in adolescent and young adult male patients with cancer. *Reproductive BioMedicine Online* 17(4): 449–453.

Van den Berg M (1998) Sample preparation. In: Elder K, Elliott T (eds.) *The Use of Epididymal and Testicular Sperm in IVF.* WorldWide Conferences on Reproduction Biology. Ladybrook Publishing, Australia, pp. 51–54.

Walmsley R, Cohen J, Ferrara-Congedo T, Reing A, Garrisi J (1999) The first births and ongoing pregnancies associated with sperm cryopreservation within evacuated egg zonae. *Human Reproduction* 13: 61–70.

Watson PF (2000) The causes of reduced fertility with cryopreserved semen. *Animal Reproduction Science* 60: 481–492.

Wyns C, Curaba M, Vanabelle B, Van Langendonckt A, Donnez J (2010) Options for fertility preservation in prepubertal boys. *Human Reproduction Update* 16(3): 312–328.

# Chapter 13

# Micromanipulation Techniques

## Introduction

Biologists and physiologists began to micromanipulate cells during the last century, using a variety of manipulator systems to dissect or record from cells. The earliest attempt to inject sperm was recorded in 1914, when G.I. Kite injected sperm cells into starfish oocytes, but with inconclusive results (Lillie, 1914). Experiments in which sperm were injected into eggs around the mid-1960s were primarily designed to investigate the early events of fertilization, i.e. the role of membrane fusion, activation of the oocyte and the formation of the pronuclei. Two series of early experiments by independent groups demonstrated major species differences. Hiramoto showed that microinjection of spermatozoa into unfertilized sea urchin oocytes did not induce activation of the oocyte or condensation of the sperm nucleus (Hiramoto, 1962), whereas others demonstrated the opposite in frog oocytes. Ryuzo Yanagimachi and his group later demonstrated that isolated hamster nuclei could develop into pronuclei after microinjection into homologous eggs, and a similar result was obtained after injecting freeze-dried human spermatozoa into a hamster egg (reviewed by Yanagimachi, 2005). These experiments indicated that membrane fusion events can be bypassed during activation of mammalian oocytes, without compromising the initiation of development. The experiments not only provided information on the mechanism of fertilization, but also led to a new technique in clinical embryology.

During the late 1980s Jacques Cohen and colleagues developed a microsurgical technique to aid fertilization of human oocytes via partial dissection of the zona pellucida (PZD) (Cohen *et al.*, 1988). This mechanical technique involves breaching the zona pellucida with a sharp glass micropipette to create a slit and subsequently placing the dissected oocyte into a suspension of spermatozoa, on the assumption that sperm entry is facilitated by the slit. Lanzendorf *et al.*

(1988) demonstrated formation of pronuclei after direct injection of sperm into human oocytes, and in 1989 S.C. Ng and colleagues in Singapore reported the first pregnancy after inserting several spermatozoa into the perivitelline space, subzonal sperm injection (SUZI). They later also reported activation of human oocytes following intracytoplasmic injection (ICSI) of human spermatozoa (Ng *et al.*, 1991).

In 1992, Palermo and colleagues in Brussels reported the first live birth from this technique of ICSI (Palermo, 1992). Since the time of these pioneering reports, ICSI is now a standard and successful assisted reproduction treatment, with >2.5 million babies born worldwide by 2012.

The technique of assisted hatching was also developed during the 1990s, using micromanipulation to cut a slit in the zona pellucida or dissolve a hole in the zona with an acid solution (zona drilling, ZD). Assisted hatching was proposed as a means of facilitating embryo implantation in selected cases. Figure 13.1 shows a diagrammatic representation of these micromanipulation procedures.

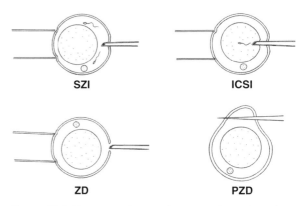

**Figure 13.1** Micromanipulation techniques include subzonal injection (SZI), intracytoplasmic sperm injection (ICSI), zona drilling (ZD) and partial zona dissection (PZD).

# ICSI – Intracytoplasmic Sperm Injection

Prior to 1992, the majority of cases of severe male infertility were virtually untreatable, and failure of fertilization was observed in up to 30% of IVF treatments for male infertility. The introduction of micromanipulation techniques such as PZD, SUZI and ZD raised the hopes of a better prognosis for these cases, but did not overall provide a substantial improvement in success rates. The introduction and successful application of ICSI by Gianpiero Palermo and colleagues at The Free University in Brussels, Belgium, produced a dramatic improvement in the treatment of severe male infertility by ART.

## Genetic Implications

The establishment of ICSI as a routine technique was quickly followed by the introduction of techniques for collecting sperm samples from the epididymis and directly from the testis, so that the whole spectrum of male infertility can now be treated, from suboptimal ejaculate samples or ejaculatory failure, to obstructive and nonobstructive causes of azoospermia. However, an increasing number of genetic defects have been found to be associated with male infertility: a higher incidence of numerical and structural chromosomal aberrations is found in infertile and subfertile men than in the general population, in particular karyotypes 47XXY, 47XYY, 46XX, 46X, derY, Robertsonian translocations, reciprocal translocations, inversions and additional marker chromosomes. Between 12% and 18% of men with azoospermia or severe oligospermia (less than 300 000 sperm in the ejaculate) have deletions in intervals 5 and 6 on the long arm of the Y chromosome. Microdeletions of the q11 region of the Y chromosome are related to the dysfunction of Deleted in Azoospermia (DAZ) and RNA-binding motif (RBM) genes, and androgen receptor (AR) gene mutations have also been reported in infertile men. In a population of approximately 3000 infertile men, the pathological (nonpolymorphic, phenotype associated) microdeletions rate, in at least one of four critical regions on the Y chromosome, was found to be as high as 22%, with an additional (as yet unknown) percentage being attributed to cryptic mosaicism. Furthermore, it appears that microdeletions will be transmitted in at least 10% of unselected father/son pairs.

The Belgian group responsible for the first ICSI births have carried out prospective follow-up studies of their first cohort of ICSI babies, born between 1992 and 1996; they confirm that this group of boys has normal pubertal development and adequate Sertoli and Leydig cell function. They then carried out a study of semen parameters in a small cohort of young adults aged between 18 and 22 years who were conceived after ICSI for male infertility with fresh ejaculated sperm; this group of young men had significantly lower median sperm concentration, total sperm count and total motile sperm count when compared with a control peer group born after spontaneous conception. Although no clear correlation was seen between the semen parameters of the young men in the study and their fathers, the study confirms the need for further investigation of transgenerational passage of male infertility (Belva *et al.*, 2016).

Three to ten per cent of infertile men present with congenital bilateral absence of the vas deferens (CBAVD), and approximately 65% of these individuals carry the gene for cystic fibrosis (CF), with defects in the cystic fibrosis conductance regulator (CFTR) gene. Many are compound heterozygous for the CFTR mutation, with an increased risk of having children with CF or CBVAD.

Although the genetic risk for couples who require ICSI treatment has yet to be fully defined, karyotyping, and preferably also Y-microdeletion analysis, is recommended as part of the pretreatment screening process for men with severe male factor infertility referred for ICSI (Qureshi *et al.*, 1996; Simoni *et al.*, 1998). The couple should also have access to professional genetic counseling to discuss potential risks, and appropriate informed consent must be obtained before treatment.

## Surgical Sperm Retrieval

In cases of obstructive azoospermia, samples can be aspirated from the epididymis. The original 'open' microsurgical technique of microepididymal sperm aspiration (MESA) was superseded by the simpler procedure of percutaneous epididymal sperm aspiration (PESA), which can be carried out by fertility specialists without microsurgical skills, and can be performed under local anesthetic or mild sedation as an outpatient procedure. Aspiration is carried out using a 25-gauge butterfly needle connected to a syringe. If sperm cannot be aspirated from the epididymis, a modification of the technique using wide-bore needle aspiration of the testis, testicular sperm aspiration (TESA) or testicular fine needle aspiration (TEFNA) often harvests sufficient testicular spermatozoa to carry out an ICSI procedure. In nonobstructive azoospermia, spermatogenesis is impaired. The epididymis is devoid of sperm, but the testis usually contains focal areas of spermatogenesis: this focal spermatogenesis makes diagnosis based upon a single biopsy unrealistic, and multiple biopsies may be required. Prepared testicular samples can also be cryopreserved for a future ICSI procedure at the time of diagnostic testicular biopsy. The biopsy is carried out either by multiple needle aspirations (TEFNA or TESA) or by open biopsy (testicular sperm extraction: TESE), and both procedures may be safely carried out with local anesthetic or mild sedation.

## Indications for ICSI

The ICSI procedure involves injecting a single immobilized spermatozoon directly into an oocyte, and therefore it can be used not only for cases in which there are extremely low numbers of sperm, but in bypassing gamete interaction at the level of the zona pellucida and the vitelline membrane it can also be used in the treatment of qualitative or functional sperm disorders.

1. Couples who have suffered recurrent failure of fertilization after IVF-ET may have one or more disorders of gamete dysfunction in which there is a barrier to fertilization at the level of the acrosome reaction, zona pellucida binding or interaction, zona penetration, or fusion with the oolemma. ICSI should be offered to patients who have unexplained failure of fertilization in a previous IVF–ET cycle.
2. Severe oligospermia can be treated with ICSI; in patients where as many normal vital sperm can be recovered as there are oocytes to be inseminated, fertilization can be achieved in approximately 90% of cases. In extreme cases of cryptozoospermia, where no sperm cells can be seen by standard microscopy, centrifugation of the neat sample at higher than usual centrifugal force (1800 g, 5 minutes) may result in the recovery of an adequate number of sperm cells.
3. Severe asthenozoospermia, including patients with sperm ultrastructural abnormalities such as Kartagener's syndrome, or '9 + 0' axoneme disorders can be treated by ICSI.
4. Teratozoospermia, including absolute teratozoospermia or globozoospermia.
5. In cases of CBAVD, vasectomy or postinflammatory obstruction of the vas, sperm samples can be retrieved by PESA, TESA or TESE.
6. Samples can be recovered by needle or open biopsy of the testis in cases of nonobstructive azoospermia.
7. In cases of ejaculatory dysfunction, such as retrograde ejaculation, a sufficient number of sperm cells can usually be recovered from the urine.
8. Paraplegic males have been given the chance of biological fatherhood using electro ejaculation and IVF; they may also be successfully treated using a combination of PESA/TESA/TESE and ICSI.
9. Immunological factors – couples in whom there may be antisperm antibodies in female sera/follicular fluid or antisperm antibodies in seminal plasma following vasectomy reversal or genital tract infection can be successfully treated by ICSI.
10. Oncology – male patients starting chemotherapy or radiotherapy should have semen samples frozen for use in the future; ICSI offers the patient an excellent chance of achieving fertilization following recovery from their disease and treatment. Testicular biopsy specimens may also be cryopreserved for these patients as a further back-up when the quality of the ejaculate is inadequate for freezing.
11. For preimplantation genetic diagnosis involving DNA amplification by PCR, ICSI should be used as the means of fertilization to prevent sperm contamination of the sample.

Although the main indication for ICSI was originally for the treatment of male factor infertility, its use has become far more widespread, with an increasing trend for its routine use in treating indications that include moderate male subfertility, advanced maternal age, low responder patients, and donor oocytes or sperm; indeed, some clinics now use ICSI as a routine for all indications. European data for 2005 showed that the proportion of ICSI cycles in different countries ranged from 58% to 67%; in the USA, 62.2% of fresh nondonor cycles used ICSI during 2006. A review of European data collected between 1997 and 2011 confirmed that the proportion of ICSI versus IVF cycles continued to increase, reaching a plateau of around 75% in 2008 (Ferraretti *et al.*, 2017), and in

2016 the International Committee for Monitoring Assisted Reproductive Technologies reported that global use of ICSI remained constant at around 66% of nondonor cycles (Dyer *et al.*, 2016). Several randomized controlled studies have compared the efficacy of IVF versus ICSI in couples with non-male factor infertility, with results that showed no difference in fertilization or pregnancy rates. A Cochrane review (van Rumste *et al.*, 2004) concluded that the use of ICSI for non-male factor infertility remains an open question, and further research should focus on live birth rates and adverse events. In their 2008 report on good clinical treatment in assisted reproduction, the European Society for Human Reproduction and Embryology (ESHRE) published an Executive Summary that concludes: 'ICSI should be considered in the presence of severe sperm abnormalities or a history of fertilization failure in conventional IVF attempts. It must be emphasized that ICSI does not represent the most suitable treatment for female pathologies such as poor ovarian response or previous implantation failure.' This conclusion continues to be reinforced by data reported up to the present day.

# Practical Aspects

ICSI demands the same meticulous attention to detail that is needed in all IVF manipulations, but the number of details requiring attention is dramatically increased. Successful results with ICSI can only be achieved with the dedication of concentrated time, effort and patience.

## Location of ICSI Set Up

The laboratory should preferably be on a ground floor, near a structural frame or wall to minimize vibrations, and must be kept dust-free. The equipment must be installed on a substantial bench top, away from distractions of traffic such as people or trolleys, etc. Any vibration will interfere with the injection procedure, and it is essential to make sure that the equipment is completely stable, using anti-vibration equipment if necessary. Subdued lighting is helpful for microscopy. Well in advance of any ICSI procedure, ensure that the microscope's optics are checked. Ensure that the tool holders and all other parts of the micromanipulation system are correctly fitted and adjusted for optimal range of movement, and that the microtools can be accurately aligned.

## Microinjection Equipment

All the major microscopy companies now supply microinjection set-ups ready for use. The essential element is an inverted microscope with ×10, ×20 and ×40 objectives, with Hoffman modulation contrast optics in order to visualize the cells on plastic Petri dishes (Nomarski optics uses polarized light and cannot be used through plastic). The micromanipulators consist of two coarse motorized manipulators and two fine mechanical, electrical or hydraulic joysticks, together with microsyringes capable of delivering minute quantities of liquid. Tables 13.1 and 13.2 compare the different types of equipment currently available. For training purposes, it is

**Table 13.1** Micromanipulator

| Manipulator type | Pros | Cons | Examples |
|---|---|---|---|
| Manual | | | |
| Fluid-filled: oil, fluorinert, distilled water | Easy control | Air bubbles render control difficult. Leakage of fluid can be messy, requires careful priming. Time-consuming to set up and flush system. Glass syringes expensive | Narashige, Eppendorf |
| Air-filled | OK for holding pipette | Good control only if set up carefully, with a bubble of oil between air and media | Research Instruments, Narashige |
| Pneumatic | Injection controlled by foot pedal | Pressure leakage | Tritech |
| Piezo Drill | Less disruption to the cytoplasm | Difficult learning curve; possible use of mercury | PrimeTech |

Comments contributed by M. Blayney, A. Burnley, L. Devlin, D. Kastelic, M. van den Berg and B. Woodward.

**Table 13.2** Joysticks

| Joystick type | Pros | Cons | Examples |
|---|---|---|---|
| Hanging joystick | Comfortable to use for short cases | Elevated hand position can be uncomfortable during long ICSI cases | Narashige |
| Standing joystick | All-in-one 3D control | May fall aside, with possible oocyte damage | Narishige, Eppendorf |
| Mechanical | Separate coarse and fine manipulators. Very little to go wrong | Usually fixed to the microscope, with possible vibration transition; 2D control separate to 'up-down' control | Research Instruments |
| Hydraulic | Smooth | System fails if there are any leaks; the oil degrades in sunlight | Narashige |
| Motorized | Very convenient if positions can be stored in memory. Movements are quick, decreasing ICSI procedure time | Some have a delay; pipette continues to move over a small distance. Potential for breakdown, difficult to repair in-house | Eppendorf, Narashige |

Comments contributed by M. Blayney, A. Burnley, L. Devlin, D. Kastelic, M. van den Berg and B. Woodward.

advisable to have a camera attached to one of the microscope optical outlets.

## Microtools

Two types of microtools are used:

1. Holding pipettes to hold and immobilize the oocyte

    Outer diameter: 0.080–0.150 mm

    Inner diameter: 0.018–0.025 mm

    Fire-polished aperture

2. Injection pipettes to immobilize, aspirate and inject the sperm cell

    Outer diameter: 0.0068–0.0078 mm

    Inner diameter: 0.0048–0.0056 mm

    Beveled tip, sometimes tipped with a spike.

Both microtools are bent to an angle of approximately 30° at the distal end in order to facilitate horizontal positioning and manipulation adjustment within culture dishes. Aspiration pipettes (of different diameters) may also be used to aspirate anucleate fragments, or to biopsy blastomeres for preimplantation diagnosis. A third type of microtool may be used for piercing or cutting the zona pellucida in assisted zona hatching techniques. Uniform microtool quality is crucial for consistent results, and specifically tooled,

sterile, ready-to-use holding and injection pipettes are commercially available. A blunt injection pipette can damage the oocyte by compression, whereas a pipette with too large a diameter will damage the oocyte by injecting too much fluid.

## Supplies

Most manufacturers of tissue culture media supply all the components necessary for micromanipulation techniques.

### Polyvinyl Pyrrolidine (PVP)

A viscous solution of 10% polyvinyl pyrrolidine can be used to reduce sperm motility prior to immobilization and aspiration into the injection pipette. Experienced operators can carry out the procedure without the use of PVP, but it is helpful in the initial stages of learning and practice. Experimental evidence has shown that PVP can interact with acrosomal and mitochondrial membranes, as well as cause chromatin deterioration after prolonged exposure, and questions have been raised about the wisdom/safety of injecting this artificial agent directly into ooplasm. Although no adverse effects have as yet been reported, PVP should be used cautiously, with attention to the time that the sperm is exposed to the polymer, and with efforts to minimize the amount that is injected into the oocyte cytoplasm.

## Hyaluronic Acid (HA)

Hyaluronic acid (HA), a natural component of the cumulus–oocyte complex, can be used as an alternative to PVP. HA has a relatively high negative charge and a high hydration capacity, so that viscous solutions can be prepared which can be used to slow sperm motility for the ICSI procedure; commercial preparations using recombinant HA are available. The motility of spermatozoa in a hyaluronate solution resembles that in the extracellular matrix of mature cumulus cells, and spermatozoa resume normal motility once returned to culture medium. Binding to HA has also been used as a marker for sperm maturity, and this offers an added benefit to its use as an alternative to PVP for moderating sperm motility (van den Bergh et al., 2009); a further advantage is that it degrades to natural sugar molecules that can be readily metabolized by cellular pathways.

## Hyaluronidase

This enzyme is used to loosen and disperse cells of the cumulus and corona, prior to their removal from the oocyte by dissection. Preparations of sheep or bovine origin were commonly used in the past, but human recombinant hyaluronidase is now used to minimize risks of disease transmission from animals.

# ICSI – Step by Step

## Selecting Sperm for Injection

As discussed in Chapter 10, there is evidence that sperm with DNA damage can have an adverse effect on the outcome of ART. Efforts have been made to develop techniques that will enhance sperm preparation methods that can be used to identify and select sperm with lesser levels of chromatin or DNA damage. Technologies that have been applied include magnetic-activated cell sorting (MACS, Said et al., 2008), electrophoretic separation of sperm on the basis of their charge and size (Fleming et al., 2008), binding to HA as an indication of sperm maturity (Huszar et al., 2007), using PICSI (Petri-dish ICSI) dishes containing HA bonded to the Petri dish, assessment of sperm head birefringence (Gianaroli et al., 2008) and the use of high-magnification microscopy (Bartoov et al., 2003).

## Magnetic-Activated Cell Sorting (MACS)

This technique aims to reduce the number of spermatozoa with fragmented DNA by eliminating those that are undergoing apoptosis. Such sperm cells may still be motile and have normal morphology. When they reach the terminal phase of apoptosis, phosphatidyl serine is externalized on the external surface of their plasma membrane, and this can be used as a biomarker for apoptosis. Annexin V is a protein that binds phospholipids, but does not pass through the plasma membrane; this molecule can be bound to magnetic microbeads that will covalently bind to phosphatidyl serine on the surface of sperm undergoing apoptosis, and these complexes can be retained in a separation column placed in a magnetic field (Mini-MACS Separator). Sperm cells that pass through the column do not express phosphatidyl serine and are therefore identified as non-apoptotic. Studies using this approach for sperm selection indicate that the number of sperm with fragmented DNA can be reduced, with an improvement in acrosome reaction and mitochondrial membrane potential, as well as increase in embryo implantation and pregnancy rates. Stimpfel et al. (2018) carried out a study in couples with teratozoospermia as the main indication for ICSI, using sibling oocytes to compare outcomes. Half of the oocytes were injected with MACS-sorted sperm, and the remainder were injected with sperm prepared by conventional methods. The overall percentage of morphologically normal sperm did not differ significantly between the ICSI and MACS–ICSI procedures, but MACS-selected sperm had more tail abnormalities. Evaluation and comparison of sperm parameters, fertilization and embryo development revealed no significant differences. However, MACS sorting apparently improved the quality of blastocysts in women over the age of 30, but not in younger women. The authors suggest that this may be explained on the basis that oocyte DNA repair capacity decreases with age, and the use of MACS sorting reduces the need for DNA repair in older oocytes. Couples with male infertility due to teratozoospermia in which the female partner is over 30 years of age could theoretically benefit from the use of MACS for sperm selection.

## Hyaluronic Acid Binding (HAB)

Hyaluronic acid is a major component of the cumulus complex surrounding human oocytes, and sperm must express HA receptors in order to traverse this complex and reach the oocyte surface. The expression of HA receptors has been reported to be an indication of normal spermatogenesis and sperm maturity, reflecting a number of upstream events that affect DNA integrity and frequency of chromosomal aneuploidies (Mokánszki *et al.*, 2014). A medium rich in HA or Petri dishes with spots of immobilized HA (PICSI dish) can be used for sperm selection. However, a systematic review and meta-analysis of data available up to June 2015 did not confirm an improvement in fertilization and clinical pregnancy rates when HA binding was used as a sperm selection technique in ICSI cycles (Beck-Fruchter *et al.*, 2016).

### Digital Holographic Microscopy (DHM)

The sperm cell is almost transparent in conventional bright-field microscopy, as its optical properties differ slightly from that of the surrounding medium. A light beam that passes through a cell undergoes a phase change which depends on the light source and the refractive index of the cell. This 'phase contrast' may be observed qualitatively using contrast interference microscopy such as Nomarski Differential Interference (DIC) microscopy and quantitively using digital holography. Digital Holographic Microscopy (DHM) is a noninvasive, label-free, high-resolution phase-contrast imaging technique that can generate automatic three-dimensional images of small cells without mechanical scanning; it has been instrumental in calculating the volume of normal and vacuolated human sperm heads (Coppola *et al.*, 2013, 2017). The volume of a normal sperm head could previously be estimated only by using linear measurements of the head; DHM measures sperm head volume as $8.03 \pm 0.75 \ \mu m^3$. DHM can also be used to track sperm in four dimensions in order to compare motility characteristics between normal and anomalous sperm cells (Di Caprio *et al.*, 2014).

DHM may be used in combination with Raman spectroscopy to identify biochemical changes in live human sperm. Current methods of DNA assessment are of limited clinical utility as the technique is invasive and generally based on fluorescence microscopy. Raman spectroscopy is based on the detection of the inelastic scattering of light and provides information on the vibrational states of the illuminated molecules. This technique does not require special dyes or culture medium, it is nondestructive and can be combined with other microscopy techniques such as contrast microscopy or holography. Raman spectroscopy has to date been used successfully to study DNA packaging in human spermatozoa, DNA fragmentation and the identification of X- and Y- bearing spermatozoa in the bovine (Ferrara *et al*, 2015).

Although these new microscopy techniques require expensive equipment, they continue to provide additional significant information, and may eventually help to identify the ideal spermatozoon for injection into the oocyte.

### IMSI (Intracytoplasmic Morphologically Selected Sperm)

Sperm morphology has long been accepted as one of the best indicators for a positive outcome in human fertilization, whether via natural fertilization, IUI, IVF or ICSI. IMSI, a technique using ultra high magnification to select 'normal sperm,' has been shown to improve pregnancy rates and decrease abortion rates in some patient categories. This procedure, originally promoted by Bartoov and colleagues (2003), consists of real-time, high magnification, motile sperm organellar morphology examination (MSOME) that uses 24 characteristics to define the normal morphology of seven sperm organelles: acrosome, postacrosomal lamina, neck, mitochondria, tail, outer dense fibers and the nucleus. MSOME is performed with an inverted light microscope equipped with high-power Nomarski optics enhanced by digital imaging that allows the embryologist to magnify sperm up to 6000 times, compared to the traditional 400 times with ICSI. Figure 13.2 shows IMSI photographs of a single normal human spermatozoon and a selection of dysmorphic spermatozoa. Males with severe oligospermia and samples dissected from testicular tissue can potentially benefit from the use of IMSI.

*Equipment and Materials for IMSI* –– Sperm observation and selection is carried out using high-magnification objectives, ranging from ×60 in air to ×100 with oil immersion. Hoffman modulation contrast optics are replaced by a system with Nomarski Differential Interference optics, which requires the use of glass-bottomed dishes or slides of 0.17-mm thickness. The optical signal is then enhanced by a video zoom and digital imaging system, giving a final magnification of up to ×10 000. The image is observed, stored and analyzed using specific software supplied by the microscopy company.

*Procedure* –– Whereas routine ICSI injection is carried out in plastic dishes with Hoffman optics, IMSI sperm identification and selection is made on glass with Nomarski optics: special glass-bottomed dishes have been designed so that the two procedures may be carried out in the same dish. In this case, the

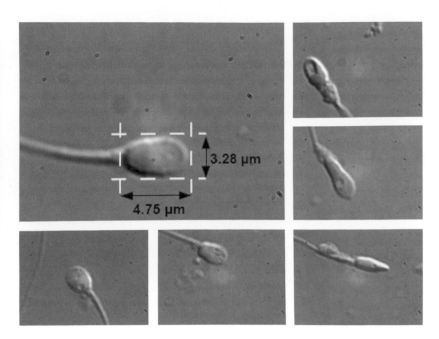

**Figure 13.2** IMSI: a single normal human spermatozoon showing true dimensions in micrometers and a selection of dysmorphic spermatozoa. Nomarski optics at ×6000 magnification.

injection procedure is carried out using Nomarski Differential Interference Contrast (DIC) optics. Tissue culture medium, PVP/HA, paraffin oil and microtools remain unchanged. Alternatively, the IMSI selection procedure can be carried out separately on a designated IMSI set up and the selected sperm then transferred to a plastic ICSI dish for microinjection on a routine ICSI micromanipulator.

Hoffman modulation optics can also be adapted/modified to allow selection of sperm at around ×600 magnification without the need for glass-bottomed dishes, but resolution is inferior to the Nomarski system. An excellent and detailed overview of all technical aspects involved in IMSI has been summarized by Vanderzwalmen *et al.* (2014).

Although IMSI can benefit a targeted group of patients, purchasing the special equipment is expensive, and its application during an ICSI procedure is very time-consuming. Selecting sperm cells on the basis of MSOME criteria can take up to 2 hours (Antinori *et al.*, 2008), and in order to reduce oocyte exposure time, IMSI sperm should be preselected in advance of the injection procedure. Since prolonged sperm handling at 37°C can also be detrimental, preselection may be carried out at room temperature rather than on a heated stage (Peer *et al.*, 2007). In general, published studies have not shown the use of IMSI to yield significant improvements in fertilization rate; studies show conflicting results, due to

differences in inclusion criteria and the numerous confounding variables that arise during IVF/ICSI treatment. It has been suggested that IMSI might be most effective in overcoming 'late' paternal effects due to sperm abnormalities at the level of DNA chromatin (Setti *et al.*, 2013).

## Oocyte Preparation and Handling

Oocyte retrieval is scheduled after programmed controlled ovarian hyperstimulation (COH), according to protocols described in Chapter 2. Oocyte identification is carried out immediately after follicle aspiration, using a dissecting microscope with heated stage. Take care to maintain stable temperature and pH of the aspirates at all times. At the end of the oocyte retrieval, note quality and assess the maturity of the oocytes, and preincubate them in the controlled atmosphere laboratory IVF incubator at 37°C until preparations are ready for cumulus–corona removal.

The incubation time before removing cumulus–corona cells can vary without significant effects but is usually carried out within 1–4 hours after oocyte retrieval. Studies using Polscope technology to examine the meiotic spindle over time suggest that oocyte aging causes the spindle to become unstable around 12 hours after OCR; injection between 9 and 11 hours post OCR resulted in very poor embryo quality (see Simopoulou *et al.*, 2016 for review). The optimal time for injection appears to be between 37 and 39 hours post hCG, but this may vary in patients with polycystic ovarian syndrome (PCOS). HEPES-buffered media can be used to allow more time for oocyte handling. If non-HEPES media is used, handling outside of the incubator must be kept to an absolute minimum; this option is open only to very experienced personnel.

### Cumulus–Corona Removal (Denudation)

1. Either add one central drop of hyaluronidase solution to the oocyte culture dish at the end of the OCR procedure, or prepare a culture dish containing one central drop of hyaluronidase solution and 5 wash drops of culture medium, covered with an overlay of equilibrated mineral oil (denudation may also be carried out in Nunc four-well dishes). Incubate at 37°C for 30–60 minutes. Note: if HEPES-buffered medium is used, this has been adjusted to pH 7.4 and usually 5 mM bicarbonate. Exposure to a $CO_2$ atmosphere will cause the pH to drop, and therefore culture dishes that contain HEPES-buffered media should be warmed to 37°C in a warming oven, and not in a $CO_2$ incubator.

2. Prepare a thin glass probe and select denudation pipettes.

3. Remove the oocyte and hyaluronidase dishes from the incubator. Place one to four oocytes together into the enzyme drop, agitating gently until the cells start to dissociate. Do not leave them in the enzyme preparation for more than 1 minute. Carefully aspirate the oocytes, leaving as much cumulus as possible behind. Wash by transferring them through at least five drops of culture medium, and change to a fine-bore tip for aspiration in order to remove all of the coronal cells.

4. Assess the quality and maturity of each oocyte under an inverted microscope. Use the glass probe to roll the oocytes around gently in order to identify the polar body, and examine the ooplasm for vacuoles or other abnormalities. Separate metaphase I or germinal vesicle (GV) oocytes from metaphase II oocytes, label them and return to the incubator until ready for the injection procedure.

5. Examine the oocytes again before starting the injection procedure to see if any more have extruded the first polar body. ICSI is carried out on all morphologically intact oocytes with first polar body extruded. Figure 13.3 illustrates different stages of egg maturity that are revealed after hyaluronidase treatment and corona dissection.

### Preparation for Injection

1. Prepare injection dishes with 4–8 droplets of 2–5 μL of HEPES-buffered culture medium for each individual oocyte, and a 5-μL droplet of PVP or HA for the sperm. The droplets can be arranged in a circle with the sperm selection drop in the center, or in parallel groups, but must be positioned so that they are not too close to the edge of the dish, where manipulation will be difficult. The oocyte droplets should not be too close to the sperm droplet, in order to avoid mixing; use an arrangement that allows quick and easy distinction between sperm and oocyte droplets, with numbers etched on the bottom of

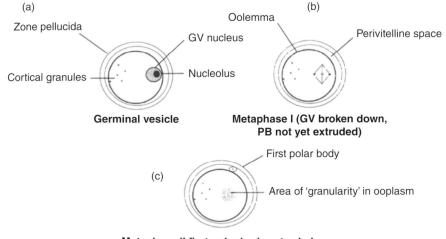

**Figure 13.3** Variations in egg maturity found after hyalase treatment and corona dissection. (a) germinal vesicle; (b) metaphase I; (c) metaphase II.

the dish if desired. Small volumes of media evaporate very quickly, and they should be covered immediately with a layer of oil. Equilibrate the dishes in the incubator for at least 20–30 minutes, and keep them in the incubator until you are ready to begin the procedure. If Falcon 1006 dishes are being used with HEPES-buffered medium, the lids must be tightly fixed if they are to be equilibrated in a $CO_2$ incubator. Dishes with HEPES medium and no lids should be warmed to 37°C without $CO_2$ atmosphere.

2. A prepared pre-equilibrated traditional culture dish should be available, to transfer and further culture the oocytes after injection.

### Micromanipulator

1. Make sure that the microscope heating stage is at a temperature that will maintain droplet temperature in the dishes at 37°C, ensure that all controls are set to neutral and can be comfortably operated and that you are confident that all parts function smoothly before you begin. It is essential to check that you can smoothly carry out very small movements. This involves not only the equipment itself, but its position on the bench in relation to your (comfortable) seating position.

2. Insert holding and injection pipettes into the pipette holders, tighten well and if an oil-filled system is being used, make sure that there are no air bubbles in the tubing system. Bubbles interfere with sensitivity when attempting to control movement with fine precision.

3. Align the pipettes so that the working tips are parallel to the microscope stage. First align the holding pipette under low magnification, then align the injection pipette, again under low magnification. Check the position of both under high magnification. It is important to begin with pipettes in accurate alignment: both working tips must be sharply in focus. If a part of the length is out of focus, the pipette is probably not parallel to the stage, but pointing upwards or downwards.

4. Adjust the injection controls: if using an oil system, the oil should just reach the distal end of the pipette; do not try to fill the needle with oil, as this will work only if you leave a tiny 5-mm gap of air between the oil and the medium. Briefly touch the tips of both pipettes in oil, and then in medium, so that the ends fill by capillary action. Apply positive pressure on the injector to hold the oil bubble at this point – the bubble of oil behind the medium acts as a buffer and should be kept in this area throughout the injection procedure. Moving the bubble further up the needle increases suction power and reduces sensitivity; moving it nearer the tip has the opposite effect and also creates a risk of injecting oil into the oocyte. The injection dish is still in the incubator, so you should be using a 'blank' dish to make these adjustments.

### Transfer of Gametes to the Injection Dish

1. Add a small aliquot of sperm suspension (0.3–0.5 mL, depending on the concentration of prepared sperm) to the edge of the central PVP/HA droplet. The viscous solution should facilitate sperm handling by slowing down their motility and also prevents the sperm cells from sticking to the injection pipette during the procedure. Be careful of sperm density: too many sperm will make selection and immobilization more difficult.

2. After the sperm droplet has been examined for the presence of debris or any other factors that might cause technical difficulties, examine all the denuded oocytes again for the presence of a first polar body; wash them with HEPES-buffered medium and transfer one oocyte into each oocyte droplet on the injection dish, taking care to avoid too much handling or cooling of the oocytes. Keep the oocytes in the incubator until you are confident that the injection procedure can proceed smoothly. Until sufficient experience of the procedure has been gained, it may be advisable to keep sperm and oocyte dishes separate, avoiding overexposure of the oocytes while selecting and immobilizing sperm.

3. Place the injection dish with central sperm droplet on the microscope stage. Using the coarse controls of the manipulator, lower the injection pipette into the drop.

### Sperm Selection and Immobilization

1. Select sperm that appear morphologically normal. Sperm can be selected and stored in the PVP drop for a limited period of time (be aware that prolonged exposure to PVP can cause damage to sperm membranes) before starting the injection procedure; this is an advantage in cases of extreme cryptozoospermia, and reduces oocyte exposure

time. If medium containing HA is being used for immobilization, the sperm become rigid and stick to the dish after approximately 30 minutes.

2. Immobilize motile spermatozoa by crushing their tails: select the sperm to be aspirated, and lower the tip of the injection needle onto the midpiece of the sperm, striking down and across, and crushing the tail against the bottom of the dish. This 'tail crushing' impairs motility and destabilizes the cell membrane; the latter may be required for sperm head decondensation. If the resulting sperm has a 'bent' tail, it will be difficult to aspirate into the needle, and will stick inside it. When this happens, abandon that sperm and repeat the procedure with another sperm. Do not strike too hard, or the sperm will stick to the bottom of the dish, also making aspiration into the needle difficult. After some practice, sperm immobilization in routine ICSI cases can be carried out quite quickly. If the preparation contains only a few sperm with barely recognizable movement and a large amount of debris, this part of the procedure can be very tedious and require great patience!

3. Aspirate the selected immobilized sperm into the injection pipette. Sperm were traditionally aspirated into the pipette tail-first, but they can be aspirated head-first (Woodward *et al.*, 2008a). Position the sperm approximately 20 μm from the tip.

4. Lift the injection needle slightly, and move the microscope stage so that the injection pipette is positioned in the first oocyte drop. If the sperm moves up the pipette (due to the difference in density between culture medium and PVP), bring it back near the tip before beginning the injection procedure.

### Injection Procedure

1. Lower the holding pipette into the first oocyte droplet, and position it adjacent to the cell. Using both microtools, slowly rotate the oocyte to locate the polar body. Aspirate gently so that the cell attaches to the pipette. The pressure should be great enough to hold the oocyte in place, but not so strong that it causes the oolemma to bulge outwards.

2. Positioning the polar body at 6 or 12 o'clock in order to minimize the possibility of damaging the meiotic spindle was thought to be important, but later evidence using polarized microscopy to visualize the spindle itself suggests that polar body positioning is of less benefit than minimizing the duration of the ICSI procedure (Woodward *et al.*, 2008b).

3. Move the injection pipette close to the oocyte, and check that it is in the same plane as the right outer border of the oolemma on the equatorial plane at the 3 o'clock position. Check that the sperm can be moved smoothly within the injection needle, and position it near the beveled tip.

4. Advance the pipette through the zona pellucida until the tip almost touches the oocyte membrane at the 9 o'clock position (Figure 13.4). If the pipette is in the wrong plane, entry into the cell will be difficult. The membrane may rupture spontaneously, or may require negative pressure, sucking the membrane into the pipette before expelling the sperm. When it breaks, there will be a sudden flux of cytoplasm into the pipette. Inject the sperm slowly into the oocyte with a minimal amount of fluid (1–2 picoliters). The sperm should be ejected past the tip of the pipette, to ensure a tight insertion among the organelles, which will hold it in place while the pipette is withdrawn. Some surplus medium may be re-aspirated to reduce the size of the breach created during perforation. If the plasma membrane is elastic and difficult to break, it may be necessary to withdraw the pipette from the first membrane invagination and slowly repeat the procedure. Oocytes do vary in their response to injection, and it is important to remain flexible and adapt technique accordingly.

5. Withdraw the injection pipette, and examine the breach area. The membrane should be funnel-shaped, pointing in toward the center. If the border of the oolemma is everted, cytoplasm may leak out, and the oocyte may subsequently cytolyze. Release the oocyte from the holding pipette.

6. Repeat the sperm aspiration and injection until all the selected metaphase II oocytes have been injected.

7. Wash all the oocytes in culture medium, transfer to the prepared, warmed culture dish and incubate overnight.

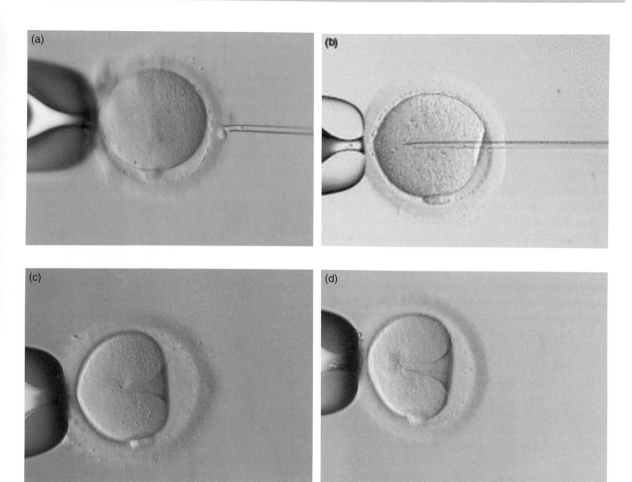

**Figure 13.4** ICSI. (a) Metaphase II oocyte with injection needle in position prior to injection. (b) Injection needle within the cytoplasm, prior to release of sperm. (c) Post-injection illustrating the typical track left following withdrawal of the needle. (d) Post-injection, oocyte with a very elastic membrane. See color plate section. With thanks to Agnese Fiorentino.

## Injection Procedure: Important Points

1. All conditions must be stable: temperature, pH, equipment properly set up, adjusted, aligned, and checked for leaks and air bubbles. Check everything, including secure and comfortable operating position, before you begin.
2. Correct immobilization of sperm.
3. Advance far enough into the ooplasm with the injection pipette.
4. Ensure that the plasma membrane is broken. (Immediate membrane rupture after introducing the injection needle results in a lower probability of fertilization.)
5. Inject a minimal volume.
6. If the sperm comes out of the ooplasm into the perivitelline space, reinject.

## Assessment of Fertilization and Cleavage

Around 16 to 18 hours after injection, assess the number and morphology of pronuclei through an inverted microscope. Polar bodies can also be counted, with reference to digynic zygotes or activated eggs; polar bodies may fragment, even in normal monospermic fertilization. Rapid cleavage (20–26 hours post-injection) can occur in ICSI zygotes (see also 'silent fertilization' in Chapter 5: 'Causes of Early Embryo Arrest').

Evaluate normally fertilized, cleaved embryos after a further 24 (or 48) hours of culture, and continue culture for transfer or freezing at cleavage or blastocyst stage according to laboratory protocols.

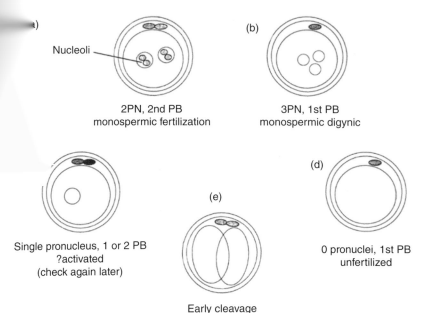

**Figure 13.5** Diagrams showing variations of fertilization after ICSI. (a) two pronuclei, two polar bodies; (b) three pronuclei, one polar body; (c) one pronucleus, two polar bodies; (d) no pronuclei, one polar body; (e) early cleavage. PN = pronuclei; PB = polar body. With thanks to Gianfranco Coppola.

### No Fertilization after ICSI

Complete failure of fertilization is rare after ICSI (reported as 1–3% of cycles), but can occur as a result of sperm defects, oocyte defects or technical problems.

Sperm defects include:

lack of motile sperm

failed sperm head decondensation

premature sperm chromatin condensation

sperm aster defects

round-headed sperm (globozoospermia)

severe oligospermia.

Fertilization rates using epididymal and testicular sperm are generally equivalent to those for ejaculated sperm, but the use of immature sperm cells results in a dramatic decrease in fertilization and pregnancy rates.

Oocyte defects include:

low oocyte numbers

abnormal oocyte morphology

spindle defects

failure of oocyte activation

fragile oocytes which are easily damaged by the trauma of the injection.

Unfertilized oocytes can show abnormal spindle and interphase microtubules, suggesting that deficiencies in ooplasmic and nuclear components may be responsible for failed fertilization.

Failure can also be due to technical problems involving incorrect injection procedure or highly elastic plasma membranes that impede complete rupture of the oocyte membrane, so that the sperm cell fails to be placed into the oocyte cytoplasm. Figure 13.5 shows the variations that can be seen on Day 1 after ICSI.

### Artificial Oocyte Activation (AOA)

As described in Chapter 4, oocyte activation is a crucial initial step in human development, orchestrated by a series of changes in intracellular calcium: activation of calcium-sensitive downstream signal transduction mechanisms initiate early events necessary for fertilization.

In IVF, the initial calcium spike is seen within a few minutes of sperm–oocyte fusion; in ICSI, the trigger is provoked when the oocyte cytoplasm is disrupted during the injection procedure, allowing an influx of calcium from the injection medium. In cases of repeated failed fertilization after ICSI, adding artificial agents (calcium ionophores such as ionomycin or calcimycin, A23187) that increase cell membrane calcium permeability has been proposed as a means of helping oocyte activation by facilitating entry of extracellular calcium into the cell cytoplasm. These agents are commercially available, and reports of their use in IVF/ICSI describe protocols that differ in ionophore concentration used and in timing, duration and number of exposures (Vanden Meerschaut *et al.*, 2014). However, the calcium rises that are artificially induced by these agents are not physiological (Santella and Dale, 2015). Generation of calcium oscillations requires reorganization of many cytoplasmic components, and the link between frequency, number, amplitude and duration of calcium signals and the kinetics of oocyte activation has not been fully elucidated. The possibility remains that imposing artificial conditions may have an effect on gene expression at this crucial stage of early development; potential effects of artificial oocyte activation (AOA) on postimplantation embryo development are unknown, and AOA cannot be considered as an established treatment until there is sufficient scientific evidence about its safety (Van Blerkom *et al.*, 2015; Ebner & Montag, 2016).

### Rescue ICSI

In cases of total failure of fertilization after IVF, 'rescue ICSI' is sometimes attempted as a last resort by injecting the oocytes on Day 1. However, it is now clear that successful embryo development is crucially dependent upon events surrounding the timing of fertilization, as well as on cytoplasmic maturity: extended culture risks numerous negative effects on the oocyte. Although fertilization can sometimes be achieved via 'rescue ICSI,' developmental potential of the embryos is very poor, with minimal chance of pregnancy. (See Beck-Fruchter *et al.*, 2014 for review.)

## Transport ICSI

In the same manner that nearby peripheral hospitals or clinics can use a central IVF laboratory to offer assisted conception treatment, a central ICSI laboratory can offer this specialized technique to peripheral hospitals that do not have the equipment or expertise. Preovulatory oocytes and prepared sperm from patients are transported from the peripheral unit by the male partner immediately after the oocyte recovery procedure. Culture tubes containing the gametes are transported in a portable incubator, as described for transport IVF in Chapter 11. On arrival at the central unit, the oocytes can be transferred to culture dishes and prepared for the ICSI procedure, and sperm preparation assessed and adjusted if necessary. Fertilized oocytes are cultured to the early cleavage or blastocyst stage, and the embryos may then be transported by the male partner back to the peripheral unit for the

embryo transfer procedure. Supernumerary embryos may also be cryopreserved at the central unit if appropriate. As with transport IVF, cooperation between participating units is particularly important in order to provide an effective service. Well-planned protocols are essential for selection, consultation and counseling of patients, the handling, preparation and transport of gametes, and communication of treatment cycle details/transport arrangements between units.

## Assisted Hatching

Jacques Cohen and colleagues postulated in the 1990s that the inability of blastocysts to hatch from the zona pellucida may be one of the factors involved in the high failure rate of human implantation after IVF procedures. The human zona becomes more brittle and loses elasticity after fertilization, and spontaneous hardening also occurs after in-vitro and in-vivo aging. Early observations from video cinematography studies suggested that embryos with a thick, even zona pellucida on Day 2 had a poor prognosis for implantation (see Chapter 11). In addition, embryos produced as a result of microsurgical fertilization had a higher implantation rate, and hatched 1 day earlier than expected (Day 5 instead of Day 6) after in-vitro culture. Original trials on assisted hatching were performed on Day 2 embryos, but studies by Dale and colleagues in Naples (Dale *et al.*, 1991; Gualtieri *et al.*, 1992) on the formation of intercellular junctions and, in particular tight junctions and desmosomes, indicated that Day 3 was a more suitable time for assisted hatching. Following these observations, a series of experiments in a mouse embryo system led to the development of a clinical protocol, with the following notable features:

1. Large holes are more efficient in supporting hatching than small holes: if the hole is too small, the embryo can become 'trapped' and fail to hatch. Zona drilling using an acid Tyrode's (AT) solution prevented 'trapping,' which occurred as a result of mechanical partial zona drilling: optimal hole size is approximately half the size of a single blastomere, 15–20 μm.

2. Embryos with these large gaps in their zonae should be transferred after the onset of compaction, on Day 3: if embryo transfer is traumatic, blastomeres may escape through the gap in the zona. Embryo transfer must therefore be gentle and atraumatic.

3. Embryos can be preselected for assisted hatching, based upon previous IVF history (repeated failed implantation), maternal age, basal FSH levels, cleavage rates and morphology of the embryos with attention to zona thickness or variation.

Breaching of the zona can be achieved by mechanical dissection, drilling with an acidic Tyrode's solution or with the use of a noncontact laser (Figure 13.6). Procedures, protocols and benefits of assisted hatching have continued to be a subject of discussion, controversy and debate since its first application in ART, more than 25 years ago. A vast number of papers and reviews have been published reporting different methods, timing, developmental stages and outcomes in different groups of patients. A recent systematic review summarizing published reports suggests that the use of laser to breach the zona is superior to mechanical or chemical methods, and reports that assisted hatching after thawing frozen/vitrified blastocysts appears to be consistently beneficial (Alteri *et al.*, 2018).

## Laser-Assisted Hatching

A few milliseconds of laser irradiation can instantly create an opening (a channel) in the zona pellucida with longitudinal apertures ranging from 3 to 25 µm. The procedure has been shown to be safe, simple and rapid. Equipment designed for the routine use of noncontact laser in ART is available from a number of different companies; manufacturer's instructions for recommended settings and set up should be followed precisely for each.

1. Depending on the application, the procedure is carried out on an embryo resting on the bottom of a culture drop, or securely held on a micromanipulator holding pipette. A pilot laser spot, target or crosshairs can typically be seen on the monitor screen to facilitate aiming.

2. Select an area in the embryo where blastomeres are furthest away from the inner edge of the zona, and fire the laser at this target; a small hole in the zona should appear.

3. Moving from the inner to the external surface of the zona, continue ablating until the zona is breached; an influx of medium may be seen. If ablation is insufficient, increase the laser pulse-width by changing the pre-set power.

4. Continue the process for all embryos to be hatched, and return the culture dish to the incubator.

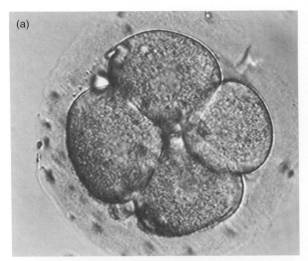

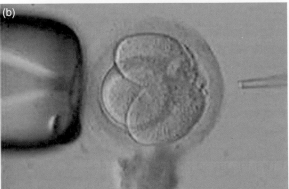

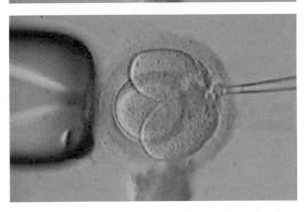

**Figure 13.6** Assisted hatching. (a) Laser-hatched four-cell embryo (see color plate section). (b) Assisted hatching with acid Tyrode's.

## Acid Tyrode's Protocol

The protocol below for assisted hatching by acid drilling of the zona pellucida is adapted from J. Cohen (2007). Tyrode's solution is acidified by titrating to pH 2.3–2.5 with HCl or can be purchased from media manufacturers.

1. Perform zona drilling with AT solution approximately 72 hours after oocyte retrieval, with embryo transfer 5–7 hours later (i.e., drill before the formation of intercellular connections, but transfer after they have been established).
2. Perform the procedure in HEPES-buffered medium.
3. Use a straight microtool with an aperture of 10–12 µm. Load the tool with AT prior to the hatching procedure.
4. Embryos are held in small microdroplets (25 µL) under mineral oil in a depression slide or shallow Falcon 1006 dish containing at least four wash droplets.
5. Hatch each embryo individually and immediately wash three to four times to remove the acidic medium.

## Assisted Hatching with Acid Tyrode's, Step by Step

The key to successful assisted hatching is to produce a gap in the zona without exposing the embryo to excessive acidified solution. Aspirating AT solution through a needle of very small diameter leaves considerable negative pressure within the needle after it is removed from the AT droplet, and this will result in culture medium being aspirated as soon as the needle enters the embryo culture droplet. This will dilute the AT solution, making it ineffective for dissolving the zona pellucida. In order to avoid this technical problem, the system should be prepared well in advance, so that the hatching needle will be precisely in the correct position relative to the embryo as soon as it is lowered into the droplet of medium. Applying slight positive pressure as soon as the needle breaks the surface of the drop will also help to counteract the residual suction.

1. Front load the microneedle with AT solution before each hatching event; the meniscus of the acidic fluid is difficult to control, and therefore precisely controlled suction is important.
2. Pre-align the embryo onto the holding pipette (syringe suction system) so that the AT-filled microneedle at the 3 o'clock area is exposed to empty perivitelline space or to extracellular fragments.
3. When the embryo is in position on the holding pipette, lower the AT-filled needle into the medium and bring it next to the target area as quickly as possible. In order to avoid diluting the AT solution with medium of normal pH, there

should be no more than a 2-second delay before the hatching begins: releasing fluid that is not sufficiently acidic will damage the embryo, without affecting the zona pellucida.
4. Expel acidic medium gently over a small (30 µm) area by holding the needle tip very close to the zona; using small circular motions can avoid excess acid in a single area.
5. If thinning is not immediately obvious, stop the procedure immediately: the total time required to breach the zona should not exceed a couple of seconds; most zona will yield within less than 5 seconds.
6. The inside of the zonae is more difficult to pierce, and the expulsion pressure may need to be increased. The optical system should be optimized for this part of the procedure, as the stream of acid will be relatively invisible, and the piercing of the inside of the zona may be almost imperceptible. Zona breakthrough should cover an area of at least 20 µm, and not a single small point.
7. As soon as the zona is breached, reverse the flow through the assisted hatching needle immediately. All of the expelled acid solution must be aspirated, paying particular attention to any solution that might have entered the PVS. Move the embryo to another area of the droplet, away from excess AT.
8. A small 'inside' hole may be widened mechanically by moving the microneedle through the opening in a tearing motion while continuing gentle suction.
9. Transfer the embryo through the wash droplets and return to culture for incubation prior to embryo transfer.

# Biopsy Procedures

The next chapter will discuss the genetic and chromosomal analysis of cells biopsied from oocytes (the polar body), cleavage stage embryos and blastocysts. The standard equipment used for embryo biopsy is a slightly modified ICSI apparatus, with specific microtools. Biopsy is carried out in two stages: the zona pellucida must be breached, and then cells are aspirated or otherwise removed from the embryo. Some of the procedures described below have now been replaced with zona breach followed by biopsy of trophectoderm (TE) cells at the blastocyst stage ('PGS v.2') and are included here for historical reference.

**Typical Clinical Protocol for Cleavage Stage Embryo Biopsy for PGS**

### Day 1 (1 Day after Oocyte Collection)

1. Set up culture dishes (one for each normally fertilized embryo): Label a four-well dish (Nunclon) with the patient's name and embryo number on the base of the dish and on the front panel. Put 0.5 mL of cleavage stage or blastocyst culture medium in each well and cover with a monolayer of washed oil. Place the dishes in the incubator to equilibrate overnight.

### Day 2 (2 Days after Oocyte Collection)

2. After scoring the embryos, transfer each embryo into blastocyst culture medium in well 1 of the appropriately labeled four-well dish, wash and transfer to well 2 and transfer to the incubator for overnight culture. The timing of the switch between cleavage stage and blastocyst culture media may differ depending on the medium used.

3. In the warming oven, place 10 mL of HEPES-buffered biopsy medium ($Ca^{2+}/Mg^{2+}$-free) and Falcon dishes (1006) for the biopsy. In the incubator, place enough washed oil for the biopsy procedure (allow 4 mL per embryo).

### Day 3 (Day of Embryo Biopsy)

4. Half an hour before the biopsy:

    (a) Set up a biopsy dish (1006 Falcon) for each embryo and label it with the patient's name and embryo number. Take a Gilson pipette set at 10 µl and a sterile yellow tip and flush the tip (×10) with the HEPES-buffered biopsy medium. Pipette three drops of HEPES-buffered biopsy medium and one drop of AT as shown in Figure 13.8; it is important that the dish is oriented as shown in relation to the 'bumps' on the outside of the dish. Immediately cover the dish with 4 mL of washed and pre-equilibrated oil to avoid evaporation and put the prepared dishes in the warming oven until required.

    (b) Set up a four-well dish for transferring the embryos into biopsy medium with 0.5 ml of HEPES-buffered biopsy medium in each of the wells, cover with oil and place in the warming oven.

5. About 15 minutes before each biopsy, take the appropriately labeled biopsy dish and the four-well transfer dish from the warming oven and carefully wash successive embryos through each well of HEPES-buffered medium, transferring

minimal medium between wells. Leave the embryo in each well for at least 1 minute: it is essential to completely remove the divalent cations from the culture medium to promote the reversal of any compaction. Place the embryo into the middle of the three droplets in the biopsy dish (the two other droplets are spare in case of difficulties during biopsy).

6. Biopsy cells.

7. At the end of the biopsy procedure, transfer the embryo into well 3 of the four-well culture dish – this is a washing stage to remove the HEPES-buffered biopsy medium. Finally, transfer the embryo with minimal medium to well 4 and return to culture.

8. Return the biopsy dish with the isolated blastomeres to the flow hood for sample preparation.

9. Repeat until all of the embryos have been biopsied.

10. When the PGD analysis result is available, assess the morphology of each embryo and count the number of cells as accurately as possible to get an indication of division post biopsy.

11. In consultation with the other members of the PGD team and finally with the couple themselves, select a maximum of two genetically unaffected embryos with the best morphology for transfer.

# Cleavage Stage Biopsy Techniques

The optimal time for cleavage stage embryo biopsy is before strong intercellular junctions are formed, which is usually Day 3. Biopsy is extremely difficult with compacted embryos, and cleavage stage embryos should be transferred to Ca/Mg-free media to facilitate the biopsy procedure. To avoid contamination with extracellular sperm that could be attached to the zona, oocytes should be fertilized using ICSI. A hole in the zona can be created using a laser, mechanically (as in PZD), or by drilling with AT solution. If using AT drilling, a pipette of 8–10 µL containing AT is placed adjacent to the zona pellucida and solution expelled from the pipette until the zona thins and eventually breaches. To biopsy, a second micropipette (fire-polished with an inner diameter of 30–40 µm) is used to aspirate a blastomere. The pipette is pushed through the breach in the zona, and the cell is drawn up into the pipette by gentle aspiration. When the cell is clearly free from the embryo, the pipette is moved sideways and the cell expelled. If the cell lyses, another cell should be aspirated.

### Aspiration (Figure 13.7a)

The embryo is held in place with a holding pipette mounted on the micromanipulator. After opening a limited spot on the surface of the zona, an aspiration micropipette is used to remove a blastomere by suction.

### Extrusion

#### (a) Stitch and Pull (Figure 13.7b)

This method involves initial zona drilling with either a laser or AT to create a hole. A stitching movement

with the microneedle is used to displace and remove a blastomere which is then pushed out of the incision by pushing the zona with a microneedle at a distance from the hole.

#### (b) Displacement (Figure 13.7c)

A beveled pipette is used to make the first incision in the zona. A second incision is then made through which one blastomere is displaced by applying a gentle flow of medium, causing the blastomere to emerge from the first incision site.

## Polar Body Biopsy

If a woman is a carrier for a genetic disease, her oocytes contain either the abnormal or the normal

(a)

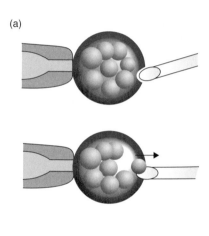

(c)

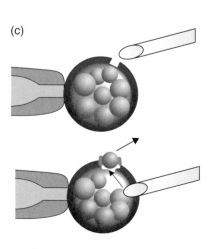

(b)

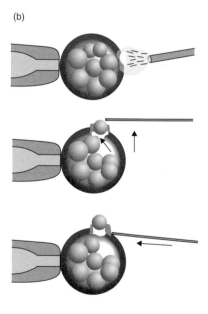

**Figure 13.7** Cleavage stage biopsy techniques: (a) aspiration; (b) stitch and pull; (c) displacement.

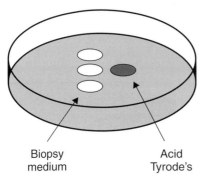

Biopsy
medium

Acid
Tyrode's

**Figure 13.8** Biopsy dish for PGD.

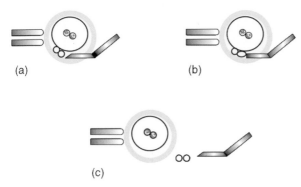

(a)

(b)

(c)

**Figure 13.9** Polar body biopsy. (a) Position the polar bodies at 5–6 o'clock position, and penetrate the zona with the biopsy pipette. (b) Gently aspirate the polar bodies from under the zona pellucida. (c) Expel the polar bodies into the medium and remove the biopsied zygote from the biopsy medium.

gene for that particular genetic disorder; analysis of the status of the gene from the polar body (PB) will indirectly determine which gene is present in the oocyte. However, for analysis of single-gene and chromosomal defects, recombination events during meiosis I require biopsy and analysis of the second polar body to confirm which allele is present in the zygote. Both polar bodies can be removed together 6–14 hours after fertilization (Figure 13.9), or PB1 can be removed soon after oocyte retrieval, and PB2 6–10 hours post-fertilization.

### Method

1. Immobilize the oocyte using a holding pipette.
2. Create a breach in the zona by mechanical, chemical or laser dissection.
3. Insert a beveled micropipette (12–15 μm in diameter) through the zona to the perivitelline space.

4. Aspirate the polar body into the pipette as it detaches from the ooplasm.

The two polar bodies are distinguished by morphology, the first having a crinkly appearance and the second being smooth, possibly with a visible interphase nucleus under interference contrast.

## Blastocyst Stage Biopsy

In recent years, many IVF centers have gradually introduced blastocyst stage biopsies into their clinical practice. Biopsy of the blastocyst TE provides a higher number of biopsied cells for molecular analysis, which increases the sensitivity and reliability of genetic analysis and increases the possibility of detecting embryo mosaicism. Embryo viability is compromised to a lesser extent than after cleavage stage biopsy, partly due to the fact that a smaller fraction of the total number of cells present in the embryo is removed. This technique requires a culture system that can reliably support blastocyst development as well as a robust program of blastocyst cryopreservation, since the time needed for genetic analysis results typically does not allow a fresh embryo transfer.

Trophectoderm biopsy of blastocysts should not affect the inner cell mass (ICM) from which the fetus later develops. However, TE cells may have diverged genetically from the ICM, as confined placental mosaicism has been observed in at least 1% of conceptions: the chromosomal status of the embryo differs from that of the placenta. Also, some studies have indicated that blastocysts may have increased levels of chromosomal mosaicism. Preferential allocation of abnormal cells to the TE could be a mechanism of early development; in that case the TE may not always be representative of the rest of the embryo, which could complicate and compromise PGS.

A biopsy technique based on the excision of TE cells from a blastocyst was first reported in 1990 (Dokras *et al.*, 1990). Blastocyst biopsy may be performed using stitch and pull, aspiration and herniation techniques; the latter technique is currently used most frequently. Emerging cells can be removed by cutting with a glass needle or scalpel blade; however, the advent of laser systems has greatly simplified excision of the biopsy sample (Veiga *et al.*, 1997).

The herniation technique for blastocyst biopsy involves creating a hole in the cleavage stage zona on day 3. Embryos are then returned to culture until Day 5 or 6, when some TE cells begin to herniate through the opening as the process of hatching is initiated. Trophectoderm biopsy can proceed once hatching begins. There is a chance that the ICM may herniate instead of the TE; in this case, a second zona breach at a different site can be created at the time of biopsy to avoid ICM disruption. Alternatively, zona drilling can be delayed until the expanded blastocyst stage, rather than on Day 3.

For laser-assisted blastocyst biopsy, a holding tool is mounted on the left and a biopsy tool of 20- or 30-μm inner diameter is mounted on the right, and both are primed similar to an ICSI setup. After setting up these tools, a blastocyst is loaded into a biopsy dish and examined under the inverted scope to clearly identify the ICM. The blastocyst is oriented so that it can be held firmly by the holding tool with the herniating TE cells facing toward the biopsy tool, and on the same focal plane as the holding tool. TE cells are then aspirated by gentle suction on the biopsy tool and pulled away from the rest of the embryo. Strategically placed laser pulses, resulting in 4 to 8 cells for the biopsy sample, are applied to the connecting TE cell 'bridge' until the sample cells can be pulled away and are fully detached, then expelled in another part of the biopsy drop.

Technical complications experienced during laser excision of TE cells can vary from one blastocyst to another. Occasionally, laser ablation to separate the selected cells from the blastocyst may be ineffective even after 4 or 5 laser pulses. The 'flicking' method can be very effective in this circumstance. The biopsy proceeds as previously described, but after laser ablation of the connecting cells, the blastocyst is released from the holding tool while maintaining gentle suction on the biopsy tool. The holding and biopsy tools should immediately be placed in parallel, overlapping each other on the same focal plane, and TE cells are detached by a quick 'flicking' movement of the biopsy tool against the holding tool. This technique can work particularly well with fully hatched blastocysts that are otherwise very difficult to biopsy.

## Aspiration (Figure 13.10a)

A number of cells are sucked from the mural TE cell layer opposite to the inner cell mass, through the aspiration micropipette. The microneedle is also used

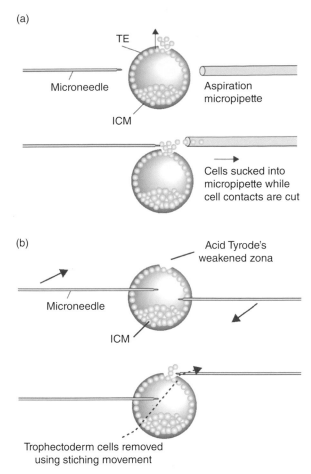

**Figure 13.10** Blastocyst biopsy techniques: (a) aspiration; (b) stitch and pull. TE = trophectoderm; ICM = inner cell mass.

to break cell–cell contacts as the TE cells herniate through the hole.

## Extrusion Technique (Figure 13.10b)

Partially dissolve a section of the zona with AT solution or with a laser, and use two siliconized glass microneedles to extrude mural TE cells with a stitch and pull motion through the zona.

# Appendix
## Equipment for ICSI

### For Microinjection

Dissecting microscope with heated stage

Inverted microscope with heated stage, attached to micromanipulators

×4 objective for locating oocytes and drops

×20 or ×40 objective for microsurgery

×15 eyepiece

Hoffman modulation contrast optics

Video monitoring facility

Bilateral micromanipulators for manipulation in three dimensions

Microtool holders

Two suction devices with steel syringes (80–100 mL) filled with light mineral oil (BDH), or appropriate alternative device for controlling holding and injection micropipettes

Incubator

Supply of 5% $CO_2$ in air

## Supplies

Shallow Falcon Petri dishes (Type 1006) Culture medium

Culture medium + HEPES

Human serum albumin (HSA)

Hyaluronidase solution

Mineral oil

PVP solution

Pasteur pipettes

Hand-pulled polished glass pipettes

Pipette bulbs

Holding pipettes

ICSI needles

## Adjustment of Manipulators for ICSI (with Thanks to Terry Leonard)

This guide refers to the Nikon/Narishige system; the same principles apply to an Olympus system, but the details are slightly different. Before attempting to fit or adjust the micromanipulators, first adjust the microscope optically, ideally using an oocyte in the same type of Petri dish to be used for ICSI. The microscope settings will influence the working distance of the microtools. The final position of the micromanipulators on the microscope will depend upon:

(a) the angle at which the tool holder is fixed

(b) the combined length of the tool holder and needle from the point where it is held in the tool holder attachment to the center of the light source.

Before finding the ideal position for the micromanipulators, they should be fitted correctly to the microscope and final adjustments made later.

## Micromanipulator Parts

1. Mounting bar: this joins the coarse manipulator to the microscope.
2. Coarse manipulator: consists of three parts, each controlling one of the three dimensions of movement. There are two types: manually operated and motor driven.
3. Fine manipulator: consists of two parts:
   (a) the driving section: attached to the coarse manipulator, controls fine movements directed by joystick.
   (b) ball joint/tool holder attachment: attached to the driving section, used both to hold the microtool holder and to vary the angle at which it is held.
4. Joystick: links to the driving section via oil-filled tubes. The movement of the joystick is scaled down and transferred to the fine manipulator.

The mounting arrangement which attaches the coarse manipulator to the microscope is L-shaped. In the Nikon/Narishige system, the mounting is fitted to the illumination pillar.

- The mounting bar position is marked with a white L-shape.
- The mounting bars have tracks into which the coarse manipulator fits, and the position of the coarse manipulator can be adjusted along these tracks. The entire mounting bar can be adjusted up and down.

## Adjusting the Coarse Manipulators

1. Set the mounting bars at 90 degrees from the microscope stage or bench top.
2. Set the second part of the mounting at 90 degrees to the first, and ensure that the track is set flat.
3. Attach the coarse micromanipulator and adjust the lower section (left/right movement) so that it is parallel with the mounting bar. Set the other two sections of the coarse manipulator at right angles to each other.

## Attaching the Fine Manipulator

The fine manipulator is attached to the coarse manipulator by a small metal rod (coupling bar). This can be screwed into one of the two holes on the driving section of the fine manipulator, depending on the side on which it is to be used. In order to fit the fine manipulator on the right-hand side, find the 'R' mark on the driving section and screw the coupling bar into the hole directly behind this mark. Attach the coupling bar/driving section to the coarse manipulator and tighten. Position the driving section so that it is parallel with the microscope or 90 degrees to the bench. Attach the left-hand side in the same manner, screwing the coupling bar into the hole directly behind the 'L' mark. Arrange the joysticks so that the 'R' and 'L' marks are facing the operator on the appropriate sides.

## Attaching the Ball Joint/Tool Holder Attachment

The ball joint/tool holder attachment has a black metal bar projecting from it. This is fitted into the V-groove of the driving unit. The ball joint is then rotated to an appropriate angle so that when a needle is held in it, the tip of the microtool will be parallel with the microscope stage. The extent to which it is rotated will depend upon the angle at which the microtool is bent. For example, for a microtool which is angled at 35 degrees from the plane of the needle, the ball joint must be rotated 35 degrees anticlockwise from the vertical position.

The manipulators should now be attached in the correct manner, but they may not be in the optimal working position. The ideal position will vary depending upon the angle of the needle and the combined length of the microtool and tool holder. It is therefore best to have a fixed tool angle, a fixed length of projection of the tool from the tool holder and a fixed (marked) point where the tool holder is clamped to the tool holding attachment. If any of these three factors change, the fine adjustments will require resetting.

## Finding the Best Position for the Micromanipulators

- Adjust the three coarse manipulators so that they are in the middle of their range of movements.
- Adjust the range of movements of the three fine manipulators on the joystick so that they are in the middle of the scales.

## Forward/Backward Movement

First ensure that the hole in the stage is positioned directly in the middle of the light path. View the micromanipulator from the side of the microscope, then align the tool holder attachment with the middle of the hole in the microscope stage. This can be adjusted by changing the position of the coupling bar on the fine manipulator, the projection from the ball joint or the two screws on the very top of the coarse manipulator, which controls the forward/backward movement.

## Left/Right Movement

Place a microtool holder together with a microtool in the tool holder attachment. Attach it at the very tip of the tool holder, and gently slide it along toward the light source. If it will not reach the light source, the entire manipulator should be moved to the left. Likewise, if it reaches it too soon (before the marked point), the entire manipulator should be shifted to the right. This adjustment is performed by loosening the bolts that attach the coarse micromanipulator to the mounting bar. After this adjustment, ensure that the micromanipulator is still parallel to the bar.

## Up/Down Movement

Adjust the manipulator so that the microtool is approximately 0.5 cm from the surface of the stage. For large adjustments, loosen the bolts that attach the mounting bar to the microscope and move up or down. Remember to ensure that it is still 90 degrees from the bench after adjustment. Fine up/down adjustments can be made by moving the small sliding section above the ball joint.

## Alignment of the ICSI Needle in the Manipulator

When using a Narishige tool holder, push the needle in so that 4–5 cm of the needle is outside the holder. Place the tool holder in the right-hand micromanipulator with the needle tip over the light source. The angle at which the tool holder is held should be such that the angled tip of the needle is parallel with the stage of the microscope. Under a very low power ($\times 4$ objective), place the tip of the ICSI needle in the field of vision of the microscope. Loosen the tool holder attachment and rotate the tool holder so that the bent portion of the needle appears to be straight. Ensure that you can focus on a good portion of the needle (from the tip). The portion of the needle after the bend will be out of focus. If the microscope has a graticule, make sure that the movement of the needle from right to left does not vary. Place the ICSI needle along the middle of the microscope field with the tip almost in the center. Align the holding pipette in the same manner so that the tips of the needle and pipette are facing each other, and then raise them up away from the stage.

Perform the final adjustment of the angle at which the tool holder is held within a sperm droplet. Find a nonmotile sperm, and then bring the ICSI needle into the same optical plane. Raise the ICSI needle off the surface of the Petri dish very slightly, move it over the top of the sperm, and try to touch the sperm by lowering the needle. If it is impossible to touch the sperm, the needle is not parallel with the surface. The end of the needle will be lower than the tip. To rectify this, raise the needle and rotate the ball point anticlockwise slightly, lower the needle, and try to touch the sperm again. If the tip of the needle can touch the sperm, but the rest of the needle is not in focus, the tip of the needle is lower than the bend. To rectify this, raise the needle and rotate the ball joint slightly in a clockwise direction.

### Ratio of Movement and Joysticks

1. Focus on the tip of the microtool.
2. Loosen the two screws on the movement adjustment rings.
3. Ignore the ratios written on the side of the joystick, and rotate the adjustment rings anticlockwise until you are satisfied with the movement as observed down the microscope.

When all of the adjustments and alignments are made, the need to repeat any of these should be minimal, unless the style of the needle or tool holder is changed. When removing the tool holder from its attachment, keep the ball joint at the same angle so that when a new needle is inserted, it will be at approximately the right angle for use. Fine adjustments will be necessary for each manipulation.

## Further Reading

### Books and Reviews

Alteri A, Vigano P, Maizar AA, Jovine L, Giacomini E, Rubino P (2018) Revisiting embryo assisted hatching approaches: a systematic review of the current protocols. *Journal of Assisted Reproduction and Genetics* 35(3): 367–391.

Beck-Fruchter R, Lavee M, Weiss A, Geslevich Y, Shalev E (2014) Rescue intracytoplasmic sperm injection: a systematic review. *Fertility and Sterility* 101(3): 690–698.

Beck-Fruchter R, Shalev E, Weiss A (2016) Clinical benefit using sperm hyaluronic acid binding technique in ICSI cycles: a review and meta-analysis. *Reproductive BioMedicine Online* 32: 286–298.

Devroey P, Van Steirteghem A (2004) A review of ten years' experience of ICSI. *Human Reproduction Update* 10(1): 19–28.

Elder K, Van den Bergh M, Woodward B (2015) *Troubleshooting and Problem-Solving in IVF.* Cambridge University Press, Cambridge, UK.

European Society of Human Reproduction and Embryology (ESHRE) (2015) Revised guidelines for good practice in IVF laboratories. Available online at: www.eshre.eu/Guidelines-and-Legal/

Montag M (ed.) (2014) *A Practical Guide to Selecting Gametes and Embryos.* Taylor & Francis Group, Boca Raton, FL

Montag M, Morbeck D (eds.) (2017) *Principles of IVF Laboratory Practice: Optimizing Performance and outcomes.* Cambridge University Press, Cambridge, UK.

Nagy ZP, Varghese AC, Agarwal A (2019) *Practical Manual of In Vitro Fertilization: Advanced Methods and Novel Devices,* 2nd edition. Springer Science & Business Media, New York.

Practice Committee of the American Society for Reproductive Medicine (2014) Role of assisted hatching in in vitro fertilization: a guideline. *Fertility and Sterility* 102(2): 348–351.

Setti AS, Ferreira Braga AP, Iaconelli A, Aoki T, Borges E (2013) Twelve years of MSOME and IMSI: a review. *Reproductive BioMedicine Online* 27: 338–352.

Simopoulou M, Giannelou P, Bakas P, *et al.* (2016) Making ICSI safer and more effective: a review of the human oocyte and ICSI practice. *In Vivo* 30: 387–400.

Simopoulou M, Gkoles L, Bakas P, *et al.* (2016) Improving ICSI: a review from the spermatozoon perspective. *Systems Biology in Reproductive Medicine* 62(6): 359–371.

van Rumste M, Evers JLH, Farquhar C (2004) Intracytoplasmic sperm injection versus conventional techniques for oocyte insemination during in vitro fertilisation in patients with non-male subfertility: A Cochrane Review. *Human Reproduction* 19(2): 223–227.

Yanagimachi R (2005) Intracytoplasmic injection of spermatozoa and spermatogenic cells: its biology and applications in humans and animals. *Reproductive Biomedicine Online* 10(2): 247–288.

### Publications

Antinori M, Licata E, Dani G, *et al.* (2008) Intracytoplasmic morphologically selected sperm injection: a prospective randomized trial. *Reproductive Biomedicine Online* 16(6): 835–841.

Antinori S, Versaci C, Dani G, *et al.* (1997) Successful fertilization and pregnancy after injection of frozen-thawed round spermatids into human oocytes. *Human Reproduction* 12: 554–556.

Barak Y, Ménézo Y, Veiga A, Elder K (2001) A physiological replacement for polyvinylpyrrolidone (PVP) in assisted reproductive technology. *Human Fertility* 4: 99–103.

Bartoov B, Berkovitz A, Eltes F, *et al.* (2003) Pregnancy rates are higher with intracytoplasmic morphologically selected sperm injection than with conventional intracytoplasmic injection. *Fertility and Sterility* 80(6): 1413–1419.

Belva F, Bonduelle M, Roelants M, *et al.* (2016) Semen quality of young adult ICSI offspring: the first results. *Human Reproduction* 31(12): 2811–2820.

Bonduelle M, Aytoz A, Wilikens A, *et al.* (1998) Prospective follow-up study of 1,987 children born after intracytoplasmic sperm injection (ICSI). In: Filicori M, Flamigni C (eds.) *Treatment of Infertility: The New Frontiers.* Communication Media for Education, Princeton Junction, NJ, pp. 445–461.

Bonduelle M, De Schrijver F, Haentjens P, Devroey P, Tournaye H (2008) Neonatal data on 530 children born after ICSI using testicular spermatozoa. Abstracts of the 24th Annual Meeting of the ESHRE, 6–8 July, 2008, Barcelona, Spain.

Bowen JR, Gibson FL, Leslie GI, Saunders DM (1998) Medical and developmental outcome at 1 year for children conceived by intracytoplasmic sperm injection. *Lancet* 351: 1553–1562.

Burmeister L, Palermo GD, Rosenwaks Z (2001) IVF: the new era. *International Journal of Fertility and Women's Medicine* 46(3): 137–144.

Chatzimeletiou K, Morrison EE, Panagiotidis Y, *et al.* (2005) Comparison of effects of zona drilling by non-contact infrared laser or acid Tyrode's on the development of human biopsied embryos as revealed by blastomere viability, cytoskeletal analysis and molecular cytogenetics. *Reproductive BioMedicine Online* 11(6): 697–710.

Cohen J (1991) Assisted hatching of human embryos. *Journal of In Vitro Fertilization and Embryo Transfer* 8(4): 179–189.

Cohen J (2007) Manipulating embryo development. In: Elder K, Cohen J (eds.) *Preimplantation Embryo Evaluation and Selection.* Informa Press, London, pp. 135–144.

Cohen J, Alikani M, Trowbridge J, Rosenwaks Z (1992) Implantation enhancement by selective assisted hatching using zona drilling of embryos with poor prognosis. *Human Reproduction* 7: 685–691.

Cohen J, Malter H, Fehilly C, *et al.* (1988) Implantation of embryos after partial opening of oocyte zona pellucida to facilitate sperm penetration. *Lancet* 2: 162.

Combelles CM (2008) What are the trade-offs between one-cell and two-cell biopsies of preimplantation embryos. *Human Reproduction* 23(3): 493–498.

Coppola G, Di Caprio G, Wilding M, et al. (2013) Digital holographic microscopy for the evaluation of human sperm structure. *Zygote* 7: 1–8.

Coppola G, Ferrara M, Di Caprio G, Coppola G, Dale B (2017) Unlabeled semen analysis by means of the holographic imaging. In: Naydenova I, Nazarova D, Babeva T (eds.) *Holographic Materials and Optical Systems.* InTech Open, London, Chapter 15. DOI: 10.5772/67552 IMTECH.

Cummins JM, Jequier AM (1995) Concerns and recommendations for Intracytoplasmic sperm injection (ICSI) treatment. *Human Reproduction* 10(Suppl.1): 138–143.

Dale B, Gualtieri R, Talevi R, *et al.* (1991) Intercellular communication in the early human embryo. *Molecular Reproduction and Development* 29: 22–28.

DeFelici M, Siracusa G (1982) "Spontaneous" hardening of the zona pellucida of mouse oocytes during in vitro culture. *Gamete Research* 6: 107–112.

de Vos A, Van Steirteghem A (2001) Aspects of biopsy procedures prior to preimplantation genetic diagnosis. *Prenatal Diagnosis* 21(9): 767–780.

Di Caprio G, El Mallahi A, Ferraro P, *et al.* (2014) 4D tracking of clinical seminal samples for quantitative characterization of motility parameters. *Biomedical Optics Express* 5(3): 690–700.

Dokras A, Sargent IL, Ross C, *et al.* (1990) Trophectoderm biopsy in human blastocysts. *Human Reproduction* 5: 821–825.

Dyer S, Chambers GM, de Mouzon J, *et al.* (2016) International Committee for Monitoring Assisted Reproductive Technologies world report: Assisted Reproductive Technology 2008, 2009 and 2010. *Human Reproduction* 31(7): 1588–1609.

Ebner T, Montag M (2016) Artificial oocyte activation: evidence for clinical readiness. *Reproductive BioMedicine Online* 32: 271–273.

Ferrara M, DeAngelis A, DeLuca A, Coppola GF, Dale B, Coppola G (2015) Simultaneous holographic microscopy and Raman spectroscopy monitoring of human spermatozoa photodegradation. *IEEE Journal of Selected Topics in Quantum Electronics.* DOI: http://10.1109/JSTQE.2015.2496265.

Ferraretti AP, Nygren K, Nyboe Andersen A, *et al.* (2017) Trends in ART in Europe: an analysis of 6 million cycles. *Human Reproduction Open* 2, ESHRE pages.

Fleming SD, Ilad RS, Griffin A-M G, *et al.* (2008) Prospective controlled trial of an electrophoretic method of sperm preparation for assisted reproduction: comparison with density gradient centrifugation. *Human Reproduction* 23(12): 2646–2651.

Germond M, Nocera D, Senn A, *et al.* (1995) Microdissection of mouse and human zona pellucida using a 1.48 m diode laser beam: efficiency and safety of the procedure. *Fertility and Sterility* 25: 604–611.

Gianaroli L, Magli MC, Collodel G, *et al.* (2008) Sperm head's birefringence: a new criterion for sperm selection. *Fertility and Sterility* 90(1): 104–112.

Gianaroli L, Magli MC, Selman HA, *et al.* (1999) Diagnostic testicular biopsy and cryopreservation of testicular tissue as an alternative to repeated surgical openings in the treatment of azoospermic men. *Human Reproduction* 14: 1034–1038.

Gossens V, De Rycke M, De Vos A, *et al.* (2008) Diagnostic efficiency, embryonic development and clinical outcome after the biopsy of one or two blastomeres for preimplantation genetic diagnosis. *Human Reproduction* 23(3): 481–492.

Gualtieri R, Santella L, Dale B (1992) Tight junctions and cavitation in the human pre-embryo. *Molecular Reproduction and Development* 32: 81–87.

Hamberger L, Sjögren A, Lundin K (1995) Microfertilization techniques: choice of correct indications. In: Hedon B, Bringer J, Mares P (eds.) *Fertility and Sterility: A Current Overview*. IFFS-95. Parthenon Publishing Group, New York, pp. 405–408.

Hardy K, Wright C, Rice S, *et al.* (2000) Future developments in assisted reproduction in humans. *Reproduction* 123(2): 171–183.

Harper J (ed.) (2009) *Preimplantation Genetic Diagnosis*, 2nd edn. Cambridge University Press, Cambridge, UK.

Hiramoto Y (1962) Microinjection of the live spermatozoa into sea urchin eggs. *Experimental Cell Research* 27: 416–426.

Hirsh AV (1999) The investigation and therapeutic options for infertile men presenting in assisted conception units. In: Brinsden PR (ed.) *A Textbook of In Vitro Fertilization and Assisted Reproduction*, 2nd edn. Parthenon Publishing Group, London, pp. 27–52.

Huszar G, Jakab A, Sakkas D, *et al.* (2007) Fertility testing and ICSI sperm selection by hyaluronic acid binding: clinical and genetic aspects. *Reproductive BioMedicine Online* 14(5): 650–663.

Jequier AM (1986) *Infertility in the Male: Current Reviews in Obstetrics and Gynaecology*. Churchill Livingstone, Edinburgh.

Kent-First M, Kol S, Muallem A (1996) Infertility in intracytoplasmic sperm injection derived sons. *Lancet* 348: 332.

Kim ED, Bischoff FZ, Lipshultz LI, Lamb DJ (1998) Genetic concerns for the sub-fertile male in the era of ICSI. *Prenatal Diagnosis* 18: 1349–1365.

Kobayashi K, Mizuno K, Hida A (1994) PCR analysis of the Y chromosome long arm in azoospermic patients: evidence for a second locus required for spermatogenesis. *Human Molecular Genetics* 3: 1965–1967.

Kurinczuk J (1997) Birth defects in infants conceived by intracytoplasmic sperm injection: an alternative interpretation. *British Medical Journal* 315: 1260–1265.

Lanzendorf SM, Slusser J, Maloney MK, et al. (1988) A preclinical evaluation of pronuclear formation by microinjection of human spermatozoa into human oocytes. *Fertility and Sterility* 49: 835–842.

Leunens L, Celestin-Westreich S, Bonduelle M, Liebaers I, Ponjaert-Kristoffersen I (2008) Follow-up of cognitive and motor development of 10-year-old singleton children born after ICSI compared with spontaneously conceived children. *Human Reproduction* 23: 105–111.

Lillie FR (1914) Studies of fertilisation IV: the mechanism of fertilization in Arbacia. *Journal of Experimental Zoology* 16: 523.

Longo FJ (1981) Changes in the zonae pellucidae and plasmalemmae of ageing mouse eggs. *Biological Reproduction* 25: 299–411.

Mansour R (1998) Intracytoplasmic sperm injection: a state of the art technique. *Human Reproduction Update* 4(1): 43–56.

Mokánszki A, Tóthné EV, Bodnár B, *et al.* (2014) Is sperm hyaluronic acid binding ability predictive for clinical success of intracytoplasmic sperm injection: PICSI vs ICSI. *Biology in Reproductive Medicine* 60(6): 348–354.

Nagy ZP, Liu J, Joris H, Devroey P, Van Steirteghem A (1993a) Intracytoplasmic single sperm injection of 1-day old unfertilized human oocytes. *Human Reproduction* 8: 2180–2184.

Nagy ZP, Janssenswillen C, Silber S, Devroey P, Van Steirteghem AC (1995) Using ejaculated, fresh, and frozen-thawed epididymal and testicular spermatozoa gives rise to comparable results after intracytoplasmic injection. *Human Reproduction* 9: 1743–1748.

Nagy ZP, Liu J, Joris H, Devroey P, Van Steirteghem A (1993b) Time-course of oocyte activation, pronucleus formation and cleavage in human oocytes fertilized by intracytoplasmic sperm injection. *Human Reproduction* 9: 1743–1748.

Ng S-C, Bongso A, Ratnam SS (1991) Microinjection of human oocytes: a technique for severe oligoasthenoteratozoospermia. *Fertility and Sterility* 56(6): 1117–1123.

Oates RD, Cobl SM, Harns DH, *et al.* (1996) Efficiency of ICSI using intentionally cryopreserved epididymal sperm. *Human Reproduction* 600: 133–138.

Palermo G, Joris H, Derde M-P, *et al.* (1993) Sperm characteristics and outcome of human assisted fertilization by subzonal insemination and intracytoplasmic sperm injection. *Fertility and Sterility* 59: 826–835.

Palermo G, Joris H, Devroey P, Van Steirteghem AC (1992) Pregnancies after intracytoplasmic injection of single spermatozoon into an oocyte. *Lancet* 340: 17–18.

Peer S, Eltes F, Berkovitz A, *et al.* (2007) Is fine morphology of the human sperm nuclei affected by in vitro incubation at 37°C? *Fertility and Sterility* 88(6): 1589–1594.

Qureshi SJ, Ross AR, Ma K, *et al.* (1996) Polymerase chain reaction screening for Y chromosome microdeletions: a first step towards the diagnosis of genetically-determined spermatogenic failure in men. *Molecular Human Reproduction* 2(10): 775–779.

Safran A, Reubinoff E, Porat-Katz A, Lewin A (1998) Assisted reproduction for the treatment of azoospermia. *Human Reproduction* 13(Suppl. 4): 41–60.

Said TM, Agarwal A, Zborowski M, *et al.* (2008) Utility of magnetic cell separation as a molecular sperm preparation technique. *Journal of Andrology* 29(2): 134–142.

Santella L, Dale B (2015) Assisted yes, but where do we draw the line. *Reproductive BioMedicine Online* 31: 476–478.

Schimmel T, Cohen J, Saunders H, Alikani M (2014) Laser-assisted zona pellucida thinning does not facilitate hatching and may disrupt the in vitro hatching process: a morphokinetic study in the mouse. *Human Reproduction* 29(12): 2670–2679.

Shimizu T, Ooki T, Suzuki M, Kamiyama H (2009) An investigation of the separation of mature spermatozoa using Sperm Slow™ for intracytoplasmic sperm injection and its clinical results. *Fertility and Sterility* 92(3): S139–S139.

Silber SJ, Johnson L (1998) Are spermatid injections of any clinical value? ROSNI and ROSI revisited: round spermatid nucleus injection and round spermatid injection. *Human Reproduction* 13: 509–515.

Silber SJ, Van Steirteghem AC, Liu J, *et al.* (1995) High fertilization and pregnancy rate after intracytoplasmic sperm injection with spermatozoa obtained from testicle biopsy. *Human Reproduction* 10: 148–152.

Simoni M, Kamischke A, Nieschlag E (1998) The current status of the molecular diagnosis of Y-chromosomal microdeletions in the work-up of male infertility. *Human Reproduction* 13(7): 1764–1768.

Sousa M, Mendoza C, Barros A, Tesarik J (1996) Calcium responses of human oocytes after intracytoplasmic injection of leucocytes, spermatocytes and round spermatids. *Molecular Human Reproduction* 11: 853–857.

Stimpfel M, Verdenik I, Zorn B, *et al.* (2018) Magnetic-activated cell sorting of non-apoptotic spermatozoa improves the quality of embryos according to female age: a prospective sibling oocyte study. *Journal of Assisted Reproduction and Genetics* 35: 1665–1674.

Sutcliffe AG, Taylor B, Li J, *et al.* (1999) Children born after intracytoplasmic sperm injection: population control study. *BMJ* 318(7185): 704–705.

Svalander P, Forsberg A-S, Jakobsson A-H, Wikland M (1995) Factors of importance for the establishment of a successful program of intracytoplasmic sperm injection treatment for male infertility. *Fertility and Sterility* 65: 828–837.

te Velde E, Van Baar A, Van Kooij R (1998) Concerns about assisted reproduction. *Lancet* 351(9115): 1524–1525.

Twigg JP, Irvine DS, Aitken RJ (1998) Oxidative damage to DNA in human spermatozoa does not preclude pronucleus formation at intracytoplasmic sperm injection. *Human Reproduction* 13(7): 1864–1871.

Wang WH, Kaskar K, Ren Y, *et al.* (2008a) Comparison of development and implantation of human embryos biopsied with two different methods: aspiration and displacement. *Fertility and Sterility* 90(S1): S343.

Wang WH, Kaskar K, Gill J, DeSplinter T (2008b) A simplified technique for embryo biopsy for preimplantation genetic diagnosis. *Fertility and Sterility* 90(2): 438–442.

Wong MYW, Ledger WL (2013) Is ICSI risky? *Obstetrics & Gynaecology International* Article ID 473289, http://dx.doi.org/10.1155/2013/473289.

Van Assche E, Bonduelle M, Tournaye H (1996) Cytogenetics of male infertility. *Human Reproduction* 11(Suppl. 4): 1–26.

Van Blerkom J, Johnson M, Cohen J (2015) A plea for caution and more research in the 'experimental' use of ionophores in ICSI. *Reproductive BioMedicine Online* 30: 323–324.

van den Bergh M, Fahy-Deshe M, Hohl MK (2009) Pronuclear zygote score following intracytoplasmic injection of hyaluronan-bound spermatozoa: a prospective randomized study. *Reproductive BioMedicine Online* 19(6): 796–801.

Vanden Meerschaut F, Nikiforaki D, Heindryckx D, De Sutter P (2014) Assisted oocyte activation following ICSI fertilization failure. *Reproductive BioMedicine Online* 28: 560–571.

Vanderzwalmen P, Bach M, Gaspard O, *et al.* (2014) Morphological selection of gametes and embryo: sperm. In: Montag M (ed.) *A Practical Guide to Selecting Gametes and Embryos.* CRC Press, Taylor & Francis Group, Boca Raton, FL, pp. 59–80.

309

Vanderzwalmen P, Nijs M, Stecher A, *et al.* (1998) Is there a future for spermatid injection? *Human Reproduction* 13(Suppl. 4): 71–84.

Van Steirteghem A (2012) Celebrating ICSI's twentieth anniversary and the birth of more than 2.5 million children: the 'how, why, when and where'. *Human Reproduction* 27: 1–2.

Van Steirteghem A, Liu J, Nagy P, *et al.* (1995) Microinsemination. In: Hebon B, Bringer J, Mares P (eds.) *Fertility and Sterility: A Current Overview.* IFFS-95. Parthenon Publishing Group, New York, pp. 295–404.

Veiga A, Sandalinas M, Benkhalifa M, *et al.* (1997) Laser blastocyst biopsy for preimplantation diagnosis in the human. *Zygote* 5: 351–354.

Woldringh GH, Janssen IM, Hehir-Kwa JY, *et al.* (2009) Constitutional DNA copy numbers in ICSI children. *Human Reproduction* 24(1): 233–240.

Woodward BJ, Campbell KH, Ramsewak SS (2008a) A comparison of headfirst and tailfirst microinjection of sperm at intracytoplasmic sperm injection. *Fertility and Sterility* 89(3): 711–714.

Woodward BJ, Montgomery S, Hartshorne G, Campbell K, Kennedy R (2008b) Spindle position assessment prior to ICSI does not benefit fertilization or early embryo quality. *Reproductive BioMedicine Online* 16(2): 232–238.

Woodward BJ, Sookram S (2010) Polar body positioning during ICSI: does it matter? *Human Fertility* 13(2): 109–111.

Worrilow K, Eid S, Matthews J, *et al.* (2007) A multi-site clinical trial evaluating PICSI® versus intracytoplasmic sperm injection (ICSI): positive clinical outcomes observed in a prospective, randomized and double-blinded study. *Fertility and Sterility* 92(3): S36–S37.

Yanagimachi R (2001) Gamete manipulation for development: new methods for conception. *Reproduction and Fertility Development* 13(1): 3–14.

Yanagimachi R (2005) Intracytoplasmic injection of spermatozoa and spermatogenic cells: its biology and applications in humans and animals. *Reproductive Biomedicine Online* 10(2): 247–288.

# Preimplantation Genetic Diagnosis

## Introduction

Preimplantation genetic diagnosis (PGD) was developed in the late 1980s to help couples who are at risk of transmitting an inherited disease to their offspring, as an alternative to prenatal diagnosis during pregnancy. Prenatal diagnosis has the disadvantage that if the diagnosis shows the fetus to be affected, the couple must decide whether they wish to terminate the pregnancy or continue with the knowledge that their child is going to be affected by the genetic disease. PGD offers some of these couples an alternative, as the diagnosis is performed on the pre-implantation embryo, and only embryos assessed as being unaffected by the genetic disease are transferred to the patient. The pregnancy is therefore initiated with the knowledge that the fetus is free from the disease, at that moment in time.

Patients referred for PGD include those who have already experienced several terminations of affected pregnancies or have experienced repeated miscarriages due to unbalanced chromosome arrangements in the fetus, those with moral or religious objections to termination, and infertility patients who carry a genetic or chromosomal abnormality.

The technology and expertise involved in PGD require the participation of, and close collaboration between, three separate disciplines: genetics, IVF and molecular biology.

## Chromosomes, Genes and the Genetics of Inherited Disease

Human cells contain 23 pairs of chromosomes, 46 in total; each parent contributes one chromosome to each of these pairs. Twenty-two of the chromosome pairs, known as autosomes (chromosomes 1–22), have the same appearance in males and females; females have two X chromosomes as the 23rd pair, and males have one X and one Y chromosome as

their 23rd pair. Reproductive cells (gametes) have 23 chromosomes, 22 autosomes and either one X (oocytes) or one Y (sperm cells) chromosome.

Autosomal genes are therefore present in two copies, one inherited from each parent; females have two gene copies on their X chromosomes, whereas males have only one copy of genes carried on their X and Y chromosomes. Genetically inherited diseases are usually caused by a mutation within a specific gene, which causes the gene to be inactive or faulty. The mutations that lead to a disease can be caused by a single change, or by more complicated changes within the gene, such as deletions, substitutions or insertions in the base sequence. A single gene may contain 'hot spots' that are prone to mutation. For example, although over 800 mutations have been identified in cystic fibrosis (CF), 70% of individuals in the United Kingdom who carry CF have the same mutation (deltaF508), caused by the deletion of three base pairs in exon 10 of the CF gene, which is located on chromosome 7.

A triplet of bases on a chromosome can sometimes be expanded, and this phenomenon leads to a group of diseases known as triplet repeat disorders. Gross chromosomal abnormalities, such as aneuploidy, translocations and inversions, can also lead to a fetus with an unbalanced chromosome complement. Age-related aneuploidy can also lead to chromosomally abnormal offspring: this is not an inherited disease, and it can occur in any pregnancy.

Single-gene defects may affect the autosomes (chromosomes 1–22) or the sex chromosomes (X and Y). Whether the disease is expressed when both or only a single copy of the gene carries a mutation is determined by the mode of inheritance: autosomal recessive, autosomal dominant or X-linked (sex-linked).

## Autosomal Recessive Disease

Autosomal recessive inheritance accounts for the majority of genetic disease; the pattern of its

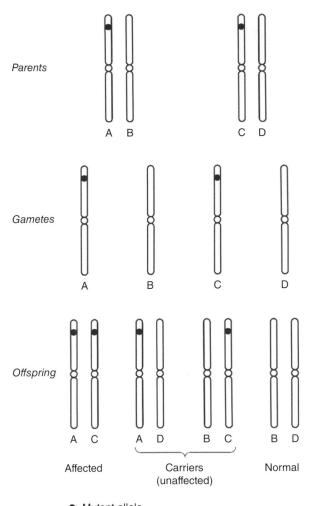

*Parents*

A  B          C  D

*Gametes*

A          B          C          D

*Offspring*

A  C      A  D      B  C      B  D

Affected        Carriers        Normal
              (unaffected)

● Mutant allele

**Figure 14.1** Autosomal recessive inheritance.

**Table 14.1** Examples of autosomal recessive diseases diagnosed by PGD

| Cystic fibrosis (various mutations) |
| Sickle cell anemia |
| Tay–Sachs disease |
| Spinal muscular atrophy |
| β-Thalassemia |
| Adrenogenital syndrome |
| Hypophosphatemia |

couples, each partner may carry a different mutation (compound heterozygotes).

Cystic fibrosis was one of the first autosomal recessive single-gene defects to be diagnosed by PGD. Since deltaF508 is a relatively common mutation, it may be carried by both partners in many couples. Table 14.1 shows examples of major autosomal single-gene defects that have been diagnosed by PGD.

## Autosomal Dominant Disorders

Disorders that are dominant in their inheritance will be expressed if a single copy of the mutated gene is present (Figure 14.2). These diseases are not as life-threatening as some recessive diseases, and therefore affected individuals can still reproduce and transmit the disease to their offspring. Many dominant disorders are late in onset, such as Huntington's disease and some inherited cancers. A large number of dominant diseases can now be diagnosed by PGD, including myotonic dystrophy, Marfan's syndrome, polyposis coli, Charcot–Marie–Tooth disease and Huntington's disease (Table 14.2).

## X-linked Diseases

X-linked diseases affect genes that are carried on the X chromosome: more than 400 X-linked diseases have been identified. They can be inherited in a recessive or dominant manner, but almost all severe types have recessive inheritance. Males inherit the X chromosome from their mother, and if this inherited X chromosome is abnormal, they will be affected with the disease (Figure 14.3). Therefore, carrier mothers transmit the disease to half of their male offspring, and half of a carrier mother's daughters will be carriers. Embryo biopsy and genetic

inheritance is outlined in Figure 14.1. If an individual has one normal and one abnormal gene for a particular disorder, he or she is a carrier of the disease and will usually be unaffected. If both parents of a child carry the same disease-causing mutation, the child will be affected by the disease. For example, if both the mother and the father are carriers of cystic fibrosis, the offspring have a 1 in 4 chance of being affected, 1 in 4 chance of being unaffected, and a 2 in 4 chance of carrying the disease without being affected.

The most common autosomal recessive single-gene defect is beta-thalassemia, which is caused by a mutation in the beta-globin gene. However, there are many different mutations for beta-thalassemia, especially between different ethnic groups: in many

**Table 14.2** Examples of autosomal dominant diseases diagnosed by PGD

| |
| --- |
| Marfan's syndrome |
| Familial adenomatous polyposis coli |
| Huntington's disease |
| Myotonic dystrophy |
| Osteogenesis imperfecta |

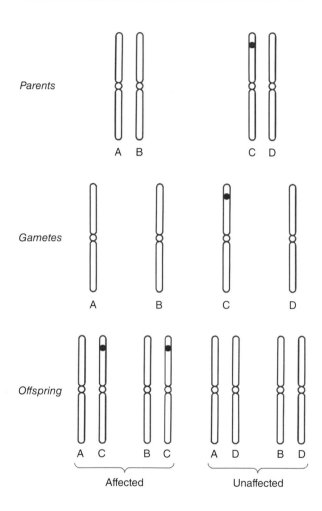

*Parents*

A   B      C   D

*Gametes*

A   B   C   D

*Offspring*

A C   B C    A D   B D

⎴ Affected     ⎴ Unaffected

● Mutant allele

**Figure 14.2** Autosomal dominant inheritance.

diagnosis can identify noncarrier female and nonaffected male embryos, which can then be selected for transfer. Some of the X-linked diseases reported as diagnosed by embryo sexing are listed in Table 14.3a, and Table 14.3b shows examples of X-linked diseases where a specific diagnosis has been performed.

# Triplet Repeat Disorders

A new class of genetic disorders was identified during the 1990s: triplet repeat disorders are caused by the expansion of a triplet of bases that are repeated within a gene, and they are usually associated with neurological disorders. Each disease has a range of repeats associated with a spectrum from normal individual to affected individuals.

For example, fragile X syndrome, which generally affects males, was originally thought to be an X-linked disease, but it has been reclassified as a triplet repeat disorder. The disease is caused by the unstable expansion of a CGG repeat in the 5′-untranslated region of the FMR1 gene, which lies on the X chromosome. This triplet expansion results in mental retardation; a normal individual will have from 6 to 54 triplet repeats, those having the 'premutation' will carry between 54 and 200 repeats, and those affected with fragile X will have over 200 repeats. Females carrying the premutation are at risk of transmitting the full mutation to their offspring, and since males inherit the X chromosome from their mothers and have a single X chromosome, their male offspring are at a 50% risk of inheriting fragile X. Females who inherit the expanded gene from their mothers will also inherit a normal X chromosome from their father, and their disease manifestation is variable. Males carrying the premutation are at risk of transmitting only the premutation to their female offspring, who will be carrier females.

Huntington's disease (HD) is a progressive neuropsychiatric disorder of late onset that is inherited in a dominant fashion. The gene is on chromosome 4 and involves a CAG triplet repeat where expansion beyond 36 results in HD. The age of onset is about 40 years and patients often die by their mid-50s. PGD has been performed for HD, but it draws some ethical discussion: many potential carriers of HD know that they have a 50% risk of being affected because one of their parents is affected, but they do not wish to know their own HD status. For prenatal testing and PGD, an exclusion test can be offered, where patients are given a risk factor without being told their actual status.

Myotonic dystrophy (DM) or Steinert's disease is a progressive muscular dystrophy. The gene is located on chromosome 19, and DM is caused by expansion of a CTG repeat at the 3′-untranslated part of the myotonic dystrophy protein kinase gene. Normal individuals have between 5 and 37

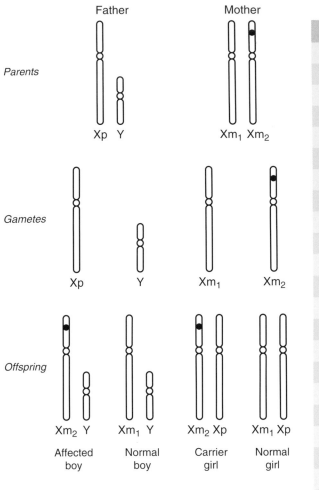

Parents — Father (Xp Y), Mother (Xm₁ Xm₂)

Gametes — Xp, Y, Xm₁, Xm₂

Offspring:
- Xm₂ Y — Affected boy
- Xm₁ Y — Normal boy
- Xm₂ Xp — Carrier girl
- Xm₁ Xp — Normal girl

● Mutant allele

**Figure 14.3** X-linked inheritance.

**Table 14.3** Examples of X-linked diseases diagnosed by PGD

| (a) Sexing |
| --- |
| Duchenne muscular dystrophy |
| Becker muscular dystrophy |
| Chronic granulomatosis |
| Hunter's syndrome |
| Hemophilia |
| Adrenoleukodystrophy |
| Barth syndrome |
| X-linked hydrocephalus |
| X-linked ataxia |
| X-linked incontinentia pigmentosa |
| X-linked mental retardation |
| X-linked Wiscott–Aldrich |
| X-linked spastic paraplegia |
| Laber's optic atrophy |
| Sensory motor neuron disease |
| Retinitis pigmentosa |
| Bruton's disease |
| Menkes disease |
| **(b) Specific diagnoses** |
| Duchenne muscular dystrophy |
| Hemophilia |
| Lesch–Nyhan syndrome |
| Charcot–Marie–Tooth disease |

repeats, and affected individuals may have anything from 50 to several thousand repeats. Intermediate numbers of repeats can give rise to a premutation. DM can be diagnosed by PGD.

## Chromosomal Abnormalities

Abnormalities that involve whole chromosomes are usually lethal. Those compatible with life include Down's syndrome (three copies of chromosome 21) and those that involve the sex chromosomes, such as Turner's syndrome (XO) and Klinefelter's syndrome (XXY).

The most common chromosome abnormality is a translocation, where two chromosomes have broken and rejoined to the opposite chromosome. If the chromosomes are still balanced, i.e., all the genetic material is still present, the patient is described as having a balanced translocation. The majority of patients carrying a balanced translocation do not realize they have abnormal chromosomes until they try to reproduce. During meiosis, the segregation of the chromosomes becomes confused, and unbalanced chromosome complements are formed in the gametes, leading to the formation of an embryo with abnormal chromosomes (unbalanced translocation). Therefore, patients carrying balanced translocations may experience infertility, repeated miscarriage or the birth of a child with abnormal chromosomes.

Robertsonian translocations involve breakages around the centromere of the 'acrocentric' chromosomes (13, 14, 15, 21, 22). These chromosomes contain a satellite region on their short arm, and loss of this area has no effect on phenotype. Since two of the acrocentric chromosomes join together, the patient has only 45 chromosomes. Robertsonian translocations can be diagnosed using PGD to identify the number of chromosomes present.

Reciprocal translocations involve breaks at any location on two chromosomes, and any chromosome can be affected. Every couple may have different chromosome breakpoints, and therefore diagnosis by PGD is difficult.

Chromosome abnormalities can also be caused by chromosome inversions, insertions, deletions or rearrangements (such as ring chromosomes).

## Age-Related Aneuploidy

Women over the age of 35 are known to be at increased risk of having a fetus with a chromosome abnormality such as Down's syndrome. However, only 20% of Down's syndrome babies are born to women over the age of 35. Screening methods have been developed to help identify those pregnancies at risk, as the use of age alone as an indication for prenatal diagnosis of age-related aneuploidy will miss the majority of affected pregnancies. Biochemical (plasma alpha-fetoprotein, hCG, unconjugated estriol) and ultrasound screening methods are therefore used to determine which pregnancies are at risk. Patients found to be at risk undergo prenatal diagnosis, with a karyotype performed to ascertain the status of the fetus. The chromosomes most commonly involved in age-related aneuploidy are 13, 16, 18, 21, X and Y.

## Prenatal Diagnosis
### Aneuploidy Screening
#### Serum Screening

During the second trimester of pregnancy (16–17 weeks) a number of markers have been found that help to identify pregnancies with chromosome abnormalities. Down's syndrome pregnancies show lower maternal serum alpha-fetoprotein (AFP) and unconjugated estriol, whereas human chorionic gonadotropin (hCG) levels are two times higher than normal. Taking into account the patient's age, a triple screening test to measure AFP, free beta-hCG and unconjugated estriol can increase the detection rate to 70%, thereby reducing the number of women who require invasive prenatal diagnosis. Pregnancy-associated plasma protein A (PAPP A) is reduced in Down's syndrome pregnancies. Noninvasive prenatal diagnosis tests (NIPD) that screen cell-free DNA in maternal serum are now also available (see below).

### Ultrasound

During the first trimester of pregnancy, ultrasound detection of nuchal translucency measuring greater than 3 mm is associated with a chromosome abnormality. This is caused by fluid accumulation at the back of the fetal neck. In conjunction with maternal age, studies have shown this to give a detection rate of 86% with a false positive rate of 4.5%. When used in combination with first and second trimester serum screening, a detection rate of over 90% has been reported.

Around one-half of all major structural abnormalities can now be detected by ultrasound in the first trimester, including acrania/anencephaly, abdominal wall defects, holoprosencephaly and cystic hygromata. Other anomalies become evident later in the second trimester, as organ systems develop: cardiac malformations, duodenal atresia, hydrops, choroid plexus cysts, nuchal edema, renal pyelectasis, omphalocele, hypoplastic midphalanx of the fifth finger, and short femur and humerus can be used to screen for aneuploidy. Digital imaging combined with computer analysis of two-dimensional ultrasound pictures can be used to create three- and four-dimensional images, which allow more in-depth assessment of cardiac and neural abnormalities, and show a clearer picture of what specific abnormalities look like.

## Diagnosis of Inherited Disorders

Couples who have already had an affected pregnancy or child, or have a family member affected with the disease, are aware that they are at risk of transmitting an inherited disease. These couples, as well as those who have a positive serum or ultrasound screen, can be offered prenatal diagnosis. Chorionic villus sampling and amniocentesis have been the traditional methods of choice for prenatal diagnosis, and more recently, new molecular biology techniques have facilitated the development of noninvasive prenatal diagnosis tests that can screen fetal DNA in the maternal circulation.

## Chorionic Villus Sampling (CVS)

CVS can be performed transcervically between 10 and 12 weeks of gestation, or from 12 weeks onwards by the transabdominal route. A sample of cells is removed from the placenta and used for diagnosis of chromosomal, metabolic and DNA analysis. The disadvantages of the procedure are that it cannot be used for neural tube and other congenital abnormalities, and some studies have suggested a risk of limb reduction deformities if it is performed too early or by inexperienced operators. There is also a 1–2% risk of miscarriage, which is a little higher than the risk after amniocentesis. In 1.5% of cases, the karyotype of the placenta is found to be different from that of the embryo (confined placental mosaicism).

## Amniocentesis

Amniocentesis for prenatal diagnosis is usually performed in the second trimester, from 15 weeks onwards. Under ultrasound guidance, 15–20 mL of amniotic fluid is aspirated; this can be used for the diagnosis of chromosome abnormalities, measurement of specific substances, detection of inborn errors of metabolism such as Tay–Sachs disease, measurement of enzyme activity and diagnosis of neural tube defects. Its disadvantages include the potential of causing fetal loss (1%) and rarely there may be continued leakage of the amniotic fluid. The main limitation of this technique is that results are available only very late in the pregnancy (17–20 weeks), so that a termination must be induced during the second trimester.

## Cell-Free Fetal DNA Screening (cfDNA)

Cell-free fetal DNA can be detected in maternal plasma as early as 7 weeks' gestation, and this has been successfully used to provide noninvasive prenatal diagnosis (NIPD) for common aneuploidies, with low false positive rates. Cell-free DNA is extracted from a maternal blood sample, and real-time polymerase chain reaction (PCR) with fluorescently labeled specific probes for target genes is used to identify and quantify fetal-specific sequences present in low copy numbers. Accuracy depends on the condition under investigation: the test can accurately diagnose Rhesus D status, and fetal sex determination can identify X-linked disorders. Sensitivity

and specificity are less for trisomy 21, 18 and 13 due to the influence of biological factors such as confined placental mosaicism (CPM). cfDNA screening is therefore currently considered as a screening test for aneuploidy, although accuracy is improving with developments in technology.

## Fetal Blood Sampling, Cordocentesis or PUBS (Percutaneous Umbilical Blood Sampling)

These techniques are used less frequently than CVS or amniocentesis; samples can be taken from 18 weeks' gestation to term. Fetal blood is taken from the cord or intrahepatic umbilical vein and used for fetal karyotyping (quick result), evaluation of fetal status (if an infection is thought to be present) and hematological abnormalities (Rh or immune hemolytic disease). The most common indication is karyotyping for single or multiple congenital abnormalities and mosaicism.

## Fetal Tissue Sampling

Using ultrasound guidance, it is possible to biopsy skin, liver, muscle and fluid collections from the urinary tract, abdomen, thorax and cystic hygroma.

# Diagnostic Testing for Prenatal Diagnosis

Tests used to establish a fetal diagnosis following CVS or amniocentesis include PCR and karyotyping. PCR analysis can detect single-gene defects and triplet repeat disorders and determine fetal gender. A karyotype is performed for any diagnosis which involves chromosome identification, i.e., in those patients carrying chromosome abnormalities or who are at risk of age-related aneuploidy. In some situations, fluorescent in-situ hybridization (FISH) or DNA microarray-based technology is used to complement the karyotype result.

## Polymerase Chain Reaction

PCR is a molecular technique developed in the 1980s that is used to amplify a portion of DNA thousands of times. For prenatal diagnosis, PCR can be used to detect the normal or mutated gene by amplifying the region around the mutation. This is achieved using primers that have a sequence which is complementary to a region of the gene. Primers that will bind to either side of the mutation are selected, and copies of the DNA sequence in between (target gene) are generated via repeated cycles of heating and cooling:

1. Heating to 96ºC to denature the DNA and create separate strands
2. Cooling to 55º C to allow primers to bind to the DNA target (primer annealing)
3. Heating to 72ºC to allow DNA synthesis (primer extension).

This PCR cycle is repeated a number of times (25–35 times) to produce billions of copies of the DNA sequence for analysis. The reaction is made possible by using a thermostable polymerase enzyme that can withstand the high temperatures needed for denaturation: the first such enzyme to be used was Taq polymerase, isolated from a heat-tolerant bacterium (*Thermus aquaticus*) that lives in hot springs and hydrothermal vents. A similar enzyme, *Pfu*DNA polymerase (from *Pyrococcus furiosus*), has superior thermostability and higher fidelity when copying DNA.

Once the DNA sequence of interest has been amplified, the PCR products are analyzed using a number of different techniques. The simplest method, which can be used to detect an insertion or deletion, is to separate the PCR products by polyacrylamide gel electrophoresis; other techniques include single-stranded conformational polymorphism (SSCP), amplification refractory mutation system (ARMS) and heteroduplex analysis, which can detect even just a single base change within a gene. The technology has further evolved over the past decade, with a range of more sophisticated DNA microarray molecular biology tools available (see Molecular Diagnosis).

### Karyotyping

Karyotype analysis examines the chromosomes of a cell. For prenatal diagnosis, the sample obtained by CVS or amniocentesis is cultured to increase the number of cells, and mitotic inhibitors are used to arrest some of the cells in metaphase. Agents which elongate the metaphase chromosomes are also used. Slide preparations of the nuclei are treated with Giemsa stain, which results in a specific banding pattern for each chromosome. Using this method, missing or extra chromosomes, translocations, inversions, etc. can be identified. Occasionally the results of a karyotype may be inconclusive, and more advanced techniques are now used to help elucidate the diagnosis. Karyotyping has also been used to check the number of chromosomes in diagnosis of age-related aneuploidy.

# Preimplantation Genetic Diagnosis

The technology required for preimplantation genetic diagnosis encompasses genetics, IVF, embryo biopsy and single-cell diagnosis. Since separate disciplines and techniques are required for embryo biopsy and diagnosis, PGD must be carried out by a genetics team in collaboration with an IVF team with access to molecular biology technology. The embryo biopsy technique should be performed by a trained embryologist, but the diagnosis must be performed by a molecular biology laboratory and confirmed by a genetics specialist.

## History

The first children born as a result of preimplantation genetic diagnoses were reported in 1990 by the group of Alan Handyside in London, studying sex-linked diseases (Handyside *et al.*, 1990). Robert Edwards had anticipated this development 22 years earlier, when he and Richard Gardner, his PhD student at the time, established a proof of principle by using blastocyst biopsy as a means of sexing rabbit embryos (Gardner & Edwards, 1968). By 2010 the number of children born in the world after screening embryos for genetic disease exceeded 10000; the HFEA in the UK currently licenses 419 genetic conditions for diagnosis by PGD.

The procedure for preimplantation genetic diagnosis involves:

1. Selection of a viable embryo
2. Collecting genetic material (embryo biopsy)
3. Preparation of the genetic material for analysis (DNA isolation and amplification)
4. Analysis of results and selection of the embryo for transfer to the mother.

Genetic analysis of embryos in fertility clinics currently has two different applications:

1. Preimplantation Genetic Diagnosis (PGD) for couples known to carry genetic disorders such as single-gene diseases or chromosomal translocations.
2. Preimplantation Genetic Selection (PGS or PGD-A), used to identify embryos with a normal karyotype.

The European Society for Human Reproduction and Embryology (ESHRE) PGD Consortium collects all European data on a regular basis, with published reports that summarize data pertaining to the cycles, from indication and methodology to cycle outcome. Their 14th Data Report (De Ryck *et al.*, 2017) confirmed that during the period 2011–2013, preimplantation diagnosis for chromosome abnormalities, single-gene disorders and sexing for X-linked diseases was performed in 17 721 IVF cycles; PGS for aneuploidy was performed in 26 737 cycles during the same period, including 705 cycles for sex selection.

## Embryo Biopsy

As outlined in Chapter 13, embryo biopsy is performed using micromanipulation equipment used for ICSI; all of the biopsy techniques involve two stages: zona drilling and aspiration (or herniation in the case of blastocyst biopsy). Cell biopsies can be taken from oocytes/embryos at three different stages:

1. Polar body biopsy in the unfertilized oocyte/zygote
2. Cleavage stage biopsy from the 6- to 8-cell embryo
3. Blastocyst stage biopsy.

Table 14.4 gives an overview of embryo biopsy methods; the techniques are discussed in detail in Chapter 13.

### Polar Body Biopsy

Biopsy of the first polar body was developed in order to overcome ethical objections to embryo biopsy, on the basis that the 'ethical status' of the unfertilized oocyte differs from that of the embryo. Some individuals opt for PGD in order to avoid termination of pregnancy, and performing the test on a preimplantation embryo may be just as objectionable as termination of pregnancy. Polar body biopsy was first used for the detection of CF; due to crossing-over events, the second polar body is also required in some situations. Polar body screening detects only maternal meiotic aneuploidies and will not identify errors that are due to paternal or postzygotic factors; biopsy of both polar bodies is recommended for PGD.

### Cleavage Stage Biopsy

Biopsies performed at the four-cell stage may alter the ratio of inner cell mass to trophectoderm (TE) cells, which may be detrimental to embryo development. Therefore, biopsy at the six- to eight-cell stage, on Day 3 post-insemination, is preferred.

Several difficulties arise from cleavage stage embryo biopsy: the first is that human embryonic cells are very fragile and easily lyse. If this occurs during the biopsy procedure, the nucleus may be lost, and another cell will have to be removed. Compaction occurs between the eight-cell and morula stage, and during compaction the cells of the embryo can no longer be distinguished as they flatten out over each other to maximize intercellular contacts. If the biopsy

**Table 14.4** Three methods of embryo biopsy used in preimplantation genetic diagnosis

|  | Day performed | Types of cells removed | Indications | Zona drilling | Cell removal | Limitations |
|---|---|---|---|---|---|---|
| Polar body (PB) | First PB Day 0 Second PB Day 1 Or simultaneously on Day 1 | First and second polar bodies | PGS Monogenics carried by mother | Laser Mechanical Beveled pipette | Aspiration | Only maternal chromosomes/ genes |
| Cleavage stage | Day 3 | Blastomeres | PGS Monogenics Sexing Chromosome abnormalities | Laser Mechanical Acid Tyrode's | Aspiration Displacement | Postzygotic mosaicism |
| Blastocyst | Day 5 | Trophectoderm | PGS Monogenics Sexing Chromosome abnormalities | Laser Mechanical Acid Tyrode's | Herniation | Postzygotic mosaicism Some embryos will arrest prior to biopsy |

Adapted from Harper *et al.* (2001), with permission.

is performed at this stage, it is very difficult to remove a blastomere, as it has established strong contact with adjacent blastomeres. Trying to remove a cell from a compacted embryo may also result in lysis of the cell. The thickness and dynamics of the zona pellucida also vary between patients and can lead to some problems during the biopsy procedure. In many cases, numerous sperm are associated with the zona pellucida, and therefore intracytoplasmic sperm injection (ICSI) should always be used with PCR techniques to reduce the risk of sperm contamination.

Studies of both cryopreserved/thawed embryos and those biopsied for PGD have shown that up to 50% of the embryo mass may be lost, and yet lead to a healthy live birth. Data from the ESHRE PGD consortium show that 97% of embryo biopsies were successful, with more than 90% of the embryos surviving. Pregnancies following embryo biopsy showed no significant developmental differences compared to controls. Deliveries, including infant birth weight and Apghar scores, were considered to be normal.

### Blastocyst Biopsy

Embryos that have reached the blastocyst stage are currently preferred for embryo biopsy, performed on Day 5 or 6 post-insemination. Vitrification is accepted as a successful method of cryopreserving blastocysts, and vitrifying blastocysts after biopsy allows more time for the diagnosis. Blastocyst biopsy has the advantage that a larger number of cells can be removed from the outer TE layer without affecting the inner cell mass from which the fetus later develops. Analysis of a larger number of cells is of benefit in diagnosis of monogenic diseases. However, TE cells may have diverged genetically from the inner cell mass (ICM): confined placental mosaicism, where the chromosome status of the embryo is different from the placenta, is observed in at least 1% of conceptions. Studies indicate that blastocysts may have high levels of chromosomal mosaicism. Preferential allocation of abnormal cells to the TE may also be a mechanism of early human development, as is seen in large farm animals. In this case the TE would not be representative of the rest of the embryo, and the analysis would complicate and compromise the outcome for the patient.

One of the limitations of blastocyst biopsy is that many embryos will not reach the blastocyst stage. Although improvements in culture conditions have increased the numbers of blastocysts available, a large number of embryos are required for PGD diagnosis to ensure that normal embryos are available for transfer; this may not be the case when embryos are cultured to the blastocyst stage.

## Analysis of Biopsied Cells

Tools and technology used to examine cellular chromosomes and genes have evolved considerably over the past decade: the original FISH/PCR methods have now been replaced by more sophisticated, complex and accurate technology to analyze all 24 chromosomes, complemented by computer software and bioinformatics for data analysis in reaching a diagnosis. Modern tests rely on initial DNA amplification (whole genome amplification, WGA) in order to supply a template sufficient for comprehensive chromosome screening (CCS). A variety of different 'kits' offering different analytical platforms for CCS are commercially available, each with its own specific advantages and disadvantages; external commercial laboratories can now carry out diagnostic tests on cells that have been biopsied and sent from an IVF laboratory. The field continues to evolve rapidly, with new technologies offering increased sensitivity in combination with automation and high throughput. The discussion below includes older and now outdated approaches as a background for historical reference, in anticipation that even those current at the time of writing may be 'outdated' by the time of publication. All of the information gained since PGD was first applied has contributed significantly to our understanding of the genetics of early development and implantation. The increased resolution of new technologies will continue to add to overall data about the health of preimplantation embryos. The biological significance of some of the new information revealed by these technologies is as yet unknown; there is a crucial need for further ongoing basic research directed toward understanding the molecular biology of preimplantation development.

### Single-Cell Diagnosis

Cells removed from the embryo after biopsy are used for diagnosis; the techniques used historically are outlined in Table 14.5. PCR can be used for the diagnosis of single-gene defects, triplet repeat disorders and embryo sexing. Karyotyping requires a metaphase spread of chromosomes, and therefore this

**Table 14.5** Methods used historically for preimplantation genetic diagnosis

| | Indications | Cell preparation | Protocol | Limitations |
|---|---|---|---|---|
| FISH | Sexing<br>Chromosome abnormalities<br>PGS | Spreading cells using methanol:acetic acid or Tween HCl | Fix<br>Denature<br>Hybridization<br>Wash off unbound probe<br>Visualize | Cumulus contamination<br>Mosaicism<br>Overlapping signals<br>Failure of probes to bind |
| PCR | Sexing<br>Monogenic disorders | Tubing cells into lysis buffer | Lyse cell<br>Cycles of denaturing, annealing, elongation<br>Detect products | Cumulus contamination<br>Sperm contamination (use ICSI)<br>Other contamination<br>Amplification failure<br>Allele dropout |
| Metaphase comparative genome hybridization | Sexing<br>Chromosome abnormalities<br>PGS | Tubing cells into lysis buffer | Lyse cell, whole genome amplification<br>Co-hybridization with control sample on to metaphase spread<br>Analysis of each chromosome using CGH software | Contamination<br>Mosaicism<br>Procedure takes several days and so currently embryos are frozen<br>Requires many skills, PCR and cytogenetics |

FISH, fluorescent in situ hybridization; PGS, preimplantation genetic selection; PCR, polymerase chain reaction; ICSI, intracytoplasmic sperm injection; CGH, comparative genomic hybridization.
Adapted from Harper *et al.* (2001), with permission.

cannot be used on single embryonic cells, as they do not divide well in culture and it is difficult to obtain metaphase spreads. In cases where a metaphase spread is obtained, the chromosomes are short and difficult to band. FISH was previously used to examine chromosomes in embryos for embryo sexing, chromosome abnormalities and aneuploidy, now replaced by techniques for CCS.

### Molecular Diagnosis

PCR can be used to diagnose single-gene defects, triplet repeat disorders and embryo sex, but it is not a simple procedure. The procedure is complicated by the major problems of contamination and allele dropout (see below). If a diagnosis is available on whole DNA, it should be possible to make such a diagnosis sensitive at the single-cell level. However, some modifications of the procedure may be required. A common method of making the PCR procedure more sensitive is the use of nested PCR, where an inner set of primers amplifies the original PCR product. Since amplification failure can occur, it is essential that PGD does not rely on a negative result. To ensure that a single-cell PCR method is accurate and sensitive, a preliminary workup is usually performed on single cells, such as buccal cells, from normal, carrier and affected individuals. PCR products have been analyzed by heteroduplex analysis, SSCP, ARMS and restriction endonuclease digestion. Fluorescent PCR is a quantitative PCR method that can also be used. For the diagnosis of some diseases, such as fragile X, polymorphic markers may be used that identify which chromosome the embryo has inherited; i.e., the normal or at-risk chromosome.

### Contamination

Single-cell PCR is so sensitive that it will amplify any DNA that may contaminate the PCR reaction, such as a stray cumulus or sperm cell that may have been released from the zona during the biopsy, cells from the atmosphere or DNA found in the air or medium. Steps must be taken to eliminate contamination in order to reduce these problems to a minimum. These include working in a positive pressure PCR room, performing ICSI for all PCR diagnosis and examining PCR products in a separate laboratory. Misdiagnoses reported after PGD probably arise from contamination. These problems can be reduced with the use of a multiplex PCR with markers that can identify all four parental alleles to ensure that the amplified product is of embryonic origin.

## Allele Dropout

Allele dropout (ADO), or preferential amplification, refers to the situation where one of the two alleles preferentially amplifies over the other. For example, for a heterozygous cell, the normal allele may preferentially amplify so that the diagnosis would only identify the normal allele; the embryo would be diagnosed as normal instead of heterozygous. This would not cause a problem for recessive conditions where both partners carry the same mutation, but would create problems for dominant disorders, or in cases where the couple carry different mutations for a recessive disorder, as affected embryos could be diagnosed as normal. To reduce this problem, methods can be built into the diagnosis to ensure that both alleles can be identified.

# Fluorescent In-Situ Hybridization

FISH was the first technique used in preimplantation diagnosis of aneuploidy (Delhanty *et al.*,1993). Munné and and coworkers subsequently applied FISH to detect chromosomal translocations (Munné *et al.*, 1998). Fluorescently labeled molecular probes are used to identify chromosomes or their fragments, with the probes binding to specific DNA regions and appearing as fluorescent spots. Three types of FISH probes have been commonly used:

1. Repeat sequences or alpha satellite probes, which can be used in interphase and metaphase chromosomes. They bind to repeat sequences, usually to the centromeres (with the exception of chromosomes 9 and Y) and can be used directly labeled with fluorochromes. They require only 1 hour for hybridization and have been cloned in plasmids and cosmids. Probes for 13/21 and 14/22 cross-hybridize.
2. Locus-specific probes can be used in interphase or metaphase chromosomes and bind to a unique sequence. They require 6–12 hours for hybridization and have been cloned in cosmids or YACs (yeast artificial chromosomes).
3. Chromosome paints can only be used in metaphase chromosomes; they paint the entire chromosome.

The FISH technique involves several stages:

1. Cell spreading.
2. Pepsin digestion to remove any protein from around the nuclei; this is especially important for blastomeres.
3. Paraformaldehyde fixation to ensure that the nuclei adhere to the slide.
4. Denaturation to make nuclear and probe DNA single-stranded.
5. Hybridization: probes find and bind to the complementary sequence.
6. Posthybridization washes to remove unbound probe.
7. Detection; for use with indirect probes.
8. Visualization.

## FISH Diagnosis

FISH has been used since 1991 to sex embryos for PGD in cases of X-linked disease. It has advantages over PCR sexing as the copy number is identified: the difference between XO and XX can be determined, and there is no risk of contamination. Probes for chromosomes X, Y and 18 are used and only embryos showing normal female chromosomes are transferred. However, specific diagnosis of the disorder using a molecular method is preferred for diagnosis of X-linked disease, as this will differentiate between affected male, unaffected male, carrier female and non-carrier female.

FISH diagnosis is performed on interphase nuclei. As outlined above, the biopsied blastomere is disrupted in hypotonic solution, digested and fixed. FISH allows every nucleus within an embryo to be examined, but the number of chromosomes that can be analyzed at one time is limited. Using two rounds of FISH on a single nucleus allows a panel of seven to nine chromosomes to be screened (commonly including X, Y, 13, 16, 18, 21, 22), but repeated denaturation leads to DNA degeneration and decreases the efficiency of the procedure.

FISH analysis has many limitations and is associated with a high risk of technical error in the preparation of the material. It is not possible to test all 24 chromosomes simultaneously; therefore, PGS–FISH diagnosis is limited to the most common abnormalities involving chromosomes 13, 15–18, 21, 22, X and Y. A study by Mastenbroek *et al.* (2007) showed that patients treated by PGD using FISH on Day 3 embryos had a lower pregnancy rate than the control group, casting doubt on the utility of PGD by this method as an adjunct to IVF.

# Comprehensive Chromosome Screening

Advances in molecular biology technology now allow all 24 chromosomes to be analyzed using a variety of techniques that have been validated for clinical application, including microarray comparative genomic hybridization (aCGH), single-nucleotide polymorphism microarrays (SNP arrays) and quantitative polymerase chain reaction (qPCR). aCGH and SNP arrays depend on first amplifying the cell DNA (whole genome amplification), and this creates a risk of allele dropout, which can potentially result in misdiagnosis of monogenic diseases. A number of different analytical platforms are available, and technology continues to evolve: aCGH has been widely used in recent years, but is now slowly being replaced by Next-Generation/Massive Parallel Sequencing (NGS/MPS).

| Acronyms/Definitions | |
|---|---|
| **aCGH:** | Array-comparative genomic hybridization; all chromosomes can be analyzed, as well as segmental abnormalities up to a certain size |
| **ADO:** | Allele Dropout, failure to successfully amplify both alleles of a locus |
| **ARMS:** | Amplification refractory mutation system, also known as allele-specific PCR or PCR amplification of specific alleles (PASA). Uses sequence-specific PCR primers that allow DNA amplification only when the target allele is contained in the sample; can discriminate among templates that differ by a single nucleotide residue |
| **CCS:** | Comprehensive Chromosome Screening |
| **CGT:** | Carrier Genetic Test, used to determine the risk of having a child with a genetic disease |
| **CNV-Seq:** | Copy number variation sequencing |
| **FISH:** | Fluorescent in-situ hybridization |
| **HDA:** | Heteroduplex analysis; detects differences between normal DNA and DNA being analyzed by showing unpaired regions, which are sites of possible mutations |
| **Massive Parallel Sequencing (MPS):** | Also known as second generation sequencing or next-generation sequencing (NGS); a high-throughput approach to DNA sequencing using miniaturized parallel platforms for sequencing |
| **mCGH:** | metaphase comparative genome hybridization; used for polar body biopsy |
| **MDA:** | Multiple Displacement Amplification: a non-PCR-based method of amplifying DNA for whole genome amplification; uses random hexamers as primers for phage DNA polymerase in an isothermal amplification reaction |
| **Multiplex PCR:** | A technique that amplifies several different DNA sequences simultaneously by using multiple primers in a reaction mixture |
| **NGS:** | Next-Generation Sequencing (see MPS, above) |
| **qPCR:** | Quantitative polymerase chain reaction; specific primers can be added for diagnosis of monogenic disease. Does not require WGA: whole chromosomes, but not segmental abnormalities, can be analyzed |
| **SSCP:** | single-stranded conformational polymorphism. Electrophoretic mobility of single-stranded DNA depends on its secondary structure, which is changed by mutations; SSCP detects variation in nucleotide sequence in amplified DNA fragments based on strand conformation, and allows nucleotide variations in DNA to be detected without sequencing |
| **WGA:** | Whole Genome Amplification: cellular DNA is randomly amplified after biopsy, increasing the amount available for testing; allows several mutations for a disease as well as aneuploidy to be examined simultaneously. WGA products can be stored for later subsequent analysis, in case of test failure or to confirm diagnosis. |

## Comparative Genomic Hybridization (CGH)

Comparative genomic hybridization, introduced in 1992 by Kallioniemi *et al.*, detects duplications or deletions of chromosome fragments. DNA labeled with a fluorescent dye from a normal control patient is placed on a slide or metaphase plate, alongside fluorescently labeled patient DNA. The two genomes, coded with different colors, are cut enzymatically into small fragments which then reorganize on chromosomes using rules of complementarity and competition for hybridization sites. All quantitative differences between them are visible as a predominance of one color over the other. The main disadvantage of the classic CGH method is its low resolution, which averages 10 Mbp; an improved version, known as array CGH (aCGH), is therefore used in preimplantation diagnosis. Array CGH is considered to be precise and highly specific, but resolution is limited in detecting translocated fragments below 6 Mbp in size.

## Single-Nucleotide Polymorphism (SNP) Analysis

Single-nucleotide polymorphisms are sites in a genome where one nucleotide in a specific *locus* is different from the others in the population. SNP markers utilize platforms/plates that allow thousands or millions of SNPs in a human population to be determined during a single DNA analysis. There are a large number of SNP methods based on hybridization, starter elongation, ligation or so-called invasive rupture. A method designed to screen 24 chromosomes for aneuploidy using SNP was developed in 2010 (Treff *et al.*, 2010).

## Next-Generation Sequencing (NGS)

Next-Generation Sequencing (also known as Massive Parallel Sequencing, MPS) uses sequencing on reaction vessels with a diameter of 3 μm to allow the parallel processing of a large number of nucleic acid molecules, up to an entire human genome. NGS has revolutionized sequencing: more than 10 NGS platforms are currently available, and technology continues to evolve. NGS can be used in fresh and frozen cycles, and can be used to analyze many types of genetic variability. It is the only method that allows aneuploidy or translocation of all chromosomes and mutations responsible for any single-gene disease to be analyzed using one biopsy: whole chromosome abnormalities, segmental abnormalities, translocations, single-gene disorders and mitochondrial disorders can potentially be diagnosed. A number of samples can be simultaneously sequenced during a single 'run,' which reduces the cost per sample.

DNA is first isolated from a single or several cells, and the whole genome is amplified. The DNA is then cut into fragments of 100–200 base pairs and placed on a 2 × 2 cm 'chip.' A sequence of each fragment is then compared to a reference sequence, and the results are analyzed using a computer. The sequencing library can be automated, reducing hands-on time, minimizing human errors and enabling higher throughput and consistency.

## Copy Number Variation Sequencing (CNV-seq)

CNV-seq is a refinement of NGS technology that can detect and quantify gene duplications or deletions. Around 99% of the variations in human gene copy number are benign, but the remainder are associated with clinically significant chromosome disease syndromes. Around 200 different chromosomal diseases are known to be caused by CNV, and these may be either inherited from parents or due to errors occurring during chromosome replication.

## Karyomapping

Karyomapping uses SNP microarray technology to map crossovers between parental haplotypes, using the principles of linkage analysis and chromosomal haploblock inheritance. The mother, father and a reference affected family member or grandparents are compared to map the origin of each chromosome inherited. Karyomap gene chips have been designed that use biomarkers within the genome to assess the probability that an embryo carries a gene variant for single-gene disorders. These can simultaneously analyze nearly 300 000 SNP loci and can be used for PGD of different monogenic diseases as well as PGS for aneuploidy.

*It is now theoretically possible to diagnose >99% of inherited single-gene disorders by PGD; the list includes more than 400 genetic diseases and continues to expand.*

# PGD of Age-Related Aneuploidy (Preimplantation Genetic Screening, PGS/PGD-A)

Up to the present decade, PGS was based primarily on biopsy of polar bodies or cleavage stage embryos with diagnosis based on FISH/PCR. This has now been replaced with blastocyst TE biopsy in combination with advanced CCS techniques +/− blastocyst vitrification, a strategy known as 'PGS 2.0'. However, considerable controversy continues about the safety, efficacy and economic effectiveness of PGS 2.0 (Geraedts & Sermon, 2016; Sermon et al., 2016). At the time of writing, the effectiveness of using PGS as an adjunct in IVF practice is still a subject for debate. Pressure from industry, competition between professionals and sometimes inflexible scientific logic have created fierce 'for or against' stances that do not help patients to make an informed choice. Whereas the benefits of using PGD for selecting healthy embryos in couples with known genetic or chromosomal problems outweighs the use of invasive techniques, the same cannot be said for PGS. Although PGS after blastocyst biopsy (counting chromosomes in an embryo) has been likened to amniocentesis (counting chromosomes in an early fetus), this is an unfortunate comparison. Blastocyst biopsy removes TE cells, part of an essential structure of the embryo: not only does this not necessarily represent the chromosomal constitution of the embryo, but the embryo is still differentiating before it implants. Amniocentesis samples cells that are external to a largely differentiated fetus. This comparison is even more irrational when we consider the tragedy of losing a fetus after amniocentesis, which occurs in about 1 in 200 cases, and the 'nonchalance' of losing a potential baby at the blastocyst stage, which occurs in up to 50% of cases in experienced hands due to damage at biopsy or technical/amplification failure.

## Current Indications for PGS

1. Patients of advanced maternal age, who tend to produce a higher number of aneuploid embryos than younger patients.
2. Patients with repeated implantation failure, recurrent miscarriage and with severe male factor infertility.
3. 'Reduced Time to Pregnancy (TTP)': patients may be told that PGS can reduce the time to achieve a normal pregnancy and may reduce the incidence of miscarriage.

There is currently no clear consensus regarding which patient groups, if any, can benefit from PGS 2.0; however, several considerations are important when a patient is counseled to undertake PGS:

1. Offering a patient PGS at the time of initial consultation, i.e., there is intention to treat, does not increase the patient's chance of pregnancy.
2. PGS does not improve an embryo but is merely a selection procedure.
3. Many embryos (up to 50% in less experienced laboratories) are lost in the diagnosis due to biopsy or amplification failure.
4. The biopsy is always invasive and leads to damage to the TE, an essential part of mammalian development.
5. Next-generation sequencing can diagnose inherited genetic disease, but it does not define embryo viability or health: it does not guarantee that genes are free from DNA breaks/errors, or that they will be expressed/transcribed correctly at the appropriate time in preimplantation development.
6. PGS cannot detect embryos whose health has been jeopardized by metabolic malfunctions due to epigenetic effects resulting from inherent gamete physiology or suboptimal in-vitro culture and handling (Swain, 2019).
7. The phenomenon of mosaicism is of crucial importance. The cells in the TE may differ from one region to another and therefore a biopsy may not be representative of the whole embryo.
8. Mosaic embryos in any case can give rise to healthy babies: mouse models show the extent of repair from mosaicism (see below).
9. A correct chromosome number does not guarantee a live birth nor, indeed, successful implantation. It has become increasingly clear that nongenomic factors, including mitochondrial activity, methylation patterns, cytoplasmic glutathione levels, or a myriad of biochemical and physiological parameters are necessary for a viable embryo and a healthy birth. For example, it has been estimated that up to 2 million DNA repair processes are carried out at the time of the first cell cycle.

Homeostasis in oocytes, as in all cells, depends on a complex interaction of cell signaling pathways which in turn are fueled by metabolic pathways, both aerobic and anaerobic. Defective signaling leads to cytoskeletal deficiencies, which lead, amongst many other cellular effects, to aneuploidy. A correct chromosome number in any cell (ploidy) is a reflection of normal cytoplasmic processes that contribute to correct cytoskeletal alignment and function, allowing the chromosomes to be evenly divided during meiosis/mitosis. Any malfunction in cell signaling/metabolic systems due to upstream cytoplasmic factors can jeopardize cytoskeletal function and result in aneuploidy; in other words, chromosome number is the gross morphological expression of cellular dysfunction – not its cause. A study by Sagawa *et al.* (2017) lends support to this principle: cytogenetic analysis of products of conception obtained from 1030 biochemical pregnancies (7–10 weeks' gestation) following ICSI and vitrified-warmed single blastocyst transfer identified 19.4% of the embryos as having a normal karyotype; no difference was found in the frequency of karyotypes compared with morphological blastocyst quality. Of the 80.6% aneuploid karyotypes, trisomy was the most frequent, with age-related significant differences for trisomy 16 in patients aged <37 years, and trisomy 20 in those >38 years. The results of this study confirm that some euploid embryos are unable to sustain a normal pregnancy; transferred embryos with serious abnormalities are probably eliminated by natural selection by the 7th week of pregnancy, or by the time the gestational sac is formed.

10. Blastocyst formation is a fundamental step in mammalian embryogenesis. An amazingly complex structure with clear developmental purpose, it is subject to regulation at the morphological, cellular, transcriptional and epigenetic levels. TE biopsy is a radical intervention involving an essential layer of cells that leads to collapse of the blastocyst cavity at a delicate moment in preimplantation development, with probable modification of epithelial elements important in cellular communication and differentiation, such as gap junctions and ion and water pumps. The TE plays a fundamental part in cross-talk with the endometrium and the production of enzymes for hatching: bovine implantation may be improved by adding trophectoderm tissue to the blastocyst (Heyman *et al.*, 1987). Introducing widespread blastocyst stage PGS screening would mean that a sizable part of the TE is eliminated in all biopsied healthy embryos that lead to birth and children born with an essential part of their preimplantation development compromised by dissection. Although the preimplantation mammalian embryo is highly regulative and may recover from such surgery, we do not know the long-term consequences of TE biopsy.

11. A three-fold increase in the risk of maternal pre-eclampsia has been found after trophectoderm biopsy for preimplantation genetic testing (Zhang *et al.*, 2019)

12. PGS may double the cost of a standard IVF treatment.

## Chromosomal Mosaicism and Embryo Repair

The phenomenon of chromosomal mosaicism in the human embryo has been known for some time. It has been estimated that the placenta has a different karyotype from the fetus (confined placental mosaicism – CPM) in 1% of conceptions. CPM was first detected when first trimester fetal karyotyping after CVS showed discrepancies between chorionic cells and the embryo proper. All of the studies performed in recent years to analyze chromosomes in embryos have been carried out using embryos generated by IVF, which may not be representative of in-vivo development. However, the classic studies of Hertig *et al.* (1956) showed that embryos from natural cycles also showed high levels of nuclear abnormalities, and studies of normally conceived pregnancies have revealed that 60% of abortions are chromosomally abnormal. The majority of human preimplantation embryos are mosaic in relation to chromosome numbers, with the embryo containing a number of both euploid and aneuploid cells. Errors in mitosis during the first cleavage divisions lead to this mosaic pattern. It was thought that the high rates of human pregnancy loss in both spontaneous and IVF cycles was due to this chromosomal inaccuracy; however, recent studies have shown that mosaic human embryos can develop into normal healthy babies.

An exciting new study on a mouse model from the laboratory of Magdalena Zernicka-Goetz in Cambridge has shown a fundamental difference in the capacity of the TE and the inner cell mass to deal with aneuploidy. The fetal lineage eliminates aneuploid cells by apoptosis, while aneuploid cells in the TE exhibit limited proliferation. Self-repair can occur in mouse blastocysts containing up to 50% aneuploid cells in the inner cell mass and lead to the birth of normal pups (Bolton *et al.*, 2016). If human embryos have the same capacity as the mouse to eliminate or repair aneuploidy, then selecting embryos on the basis of chromosomal number in human IVF makes little sense.

Studies on embryos donated for research and those with abnormal fertilization (such as polyspermic embryos) have shown that the latter were highly abnormal, in agreement with karyotype data. Mosaicism was observed in the majority of cases, but normal diploid embryos from supposedly polyspermic embryos were sometimes identified; this may have been due to misidentification of a vacuole as a pronucleus. As expected, embryos from older women show high levels of chromosome abnormalities, but, interestingly, normally fertilized, normally developing embryos also show high levels of chromosomal abnormalities. Patterns have been categorized into four groups:

(a) uniformly diploid,
(b) uniformly abnormal, such as Down's syndrome or Turner's,
(c) mosaic, where usually both diploid cells and aneuploid, haploid or polyploid nuclei are present or
(d) chaotic embryos, where every nucleus shows a different chromosome complement.

The data from FISH and CGH analysis show a higher rate of abnormalities than has previously been reported from karyotyping data. However, since mosaic and chaotic embryos are common, if only one or two cells are analyzable from an embryo, then karyotyping would underestimate the level of chromosome abnormalities.

Normal, abnormal and mosaic embryos have all been observed in fetal development; as mentioned previously, confined placental mosaicism has been found in an estimated 1% of conceptions. The presence of two cell lines could arise due to an abnormal chromosome arrangement caused by a postzygotic event, or the chromosome loss from a trisomic embryo, which restores the diploid state (trisomic rescue). Several mechanisms would indicate that these abnormal cells are more likely to be found in the TE, and hence the placenta. First, only a few cells from a blastocyst give rise to the embryo, and it would be unlikely that the abnormal cells would be found in the embryo; second, in most cases a fetus with abnormal chromosomes will not be compatible with life. The chaotic group of embryos was an unexpected finding, as such embryos have not been observed in later stages of embryonic development, probably because these embryos would arrest and fail to implant.

Multinucleated blastomeres have been reported and confirmed from both karyotyping and FISH analysis. The presence of such blastomeres may be more common in arrested embryos and may occur more readily in some patients. Binucleate blastomeres have been observed in mouse embryos at the morula stage, and it has been suggested that these blastomeres might be the precursors for mural TE giant cells. However, in human embryos the binucleate cells appear at cleavage stages before TE differentiation. Binucleate cells may arise from asymmetrical cytokinesis so that one daughter cell contains two nuclei and the other is anucleate. In addition, aneuploidy can activate a spindle-apparatus checkpoint in different types of cells, causing multinucleation in that cell; it is possible that blastomere multinucleation may be the equivalent of a cell cycle checkpoint, which can convert a mosaic embryo to one that is euploid (Tesarik, 2018).

Embryos containing tetraploid cells may be a normal part of development of the TE. Such cells have also been found in cattle, pig and sheep. Overall, extrapolation of this data would suggest that few embryos are completely chromosomally normal at early cleavage stage. However, various models for which there are experimental data may help to explain the observation that pregnancies following IVF do not result in an increased incidence of chromosomally abnormal infants. Few cells (possibly a single cell from an eight-cell embryo) differentiate to the embryo proper – the majority contribute to the cytotrophoblast and fetal membranes. Data accumulated on the chromosomal constitution of surplus non-transferred embryos from PGD cycles have revealed that, despite the fact that these embryos are from women of proven fertility, the incidence of postzygotic chromosomal anomalies is similar to that in embryos from routine IVF patients. This finding may provide one explanation for the apparently poor success rate of IVF procedures. A second significant finding is that the incidence of the most bizarre type of anomaly, chaotically dividing embryos, is strongly patient-related. In repeated cycles, certain women regularly produced 'chaotic' embryos while others did not, although the frequency of diploid mosaics was similar in both groups.

A study by Lagalla *et al.* (2017) presents interesting evidence of self-correction during preimplantation development in human embryos. This group analyzed blastocyst TE biopsies by array CGH after blastocyst TE biopsy, as well as excluded cells of 18 blastocysts that developed from partially compacted morulas. These results were compared with retrospective time-lapse morphokinetic data for the same embryos, in order to identify whether embryos from irregular cleavage divisions, which are presumed to have an abnormal chromosome complement, could develop into euploid blastocysts. Although embryos identified as having irregular cleavage were at increased risk of developmental arrest, some of them did reach blastocyst stage, producing chromosomally normal embryos. Some of these embryos were also observed to have incomplete compaction at the morula stage, with exclusion of some cells, and the authors hypothesize that this cell exclusion might represent a 'correction' mechanism, rescuing embryos from chromosomal aneuploidy after abnormal cleavage by preferentially eliminating anomalous cells. Their results further suggested that this hypothetical self-correction mechanism is less efficient in embryos from older women (age >39 years).

## Mosaicism and PGD

Chromosomal mosaicism may confound PGD for some diseases, namely dominant disorders and chromosome abnormalities. A misdiagnosis of embryo sex would be unlikely to occur as an XX cell would have to be found in an XY embryo. XO cells have been identified in male embryos, but XO embryos should never be considered for transfer; if the offspring have Turner's syndrome, they would have the same risk of suffering the X-linked disease as would a male. For recessive disorders, the presence of extra chromosomes or a haploid cell would not lead to a misdiagnosis. A carrier embryo with a haploid cell would be diagnosed as normal or affected depending on which gene was present in the cell: this would be the same situation if allele dropout had occurred. For dominant disorders, a haploid cell could lead to a misdiagnosis; if a cell from an affected embryo carried only the unaffected gene, the cell would be diagnosed as normal. Therefore, the same precautions as for allele dropout would have to be applied. For chromosome abnormalities, mosaic embryos containing some normal and some abnormal cells have been identified, such as in cases where a few normal cells arise in an embryo which otherwise carried trisomy 21. If the normal cells are biopsied, the embryo would be diagnosed as normal, resulting in misdiagnosis. As with confined placental mosaicism, this problem cannot be solved. Patients undergoing PGD for chromosomal abnormalities have to be aware that chromosomal mosaicism can lead to a misdiagnosis, but that this is a rare event.

## Ethics and Laws

The law governing PGD varies worldwide. Some countries have legislation regulating PGD, or PGD and embryo research, and others have no legislation. Although a few countries banned cleavage stage biopsy, blastocyst biopsy means that this is no longer of any relevance. Some of the arguments against PGD include the fact that it may be abused, as in the case of embryo sex selection for family balancing, or for choosing certain characteristics, the so-called 'Designer Baby.' Prenatal diagnosis has been abused for fetal sex selection in several countries for many years, but, as with all medical practices, the good should outweigh the bad: such practices should not be banned just because they could be abused. Legislation governing the use of PGD should eliminate such problems. In the United Kingdom, the Human Fertilisation and Embryology Authority (HFEA), which licenses all IVF practices, licenses PGD centers separately, and has banned embryo sexing for family balancing. It must be remembered that undertaking PGD is a significant ordeal for couples, as the IVF procedure is so invasive, and the pregnancy rate is low. If couples wished to select their baby, the cheaper and simpler route would be prenatal diagnosis, where many diseases could be diagnosed at one time.

## The Future of PGD

PGD is more complicated than originally thought: the concept that a single cell would be representative of the rest of the embryo has been confused and compounded by the discovery of high levels of chromosomal mosaicism in human embryos, as well as by an increased understanding of the numerous complexities surrounding preimplantation development. Although techniques and technology have significantly reduced the incidence of misdiagnosis, unfortunately this can still occur, due to chromosomal mosaicism, allele dropout or contamination (possible from cumulus or sperm cells).

Cost is also an important consideration, as some single-cell diagnoses are expensive techniques, and array technology is currently very expensive. For example, the cost of diagnostic technology can equal the cost of an IVF treatment cycle, which makes PGD a very expensive technique. In the United Kingdom, some health authorities have paid for PGD cycles, and in other countries government or health insurance funds are available; if patients have to meet the cost themselves, they may opt for prenatal diagnosis.

Data from the ESHRE PGD consortium shows that the delivery rate per cycle for PGD is similar to that seen in IVF, even though PGD patients are normally fertile. Therefore, any center or patient embarking on PGD has to be aware that the diagnosis may not be 100% accurate due to mosaicism and technical problems, and that the chance of an unaffected baby after one cycle is low. The patients also have to decide whether undertaking an IVF cycle is more or less traumatic than natural conception and prenatal diagnosis. The natural pregnancy rate for patients registered for PGD may be high, as most of them have the alternative of prenatal diagnosis.

Patients who carry chromosome abnormalities are one of the most difficult groups of patients to treat, due to the high levels of abnormal embryos they produce.

Many couples around the world opt for PGD as an alternative to prenatal diagnosis, and several thousand babies have been born. Although it is a demanding technique that requires a fully equipped molecular biology laboratory, highly skilled molecular biologists and close collaboration with clinical geneticists, technical breakthroughs over the past decade continue to make PGD a very real alternative for couples at risk. Hopefully, improvements in IVF and single-cell diagnosis will increase the range of diseases that can be diagnosed at the single-cell level in order to help as many couples who carry genetic disease as possible.

# Further Reading

## Books and Reviews

Elder K, Cohen J (eds.) (2007) *Human Preimplantation Embryo Evaluation and Selection.* Informa Press, London.

Dale B, Ménézo Y, Coppola G (2015) Trends, Fads and Art. *Journal of Assisted Reproduction and Genetics* 32: 489–493.

Dale B, Ménézo Y, Elder K (2016) Who benefits from PGS? *Austin Journal of IVF* 3: 1026.

Dahdouh EM, Balayla J, Audibert F, Genetics Committee (2015) Technical update: preimplantation genetic diagnosis and screening. *Journal of Obstetrics and Gynaecology Canada* 37(5): 451–463.

De Ryck M, Goossens V, Kokkali G, *et al.* (2017) ESHRE PGD Consortium data collection XIV–XV: cycles from January 2011 to December 2012 with pregnancy follow-up to October 2013. *Human Reproduction* 32(10): 1974–1994.

Fauser B (2006) Pre-implantation genetic screening: the end of an affair? *Human Reproduction* 23: 2622–2625.

Geraedts J, Sermon K (2016) Preimplantation genetic screening 2.0: the theory. *Molecular Human Reproduction* 22(8): 539–544.

Gleicher N, Orvieto R (2017) Is the hypothesis of pre-implantation genetic screening (PGS) still supportable? A review. *Journal of Ovarian Research* 10: 1–7.

Harper J, Delhanty JDA, Handyside AH (2001) *Preimplantation Genetic Diagnosis.* Cambridge University Press, Cambridge, UK.

Harper J (2009) *Preimplantation Genetic Diagnosis*, 2nd edn. Cambridge University Press, Cambridge, UK.

Hayward J, Chitty L (2018) Beyond screening for chromosomal abnormalities: advances in non-invasive diagnosis of single gene disorders and fetal exome sequencing. *Seminars in Fetal and Neonatal Medicine* 23(2): 94–101.

Mastenbroek S, Repping S (2014) Preimplantation genetic screening: back to the future. *Human Reproduction* 29: 1846–1850.

Meaney C, Norbury G (2011) Non-invasive prenatal diagnosis. In: Theophilus B, Rapley R (eds.) *PCR Mutation Detection Protocols*. Methods in Molecular Biology (Methods and Protocols), vol 688. Humana Press, Springer Science + Business Media, London, pp. 155–172.

Munné S (2018) Status of preimplantation genetic testing and embryo selection. *Reproductive BioMedicine Online* 28(4): 393–396.

Sanders KD, Griffin KD (2017) Chromosomal preimplantation genetic diagnosis: 25 years and counting. *Journal of Fetal Medicine* 4(2): 51–56.

Sermon K, Capalbo A, Cohen J, *et al.* (2016) The why, the how and the when of PGS 2.0: current practices and expert opinions of fertility specialists, molecular biologists and embryologists. *Molecular Human Reproduction* 22(8): 545–557.

## Research Articles

Bolton H, Graham S, Van de Aa N (2016) Mouse model of a chromosome mosaicism reveals lineage-specific depletion of aneuploid cells and normal developmental potential. *Nature Communications* 7: 11165.

Coonen E, Harper JC, Ramaekers FCS, *et al.* (1994) Presence of chromosomal mosaicism in abnormal preimplantation embryos detected by fluorescent in situ hybridisation. *Human Genetics* 54: 609–615.

Delhanty JDA, Griffin DK, Handyside AH, *et al.* (1993) Detection of aneuploidy and chromosomal mosaicism in human embryos during preimplantation sex determination by fluorescent in situ hybridization (FISH). *Human Molecular Genetics* 2(8): 1183–1185.

Delhanty JDA, Harper JC, Ao A, Handyside AH, Winston RML (1997) Multicolour FISH detects frequent chromosomal mosaicism and chaotic division in normal preimplantation embryos from fertile patients. *Human Genetics* 99: 755–760.

Gardner RL, Edwards RG (1968) Control of the sex ratio at full term in the rabbit by transferring sexed blastocysts. *Nature* 218: 346–349.

Gianaroli L, Magli MC, Ferraretti AP, Munné S (1999) Preimplantation diagnosis for aneuploidies in patients undergoing in-vitro fertilization with a poor prognosis: identification of the categories for which it should be proposed. *Fertility and Sterility* 72(5): 837–844.

Handyside AH, Kontogianni EH, Hardy K, Winston RM (1990) Pregnancies from biopsied human preimplantation embryos sexed by Y-specific DNA amplification. *Nature* 344(6268): 768–770.

Harper JC, Coonan E, Handyside AH, *et al.* (1995) Mosaicism of autosomes and sex chromosomes in morphologically normal, monospermic preimplantation human embryos. *Prenatal Diagnosis* 15: 41–49.

Harper J, Jackson E, Sermon K, *et al.* (2017) Adjuncts in the IVF laboratory: where is the evidence for add-on interventions. *Human Reproduction* 32(3): 485–449.

Hertig AT, Rock J, Adams EC (1956) A description of 34 human ova within the first 17 days of development. *American Journal of Anatomy* 98: 435.

James RM, West JD (1994) A chimaeric animal model for confined placental mosaicism. *Human Genetics* 93: 603–604.

Heyman Y, Chesné P, Chupin D, Ménézo Y (1987) Improvement of survival rate of frozen cattle blastocysts after transfer with trophoblastic vesicles. *Theriogenology* 27: 477–484.

Kallioniemi A, Kallioniemi OP, Sudar D, *et al.* (1992) Comparative genomic hybridization for molecular cytogenetic analysis of solid tumors. *Science* 258: 818–821.

Lagalla C, Tarozzi N, Sciajno R, *et al.* (2017) Embryos with morphokinetic abnormalities may develop into euploid blastocysts. *Reproductive BioMedicine Online* 34(2): 137–146.

Liss J, Chromik I, Szczyglinska J, Jagiello M, Lukaszuk A, Lukaszuk K (2016) Current methods for pre-implantation genetic diagnosis. *Ginekologia Polska* 87: 522–526.

Mackie FL, Hemming K, Allen S, Morris RK, Kilby MD (2017) The accuracy of cell-free fetal DNA-based non-invasive prenatal testing in singleton pregnancies: a systematic review and bivariate meta-analysis. *British Journal of Obstetrics and Gynaecology* 124: 32–46.

Mastenbroek S, Twisk M, van Echten-Arends J, *et al.* (2007) In vitro fertilization with preimplantation genetic screening. *New England Journal of Medicine* 357: 9–17.

Munné S, Scott R, Sable D, Cohen J (1998) First pregnancies after preconception diagnosis of translocations of maternal origin. *Fertility and Sterility* 69(4): 675–681.

Munné S, Wells D (2003) Questions concerning the suitability of comparative genomic hybridization for preimplantation genetic diagnosis. *Fertility and Sterility* 80(4): 871–872; discussion 875.

Munné S, Grifo J, Wells D (2016) Mosaicism: survival of the fittest vs no embryo left behind. *Fertility and Sterility* 105: 1146–1149.

Platteau P, Staessen C, Michiels A, *et al.* (2006) Which patients with recurrent implantation failure after IVF benefit from PGD for aneuploidy screening? *Reproductive BioMedicine Online* 12(3): 334–339.

Sagawa T, Kuroda T, Kato K, *et al.* (2017) Cytogenetic analysis of the retained products of conception after missed abortion following blastocyst transfer: a retrospective, large-scale, single-centre study. *Reproductive BioMedicine Online* 34(2): 203–210.

Schattman G (2018) Chromosomal mosaicism in human pre-implantation embryos: another fact that cannot be ignored. *Fertility and Sterility* 109: 54–55.

Schrurs BM, Winston RM, Handyside AH (1993) Preimplantation diagnosis of aneuploidy using fluorescent in-situ hybridization: evaluation using a chromosome 18-specific probe. *Human Reproduction* 8: 296–301.

Sermondade N, Mandelbaum J (2009) Mastenbroek controversy or how much ink is spilled on preimplantation genetic screening subject? *Gynécologie Obstétrique & Fertilité* 37(3): 252–256.

Swain J (2019) Controversies in ART: can the IVF laboratory influence preimplantation embryo aneuploidy? *Reproductive BioMedicine Online* 39(4), published online September 2019.

Tesarik J (2018) Is blastomere multinucleation a safeguard against embryo aneuploidy? Back to the future. *Reproductive BioMedicine Online* 37(4): 506–507.

Treff NR, Su J, Tao X, *et al.* (2010) Accurate single cell 24 chromosome aneuploidy screening using whole genome amplification and single nucleotide polymorphism microarrays. *Fertility and Sterility* 94: 2017–2021.

Vanneste E, Voet T, Melotte C, *et al.*(2009) What next for pre-implantation genetic screening: high mitotic chromosome instability rate provides the biological basis for the low success rate. *Human Reproduction* 24: 2679–2682.

Verlinsky Y, Cieslak J, Freidine M, *et al.* (1995) Pregnancies following pre-conception diagnosis of common aneuploidies by fluorescent in situ hybridisation. *Molecular Human Reproduction* 10: 1927–1934.

Verlinsky Y, Strom C, Cieslak J, *et al.* (1996) Birth of healthy children after preimplantation diagnosis of common aneuploidies by polar body fluorescent in situ hybridisation analysis. *Fertility and Sterility* 66: 126–129.

Wells D (2007) Future genetic and other technologies for assessing embryos. In: Elder K, Cohen J (eds.) *Human Preimplantation Embryo Evaluation and Selection*. Informa Press, London, pp. 287–300.

Zhang WY, von Versen-Höynck F, Kapphahn KL, *et al.*, (2019) Maternal and neonatal outcomes associated with trophectoderm biopsy. *Fertility and Sterility*. 112(2): 283–290.e2.

# Chapter 15

# Epigenetics and Human Assisted Reproduction

John Huntriss

## Introduction

During mammalian development the growth of the fetus is regulated by genetic information that is inherited from both the sperm and the oocyte. Apart from the clear differences that are associated with the X and Y chromosomes, the parental genetic contributions to the embryo also differ via a system of 'epigenetic' marks. The differences in function between the parental genomes, how gametes and preimplantation embryos are reprogrammed, and how these delicate processes may be affected by ART and infertility will be described in this chapter. A full understanding of the cellular and molecular biology of human reproduction must include a study of epigenetics and genomic imprinting.

## Epigenetics

Epigenetics is an additional 'layer' of information that complements the information in the genomic DNA sequence; it is essentially a marking system that regulates gene expression and hence the phenotype of the cell. An epigenetic mark either modifies a DNA base sequence chemically, or modifies another molecule (e.g., histone) that leads to a change in chromatin structure. These modifications influence the way that DNA interacts with transcription complexes and other regulatory factors, altering the sequence information that is read by the cell. This level of gene expression is known as the 'epigenotype'; an incorrect representation of the information, such as occurs in an epigenetic disease, is an 'epimutation.' An epigenetic marking system is essential for normal mammalian development, and disruption of the process can lead to disease. Epigenetic marks are extensively reprogrammed during gametogenesis and preimplantation development, subsequently instructing the growth and development of the conceptus. It is therefore crucial to ensure that these intricate processes are adequately

supported during ART pathways and manipulations. The biological mechanisms that are regulated via epigenetic modification include X chromosome inactivation and parent-of-origin effects of genomic imprinting, as well as tissue-specific and age-dependent DNA modification. Epigenetic information is also responsible for the phenotypic variability of somatic cells within an organism, controlling how tissues and cells in the body define themselves. For example, within a human individual, the genotype (the gene complement) is the same for different types of cells (e.g., a muscle cell or a liver cell), yet the cellular functions and phenotypes are very different. Although the DNA sequence within these different cells is identical, the repertoire of expressed genes differs greatly between cell types, a difference that is essential in determining the specific functions of different cells.

## Epigenetic Marks

The mechanisms that contribute to imprinting include DNA methylation, histone modification and RNA-mediated (transcriptional) mechanisms. DNA methylation is stable but reprogrammable, heritable and affects the regulation of gene expression. This type of epigenetic mark involves methylation of CpG dinucleotides around certain genes. For example, a gene whose active expression is required in a liver cell may be unmethylated across the majority of CpG sites in the promoter area of its sequence, whereas a gene that needs to be silenced in the liver may be heavily methylated, repressing transcription by 'locking' the genes within an inaccessible heterochromatin structure.

Histone proteins are important in DNA packaging; they can be covalently modified by a number of post-translational modifications that significantly affect whether chromatin conformation is open or closed. 'Open' chromatin is accessible to DNA replication and transcription (gene expression), and 'closed' chromatin is not accessible. Chromatin conformation is affected by modification of histone tails via methylation, acetylation, phosphorylation etc., especially those of H3 and H4 histones. Each different modification or combination of modifications affects chromatin structure, and thus gene expression, differently. In many situations, both DNA methylation and the histone modification 'code' probably contribute to the overall process of epigenetic regulation.

RNA is increasingly recognized as an important epigenetic regulator, including small noncoding RNA (sncRNA) classes that are expressed in oocytes and preimplantation embryos. For example, microRNAs (miRNAs) are short, noncoding RNA molecules 21 to 24 nucleotides in length that can contribute to an RNA-induced silencing complex; this complex can regulate gene expression by post-transcriptional mechanisms that silence a gene. Surprisingly, mammalian spermatozoa carry sncRNAs: these may be involved in epigenetic processes that are important for the early stages of fertilization (Rivera & Ross, 2013; Yuan *et al.*, 2016).

---

### Histone Nomenclature

Histone modifications are named by using:

- the name of the histone (e.g., H3)
- the abbreviation for the amino acid and its position within the modified histone protein (e.g., K9 for lysine at position 9)
- the type of epigenetic modification (e.g., 'me' for methylation)
- the extent of the particular modification (e.g., mono, di or tri-methylation: me1, me2, me3).

---

# Genomic Imprinting

Genomic imprinting is the exclusive expression of only one of the parental alleles of a gene, a unique mode of gene expression that affects the growth and development of the fetus according to whether an allele of a particular imprinted gene is inherited paternally or maternally. In normal circumstances, imprinting exerts fine control over the growth of the developing conceptus via the placenta. A number of human diseases involve abnormal regulation of imprinted genes or 'parent of origin' effects, and disruption of imprinting can lead to cancer (Walter and Paulsen, 2003; Holm *et al.*, 2005). Genomic imprinting is particularly susceptible to disruption during early preimplantation

development, and is therefore vulnerable to potential aberrations that may be introduced through certain ART procedures.

Over 200 genes that show imprinted monoallelic expression have been described to date in humans (Morison & Reeve, 1998; Skaar *et al.*, 2012). Genomic imprinting is regulated by imprinting control regions or imprinting centers (ICRs or ICs) that acquire epigenetic marks such as DNA methylation upon passage through the germline. Imprinted genes on maternal and paternal alleles have different methylation patterns (differentially methylated regions, DMRs) that are important in regulating gene expression. DMRs typically consist of stretches of differentially methylated CpG sites that are close to an imprinted gene, and this epigenetic information regulates allele-specific gene expression. A germline DMR will therefore have a different methylation pattern in the sperm than in the oocyte, and this differential marking will be recognized in the zygote and preimplantation embryo. The majority of imprinted genes are located in clusters within the genome and are regulated by ICRs that instruct all or most of the imprinted genes in a cluster.

Figure 15.1 shows a simplified representation of differential allele marking of an imprinted gene in the germline, which leads to monoallelic expression in somatic tissue of the offspring. The paternal allele is not methylated in sperm (left), whilst the maternal allele is methylated in the oocyte (right). This differential methylation imprint persists after fertilization and early development. The epigenetic mark (methylation) placed on the allele during oogenesis silences the maternal allele in the offspring, and only the paternal allele is transcribed to mRNA (bent arrow). The correct dosage of imprinted gene transcripts is critical in early development (Charalambous *et al.*, 2012). Imprinted genes are also believed to play a role in the parent–offspring conflict model (Moore and Haig, 1991), a theory proposing that the parental alleles of these loci have different interests with respect to regulation of fetal, placental and neonatal growth; i.e., the paternal genome will fight for the biggest size and health of the current litter (his litter), whereas the maternal genome will try to counter or moderate this effect in order to reduce current nutritional strain on herself and ensure that she will be able to raise future litters. This hypothesis is reinforced by the fact that many imprinted genes regulate growth of the fetus and placenta. Imprinting may also prevent

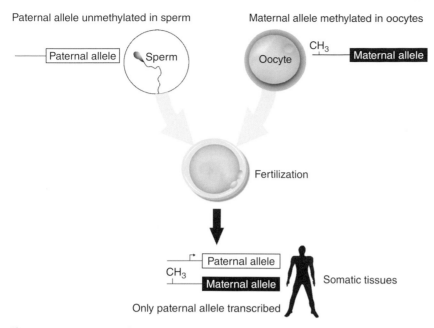

Paternal allele unmethylated in sperm

Maternal allele methylated in oocytes

Paternal allele · Sperm

Oocyte · $CH_3$ · Maternal allele

Fertilization

Paternal allele

$CH_3$ · Maternal allele

Somatic tissues

Only paternal allele transcribed

**Figure 15.1** Epigenetic information from the germline regulates genomic imprinting.

parthenogenesis, since it ensures that both parental genomes are necessary for an embryo to develop to term (Kono, 2009).

# Epigenetic Reprogramming in the Germline

The mature oocyte and sperm are highly specialized cells, and this means that their cellular specialization needs a significant amount of epigenetic information. Information inherited from the previous generation must be erased in primordial germ cells, so that new epigenetic information may be subsequently added according to whether the primordial germ cell is destined to become an oocyte or a sperm cell (Figure 15.2). Extensive epigenetic reprogramming is therefore required in the primordial germ cells (erasure) and during gametogenesis (establishment) (see Morgan et al., 2005 for review). The most complete information available for reprogramming is via DNA methylation, but other epigenetic marks (e.g., the histone code) are also reprogrammed in primordial germ cells and during gametogenesis.

## Erasure

Reprogramming events have been studied extensively in the mouse (reviewed in Constância et al., 1998). Mouse primordial germ cells are identifiable by embryonic Day E7.5, and they then migrate to the genital ridge by Day E10.5–11.5, where they form the gonadal primordia. At

this stage, primordial germ cells still retain methylation patterns derived from the oocyte and sperm, and any of their respective modifications from early development. At Day E13.5, male germ cells enter into mitotic arrest and female germ cells enter meiotic prophase. Between Days E10.5 and E13.5 DNA at imprinted genes is globally demethylated in the primordial germ cells of both sexes, as well as at many DNA elements including Intracisternal A Particles, AIPS (retroviral elements containing long terminal repeats), Line 1 sequences (long interspersed nucleotide elements), direct repeats and non-CpG island genes. Each element displays a unique erasure profile, and different degrees of demethylation occur between the various elements (see Lees-Murdock and Walsh, 2008 for review).

## Establishment

After methylation has been erased, the germ cells that are still diploid undergo de novo methylation. In mouse gametogenesis, the majority of DNA remethylation occurs around Day E15.5 in both sexes, although timing does vary between the various elements; timing also differs between the male germline and female germline (Lees-Murdock and Walsh, 2008). IAPs, Line 1 sequences and other elements are fully methylated in mature sperm. Certain genes escape this remethylation, for example those containing CpG islands (genomic regions with high

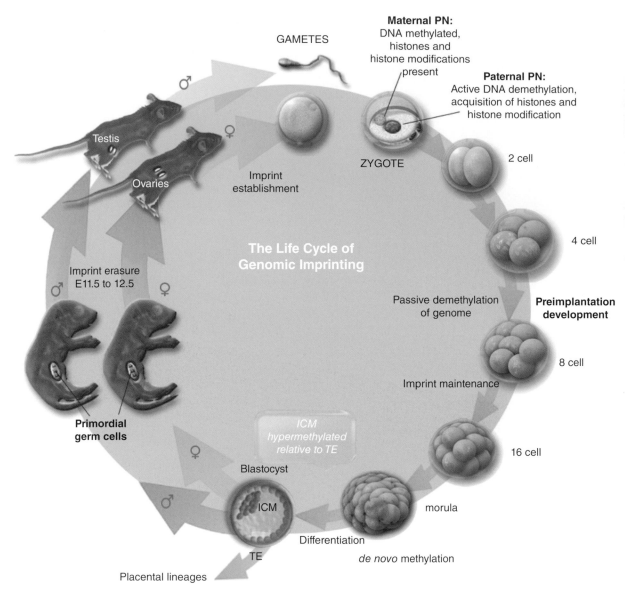

**Figure 15.2** The life cycle of genomic imprinting (adapted with permission from Morgan *et al.*, 2005). Imprint erasure, establishment and maintenance are all features of the epigenetic reprogramming cycle that is required for genomic imprinting. In this figure, the imprint is via DNA methylation. Extensive reprogramming occurs in the primordial germ cells, erasing the imprints from the previous generation. Imprints are re-established during gametogenesis according to the sex of the embryo, maintained in the embryo, and translated into stable functional differences between the parental alleles in the developing conceptus. Extensive epigenetic reprogramming of the paternal pronucleus occurs in zygotes.

densities of CpG nucleotides, which are distinct from the smaller differentially methylated CpG sites of imprinted genes).

Imprinting marks are established according to the sex of the individual (i.e., whether the germ cell is an oogonium or spermatogonium), and most of the imprinted genes acquire methylation in the female germline. The H19 imprinted gene is methylated in the male germline. Despite the fact that epigenetic information has been erased in the primordial germ cells, sufficient underlying epigenetic information remains so that the parental origin of all of the alleles can still be distinguished: for H19 in the male germline, the DMR on the paternal allele is completely remethylated by E15.5, whilst the maternal DMR is remethylated around birth.

In the female germline, maternal DMRs remain hypomethylated until the pachytene stage of meiosis I in the postnatal growing oocyte. Maternal methylation imprints are acquired during oocyte growth, and the DMRs for different imprinted genes appear to be remethylated at different times. Thus, imprinted genes *Snrpn*, *Znf127*, and *Ndn* are methylated by the primary follicle stage, *Peg3* and *Igf2r* genes are methylated by the secondary follicle stage, and the *Impact* gene is methylated by the antral follicle stage. As in the male germline, some underlying epigenetic signal is retained since the maternally inherited alleles of *Snrpn*, *Zac1* and *Peg1* genes are methylated before the paternally inherited alleles (Obata and Kono, 2002; Lucifero *et al.*, 2004; Hiura *et al.*, 2006).

The DNA methyltransferases (Dnmts) play a major role in the establishment of methylation imprints during gametogenesis; the de novo methyltransferases Dnmt3a, Dnmt3b and the related protein Dnmt3L are expressed coordinately and work together to establish methylation imprints during oogenesis. Methylation at imprinted genes in oocytes appears to be dependent on the size of the oocyte, and it has been suggested that methylation is linked to the accumulation of DNA methyltransferases during the growth phase. In oocytes, histone H3K4 must be demethylated (via KDM1B histone demethylase) before the DNA methylation imprints are established; transcription through imprinted gene DMRs keeps chromatin domains open and accessible for methylation (Figure 15.3).

# Epigenetic Events during Fertilization and Preimplantation Development

Parental genomes are packaged differently in the gametes and during the first stages of fertilization. The maternal genome from the oocyte is nucleosomal, whilst the paternal genome from the sperm is condensed and packaged mostly by protamines, which are quickly lost and replaced by histones after sperm entry into the oocyte. During pronuclear maturation, the paternal pronucleus undergoes significant chromatin reorganization, with active demethylation during the transition from PN0 to PN5 and metaphase, followed by histone acquisition toward the end of PN maturation. The male pronucleus gathers epigenetic marks such as H3K9me1 and me2, and H3K27me2/3, whilst the maternal pronucleus, largely rich in histone epigenetic marks, remains relatively unchanged from PN0 to PN5. This difference between male and female pronuclei is referred to as 'epigenetic asymmetry.' By the end of pronuclear maturation (PN4/PN5), DNA methylation (5MeC) is removed from the male pronucleus. Active demethylation is mediated by the ten-eleven translocation (TET) family of enzymes, which hydroxylate 5-methylcytosine to 5-hydroxymethylcytosine (5-hmC) (Hill *et al.*, 2014; see also Chapter 1, DNA methylation). Differential histone modifications between the parental genomes are observed in the early embryo (reviewed in Corry *et al.*, 2009).

DNA methylation is again reprogrammed during preimplantation development (reviewed in Reik *et al.*,

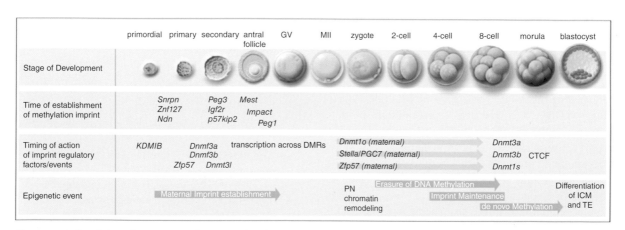

**Figure 15.3** Regulation of imprinting in the mouse female germline. The approximate sequence of gene-specific imprint establishment in the mouse female germline is illustrated, showing factors that are relevant to the reprogramming events. Imprinted genes receive methylation imprints at different times during the oocyte growth phase. The lower panel shows key reprogramming phases that occur at imprinted genes and in the genome as a whole. GV = germinal vesicle; MII = metaphase II; PN = pronuclear; ICM = inner cell mass; TE = trophectoderm.

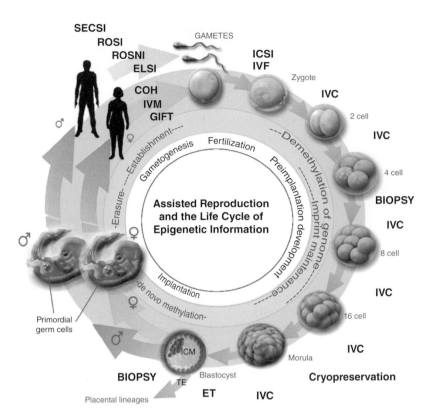

**Figure 15.4** Assisted reproduction procedures associated with epigenetic errors, based on animal and/or human studies, superimposed on the main events in the epigenetic reprogramming cycle. SECSI = secondary spermatocyte injection; ROSI = round spermatid injection; ROSNI = round spermatid nucleus injection; COH = controlled ovarian hyperstimulation; IVM = in-vitro maturation (of oocytes); GIFT = gamete intrafallopian transfer; ICSI = intracytoplasmic sperm injection; IVF = in-vitro fertilization; IVC = in-vitro culture; ET = embryo transfe; ELSI = elongated sperm injection.
Adapted from Huntriss (2011) and with permission from Hiura *et al.* (2014), Imprinting Methylation Errors in ART, *Reprod Med Biol* 13(4): 193–202, licensed under CCL/by/4.0.

2001), with initial erasure and then de novo DNA methylation toward the end of the preimplantation period as differentiation occurs. The inner cell mass (ICM) and trophectoderm of the blastocyst show epigenetic differences: H3K27me1, me2 and me3 are present predominantly in the ICM (reviewed in Morgan *et al.*, 2005). The ICM and trophectoderm cell lineages of the mouse blastocyst are differentially marked by histone H3 lysine 27 methylation at key developmental genes.

Genome-wide analysis of methylation can now be carried out via methods based on next-generation sequencing, including whole genome bisulfide sequencing (WGBS) and reduced representation bisulfite sequencing (RRBS). These methods have been used to report comprehensive methylation landscapes in mouse oocytes and preimplantation embryos (Smallwood *et al.*, 2011), and more recently in human gametes and preimplantation embryos (Guo *et al.*, 2014). Results from these novel sequencing-based methods generally support earlier observations based on immunofluorescent methods, i.e., a general decrease in methylation is observed during human preimplantation development. The increased sensitivity of the

sequencing-based methods allows the sequences themselves to be identified and has also revealed additional interesting observations during human preimplantation development. Most significantly, despite a decrease in DNA methylation overall, there are two short bursts of remethylation: (i) in the zygote and (ii) at the four- to eight-cell stage. In addition, sensitive single-cell analysis has shown that individual embryonic blastomeres can be traced back to the cell of origin by DNA methylation patterns (Figure 15.4).

### Species-Specific Differences in Mammalian Reprogramming

Assessment of 5-methylcytosine immunostaining in different mammalian zygotes shows:

- The paternal pronucleus undergoes demethylation in mouse, human and bovine zygotes, but not in sheep and rabbit zygotes.
- Demethylation of the male pronucleus occurs more slowly in rat than in mouse.
- The male pronucleus is completely demethylated within 4 hours of fertilization in the mouse, and passive loss of methylation in the embryo continues up to the morula stage.

## Imprint Maintenance during Preimplantation Development

Dynamic changes take place in the level of genomic DNA methylation during preimplantation development. The imprints that were established in the male and female germline must be recognized and maintained during global DNA demethylation in the early embryo, so that the imprinting mark may be propagated during later development in order to allow expression of the appropriate allele.

# Epigenetic Modification and Assisted Reproductive Technologies

Handling human gametes and embryos outside the human body could potentially introduce stresses that might later be manifested during development. In addition, ART procedures are performed during a period when dynamic and essential epigenetic reprogramming events are occurring on the genome of the gamete or embryo during normal development. Not surprisingly, data surrounding the subject is fragmented and incomplete, fraught with differences in sample size and selection criteria. At the time of writing, an estimated 8 to 10 million healthy children have been born after ART, bearing testimony to this remarkable technology of the twentieth century. However, developmental abnormalities must be rigidly monitored, and research on the epigenetic regulation of human gametes and embryos is fundamental. A summary of some of the syndromes that have been noted in ART children is presented below, together with examples of potential ART pathways that might possibly induce epigenetic mistakes.

# Disorders of Genomic Imprinting and Human ART

Several congenital disorders occurring after natural conception that feature disrupted expression of imprinted genes have been recognized as imprinting disorders. Examples of imprinting disorders include Beckwith–Wiedemann syndrome (BWS), Silver–Russell syndrome (SRS) and Angelman syndrome (Odom and Segars, 2010; Eggerman et al., 2015). These disorders can be caused by a variety of mechanisms, including chromosomal causes (e.g., disomy), gene mutations or defects in epigenetic mechanisms. In rare cases, it appears that assisted reproduction may affect epigenetic mechanisms that may result in imprinting disorders. The association between disorders of genomic imprinting and human ART has been extensively summarized (Hiura et al., 2014). A survey of the registries for each of the disorders of genomic imprinting as well as data from case studies of affected individuals were used in order to propose conclusions. A systematic review and meta-analysis of the existing literature on the connection between ART and imprinting disorders published in 2014 indicated that the risk of imprinting disorders is higher in children conceived through ART compared with those who are conceived naturally (Lazaraviciute et al., 2014). Current data indicate that BWS is more prevalent with the use of assisted reproduction. SRS has also been reported as more prevalent with the use of ART. It is important to state that these cases of ART-associated imprinting disorders are rare. However, it is of paramount importance to understand the mechanism and the ART conditions that can cause epigenetic disruption in order to minimize the risk to children born after ART. Earlier publications reported possible associations between the use of ART and Angelman syndrome (AS) and Prader–Willi syndrome (PWS); however, more recent assessments indicate that children with AS and PWS are more likely to be born to parents with a fertility problem, rather than being caused by ART procedures themselves (Vermeiden & Bernardus, 2013).

### Beckwith–Wiedemann Syndrome

BWS is caused by faulty expression of the imprinted genes on chromosome 11q15.5 and occurs sporadically after natural conception at an approximate rate of 1 in 15000 births. The syndrome is associated with large pre/postnatal growth (approximately 160% increase), childhood tumors (commonly Wilms' tumor), macroglossia, exomphalos, organomegaly, hypoglycemia and hemihypertrophy. Approximately 20% of cases show paternal uniparental disomy of the 11q15.5 chromosome, and overexpression of the imprinted gene *IGF2* is found in 80% of cases.

BWS registries reveal that the syndrome has been observed in children conceived after assisted reproduction. The major epimutation identified in these children is hypomethylation of the *KvDMR1*, a methylated imprinting control element on maternal (oocyte) chromosome 11p15.5, at the promoter region of the *KCNQ1OT1* gene; 24 out of 25 ART children with BWS presented with hypomethylation at *KvDMR1* (Lim *et al.*, 2009). The cause of the BWS epimutation could not be linked to any particular aspect of ART or infertility, but a study that identified 19 ART-conceived children from a BWS registry found the use of ovarian stimulation to be the only common parameter identified (Chang *et al.*, 2005). This aspect will be covered in more detail later in this chapter. Summarizing the data in 2013, Vermeiden and Bernardus described a significant positive association between IVF/ICSI treatment and BWS, with a relative risk of 5.2 (95% confidence interval 1.6–7.4). Mussa *et al.* (2017) assessed the prevalence of the syndrome in a large group of naturally conceived patients born with BWS in Piemonte, Italy, between 2005 and 2014. A comparison with BWS prevalence in children reported in the corresponding regional ART registry revealed that ART leads to a 10-fold increased risk of BWS compared to the naturally conceived population; however, the report included some BWS cases with nonepigenetic aetiology. Tenorio *et al.* (2016 ) observed that 88% of BWS patients born after ART had hypomethylation of *KvDMR1*, compared to 49% for patients with BWS that were conceived naturally.

## Silver-Russell Syndrome

SRS is a genetically heterogeneous condition that features growth retardation and learning disabilities. Some cases of SRS are caused by hypomethylation of the *IGF2/H19* imprinting center region (ICR1). Several cases of SRS have been described in children conceived by ART, but more studies are required to establish whether there is a true association. Chopra *et al.* (2010) reported a female child conceived by ICSI who showed hypomethylation of the paternally derived *H19/IGF2* locus. The same paper also presented details of six earlier cases of ART-related SRS compiled from other studies. In 2012, a Japanese nationwide epidemiological study reported five cases of ART-related SRS with hypomethylation of the *H19/IGF2* locus, but noted that other imprinted loci were also affected (Hiura *et al.*, 2012). Kagami *et al.* (2007) documented a case of SRS in a child conceived via IVF who showed hypermethylation at

the *PEG1/MEST* DMR, although this particular case had normal methylation at the *H19* DMR, the region that is most typically implicated in SRS. Vermeiden and Bernardus (2013) summarized data from several studies, with the conclusion that a significant positive association between SRS and IVF/ICSI treatment is likely.

## Angelman Syndrome

AS is a rare disease that affects approximately 1 in 15000 newborns, caused by a spectrum of genetic defects, including a defect in the *SNRPN* gene on the chromosome 15 imprinting center. An increased incidence of AS has been reported following the use of ICSI (Cox *et al.*, 2002; Ørstavik *et al.*, 2003; Ludwig *et al.*, 2005; Sutcliffe *et al.*, 2006); it has been suggested that some aspects of the ICSI technique might be responsible for the epigenetic abnormality, for example introduction of the sperm acrosome and its digestive enzymes into the ooplasm, ICSI-induced mechanical stress on the oocyte, or disruption of cellular factors or structures required for correct imprinting of chromosome 15. Paternal RNA-mediated mechanisms must also be considered. Loss of methylation at the *SNRPN* imprinting control region was observed in three cases (normally accounting for less than 5% of all AS cases, occurring in only 1 in 300 000 newborns). Conversely, no *SNRPN* methylation defects were observed in a study of 92 children born after ICSI (Manning *et al.*, 2000). Sanchez-Albisua *et al.* (2007) described one AS case born via ICSI with an imprinting defect; Johnson *et al.* (2018) documented a case of AS with an imprinting defect at *SNRPN* after IVF. A study by Doornbos *et al.* (2007) suggests a significant association between fertility problems and AS, but not between fertility treatments (IVF or ICSI) and AS. Vermeiden and Bernardus (2013) also concluded that there is probably a positive association between fertility problems and AS, but no significant association with fertility treatments *per se*. At the present time, data suggest that AS may be associated with infertility, but are in conflict regarding its association with ART pathways.

## *Do BWS and SRS Cases Point to Generalized Disruption of Imprinting?*

The molecular genetic information from the above examples suggests that a more generalized epigenetic defect may be associated with ART in some cases (e.g., inefficient maintenance of imprints in the preimplantation embryo). In a small number of ART-conceived BWS patients, epigenetic defects outside of KvDMR1 were identified at the DMRs for the imprinted genes *IGF2R*, *SNRPN* and *PEG1/MEST* (Rossignol *et al.*, 2006). However, widespread epigenetic errors are also seen in naturally conceived BWS patients. Hypomethylation at *KvDMR1* has also been observed in 3 out of 18 normal children that were conceived by ART (Gomes *et al.*, 2009), supporting the idea that epigenetic defects associated with ART may be more 'global' in nature, perhaps insufficient to cause BWS in these cases. Tee *et al.* (2013) reported that the subgroup of BWS cases with multiple epimutations are preferentially, but not exclusively, conceived with ART.

# Epigenetic Changes in Human ART Embryos and ART Cohorts

Epigenetic programming essentially acts as the interface between the environment and the genome, and therefore epigenetic signatures associated with an artificial environment may be evident in preimplantation IVF/ICSI embryos. A legacy of these epigenetic changes may be retained through to adulthood. Despite significant recent advancements, assessing the epigenetic health status of the human ART embryo is not currently practical. With perhaps the exception of the rare cases of imprinting disorders described above, it is not possible to determine with certainty whether any epigenetic changes that may be induced as a result of ART and/or infertility will go on to cause disease in the infant at birth, or lead to long-term developmental consequences. Although our understanding of epigenetic programming in human preimplantation development has improved markedly in recent years, much information is still missing with regard to how this information is regulated during subsequent postimplantation development of the human conceptus. Current data indicate that epigenetic signatures of ART cohorts may differ from naturally conceived cohorts. There have also been reports that human ART embryos themselves may harbor epigenetic changes; however, the major restriction to these studies is that comparison with the epigenetic status of the naturally conceived embryo is not possible. At present we are unable to elucidate whether the epigenetic errors reported in ART cohorts and human ART embryos are the result of the ART procedures, the underlying infertility or a combination of these.

## Epigenetic Changes in ART Cohorts

A number of research groups have assessed either gene methylation and/or gene expression differences between cohorts of children born after ART and natural conception (summarized by Batcheller *et al.*, 2011 and Mainigi *et al.*, 2016). Out of 10 studies reported by Mainigi *et al.* (2016), 7 observed epigenetic differences in ART cohorts. Data as to whether epigenetic signatures of ART cohorts differ from naturally conceived cohorts are currently in conflict. It is important to note that conclusions for some studies will be limited if they were performed using earlier PCR-based DNA methylation analysis of a restricted number of imprinted genes, thought to be the most likely to be susceptible to epigenetic perturbation. More recent studies have used more comprehensive genome-wide assessment of DNA methylation. Using a methylation array-based approach, Melamed *et al.* (2015) observed hypomethylation and significantly higher variation in DNA methylation in the assisted reproduction group, compared with naturally conceived cohorts. Newly developed methods of methylation analysis such as pyrosequencing allow quantitative assessment of methylation, albeit at a restricted number of loci. Using this method, Whitelaw *et al.* (2014) indicated that the use of ICSI was associated with a higher level of *SNRPN* methylation when compared to spontaneous conceptions or IVF offspring. Epigenetic changes induced by ART or infertility may also have detrimental effects on the placenta, although data are again conflicting. Choufani *et al.* (2018) used genome-wide profiling to reveal methylation loss of several imprinted genes in a subset of ART placentas, and also identified epigenetic profiles in IVF/ICSI placentas that were distinct from those derived from other less invasive ART procedures. Using two different surrogate measures of global DNA methylation (sequence-specific LINE1 assay and Luminometric methylation assay, LUMA), Ghosh *et al.* (2017) showed that global DNA methylation in IVF placentas differs from that of placentas obtained from natural conceptions. The same study showed that placental DNA methylation was affected by two clinical procedures: oxygen tension and fresh versus frozen embryo transfer. Song *et al.* (2015) also described differences in placental DNA methylation in children conceived using ART compared to natural conception, and attributed these changes to the ART procedure rather than to a predisposing parental effect. In contrast, Camprubi *et al.* (2013), using focused methods to assess DNA methylation as well as allelic expression of the imprinted genes, did not identify any defects in placental genomic imprinting after ART.

### Epigenetic Changes in ART Embryos

Comprehensive DNA methylation data for human preimplantation embryos has only recently become available. Human studies have been restricted not only by technology, but also because obtaining ART embryos for research is difficult (consent for research and ethical permission). Moreover, human embryos from natural conceptions are not available for use as a control for the investigations that are performed in ART-derived embryos. Studies are also complicated by genetic heterogeneity between human preimplantation embryos. Methylation defects in human ART preimplantation embryos have been identified at DMRs of imprinted genes, but we will never know the naturally occurring rates of these defects in in-vivo conceptions. Geuns *et al.* (2003) characterized DNA methylation at the imprint control (IC) region of the *SNRPN* gene in human preimplantation embryos, reporting that the status of a number of embryos appeared to be mainly methylated or mainly unmethylated, possibly indicating an abnormal imprint in these embryos, with a normal imprint in other embryos. White *et al.* (2015) used traditional bisulfite mutagenesis and sequencing to study imprinted genes in Day 3 and blastocyst stage embryos. Abnormal methylation of imprinted genes/regions *SNRPN*, KvDMR1/*KCNQ1OT1* and *H19* was observed at both developmental stages; however, the authors suggest that extended culture to blastocyst stage did not result in embryos with a greater number of epigenetic defects. Khoueiry *et al.* (2012) reported aberrant methylation of KvDMR1 in abnormal and developmentally delayed embryos that had been fertilized by intracytoplasmic sperm injection (ICSI). In contrast, the same study indicated that the *H19* imprint was not affected by embryo grade or developmental delay. Ibala-Romdhane *et al.* (2011) identified significant hypomethylation as well as hypermethylation of the *H19* DMR in arrested pre-implantation embryos, whereas methylation of the *H19* DMR was normal in embryos that were deemed suitable for transfer. Huntriss *et al.* (2013) observed

contrasting imprinting states for the *PEG1/MEST* gene in human ART embryos: *PEG1/MEST* expression was strictly monoallelic in some embryos, and other embryos had bi-allelic *PEG1/MEST* expression. Therefore, although several studies apparently provide evidence for detection of abnormal methylation and/or expression of imprinted genes in ART-derived embryos, it is important to reiterate the lack of current understanding about the frequency/prevalence of these errors in natural conceptions.

The data described above indicate that it may be interesting to further explore connections between epigenetics and embryo quality/developmental potential. Earlier publications that used immunohistochemical assessment of 5-methyl cytosine also described epigenetic errors in arrested human embryos (Santos *et al.*, 2010). The largest study to date carried out a comprehensive analysis of 57 human blastocysts by WGBS, revealing significant differences in DNA methylation levels between high-quality, middle-quality and low-quality blastocysts; lower quality blastocysts showed more variation in DNA methylation (extremes). The authors also observed an association between the DNA methylome status of the blastocyst and live birth rates (Li *et al.*, 2017).

## Epigenetic Changes Attributed to ART Procedures

Elucidating mechanisms that may be detrimental to epigenetic processes is an important goal in order to minimize risk to ART cohorts, with experimental assessment of ART techniques and protocols. Evidence from both human and other mammalian studies suggests that different ART procedures may cause epigenetic changes. Importantly, animal studies are performed in fertile animals, which allows the effect of the ART protocol to be studied in a fertile background with suitable in-vivo-derived controls. In human ART patients, it is difficult to determine whether any detrimental effects are due to the effects of the ART protocols or to infertility itself; furthermore, control embryos are not available from natural conceptions. Current evidence indicates that a number of ART pathways have the potential to cause suboptimal epigenetic programming (see Figure 15.4), but in-depth discussion of all of these areas is beyond the scope of this chapter. ART protocols with potential consequences identified include embryo culture media (formulation, age, addition of growth factors), culture conditions (pH, oxygen tension, build up of waste products), culture period, use of controlled ovarian stimulation/superovulation, embryo transfer, ICSI, embryo biopsy, cryopreservation, in-vitro maturation of oocytes and in-vitro growth. The evidence for epigenetic changes caused by cell culture, controlled ovarian stimulation/superovulation and cryopreservation are discussed in more detail below.

## Culture Media and Culture Environment

The preimplantation embryo develops in an artificial environment during ART, and culture media must be suitable and sufficient to support early development, including the capacity to support dynamic epigenetic processes during fertilization and preimplantation development. Our knowledge of how in-vitro culture (IVC) influences the human epigenome is at an early stage. Given the difficulties of using human embryos for research, much of our understanding of how IVC may affect embryo development comes from other mammals, particularly bovine, ovine and mouse data. However, it must be appreciated that not all findings from these studies are immediately relevant to humans, due to species-specific differences in epigenetic programming. A large body of literature has described the effects of IVC on gene expression in preimplantation embryos from several mammalian species (Khosla et al., 2001; Huntriss & Picton, 2008; Denomme & Mann, 2012). Sasaki et al. (1995) showed that IVC mouse embryos experience a loss in H19 imprinting compared to in-vivo-derived embryos. Doherty et al. (2000) and Khosla et al. (2001) concluded that culture conditions can affect the expression of the H19 imprinted gene. Further studies revealed that some types of culture media could alter the expression and/or methylation of a number of imprinted genes in the embryo as well as the placenta (Mann et al., 2004; Market-Velker et al., 2010; Fauque et al., 2007). Earlier studies were restricted by the molecular techniques available at the time, and thus could assess only a small number of genes. More recent data suggest that non-imprinted genes may also be susceptible, indicating that 'global' epigenetic changes may be manifested during cell culture. A comprehensive assessment of the effects of culture media was reported by Schwarzer et al. (2012). Mouse preimplantation embryos were exposed to 13 commercially available embryo media used for human ART, and a wide range of cellular and developmental effects on the embryos

was assessed. In particular, large-scale assessment of preimplantation embryo gene expression indicated that IVC induced effects on metabolic pathways, suggesting that the embryos might modify their metabolism to accommodate/adapt to the media type used.

It is extremely difficult to perform similar experiments in human preimplantation embryos, and accordingly, only a small number of studies have directly investigated the effects of culture media in human embryos. Kleijkers et al. (2015a) used microarray analysis to compare embryonic gene expression patterns after exposure to either G5 medium or human tubal fluid medium. This study showed that several pathways, including metabolic pathways, were differentially expressed between the two different media. Mantikou et al. (2016) observed differences in the expression of 174 genes when human embryos cultured in G5 medium or HTF medium were compared. This study also reported that the developmental stage of the embryo and maternal age had a greater effect on gene expression than the type of culture media used. Kimber et al. (2008) showed that single growth factors added to human embryo culture media caused unexpected changes in embryonic gene expression profiles.

Numerous animal studies indicate that IVC can potentially cause genome-wide changes in gene regulation. In ruminants, IVC can lead to large offspring syndrome (LOS) in some cases, a condition that causes the fetus to grow excessively large in the womb. LOS offspring have developmental defects, and the large size of the conceptus can cause danger to the mother (Young et al., 1998). Earlier studies of the underlying mechanisms indicated that IVC led to detrimental epigenetic changes at Igf2r (Insulin-like growth factor 2 receptor), and were attributed to the use of serum in the media. More recently, with the benefit of genome-wide transcriptome RNA sequencing analysis, it appears that multiple imprinted loci are affected by IVC in LOS offspring, with loss of imprinting observed across a range of tissues (Chen et al., 2015).

The mechanisms that may cause epigenetic disruption during embryo culture are not fully understood; however, exposure to suboptimal culture media and/or culture environments can lead to alterations in metabolic pathways (Schwarzer et al., 2012; Gad et al., 2012; Kleijkers et al., 2015). It is possible that embryo culture could cause disturbances/deficiencies in 1-carbon metabolic pathways that may affect

341

*S*-adenosyl methionine-mediated epigenetic regulation during embryonic development (see Chapter 1).

It is important to note that factors in the in-vitro environment other than type of media can affect the epigenetic profile of preimplantation embryos, including oxygen (oxidative stress), temperature, pH and the presence of specific chemicals and additives in culture media and build up of waste products such as ammonia (Lane & Gardner, 1994; Gardner & Kelly, 2017).

The effect of culture media on human birthweight has been the subject of considerable debate, with conflicting results published. Human birthweight data is a useful surrogate for fetal growth, and is used to predict early postnatal growth and long-term risk of cardiometabolic disease. Initially, Dumoulin *et al.* (2010) observed a significant increase in birthweight after IVC of human embryos in one of two commercially available media tested. Birthweight differences were described in subsequent studies by the same group (Nelissen *et al.*, 2012; Zandstra *et al.*, 2018), and offspring were reported to remain heavier during the first 2 years of life. In contrast, however, a number of other studies found no significant correlation between culture media and birthweight (Lin *et al.*, 2013). Zandstra *et al.* (2015) described differences in birthweight in 6 out of 11 media comparison studies. In a 2018 follow-up study of 9-year-old children born after IVF/ICSI with two different media, the same authors reported significant differences in body weight, BMI and waist circumference. Reassuringly, no significant differences in cardiovascular development were detected (Zandstra *et al.*, 2018). Several factors that might be implicated in birthweight must be considered, including duration of culture, age of the media and its protein source (Zhu *et al.*, 2014a, 2014b). In contrast, Maas *et al.* (2016) observed that birthweight was not affected by a number of clinical and laboratory changes over an 18-year period, reporting no differences in birthweight when variables such as different media, laboratory location, use of gonadotrophins, IVF or ICSI, and day of transfer were compared. A significant difference in birthweight was observed only between fresh and frozen transfers. Clearly, more research is required to determine whether different media formulations can affect birthweight, subsequent development and long-term health. In 2016, an ESHRE working party called for tracking of culture media use in ART registries with long-term assessment of health risks, together with a call for disclosure of media composition by commercial manufacturers (Sunde *et al.*, 2016). These and other recommendations were echoed by others (Ménézo *et al.*, 2018; Huntriss *et al.*, 2018).

## Controlled Ovarian Hyperstimulation (COH)/Superovulation

Animal and human studies both suggest that superovulation can cause epigenetic errors in the oocyte, the embryo and the placenta (Fauque *et al.*, 2013). Ovarian stimulation may drive oocyte maturation within an inappropriate time frame, or in a cellular and developmental context that is incompatible with achieving complete epigenetic programming of the oocyte. It is possible that ovarian stimulation may override the progressive processes of epigenetic maturation and imprint establishment that are connected with oocyte growth and size (Obata and Kono, 2002; O'Doherty *et al.*, 2012). Superovulation could interfere with this stepwise process, recruiting young follicles that have not correctly established their imprinting during maturation. Alternatively, ovarian stimulation may lead to the recruitment of poor quality oocytes that would not be selected to ovulate under normal circumstances, pushing lower quality oocytes to maturity (Market-Velker *et al.*, 2010; Van der Auwera and D'Hooghe, 2001). Due to the difficulties intrinsic to determining the epigenetic status of human oocytes, there are few reports to date; however, controlled ovarian hyperstimulation has been associated with epigenetic changes at a small number of loci (Sato *et al.*, 2007; Khoueiry *et al.*, 2008). As described above, COH was found to be the common treatment in 19 children with BWS that had been conceived through ART (Chang *et al.*, 2005).

Mouse studies have been particularly important in assessing effects of superovulation, but these findings might not necessarily translate between the differing reproductive physiologies of mice and humans. Ovarian stimulation may have transgenerational effects, *i.e.*, induced epigenetic changes can persist in the sperm of second generation male offspring that are born from superovulated female mice (Stouder *et al.*, 2009). Mouse experiments have shown that superovulation can cause aberrant genomic imprinting of both maternally and paternally expressed genes in the embryo and placenta (Fortier *et al.*, 2008; Market-Velker *et al.*, 2010). Disruption of paternally imprinted genes in addition to maternally imprinted genes indicates that ovarian stimulation has the capacity to disrupt key epigenetic 'master' regulators, or perhaps other epigenetic processes or related oocyte/early embryonic structures that are required for maintenance of genomic imprinting during preimplantation development (Nakamura *et al.*, 2007; Denomme *et al.*, 2011; Huffman *et al.*, 2015). The effects of superovulation assessed at later time points after implantation indicated that superovulation can affect oocytes sufficiently to cause abnormal imprinted gene expression (*Igf2*) in the placenta (Fortier *et al.*, 2014).

### Cryopreservation

Experimental data suggest that cryopreservation can alter epigenetic marks in mammalian cells (Kobayashi *et al.*, 2009), although the mechanisms causing this damage are unclear at present. These could include general cell damage and/or damage to structures associated with epigenetic programming in oocytes/embryos, or perhaps damage to the spindle. As with all studies of this nature, reports of potentially detrimental consequences are in conflict. Table 15.1 shows a summary of epigenetic consequences observed in several species after vitrification.

# Infertility and Epigenetics

Chapter 3 outlines the fact that gametogenesis is a complex process, requiring coordination of numerous cellular and molecular events over extended periods of time. Some cases of infertility may be due to suboptimal gametogenesis, and there may be disruption of important epigenetic processes, causing the gamete itself to carry epigenetic defects. Further research is required to fully understand the impact of any gamete-borne epigenetic changes on the process of fertilization and subsequent embryo development – an area that remains a subject of debate. For example, some studies have shown that epigenetic errors may be inherited from the sperm (Kobayashi *et al.*, 2009). However, other studies suggest that epigenetic defects are due to the assisted reproduction procedures rather than defects present in the gametes (Song *et al.*, 2015). It is possible that epigenetic defects present in the gametes could be exacerbated by suboptimal conditions in assisted reproduction.

The cause of these epigenetic defects in the infertile patient may be a result of general defects in gene expression patterns impacting on epigenetic

processes, a legacy of the defective process of gametogenesis. A small number of cases could be caused by a genetic mutation in the gamete's epigenetic machinery. For example, an association has been found between DNA methylation defects observed at imprinted loci in ART concepti and mutations in the gene encoding *DNMT3L*, a gene that is important in imprint establishment. These mutations were also present in parental sperm (Kobayashi *et al.*, 2009). However, many factors can influence epigenetic programming in the mammalian germline, some of which will influence the physiology of the offspring, including diet and dietary supplements, body composition, advanced age and use of medicines. Environmental exposures and lifestyle factors such as smoking are also important. Finally, genetic/epigenetic variation will also influence gametic programming (Rajender *et al.*, 2011; Boissonnas *et al.*, 2013; Ge *et al.*, 2014; Jenkins *et al.*, 2014; Soubry *et al.*, 2014; Shea *et al.*, 2015; Stuppia *et al.*, 2015; de Castro *et al.*, 2016).

# Epigenetic Signatures of Infertility
## DNA Methylation

Defective epigenetic signatures associated with a number of different classes of human male infertility are now well documented. Equivalent epigenetic defects in the female germline may be associated with female infertility, but oocytes are far less amenable to epigenetic research than sperm. Many research groups have compared DNA methylation marks at a number of key genes in sperm from infertile males with those from fertile controls, with significant focus on imprinted genes, revealing perturbed sperm DNA methylation signatures at imprinted genes as well as other sequences in cases of male infertility. A meta-analysis including 24 of these studies concluded that male infertility is associated with altered sperm methylation at three imprinted genes (*H19*, *SNRPN*, *MEST*) (Santi *et al.*, 2017). Although imprinted genes are a particularly important group of genes to study, it is likely that infertility can lead to genome-wide changes in DNA methylation compared to that observed in the typical fertile gamete. Modern methods of epigenetic screening, particularly DNA methylation arrays or analysis based on next-generation sequencing, now facilitate understanding this bigger picture, allowing epigenetic marks present in mature, functional gametes and those affected in infertile gametes to be

**Table 15.1** Epigenetic consequences observed after vitrification

| Species | Method | Cells | Mark | Method | Difference? | Reference |
|---------|--------|-------|------|--------|-------------|-----------|
| **Human** | Oocyte vitrification | Day 3 embryos | 5mC/ 5hmc | Immunofluorescence | No difference | De Munck et al., 2015 |
| **Mouse** | Oocyte vitrification (Preantral follicle) | | 5mC | Pyrosequencing (Snrpn, Igf2r) | No difference in imprinted DMR but differences at sporadic CpGs | Trapphoff et al., 2010 |
| **Mouse** | Oocyte vitrification | Oocytes and embryos | 5mC | Immunofluorescence | Lower global DNA methylation | Liang et al., 2014 |
| **Rabbit** | Embryo vitrification | Embryo | 5mC | Bisulfite sequencing OCT4 promoter | No difference | Saenz-de Juano et al., 2014 |
| **Mouse** | Oocyte vitrification | Oocytes and embryos | 5mC | Bisulfite sequencing H19, Peg3, Snrpn | Lower DNA methylation +Dnmt expression lower | Cheng et al., 2014 |
| **Mouse** | Embryo vitrification | Embryo | 5mC | Bisulfite sequencing Grb10 Immunofluorescence | Lower *Grb10* DNA methylation Lower *Grb10* expression Lower global DNA methylation | Yao et al., 2017 |
| **Mouse** | Oocyte vitrification | Oocytes | 5mC | Bisulfite sequencing Dnmt1o, Hdac1, Hat1 | No difference in DNA methylation but Decreased Dnmt1o expression | Zhao et al., 2013 |
| **Bovine** | Oocyte vitrification | Oocyte | 5mC and histone marks | Bisulfite sequencing Immunofluorescence | Difference in one epigenetic mark in TE only Difference in imprinted gene expression in blastocysts | Chen H et al., 2016 |
| **Mouse** | Oocyte vitrification | Oocyte | Histone marks | Immunofluorescence | H3K9 methylation increased H4K5 acetylation increased | Yan et al., 2010 |
| **Mouse** | Embryo vitrification | Fetus and placenta | 5mC | Bisulfite sequencing H19/Igf2 | Loss of H19 methylation Altered H19 expression | Wang et al., 2010 |
| **Human** | Embryo vitrification | Embryo | 5mC | Bisulfite sequencing H19/Igf2 | No difference | Derakhshan-Horeh et al., 2016 |

recognized. Global DNA methylation analysis methods indicate that poor quality human sperm may be due to defects in the process of DNA methylation erasure (Houshdaran et al., 2007). Genome-wide DNA methylation analysis by sequencing and array methods has also been used to identify potential epigenetic markers of male infertility for inclusion in infertility screening panels (Sujit et al., 2018).

## Protamines

The epigenetic status of a gamete is dictated by systems other than DNA methylation. During human spermiogenesis, the transition from histones to protamines is an important step. The ratio of Protamine 1 to Protamine 2 (P1/P2) is normally 0.8–1.2, and this ratio appears to be important in fertility; disruption of this ratio may be associated with decreased embryo quality and poor IVF outcomes (Aoki et al., 2005, 2006a, 2006b). Abnormal P1/P2 ratios and low protamine levels are associated with increased DNA fragmentation, suggesting that incorrect compaction exposes DNA to oxidative stress and damage (Aoki et al., 2006b; Torregrosa et al., 2006). Histones are not completely replaced by protamines, being retained at a small number of places in the sperm genome, e.g., at key regulatory regions of the genome kept 'poised' for activation in early embryonic development. These marks may be major determinants of embryo developmental outcome (Denomme et al., 2017).

## Histone Modification

Histone modification plays a crucial role in spermatogenesis. Histone tails are subjected to post-translational modification (methylation, acetylation, phosphorylation and ubiquitination) on different amino acid residues. Histone acetyl transferases (HATs) acetylate lysine residues (K), particularly on histones H3 and H4. This has the effect of relaxing chromatin and making it accessible to transcription factors, and histone acetylation is thus generally associated with gene activation. In contrast, deacetylation by histone deacetylases (HDACs) often leads to gene silencing. The disruption of histone acetylation in spermatogenesis can lead to severe male infertility (Fenic et al., 2004, 2008; Ge et al., 2014). Histone methylation patterns are dynamic during spermatogenesis; the timing of their establishment and removal is critical, controlled by a number of specific enzymes, including histone methyltransferases (HMTs) and histone demethylases (HDM). Generally, methylation

of H3K4 is associated with gene expression whilst methylation of H3K9 and H3K27 is linked to gene silencing (Okada et al., 2007; Sikienka et al., 2015).

### RNA-Mediated Epigenetic Processes As a Major Epigenetic Determinant of Fertility

RNAs play an important role in germline epigenetic regulation. Human sperm RNA profiles have been shown to differ between fertile and infertile men (Ostermeier et al., 2002). Surprisingly, the sperm nucleus contains many RNAs – not only messenger RNAs (mRNAs), but also sncRNAs, such as miRNAs, piRNAs and sperm tRNA-derived small RNAs (tsRNAs) (Chen Q et al., 2016; Sharma et al., 2016). Some of these RNA species may be particularly important during fertilization (Gross et al., 2017). RNAs play an important role in the epigenetic control of retrotransposons in the germline. Approximately 45% of the human genome is derived from transposable elements, the majority of which originate from retrotransposons, and these can drive their own genomic replication. Insertional mutagenesis results in uncontrolled retrotransposon activity, causing genomic instability and cell death - this must be suppressed in the germline. Retrotransposons are suppressed by DNA methylation in somatic cells. However, DNA methylation is being reprogrammed and is temporarily lost from most of the sperm genome during germline epigenetic reprogramming, and a different mechanism for retrotransposon suppression is employed. piRNAs, together with other factors, facilitate DNA methylation at these elements (Aravin & Hannon, 2008; Frost et al., 2010; Pastor et al., 2014).

# Looking to the Future: Epigenetics and the ART Laboratory

Severe technical limitations have hampered epigenetic studies of human preimplantation embryos to date, limiting investigations to a restricted number of loci. These have recently been largely overcome, and refinement of these and other techniques that facilitate work on single embryos, oocytes and even single cells has considerably expanded our ability to understand epigenetic regulation in early human development. Mapping the origins and mechanisms that underlie ART-induced epigenetic defects on a patient-specific basis is now on the horizon.

Sampling of embryonic DNA methylation (for example through trophectoderm biopsy and single-cell sensitive WGBS) remains of debatable predictive value in human ART without further research; however, the technologies to enable this at least for DNA methylation analysis are effectively in place.

The most immediate and practical use of epigenetic screening methods may be their application in the diagnosis of male infertility. A number of groups advocate diagnostic epigenetic screening of sperm for cases of male infertility (Aston & Carrell, 2014; Hotaling & Carrell, 2014; Klaver & Gromoll, 2014). This approach is likely to require extensive validation, as well as further research on human developmental epigenetics.

Research goals for the future include assessing epigenetic marks associated with low pregnancy rates, poor embryo development, potential risks of disease transfer to the offspring and better categorization of infertility aetiologies in order to optimize the treatment path.

## Summary

The human embryo is exquisitely sensitive to changes in its environment; ART protocols have been evolving

and changing rapidly over the past 40 years, and the fact that so many healthy children have been born despite numerous differences in in-vitro embryo culture is a testament to human developmental plasticity. This biological phenomenon is crucial in ART practice: although it is clear that techniques and protocols can have an effect at the molecular and cellular level, optimal conditions are not yet defined, and the extent of effects on health in the short or long term are unclear (Roseboom, 2018). An association between ART and an increased risk of at least some epigenetic disorders must clearly be considered (Figure 15.5), and sophisticated molecular studies that compare the 'global' epigenetic status of children born in vivo and those born in vitro are now emerging. Studies such as these will help us to understand the molecular processes that are affected by ART, and the potential risks associated with each technique. Research techniques have now been developed that allow the epigenetic effects of ART technologies to be rigorously tested to precisely gauge their effect upon the epigenetic development of human gametes and preimplantation embryos so that ART protocols can be adapted to avoid potential problems. Animal

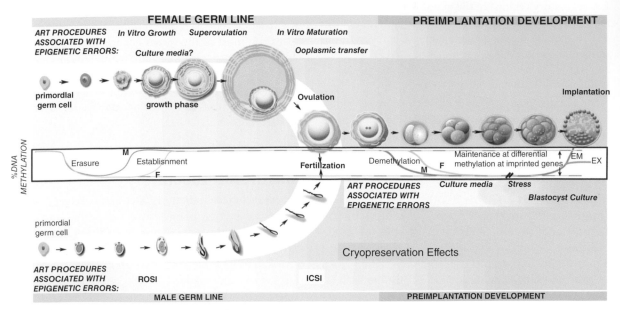

**Figure 15.5** Major DNA methylation reprogramming events during mammalian gametogenesis and preimplantation development shown together with a summary of the assisted reproductive technology (ART) procedures that are associated with epigenetic errors. The methylation reprogramming panel (center panel, adapted from Reik *et al.*, 2001) indicates the level of methylation in male (M) and female (F) gametes (left side), and also in the paternally inherited (M) and the maternally inherited genomes (F) after fertilization, during preimplantation development (right side). The timing and nature of these reprogramming events varies between species. The dashed lines indicate the maintenance of differential methylation at imprinted genes during preimplantation development. The genome is remethylated differentially within the blastocyst in the embryonic (EM) and extraembryonic lineages (EX). Reprinted with permission from Huntriss and Picton (2008).

studies are useful in highlighting problems associated with particular ART methods, but there are significant differences between humans and other mammals with respect to epigenetic regulation, and in the regulation of imprinting during gametogenesis and early development. Further research on the epigenetic regulation of human gametes and preimplantation embryos is urgently needed in order to understand how infertility, as well as lifestyle factors, impact the epigenome of the gametes, and whether ART can exacerbate these errors. A focus on safety aspects of existing and emerging ART treatments is essential, together with long-term follow-up studies of children born as a result of ART.

# Further Reading

## Reviews

Amor DJ, Halliday J (2008) A review of known imprinting syndromes and their association with assisted reproduction technologies. *Human Reproduction* 23(12): 2826–2834.

ASRM Practice Committee Pages (2013) Blastocyst culture and transfer in clinical assisted reproduction: a committee opinion. *Fertility and Sterility* 99(3): 0015–0282.

Gosden R, Trasler J, Lucifero D, Faddy M (2003) Rare congenital disorders, imprinted genes, and assisted reproductive technology. *Lancet* 361(9373): 1975–1977.

Huntriss J, Picton HM (2008) Epigenetic consequences of assisted reproduction and infertility on the human preimplantation embryo. *Human Fertility* 11(2): 85–94.

Maher ER, Afnan M, Barratt CL (2003) Epigenetic risks related to assisted reproductive technologies: epigenetics, imprinting, ART and icebergs? *Human Reproduction* 18(12): 2508–2511.

Manipalviratn S, DeCherney A, Segars J (2009) Imprinting disorders and assisted reproductive technology. *Fertility and Sterility* 91(2): 305–315.

Roseboom TJ (2018) Developmental plasticity and its relevance to assisted human reproduction. *Human Reproduction* 33(4): 546–552.

## Publications

Abeyta MJ, Clark AT, Rodriguez RT, *et al.* (2004) Unique gene expression signatures of independently-derived human embryonic stem cell lines. *Human Molecular Genetics* 13: 601–608.

Adewumi O, Aflatoonian B, Ahrlund-Richter L, *et al.* (2007) Characterization of human embryonic stem cell lines by the International Stem Cell Initiative. *Nature Biotechnology* 25: 803–816.

Albert M, Peters AH (2009) Genetic and epigenetic control of early mouse development. *Current Opinion in Genetics and Development* 19(2): 113–121.

Allegrucci C, Wu YZ, Thurston A, *et al.* (2007) Restriction landmark genome scanning identifies culture-induced DNA methylation instability in the human embryonic stem cell epigenome. *Human Molecular Genetics* 16: 1253–1268.

Anckaert E, Adriaenssens T, Romero S, Dremier S, Smitz J (2009a) Unaltered imprinting establishment of key imprinted genes in mouse oocytes after in vitro follicle culture under variable follicle-stimulating hormone exposure. *International Journal of Developmental Biology* 53(4): 541–548.

Anckaert E, Adriaenssens T, Romero S, Smitz J (2009b) Ammonium accumulation and use of mineral oil overlay do not alter imprinting establishment at three key imprinted genes in mouse oocytes grown and matured in a long-term follicle culture. *Biology of Reproduction* 81(4): 666–673.

Anteby I, Cohen E, Anteby E, BenEzra D (2001) Ocular manifestations in children born after in vitro fertilization. *Archives of Ophthalmology* 119(10): 1525–1529.

Aoki VW, Emery BR, Liu L, Carrell DT (2006a) Protamine levels vary between individual sperm cells of infertile human males and correlate with viability and DNA integrity. *Journal of Andrology* 27: 890–898.

Aoki VW, Liu L, Jones KP, *et al.* (2006b) Sperm protamine 1/protamine 2 ratios are related to in vitro fertilization pregnancy rates and predictive of fertilization ability. *Fertility and Sterility* 86: 1408–1415.

Aoki VW, Moskovtsev SI, Willis J, *et al.* (2005) DNA integrity is compromised in protamine-deficient human sperm. *Journal of Andrology* 26: 741–748.

Apostolidou S, Abu-Amero S, O'Donoghue K, *et al.* (2007) Elevated placental expression of the imprinted PHLDA2 gene is associated with low birth weight. *Journal of Molecular Medicine* 85: 379–387.

Aravin AA, Hannon GJ (2008) Small RNA silencing pathways in germ and stem cells. *Cold Spring Harbor Symposia on Quantitative Biology* 73: 283–290.

Aston KI, Carrell DT (2014) Prospects for clinically relevant epigenetic tests in the andrology laboratory. *Asian Journal of Andrology* 16(5): 782.

Batcheller A, Cardozo E, Maguire M, DeCherney AH, Segars JH (2011) Are there subtle genome-wide epigenetic alterations in normal offspring conceived by assisted reproductive technologies? *Fertility and Sterility* 96(6):1306–1311.

Beaujean N, Hartshorne G, Cavilla J, *et al.* (2004) Non-conservation of mammalian preimplantation methylation dynamics. *Current Biology* 14(7): R266–267.

Bell AC, Felsenfeld G (2000) Methylation of a CTCF-dependent boundary controls imprinted expression of the Igf2 gene. *Nature* 405(6785): 482–485.

Benchaib M, Braun V, Ressnikof D, *et al.* (2005) Influence of global sperm DNA methylation on IVF results. *Human Reproduction* 20: 768–773.

Bliek J, Terhal P, van den Bogaard MJ, *et al.* (2006) Hypomethylation of the H19 gene causes not only Silver–Russell syndrome (SRS) but also isolated asymmetry or an SRS-like phenotype. *American Journal of Human Genetics* 78: 604–614.

Blondin P, Farin PW, Crosier AE, Alexander JE, Farin CE (2000) In vitro production of embryos alters levels of insulin-like growth factor-II messenger ribonucleic acid in bovine fetuses 63 days after transfer. *Biology and Reproduction* 62(2): 384–389.

Boissonnas CC, Abdalaoui HE, Haelewyn V, *et al.* (2010) Specific epigenetic alterations of IGF2-H19 locus in spermatozoa from infertile men. *European Journal of Human Genetics* 18(1): 73–80.

Boissonnas CC, Jouannet P, Jammes H (2013). Epigenetic disorders and male subfertility. *Fertility and Sterility* 99(3): 624–631.

Boonen SE, Porksen S, Mackay DJ, *et al.* (2008) Clinical characterisation of the multiple maternal hypomethylation syndrome in siblings. *European Journal of Human Genetics* 16: 453–461.

Borghol N, Blachère T, Lefèvre A (2008) Transcriptional and epigenetic status of protamine 1 and 2 genes following round spermatid injection into mouse oocytes. *Genomics* 91(5): 415–422.

Borghol N, Lornage J, Blachere T, Sophie Garret A, Lefevre A (2006) Epigenetic status of the H19 locus in human oocytes following in vitro maturation. *Genomics* 87: 417–426.

Bourc'his D, Xu GL, Lin CS, Bollman B, Bestor TH (2001) Dnmt3L and the establishment of maternal genomic imprints. *Science* 294(5551): 2536–2539.

Bourque DK, Avila L, Peñaherrera M, von Dadelszen P, Robinson WP (2010) Decreased placental methylation at the H19/IGF2 imprinting control region is associated with normotensive intrauterine growth restriction but not preeclampsia. *Placenta* 31(3): 197–202.

Camprubi C, Iglesias-Platas I, Martin-Trujillo A, *et al.* (2013) Stability of genomic imprinting and gestational-age dynamic methylation in complicated pregnancies conceived following assisted reproductive technologies. *Biology of Reproduction* 89(3): 50.

Carlone DL, Lee JH, Young SR, *et al.* (2005) Reduced genomic cytosine methylation and defective cellular differentiation in embryonic stem cells lacking CpG binding protein. *Molecular and Cellular Biology* 25(12): 4881–4891.

Carlone DL, Skalnik DG (2001) CpG binding protein is crucial for early embryonic development. *Molecular and Cellular Biology* 21(22): 7601–7606.

Carrasco B, Boada M, Rodriguez I, Coroleu B, Barri PN, Veiga A (2013) Does culture medium influence offspring birth weight? *Fertility and Sterility* 100(5): 1283–1288.

Carrell DT (2012) Epigenetics of the male gamete. *Fertility and Sterility* 97(2): 267–274.

Carrell DT, Emery BR, Hammoud S (2007) Altered protamine expression and diminished spermatogenesis: what is the link? *Human Reproduction Update* 13: 313–327.

Cetin I, Cozzi V, Antonazzo P (2003) Fetal development after assisted reproduction – a review. *Placenta* 24(Suppl. B): S104–113.

Chang AS, Moley KH, Wangler M, Feinberg AP, Debaun MR (2005) Association between Beckwith-Wiedemann syndrome and assisted reproductive technology: a case series of 19 patients. *Fertility and Sterility* 83: 349–354.

Charalambous M, Ferron SR, da Rocha ST, *et al.* (2012) Imprinted gene dosage is critical for the transition to independent life. *Cell Metabolism* 15(2): 209–221.

Chatterjee A, Saha D, Niemann H, Gryshkov O, Gismacher B, Hofmann N (2017) Effects of cryopreservation on the epigenetic profile of cells. *Cryobiology* 74: 1–7.

Chen Z, Hagen DE, Elsik CG, *et al.* (2015) Characterization of global loss of imprinting in fetal overgrowth syndrome induced by assisted reproduction. *Proceedings of the National Academy of Sciences of the USA* 112(15): 4618–4623.

Chen Q, Yan M, Cao Z, *et al.* (2016) Sperm tsRNAs contribute to intergenerational inheritance of an acquired metabolic disorder. *Science* 351(6271): 397–400.

Chen H, Zhang L, Deng T, *et al.* (2016) Effects of oocyte vitrification on epigenetic status in early bovine embryos. *Theriogenology* 86(3): 868–878.

Cheng KR, Fu XW, Zhang RN, Jia GX, Hou YP, Zhu SE (2014) Effect of oocyte vitrification on deoxyribonucleic acid methylation of H19, Peg3, and Snrpn differentially methylated regions in mouse blastocysts. *Fertility and Sterility* 102(4): 1183–1190.

Chopra M, Amor DJ, Sutton L, Algar E, Mowat D (2010) Russell-Silver syndrome due to paternal H19/IGF2 hypomethylation in a patient conceived using intracytoplasmic sperm injection. *Reproductive Biomedicine Online* 20(6): 843–847.

Chotalia M, Smallwood SA, Ruf N, *et al.* (2009) Transcription is required for establishment of germline methylation marks at imprinted genes. *Genes and Development* 23(1): 105–117.

Choufani S, Turinsky AL, Melamed N, *et al.* (2018) Impact of assisted reproduction, infertility, sex, and paternal factors on the placental DNA methylome. *Human Molecular Genetics* 28(3): 372–385.

Ciccone DN, Su H, Hevi S, *et al.* (2009) KDM1B is a histone H3K4 demethylase required to establish maternal genomic imprints. *Nature* 461(7262): 415–418.

Coan PM, Burton GJ, Ferguson-Smith AC (2005) Imprinted genes in the placenta; a review. *Placenta* 26: S10–20.

Constância M, Pickard B, Kelsey G, Reik W (1998) Imprinting mechanisms. *Genome Research* 8(9): 881–900.

Corry GN, Tanasijevic B, Barry ER, Krueger W, Rasmussen TP (2009) Epigenetic regulatory mechanisms during preimplantation development. *Birth Defects Research Part C Embryo Today* 87(4): 297–313.

Cox GF, Burger J, Lip V, *et al.* (2002) Intracytoplasmic sperm injection may increase the risk of imprinting defects. *American Journal of Human Genetics* 1(1): 162–164.

Dahl JA, Reiner AH, Klungland A, Wakayama T, Collas P (2010) Histone H3 lysine 27 methylation asymmetry on developmentally-regulated promoters distinguish the first two lineages in mouse preimplantation embryos. *PLoS One* 5(2): e9150.

DeBaun MR, Niemitz EL, Feinberg AP (2003) Association of in vitro fertilization with Beckwith-Wiedemann syndrome and epigenetic alterations of LIT1 and H19. *American Journal of Human Genetics* 72: 156–160.

De Munck N, Petrussa L, Verheyen G, *et al.* (2015) Chromosomal meiotic segregation, embryonic developmental kinetics and DNA (hydroxy)methylation analysis consolidate the safety of human oocyte vitrification. *Molecular Human Reproduction* 21(6): 535–544.

Denomme MM, Mann MR (2012) Genomic imprints as a model for the analysis of epigenetic stability during assisted reproductive technologies. *Reproduction* 144(4): 393–409.

Denomme MM, McCallie BR, Parks JC, Schoolcraft WB, Katz-Jaffe MG (2017) Alterations in the sperm histone retained epigenome are associated with unexplained male factor infertility and poor blastocyst development in donor oocyte IVF cycles. *Human Reproduction* 32(12): 2443–2455.

Denomme MM, Zhang L, Mann MR (2011) Embryonic imprinting perturbations do not originate from superovulation-induced defects in DNA methylation acquisition. *Fertility and Sterility* 96(3): 734–738.e2.

de Castro Barbosa T, Ingerslev LR, Alm PS, *et al.* (2016) High-fat diet reprograms the epigenome of rat spermatozoa and transgenerationally affects metabolism of the offspring. *Molecular Metabolism* 5(3): 184–197.

De Vos A, Janssens R, Van de Velde H, *et al.* (2015) The type of culture medium and the duration of in vitro culture do not influence birthweight of ART singletons. *Human Reproduction* 30(1): 20–27.

Derakhshan-Horeh M, Abolhassani F, Jafarpour F, *et al.* (2016) Vitrification at Day 3 stage appears not to affect the methylation status of H19/IGF2 differentially methylated region of in vitro produced human blastocysts. *Cryobiology* 73(2): 168–174.

Doherty AS, Mann MR, Tremblay KD, Bartolomei MS, Schultz RM (2000) Differential effects of culture on imprinted H19 expression in the preimplantation mouse embryo. *Biology of Reproduction* 62(6): 1526–1535.

Doornbos ME, Maas SM, McDonnell J, Vermeiden JP, Hennekam RC (2007) Infertility, assisted reproduction technologies and imprinting disturbances: a Dutch study. *Human Reproduction* 22: 2476–2480.

Dumoulin JC, Land JA, Van Montfoort AP, *et al.* (2010) Effect of in vitro culture of human embryos on birthweight of newborns. *Human Reproduction* 25(3): 605–612.

Eggermann T, Perez de Nanclares G, Maher ER, *et al.* (2015) Imprinting disorders: a group of congenital disorders with overlapping patterns of molecular changes affecting imprinted loci. *Clinical Epigenetics* 7: 123.

Eskld A, Monkerud L, Tanbo T (2013) Birthweight and placental weight; do changes in culture media used for IVF matter? Comparisons with spontaneous pregnancies in the corresponding time periods. *Human Reproduction* 28(12): 3207–3214.

Fauque P (2013) Superovulation: ovulation induction and epigenetic anomalies. *Fertility and Sterility* 99(3): 616–623.

Fauque P, Jouannet P, Lesaffre C, *et al.* (2007) Assisted reproductive technology affects developmental kinetics, H19 imprinting control region methylation and H19 gene expression in individual mouse embryos. *BMC Developmental Biology* 7: 116.

Fauque P, Mondon F, Letourneur F, *et al.* (2010b) In vitro fertilization and embryo culture strongly impact the placental transcriptome in the mouse model. *PLoS One* 5(2): e9218.

Fauque P, Ripoche MA, Tost J, *et al.* (2010a) Modulation of imprinted gene network in placenta results in normal development of in vitro manipulated mouse embryos. *Human Molecular Genetics* 19(9): 1779–1790

Fenic I, Hossain HM, Sonnack V, *et al.* (2008) In vivo application of histone deacetylase inhibitor trichostatin-a impairs murine male meiosis. *Journal of Andrology* 29: 172–185.

Fenic I, Sonnack V, Failing K, Bergmann M, Steger K (2004) In vivo effects of histone-deacetylase inhibitor trichostatin-A on murine spermatogenesis *Journal of Andrology* 25: 811–818.

Fernandez-Gonzalez R, Moreira P, Bilbao A, *et al.* (2004) Long-term effect of in vitro culture of mouse embryos with serum on mRNA expression of imprinting genes, development, and behavior. *Proceedings of the National Academy of Sciences of the USA* 101: 5880–5885.

Fortier AL, Lopes FL, Darricarrère N, Martel J, Trasler JM (2008) Superovulation alters the expression of imprinted genes in the midgestation mouse placenta. *Human Molecular Genetics* 17(11): 1653–1665.

Fortier AL, McGraw S, Lopes FL, *et al.* (2014) Modulation of imprinted gene expression following superovulation. *Molecular and Cellular Endocrinology* 388(1–2): 51–57.

Frost RJ, Hamra FK, Richardson JA, Qi X, BAssel-Duby R, Olson EN (2010) MOV10L1 is necessary for protection of spermatocytes against retrotransposons by Piwi-interacting RNAs. *Proceedings of the National Academy of Sciences of the USA* 107: 11847–11852.

Gad A, Schellander K, Hoelker M, Tesfaye D (2012) Transcriptome profile of early mammalian embryos in response to culture environment. *Animal Reproduction Science* 134(1–2): 76–83.

Galli-Tsinopoulou A, Emmanouilidou E, Karagianni P, *et al.* (2008) A female infant with Silver Russell Syndrome, mesocardia and enlargement of the clitoris. *Hormones (Athens)* 7: 77–81.

Gardner DK, Kelly RL (2017) Impact of the IVF laboratory environment on human preimplantation embryo phenotype. *Journal of Developmental Origins of Health and Disease* 8(4): 418–435.

Ge ZJ, Liang QX, Hou Y, *et al.* (2014) Maternal obesity and diabetes may cause DNA methylation alteration in the spermatozoa of offspring in mice. *Reproductive Biology and Endocrinology* 12: 29.

Geuns E, De Rycke M, Van Steirteghem A, Liebaers I (2003) Methylation imprints of the imprint control region of the SNRPN-gene in human gametes and preimplantation embryos. *Human Molecular Genetics* 12(22): 2873–2879.

Ghosh J, Coutifaris C, Sapienza C, Mainigi M (2017) Global DNA methylation levels are altered by modifiable clinical manipulations in assisted reproductive technologies. *Clinical Epigenetics* 9: 14.

Gicquel C, Gaston V, Mandelbaum J, *et al.* (2003) In vitro fertilization may increase the risk of Beckwith-Wiedemann syndrome related to the abnormal imprinting of the KCN1OT gene. *American Journal of Human Genetics* 72: 1338.

Ginsburg M, Snow MH, McLaren A (1990) Primordial germ cells in the mouse embryo during gastrulation. *Development* 110: 521–528.

Gomes MV, Huber J, Ferriani RA, Amaral Neto AM, Ramos ES (2009) Abnormal methylation at the KvDMR1 imprinting control region in clinically normal children conceived by assisted reproductive technologies. *Molecular and Human Reproduction* 15(8): 471–477.

Gross N, Kroop J, Khatib H (2017) MicroRNA signaling in embryo development. *Biology (Basel)* 6(3): pii:E34.

Guo H, Zhu P, Yan L, *et al.* (2014) The DNA methylation landscape of human early embryos. *Nature* 511: 606–610.

Halliday J, Oke K, Breheny S, Algar EJ Amor D (2004) Beckwith-Wiedemann syndrome and IVF: a case-control study. *American Journal of Human Genetics* 75: 526–528.

Hammoud SS, Purwar J, Pflueger C, Cairns BR, Carrell DT (2010) Alterations in sperm DNA methylation patterns at imprinted loci in two classes of infertility. *Fertility and Sterility* 94(5): 1728–1733.

Hammoud SS, Nix DA, Hammoud AO, Gibson M, Cairns BR, Carrell DT (2011) Genome-wide analysis identifies changes in histone retention and epigenetic modifications at developmental and imprinted gene loci in the sperm of infertile men. *Human Reproduction* 26: 2558–2569.

Hammoud SS, Nix DA, Zhang H, Purwar K, Carrell DT, Cairns BR (2009) Distinctive chromatin in human sperm packages genes for embryo development. *Nature* 460: 473–478.

Hata K, Okano M, Lei H, Li E (2002) Dnmt3L cooperates with the Dnmt3 family of de novo DNA methyltransferases to establish maternal imprints in mice. *Development* 129(8): 1983–1993.

Hayashi S, Yang J, Christenson L, Yanagimachi R, Hecht NB (2003) Mouse preimplantation embryos developed from oocytes injected with round spermatids or spermatozoa have similar but distinct patterns of early messenger RNA expression. *Biology of Reproduction* 69: 1170–1176.

Hiendleder S, Mund C, Reichenbach HD, *et al.* (2004) Tissue-specific elevated genomic cytosine methylation levels are associated with an overgrowth phenotype of bovine fetuses derived by in vitro techniques. *Biology of Reproduction* 71(1): 217–223.

Hill PW, Amouroux R, Hajkova P (2014) DNA demethylation, Tet proteins and 5-hydroxymethylcytosine in epigenetic reprogramming: an emerging complex story. *Genomics* 104(5): 324–333.

Hirasawa R, Chiba H, Kaneda M, *et al.* (2008) Maternal and zygotic Dnmt1 are necessary and sufficient for the maintenance of DNA methylation imprints during preimplantation development. *Genes and Development* 22(12): 1607–1616.

Hiura H, Obata Y, Komiyama J, Shirai M, Kono T (2006) Oocyte growth-dependent progression of maternal imprinting in mice. *Genes to Cells* 11(4): 353–361.

Hiura H, Okae H, Chiba H, *et al.* (2014) Imprinting methylation errors in ART. *Reproductive Medicine and Biology* 13(4): 193–202.

Hiura H, Okae H, Miyauchi N, *et al.* (2012) Characterization of DNA methylation errors in patients with imprinting disorders conceived by assisted reproduction technologies. *Human Reproduction* 27(8): 2541–2548.

Holm TM, Jackson-Grusby L, Brambrink T, *et al.* (2005) Global loss of imprinting leads to widespread tumorigenesis in adult mice. *Cancer Cell* 8: 275–285.

Hotaling J, Carrell DT (2014) Clinical genetic testing for male factor infertility: current applications and future directions. *Andrology* 2(3): 339–350.

Houshdaran S, Cortessis VK, Siegmund K, *et al.* (2007) Widespread epigenetic abnormalities suggest a broad DNA methylation erasure defect in abnormal human sperm. *PLoS One* 2(12): e1289.

Huffman SR, Pak Y, Rivera RM (2015) Superovulation induces alterations in the epigenome of zygotes, and results in differences in gene expression at the blastocyst stage in mice. *Molecular Reproduction and Development* 82(3): 207–217.

Huntriss J (2011) Epigenetics and assisted reproduction. In: Elder K, Dale B (eds.) *In-Vitro Fertilization*, 3rd edn. Cambridge University Press, Cambridge, UK, pp. 252–267.

Huntriss J, Balen AH, Sinclair KD, Brison DR, Picton HM; Royal College of Obstetricians Gynaecologists (2018) Epigenetics and Reproductive Medicine: Scientific Impact Paper No. 57. *BJOG* 125(13): e43–e54.

Huntriss JD, Hemmings KE, Hinkins M, *et al.* (2013) Variable imprinting of the MEST gene in human preimplantation embryos. *European Journal of Human Genetics* 21(1): 40–47.

Huntriss J, Picton HM (2008) Epigenetic consequences of assisted reproduction and infertility on the human preimplantation embryo. *Human Fertility (Cambridge)* 11(2): 85–94.

Ibala-Romdhane S, Al-Khtib M, Khoueiry R, Blachére T, Guerin JF, Lefévre A (2011) Analysis of H19 methylation in control and abnormal human embryos, sperm and oocytes. *European Journal of Human Genetics* 19(11): 1138–1143.

Imamura T, Kerjean A, Heams T, *et al.* (2005) Dynamic CpG and non-CpG methylation of the Peg1/Mest gene in the mouse oocyte and preimplantation embryo. *Journal of Biological Chemistry* 280: 20171–20175.

Isles AR, Holland AJ (2005) Imprinted genes and mother-offspring interactions. *Early Human Development* 81: 73–77.

Jenkins TG, Aston KI, Pflueger C, Cairns BR, Carrell DT (2014) Age-associated sperm DNA methylation alterations: possible implications in offspring disease susceptibility. *PLoS Genetics* 10(7): e1004458.

Jenkins TG, James ER, Alonso DF, *et al.* (2017) Cigarette smoking significantly alters sperm DNA methylation patterns. *Andrology* 5(6): 1089–1099.

Johnson JP, Schoof J, Beischel L, *et al.* (2018) Detection of a case of Angelman syndrome caused by an imprinting error in 949 pregnancies analyzed for AS following IVF. *Journal of Assisted Reproduction and Genetics* 35(6): 981–984.

Kagami M, Nagai T, Fukami M, Yamazawa K, Ogata T (2007) Silver-Russell syndrome in a girl born after in vitro fertilization: partial hypermethylation at the differentially methylated region of PEG1/MEST. *Journal of Assisted Reproduction and Genetics* 24: 131–136.

Källén B, Finnström O, Lindam A, *et al.* (2010) Congenital malformations in infants born after in vitro fertilization in Sweden. *Birth Defects Research A: Clinical and Molecular Teratology* 88(3): 137–143.

Källén B, Finnström O, Nygren KG, Olausson PO (2005) In vitro fertilization (IVF) in Sweden: infant outcome after different IVF fertilization methods. *Fertility and Sterility* 84: 611–617.

Kanber D, Berulava T, Ammerpohl O, *et al.* (2009a) The human retinoblastoma gene is imprinted. *PLoS Genetics* 5(12): e1000790.

Kanber D, Buiting K, Zeschnigk M, Ludwig M, Horsthemke B (2009b) Low frequency of imprinting defects in ICSI children born small for gestational age. *European Journal of Human Genetics* 17(1): 22–29.

Kerjean A, Couvert P, Heams T, *et al.* (2003) In vitro follicular growth affects oocyte imprinting establishment in mice. *European Journal of Human Genetics* 11: 493–496,

Khosla S, Dean W, Brown D, Reik W, Feil R (2001) Culture of preimplantation mouse embryos affects fetal development and the expression of imprinted genes. *Biology of Reproduction* 64: 918–926.

Khoueiry R, Ibala-Rhomdane S, Al-Khtib M, *et al.* (2012) Abnormal methylation of KCNQ1OT1 and differential methylation of H19 imprinting control regions in human ICSI embryos. *Zygote* 21: 1–10.

Khoueiry R, Ibala-Rhomdane S, Méry L, *et al.* (2008) Dynamic CpG methylation of the KCNQ1OT1 gene during maturation of human oocytes. *Journal of Medical Genetics* 45(9): 583–588.

Kim KP, Thurston A, Mummery C, *et al.* (2007) Gene-specific vulnerability to imprinting variability in human embryonic stem cell lines. *Genome Research* 17: 1731–1742.

Kimber SJ, Sneddon SF, Bloor DJ, *et al.* (2008) Expression of genes involved in early cell fate decisions in human embryos and their regulation by growth factors. *Reproduction* 135(5): 635–647.

Kishigami S, Van Thuan N, Hikichi T, *et al.* (2006) Epigenetic abnormalities of the mouse paternal zygotic genome associated with microinsemination of round spermatids. *Developmental Biology* 289: 195–205.

Klaver R, Gromoll J (2014) Bringing epigenetics into the diagnostics of the andrology laboratory: challenges and perspectives. *Asian Journal of Andrology* 16(5): 669–674.

Kleijkers SH, Eijssen LM, Coonen E, *et al.*(2015a) Differences in gene expression profiles between human preimplantation embryos cultured in two different IVF culture media. *Human Reproduction* 30(10): 2303–2311.

Kleijkers SH, van Montfoort AP, Smits LJ, *et al.* (2015b) Age of G-1 PLUS v5 embryo culture medium is inversely associated with birthweight of the newborn. *Human Reproduction* 30(6): 1352–1357.

Kobayashi H, Hiura H, John RM, *et al.* (2009) DNA methylation errors at imprinted loci after assisted conception originate in the parental sperm. *European Journal of Human Genetics* 17(12): 1582–1591.

Kobayashi H, Sato A, Otsu E, *et al.* (2007) Aberrant DNA methylation of imprinted loci in sperm from oligospermic patients. *Human Molecular Genetics* 16: 2542–2551.

Kono T (2009) Genetic modification for bimaternal embryo development. *Reproduction and Fertility Development* 21(1): 31–36.

Kurihara Y, Kawamura Y, Uchijima Y, *et al.* (2008) Maintenance of genomic methylation patterns during preimplantation development requires the somatic form of DNA methyltransferase 1. *Developmental Biology* 313(1): 335–346.

Lane M, Gardner DK (1994) Increase in postimplantation development of cultured mouse embryos by amino acids and induction of fetal retardation and exencephaly by ammonium ions. *Journal of Reproduction & Fertility* 102(2): 305–312.

Lane M, Gardner DK (2003) Ammonium induces aberrant blastocyst differentiation, metabolism, pH regulation, gene expression and subsequently alters fetal development in the mouse. *Biology of Reproduction* 69: 1109–1117.

Lazaraviciute G, Kauser M, Bhattacharya S, Haggarty P (2014) A systematic review and meta-analysis of DNA methylation levels and imprinting disorders in children conceived by IVF/ICSI compared with children conceived spontaneously. *Human Reproduction Update* 20(6): 840–852.

Lee I, Finger PT, Grifo JA, *et al.* (2004) Retinoblastoma in a child conceived by in vitro fertilisation. *British Journal of Ophthalmology* 88(8): 1098–1099.

Lee MG, Wynder C, Cooch N, Shiekhattar R (2005) An essential role for CoREST in nucleosomal histone-3-lysine-4 demethylation. *Nature* 437: 432–435.

Lee YS, Latham KE, Vandevoort CA (2008) Effects of in vitro maturation on gene expression in rhesus monkey oocytes. *Physiological Genomics* 35(2): 145–158.

Lees-Murdock DJ, Lau HT, Castrillon DH, De Felici M, Walsh CP (2008) DNA methyltransferase loading, but not de novo methylation, is an oocyte-autonomous process stimulated by SCF signalling. *Developmental Biology* 321(1): 238–250.

Lees-Murdock DJ, Walsh CP (2008) DNA methylation reprogramming in the germ line. *Advances in Experimental Medicine and Biology* 626: 1–15.

Li G, Yu Y, Fan Y, *et al.* (2017) Genome wide abnormal DNA methylome of human blastocyst in assisted reproductive technology. *Journal of Genetics and Genomics* 44(10): 475–481.

Li T, Vu TH, Ulaner GA, *et al.* (2005) IVF results in de novo DNA methylation and histone methylation at an Igf2-H19 imprinting epigenetic switch. *Molecular Human Reproduction* 11: 631–640.

Li X, Ito M, Zhou F, *et al.* (2008) A maternal-zygotic effect gene, Zfp57, maintains both maternal and paternal imprints. *Developmental Cell* 15(4): 547–557.

Liang XW, Zhu JQ, Miao YL, *et al.* (2008) Loss of methylation imprint of Snrpn in postovulatory aging mouse oocyte. *Biochemical and Biophysical Research Communications* 371(1): 16–21.

Liang Y, Fu XW, Li JJ, Yuan DS, Zhu SE (2014) DNA methylation pattern in mouse oocytes and their in vitro fertilized early embryos: effect of oocyte vitrification. *Zygote* 22(2): 138–145.

Lim D, Bowdin SC, Tee L, *et al.* (2009) Clinical and molecular genetic features of Beckwith-Wiedemann syndrome associated with assisted reproductive technologies. *Human Reproduction* 24(3): 741–747.

Lin S, Li M, Lian Y, Chen L, Liu P (2013) No effect of embryo culture media on birthweight and length of newborns. *Human Reproduction* 28(7): 1762–1767.

Lucifero D, La Salle S, Bourc'his D, *et al.* (2007) Coordinate regulation of DNA methyltransferase expression during oogenesis. *BMC Developmental Biology* 7: 36.

Lucifero D, Mann MR, Bartolomei MS, Trasler JM (2004) Gene-specific timing and epigenetic memory in oocyte imprinting. *Human Molecular Genetics* 13(8): 839–849.

Ludwig M, Katalinic A, Gross S, *et al.* (2005) Increased prevalence of imprinting defects in patients with Angelman syndrome born to subfertile couples. *Journal of Medical Genetics* 42: 289–291.

Luedi PP, Dietrich FS, Weidman JR, *et al.* (2007) Computational and experimental identification of novel human imprinted genes. *Genome Research* 17(12): 1723–1730.

Maas K, Galinka E, Thornton K, Penzias AS, Sakkas D (2016) No change in live birthweight of IVF singleton deliveries over an 18-year period despite significant clinical and laboratory changes. *Human Reproduction* 31(9): 1987–1996.

Mackay DJ, Boonen SE, Clayton-Smith J, *et al.* (2006) A maternal hypomethylation syndrome presenting as transient neonatal diabetes mellitus. *Human Genetics* 120: 262–269.

Maher ER, Brueton LA, Bowdin SC, *et al.* (2003) Beckwith-Wiedemann syndrome and assisted reproduction technology (ART). *Journal of Medical Genetics* 40: 62–64.

Maher ER, Reik W (2000) Beckwith-Wiedemann syndrome: imprinting in clusters revisited. *Journal of Clinical Investigation* 105(3): 247–252.

Mainigi MA, Sapienza C, Butts S, Coutifaris C (2016) A molecular perspective on procedures and outcomes with assisted reproductive technologies. *Cold Spring Harbor Perspectives in Medicine* 6(4): a023416.

Malter HE, Cohen J (2002) Ooplasmic transfer: animal models assist human studies. *Reproductive Biomedicine Online* 5(1): 26–35.

Mann MR, Lee SS, Doherty AS, *et al.* (2004) Selective loss of imprinting in the placenta following preimplantation development in culture. *Development* 131: 3727–3735.

Manning M, Lissens W, Bonduelle M, *et al.* (2000) Study of DNA-methylation patterns at chromosome 15q11-q13 in children born after ICSI reveals no imprinting defects. *Molecular Human Reproduction* 6: 1049–1053.

Manning M, Lissens W, Liebaers I, Van Steirteghem A, Weidner W (2001a) Imprinting analysis in spermatozoa prepared for intracytoplasmic sperm injection (ICSI). *International Journal of Andrology* 24(2): 87–94.

Manning M, Lissens W, Weidner W, Liebaers I (2001b) DNA methylation analysis in immature testicular sperm cells at different developmental stages. *Urology International* 67(2): 151–155.

Mantikou E, Jonker MJ, Wong KM, *et al.* (2016) Factors affecting the gene expression of in vitro cultured human preimplantation embryos. *Human Reproduction* 31(2): 298–311.

Marees T, Dommering CJ, Imhof SM, *et al.* (2009) Incidence of retinoblastoma in Dutch children conceived by IVF: an expanded study. *Human Reproduction* 24(12): 3220–3224.

Market-Velker BA, Fernandes AD, Mann MR (2010) Side-by-side comparison of five commercial media systems in a mouse model: suboptimal in vitro culture interferes with imprint maintenance. *Biology of Reproduction* 83(6): 938–950.

Market-Velker BA, Zhang L, Magri LS, Bonvissuto AC, Mann MR (2010) Dual effects of superovulation: loss of maternal and paternal imprinted methylation in a dose-dependent manner. *Human Molecular Genetics* 19(1): 36–51.

Marques CJ, Carvalho F, Sousa M, Barros A (2004) Genomic imprinting in disruptive spermatogenesis. *Lancet* 363: 1700–1702.

Marques CJ, Costa P, Vaz B, *et al.* (2008) Abnormal methylation of imprinted genes in human sperm is associated with oligozoospermia. *Molecular Human Reproduction* 14(2): 67–74.

Marques CJ, Francisco T, Sousa S, *et al.* (2010) Methylation defects of imprinted genes in human testicular spermatozoa. *Fertility and Sterility* 94(2): 585–594.

McMinn J, Wei M, Schupf N, *et al.* (2006) Unbalanced placental expression of imprinted genes in human intrauterine growth restriction. *Placenta* 27: 540–549.

Melamed N, Choufani S, Wilkins-Haug LE, Koren G, Weksberg R (2015) Comparison of genome-wide and gene-specific DNA methylation between ART and naturally conceived pregnancies. *Epigenetics* 10(6): 474–483.

Ménézo Y, Elder K, Benkhalifa M, Dale B (2010) DNA methylation and gene expression in IVF. *Reproductive Biomedicine Online* 20(6): 709–710.

Ménézo Y, Dale B, Elder K (2018) Time to re-evaluate ART protocols in the light of advances in knowledge about methylation and epigenetics: an opinion paper. *Human Fertility (Cambridge)* 21(3): 156–162.

Meschede D, De Geyter C, Nieschlag E, Horst J (1995) Genetic risk in micromanipulative assisted reproduction. *Human Reproduction* 10: 2880–2886.

Moll AC, Imhof SM, Cruysberg JR, *et al.* (2003) Incidence of retinoblastoma in children born after in-vitro fertilisation. *Lancet* 361(9354): 309–310.

Monk M, Boubelik M, Lehnert S (1987) Temporal and regional changes in DNA methylation in the embryonic, extraembryonic and germ cell lineages during mouse embryo development. *Development* 99(3): 371–382.

Moore T, Haig D (1991) Genomic imprinting in mammalian development: a parental tug of war. *Trends in Genetics* 7: 45–49.

Morgan HD, Santos F, Green K, Dean W, Reik W (2005) Epigenetic reprogramming in mammals. *Human Molecular Genetics* 14(Spec No 1): R47–58.

Morison IM, Ramsay JP, Spencer HG (2005) A census of mammalian imprinting. *Trends in Genetics* 21: 457–465.

Morison IM, Reeve AE (1998) A catalogue of imprinted genes and parent-of-origin effects in humans and animals. *Human Molecular Genetics* 7: 1599–1609.

Mussa A, Molinatto C, Cerrato F, *et al.* (2017) Assisted reproductive techniques and risk of Beckwith-Wiedemann Syndrome *Pediatrics* 140(1): pii e20164311.

Nakamura T, Arai Y, Umehara H, *et al.* (2007) PGC7/Stella protects against DNA demethylation in early embryogenesis. *Nature Cell Biology* 9(1): 64–71.

Nelissen EC, Van Montfoort AP, Coonen E, *et al.* (2012) Further evidence that culture media affect perinatal outcome: findings after transfer of fresh and cryopreserved embryos. *Human Reproduction* 27(7): 1966–1976.

Obata Y, Kaneko-Ishino T, Koide T, *et al.* (1998) Disruption of primary imprinting during oocyte growth leads to the modified expression of imprinted genes during embryogenesis. *Development* 125: 1553–1560.

Obata Y, Kono T (2002) Maternal primary imprinting is established at a specific time for each gene throughout oocyte growth. *Journal of Biological Chemistry* 277: 5285–5289.

O'Doherty AM, O'Shea LC, Fair T (2012) Bovine DNA methylation imprints are established in an oocyte size-specific manner, which are coordinated with the expression of the DNMT3 family proteins. *Biology of Reproduction* 86(3): 67.

Odom LN, Segars J (2010) Imprinting disorders and assisted reproductive technology. *Current Opinion in Endocrinology, Diabetes, and Obesity* 17(6): 517–522.

Ohno M, Aoki N, Sasaki H (2001) Allele-specific detection of nascent transcripts by fluorescence in situ hybridization reveals temporal and culture-induced changes in Igf2 imprinting during pre-implantation mouse development. *Genes to Cells* 6: 249–259.

Okada Y, Scott G, Ray MK, Mishina Y, Zhang Y (2007) Histone demethylase JHDM2A is critical for Tnp1 and Prm1 transcription and spermatogenesis. *Nature* 450(7166):119–123.

Okae H, Chiba H, Hiura H, *et al.* (2014) Genome-wide analysis of DNA methylation dynamics during early human development. *PLoS Genetics* 10(12): e1004868.

Omisanjo OA, Biermann K, Hartmann S, *et al.* (2007) DNMT1 and HDAC1 gene expression in impaired spermatogenesis and testicular cancer. *Histochemistry and Cell Biology* 127: 175–181.

Ørstavik KH, Eiklid K, van der Hagen CB, *et al.* (2003) Another case of imprinting defect in a girl with Angelman syndrome who was conceived by intracytoplasmic semen injection. *American Journal of Human Genetics* 72: 218–219.

Ostermeier GC, Dix DJ, Miller DD, Khatri P, Krawetz SA (2002) Spermatozoal RNA profiles of normal fertile men. *Lancet* 360(9335): 772–777.

Pantoja C, de Los Rios L, Matheu A, Antequera F, Serrano M (2005) Inactivation of imprinted genes induced by cellular stress and tumorigenesis. *Cancer Research* 65: 26–33.

Pastor WA, Stroud H, Nee K, *et al.* (2014) MORC1 represses transposable elements in the mouse male germline. *Nature Communications* 12(5): 5795.

Poplinski A, Tüttelmann F, Kanber D, Horsthemke B, Gromoll J (2010) Idiopathic male infertility is strongly associated with aberrant methylation of MEST and IGF2/H19 ICR1. *International Journal of Andrology* 33(4): 642–649.

Probst AV, Santos F, Reik W, Almouzni G, Dean W (2007) Structural differences in centromeric heterochromatin are spatially reconciled on fertilisation in the mouse zygote. *Chromosoma* 116(4): 403–415.

Qiao J, Chen Y, Yan LY, *et al.* (2009) Changes in histone methylation during human oocyte maturation and IVF- or ICSI-derived embryo development. *Fertility and Sterility* 93(5): 1628–1636.

Rajender S, Avery K, Agarwal A (2011) Epigenetics, spermatogenesis and male infertility. *Mutation Research* 727: 62–71.

Reik W, Dean W, Walter J (2001) Epigenetic reprogramming in mammalian development. *Science* 293(5532): 1089–1093.

Reik W, Maher ER (1997) Imprinting in clusters: lessons from Beckwith-Wiedemann syndrome. *Trends in Genetics* 13(8): 330–334.

Reik W, Walter J (2001) Genomic imprinting: parental influence on the genome. *Nature Reviews (Genetics)* 2: 21–32.

Renard JP, Baldacci P, Richouxduranthon V, Pournin S, Babinet C (1994) A maternal factor affecting mouse blastocyst formation. *Development* 120: 797–802.

Rivera RM, Ross JW (2013) Epigenetics in fertilization and preimplantation development. *Prog Biophys Mol Biol* 113(3): 423–432.

Rossignol S, Steunou V, Chalas C, *et al.* (2006) The epigenetic imprinting defect of patients with Beckwith-Wiedemann syndrome born after assisted reproductive technology is not restricted to the 11p15 region. *Journal of Medical Genetics* 43: 902–907.

Rugg-Gunn PJ, Ferguson-Smith AC, Pedersen RA (2005) Epigenetic status of human embryonic stem cells. *Nature Genetics* 37: 585–587.

Sagirkaya H, Misirlioglu M, Kaya A, *et al.* (2006) Developmental and molecular correlates of bovine preimplantation embryos. *Reproduction* 131: 895–904.

Sagirkaya H, Misirlioglu M, Kaya A, *et al.* (2007) Developmental potential of bovine oocytes cultured in different maturation and culture conditions. *Animal Reproduction Science* 101: 225–240.

Saenz-de-Juano MD, Peñaranda DS, Marco-Jiménez F, Vicente JS (2014) Does vitrification alter the methylation pattern of OCT4 promoter in rabbit late blastocyst? *Cryobiology* 69(1): 178–180.

Sanchez-Albisua I, Borell-Kost S, Mau-Holzmann UA, Licht P, Krägeloh-Mann I (2007) Increased frequency of severe major anomalies in children conceived by intracytoplasmic sperm injection. *Developments in Medical Child Neurology* 49(2): 129–134.

Santi D, De Vincentis S, Magnani E, Spaggiari G (2017) Impairment of sperm DNA methylation in male infertility: a meta-analytic study. *Andrology* 5(4): 695–703.

Santos F, Hendrich B, Reik W, Dean W (2002) Dynamic reprogramming of DNA methylation in the early mouse embryo. *Developmental Biology* 241(1): 172–182.

Santos F, Hyslop L, Stojkovic P, *et al.* (2010) Evaluation of epigenetic marks in human embryos derived from IVF and ICSI. *Human Reproduction* 25(9): 2387–2395.

Sasaki H, Ferguson-Smith AC, Shum AS, Barton SC, Surani MA (1995) Temporal and spatial regulation of H19 imprinting in normal and uniparental mouse embryos. *Development.*121(12): 4195–4202.

Sato A, Otsu E, Negishi H, Utsunomiya T, Arima T (2007) Aberrant DNA methylation of imprinted loci in superovulated oocytes. *Human Reproduction* 22: 26–35.

Schwarzer C, Esteves TC, Arauzo-Bravo MJ, *et al.* (2012) ART culture conditions change the probability of mouse embryo gestation through defined cellular and molecular responses. *Human Reproduction* 27(9): 2627–2640.

Shamanski FL, Kimura Y, Lavoir MC, Pedersen RA, Yanagimachi R (1999) Status of genomic imprinting in mouse spermatids. *Human Reproduction* 14: 1050–1056.

Sharma U, Conine CC, Shea JM, *et al.* (2016) Biogenesis and function of tRNA fragments during sperm maturation and fertilization in mammals. *Science* 351(6271): 391–396.

Shea JM, Serra RW, Carone BR, *et al.*(2015) Genetic and epigenetic variation, but not diet, shape the sperm methylome. *Developmental Cell* 35(6): 750–758.

Shi W, Haaf T (2002) Aberrant methylation patterns at the two-cell stage as an indicator of early developmental failure. *Molecular Reproduction and Development* 63: 329–334.

Shi Y, Lan F, Matson C, *et al.*(2004) Histone demethylation mediated by the nuclear amine oxidase homolog LSD1. *Cell* 119: 941–953.

Sikienka K, Erek S, Godmann M, *et al.* (2015) Disruption of histone methylation in developing sperm impairs offspring health transgenerationally. *Science* 350(6261): aab2006.

Skaar DA, Li Y, Bernal AJ, Hoyo C, Murphy SK, Jirtle RL (2012) The human imprintome: regulatory mechanisms, methods of ascertainment, and roles in disease susceptibility. *ILAR Journal/National Research Council, Institute of Laboratory Animal Resources* 53(3–4): 341–358.

Smallwood SA, Kelsey G (2012) Genome-wide analysis of DNA methylation in low cell numbers by reduced representation bisulfite sequencing. *Methods in Molecular Biology* 925: 187–197.

Smallwood SA, Tomizawa S, Krueger F, *et al.* (2011) Dynamic CpG island methylation landscape in oocytes and preimplantation embryos. *Nature Genetics* 43(8): 811–814.

Smith ZD, Chan MM, Humm KC, *et al.* (2014) DNA methylation dynamics of the human preimplantation embryo. *Nature* 511: 611–615.

Song S, Ghosh J, Mainigi M, *et al.* (2015) DNA methylation differences between in vitro- and in vivo-conceived children are associated with ART procedures rather than infertility. *Clinical Epigenetics* 7: 41.

Soubry A, Hoyo C, Jirtle RL, Murphy SK (2014) A paternal environmental legacy: evidence for epigenetic inheritance through the male germ line. *BioEssays: News and Reviews in Molecular, Cellular And Developmental Biology* 36(4): 359–371.

Stouder C, Deutsch S, Paoloni-Giacobino A (2009) Superovulation in mice alters the methylation pattern of imprinted genes in the sperm of the offspring. *Reproductive Toxicology* 28(4): 536–541.

Stuppia L, Franzago M, Ballerini P, Gatta V, Antonucci I (2015) Epigenetics and male reproduction: the consequences of paternal lifestyle on fertility, embryo development, and children lifetime health. *Clinical Epigenetics* 7: 120

Sujit KM,Sarkar S, Singh V, *et al* (2018) Genome-wide differential methylation analyses identifies methylation signatures of male infertility. *Human Reproduction* 33(12): 2256–2267.

Sun BW, Yang AC, Feng Y, *et al.* (2006) Temporal and parental-specific expression of imprinted genes in a newly derived Chinese human embryonic stem cell line and embryoid bodies. *Human Molecular Genetics* 15: 65–75.

Sunde A, Brison D, Dumoulin J, *et al.* (2016) Time to take human embryo culture seriously. *Human Reproduction* 31(10): 2174–2182.

Sutcliffe AG, Peters CJ, Bowdin S, *et al.* (2006) Assisted reproductive therapies and imprinting disorders: a preliminary British survey. *Human Reproduction* 21: 1009–1011.

Suzuki J Jr, Therrien J, Filion F, *et al.* (2009) In vitro culture and somatic cell nuclear transfer affect imprinting of SNRPN gene in pre- and post-implantation stages of development in cattle. *BMC Developmental Biology* 9: 9.

Svensson J, Bjornstahl A, Ivarsson SA (2005) Increased risk of Silver–Russell syndrome after in vitro fertilization? *Acta Paediatrica* 94: 1163–1165.

Tee L, Lim DH, Dias RP, *et al.* (2013) Epimutation profiling in Beckwith-Wiedemann syndrome: relationship with assisted reproductive technology. *Clinical Epigenetics* 5(1): 23.

Tenorio J, Ramanelli V, Martin-Trujillo A, *et al.* (2016) Clinical and molecular analyses of Beckwith-Wiedemann syndrome: Comparison between spontaneous conception and assisted reproduction techniques. *American Journal of Medical Genetics* 170(10): 2740–2749.

Torregrosa N, Dominguez-Fandos D, Camejo MI, *et al.* (2006) Protamine 2 precursors, protamine 1/protamine 2 ratio, DNA integrity and other sperm parameters in infertile patients. *Human Reproduction* 21: 2084–2089.

Trapphoff T, El Hjj N, Zechner U, Haaf T, Eichenlaub-Ritter U (2010) DNA integrity, growth pattern, spindle formation, chromosomal constitution and imprinting patterns of mouse oocytes from vitrified pre-antral follicles. *Human Reproduction* 25(12): 3025–3042.

Van der Auwera I, D'Hooghe T (2001) Superovulation of female mice delays embryonic and fetal development. *Human Reproduction* 16(6):1237–1243.

Vermeiden JP, Bernardus RE (2013) Are imprinting disorders more prevalent after human in vitro fertilization or intracytoplasmic sperm injection? *Fertility and Sterility* 99(3): 642–651.

Walter J, Paulsen M (2003) Imprinting and disease. *Seminars in Cell and Developmental Biology* 14: 101–110.

Wang Z, Xu L, He F (2010) Embryo vitrification affects the methylation of the H19/Igf2 differentially methylated domain and the expression of H19 and Igf2. *Fertility and Sterility* 93(8): 2729–2733.

White CR, Denomme MM, Tekpetey FR, Feyles V, Power SG, Mann MR (2015) High frequency of imprinted methylation errors in human preimplantation embryos. *Scientific Reports* 5: 17311.

Whitelaw N, Bhattacharya S, Hoad G, Horgan GW, Hamilton M, Haggarty P (2014) Epigenetic status in the offspring of spontaneous and assisted conception. *Human Reproduction* 29(7): 1452–1458.

Yamazaki T, Yamagata K, Baba T (2007) Time-lapse and retrospective analysis of DNA methylation in mouse preimplantation embryos by live cell imaging. *Developmental Biology* 304: 409–419.

Yan LY, Yan J, Qiao J, Zhao PL, Liu P (2010) Effects of oocyte vitrification on histone modifications. *Reproduction Fertility and Development* 22(6): 920–925.

Yao J, Geng L, Huang R, *et al.* (2017) Effect of vitrification on in vitro development and imprinted gene Grb10 in mouse embryos. *Reproduction* 154(3): 97–105.

Young LE, Fernandes K, McEvoy TG, *et al.* (2001) Epigenetic change in IGF2R is associated with fetal overgrowth after sheep embryo culture. *Nature Genetics* 27: 153–154.

Young LE, Sinclair KD, Wilmut I (1998) Large offspring syndrome in cattle and sheep. *Reviews of Reproduction* 3(3): 155–163.

Yuan S, Schuster A, Tang C, *et al.* (2016) Sperm-borne miRNAs and endo-siRNAs are important for fertilization and preimplantation embryonic development. *Development* 143(4): 635–647.

Zaitseva I, Zaitsev S, Alenina N, Bader M, Krivokharchenko A (2007) Dynamics of DNA-demethylation in early mouse and rat embryos developed in vivo and in vitro. *Molecular Reproduction and Development* 74(10): 1255–1261.

Zandstra H, Brentjens LBPM, Spauwen B, Touwslager RNH (2018) Association of culture medium with growth, weight and cardiovascular development of IVF children at the age of 9 years. *Human Reproduction* 33(9): 1645–1656.

Zandstra H, Van Montfoort AP, Dumoulin JC (2015) Does the type of culture medium used influence birthweight of children born after IVF? *Human Reproduction* 30(11): 2693.

Zhao XM, Du WH, Hao HS, *et al.* (2012) Effect of vitrification on promoter methylation and the expression of pluripotency and differentiation genes in mouse blastocysts. *Molecular Reproduction and Development* 79(7): 445–450.

Zhao XM, Ren JJ, Du WH, *et al.* (2013) Effect of vitrification on promoter CpG island methylation patterns and expression levels of DNA methyltransferase 1o, histone acetyltransferase 1, and deacetylase 1 in metaphase II mouse oocytes. *Fertility and Sterility* 100(1): 256–261.

Zhu J, Li M, Chen L, Liu P, Qiao J (2014b) The protein source in embryo culture media influences birthweight: a comparative study between G1 v5 and G1-PLUS v5. *Human Reproduction* 29(7): 1387–1392.

Zhu J, Lin S, Li M, *et al.* (2014a) Effect of in vitro culture period on birthweight of singleton newborns. *Human Reproduction* 29(3): 448–454.

Zhu P, Guo H, Ren Y, *et al.* (2018) Single-cell DNA methylome sequencing of human preimplantation embryos. *Nature Genetics* 50(1): 12–19.

Ziyyat A, Lefevre A (2001) Differential gene expression in pre-implantation embryos from mouse oocytes injected with round spermatids or spermatozoa. *Human Reproduction* 16: 1449–1456.

# Index